Controlled Experimentation of Digital Forensics

Edson OliveiraJr • Thiago J. Silva •
Charles V. Neu • Avelino F. Zorzo • Ana H. Mazur

Controlled Experimentation of Digital Forensics

Towards Formalization for Strengthening Evidence Reproducibility, Reliability, and Transparency

Springer

Edson OliveiraJr
State University of Maringá
Maringá, Brazil

Charles V. Neu
University of Santa Cruz do Sul (UNISC)
Santa Cruz, Brazil

Ana H. Mazur
State University of Maringá
Maringá, Brazil

Thiago J. Silva
AmbevTech
Maringá, Brazil

Avelino F. Zorzo
PUCRS
Porto Alegre, Brazil

ISBN 978-3-032-19950-8 ISBN 978-3-032-19951-5 (eBook)
https://doi.org/10.1007/978-3-032-19951-5

This Springer imprint is published by the registered company Springer Nature Switzerland AG
The registered company address is: Gewerbestrasse 11, 6330 Cham, Switzerland

To my not-so-little bear, ***Beatriz****, whose laughter fills my heart and gives meaning to every page.*
Daddy Edson Jr.

Foreword

Trust is the bedrock of forensic science, and trust is earned through reproducibility. In legal, corporate, and policy settings alike, digital evidence carries weight only when others can verify that the findings are repeatable, well-founded, and transparent. Over the past decades, digital forensics has become integral to everything from incident response to criminal prosecution. Yet the field still grapples with a fundamental scientific challenge: how to elevate a practice often driven by proprietary tools and case-by-case improvisation into one grounded in controlled, rigorous experimentation. This book, *Controlled Experimentation of Digital Forensics: Towards Formalization for Strengthening Evidence Reproducibility, Reliability, and Transparency*, directly addresses that challenge.

The authors argue persuasively that in digital forensics, methodology matters as much as technology. They reposition forensic investigations within the framework of empirical science, where one plans carefully, controls variables, makes procedures explicit, analyzes data with statistical rigor, and reports results for independent verification. In doing so, the book provides a path to transition from anecdotal "one-off" findings to results that anyone can reproduce. This shift is more than academic; it is what transforms a subjective expert opinion into an objective scientific finding that can withstand scrutiny and be replicated by others.

The book's five-part structure reinforces this theme. Part I—Fundamentals of Digital Forensics and Controlled Experimentation—situates digital forensics within its historical, technical, and scientific context. It revisits the investigative process and the field's main and emerging branches, while also introducing the broader landscape of empirical methods drawn from computer science and software engineering. By treating controlled experimentation and reproducibility as core pillars, Part I connects digital forensics to ongoing discussions about evidence-based practice and the wider Open Science movement, emphasizing that rigorous design, transparent documentation, and repeatable procedures are prerequisites for credible forensic knowledge.

Part II—Conceptual Modeling of Digital Forensics Controlled Experiments—introduces a unifying solution to these needs. It first surveys the role and history of conceptual modeling as a means to structure and clarify complex domains, and then presents ExperDF-CM (Experimentation in Digital Forensics—Conceptual Model), a comprehensive model for designing and conducting controlled experiments in digital forensics. ExperDF-CM breaks an experiment into five defined phases—Planning, Pre-Operation, Operation, Analysis and Interpretation, and Dissemination—mirroring the entire research lifecycle from hypothesis to published result. Each phase is detailed with its objectives, inputs, and outputs, giving practitioners and researchers a common vocabulary and structure for experimentation. For example, the Planning phase involves formulating research questions, hypotheses, and variables, and considering ethical and legal constraints, while the Operation phase focuses on data collection under controlled conditions. The Dissemination phase ensures that data sets, code, and results are openly shared for verification. This model doesn't remain theoretical: the book demonstrates how to apply ExperDF-CM step by step, including support for modern practices such as Registered Reports and the preparation of ethics and approval documentation. In short, Part II delivers an actionable blueprint that any lab or researcher can adopt immediately to enhance the scientific rigor of their forensic experiments.

Part III—Formal Representation and Semantic Integration of Digital Forensics Controlled Experiments—extends the discussion into the realm of knowledge representation, interoperability, and machine reasoning. It begins with an accessible primer on ontology design and SPARQL querying, and introduces the ExperDF-Portal as a digital environment for managing and querying experimental information. Building on this foundation, the authors present ExperDF-Onto, an ontology that formalizes the key entities and relationships of a digital forensics experiment (cases, artifacts, tools, procedures, results, and more) using established standards such as RDF/OWL for specification and SPARQL for querying. ExperDF-Onto is aligned with metadata and provenance standards, including Dublin Core and the PROV family, to capture how evidence and results are generated and transformed. By encoding experiment details semantically, the book enables machines (and researchers) to interpret and reuse experimental data in ways that were previously impossible. Concrete SPARQL queries are provided for each phase of ExperDF-CM—for instance, retrieving all experiments that used a certain tool or checking whether all required steps of an analysis were documented. This semantic layer makes experiments discoverable, comparable, and interoperable, enabling them to be combined into a growing, machine-readable body of forensic knowledge rather than remaining isolated narratives.

Part IV—ExperDF-Onto Walkthroughs of Exemplary Digital Forensics Experiments—moves from theory to practice. Through a set of carefully chosen case studies, it shows how ExperDF-CM and ExperDF-Onto can be instantiated to model real-world forensic experiments end-to-end. These walkthroughs span diverse scenarios, including memory acquisition, smartphone extraction and lock bypass, cloud log tampering, IoT intrusion detection, and blockchain-based provenance. Each example traces the five phases of ExperDF-CM, illustrates how variables and procedures are represented semantically, and demonstrates how SPARQL queries can be used to verify coverage, check provenance, and support teaching. The inclusion of "minimal reproducibility kits," coverage analyses, and teaching notes in these examples underscores the authors' commitment to making the frameworks not only conceptually sound but also concretely usable in research, education, and practice.

Finally, Part V—Integration, Reflection, and Future Directions—synthesizes the previous parts and articulates a vision for the discipline's future. It describes a path toward a more scientifically grounded, transparent, and collaborative digital forensics. Crucially, it emphasizes that emerging realities make this shift imperative. Today's investigators contend with phenomena like cloud services spreading data across jurisdictions and multi-tenant infrastructures, IoT ecosystems where evidence is fragmented across device firmware, mobile apps, gateways, and cloud back-ends, fileless malware that resides only in volatile memory, encrypted communication channels that thwart traditional analysis, and AI- and machine-learning-driven systems that introduce new forms of evidence while obscuring decision processes. The concluding discussion argues that only by embracing formalized experimentation, semantic consistency, and open sharing of results will digital forensics keep pace with these challenges. The authors stop short of utopian predictions, but they clearly make the case that the methodologies presented—controlled experimentation via ExperDF-CM and knowledge integration via ExperDF-Onto and its supporting portal—can raise both the floor and the ceiling of forensic science practice. Higher minimum standards of evidence validity and reproducibility will increase confidence in everyday investigations, while richer datasets and interoperable tools will open new frontiers of research and capability.

The value of this work is broad. For researchers, it provides a clear framework for designing robust experiments and a means to disseminate results so others can query and extend them. Adopting ExperDF-CM, ExperDF-Onto, and the associated tooling could significantly improve the comparability of studies in academic digital forensics, making it easier to build on each other's work rather than reinventing setups. For practitioners and forensic tool developers, the controlled experimentation approach provides a means to empirically evaluate and verify tools, procedures, and analytical techniques across various conditions. Using these methods, one can quantify the accuracy and error rates of forensic tools, establish statistical confidence in their results, and maintain detailed provenance for how conclusions were reached—all of which strengthen the evidentiary value and defensibility of digital forensic findings. For educators and training programs, the content in this book can modernize curricula. Students can be taught to follow the ExperDF-CM phases in classroom labs and document their projects in ExperDF-Onto (and through the portal), ingraining in them a mindset of scientific rigor, reproducibility, and semantic precision from the start. This could help cultivate the next generation of forensic professionals who are as comfortable designing an experiment or writing a SPARQL query as they are collecting a disk image.

Beyond its immediate practicality, this volume advances a subtle but essential cultural shift in digital forensics. It shows that being more open, systematic, and precise in our methods need not slow us down—in fact, it can make our work more efficient and impactful. It demonstrates that we can achieve semantic clarity (through formal models, ontologies, and machine-actionable representations) without sacrificing hands-on problem solving. Perhaps most importantly, it reinforces the idea that digital forensics can evolve into a truly cumulative science: one in which results accumulate, interconnect, and drive the field forward, rather than dissipate into isolated case reports. In that sense, this book is not just a compilation of knowledge, but an invitation and a roadmap to improve our collective practice. It is an invitation to design investigations with greater intent, to rigorously measure and evaluate our forensic techniques, and to share our findings in a structured way so that others can build upon them openly.

I congratulate the authors for devising and delivering this much-needed framework for the community. Controlled Experimentation of Digital Forensics is both a call to action and a tangible toolkit. Taken to heart, the approaches in this book could dramatically enhance the credibility and scientific maturity of digital forensic investigations. The payoff will likely be seen not only in stronger research publications but also in everyday practice: more reliable tools, more consistent procedures, and ultimately more trustworthy justice when digital evidence is at play.

Professor & Canada Research Chair in,
Cybersecurity & Threat Intelligence, University
of Guelph, Guelph, ON, Canada
December 2025

Ali Dehghantanha

Preface

What Is This Book About?

This book represents the culmination of years of collaborative research, reflection, and shared vision between two leading Brazilian research groups in Digital Forensics: the **Computer Science Investigation in Digital Forensics (CSI-DIN)** and the **Research Group on Systematic Software Reuse and Continuous Experimentation (GReater)** at the State University of Maringá (UEM), coordinated by Prof. Edson OliveiraJr, and the **Dependable and Secure Systems Group (CONSEG)** at the Pontifical Catholic University of Rio Grande do Sul (PUCRS), led by Prof. Avelino F. Zorzo. This partnership was nurtured within the framework of the Brazilian National Institute of Science and Technology on Forensic Sciences (INCT-CF), which has played a pivotal role in promoting interdisciplinary collaboration and advancing scientific approaches to the analysis of digital evidence.

The book provides a comprehensive reflection on the scientific foundations of **Evidence-based Digital Forensics** as an emerging discipline. It goes beyond the practice-oriented roots of Digital Forensics to present a mature field grounded in reproducible, systematic, and transparent research methods. Its title, *Controlled Experimentation of Digital Forensics: Towards Formalization for Strengthening Evidence Reproducibility, Reliability, and Transparency*, encapsulates this ambition, emphasizing both the need to formalize experimental processes and the commitment to foster openness and rigor in forensic science.

Through conceptual models (*ExperDF-CM*) and semantic frameworks (*ExperDF-Onto*), the book proposes practical mechanisms for structuring, documenting, and validating experiments in Digital Forensics. It ultimately situates the discipline within the broader movement of Open Science, aligning its principles with the UNESCO Recommendation on Open Science and the pursuit of socially responsible research.

Who Should Read This Book?

This book is written for a broad and interdisciplinary audience that includes not only researchers and professionals in Digital Forensics but also those interested in the foundations of scientific inquiry, empirical research, and Open Science. Its contents are designed to support both academic reflection and practical application, bridging the gap between theoretical principles and operational challenges.

For **researchers**, the book offers a solid methodological and conceptual foundation for designing, conducting, and publishing controlled experiments in a reproducible and transparent manner. It provides models, ontologies, and semantic structures that formalize experimental reasoning and ensure that results can be independently verified, compared, and reused. Researchers will find in it a roadmap for producing cumulative and interoperable scientific knowledge in a field that increasingly depends on collaboration and data integration.

For **practitioners**, the book serves as a practical guide to improving the reliability, traceability, and defensibility of forensic analyses. It presents conceptual models and documentation standards that allow experts to structure their investigations systematically, making their findings more robust in both scientific and judicial contexts. The emphasis on reproducibility and transparency helps practitioners align their technical work with the growing expectations of accountability and quality assurance in forensic science.

For **educators**, it functions as a didactic resource for introducing students to the principles of experimental design, empirical reasoning, and scientific openness. The conceptual and ontological models presented here can be used to teach how evidence, hypotheses, and experimental variables interrelate, helping learners develop a critical understanding of scientific rigor in Digital Forensics. In this sense, the book supports both curricular innovation and the training of future professionals capable of integrating ethical awareness with methodological discipline.

For **policymakers** and **funding agencies**, it provides conceptual grounding for establishing evaluation criteria, standards, and incentives that promote transparency, reliability, and trust in Digital Forensics research. By translating the principles of Open Science into concrete methodological and semantic instruments, the book offers a foundation for shaping policies that encourage reproducibility, data sharing, and responsible research practices.

Beyond academic and professional communities, this work also speaks to a wider audience concerned with the integrity of digital evidence and its role in safeguarding citizens' rights. As societies become increasingly digitalized, the credibility of forensic evidence directly influences public trust in institutions, judicial decisions, and democratic governance. By reinforcing the evidential foundation of Digital Forensics, this book contributes to building a more accountable, transparent, and equitable justice system in which scientific rigor serves both truth and society.

How Is This Book Organized?

The organization of this book follows a logical progression that moves from theoretical foundations to applied instantiation and reflection, guiding the reader through the conceptual, semantic, and empirical dimensions of controlled experimentation in Digital Forensics. Each part builds upon the previous one, creating an integrated framework that combines scientific rigor, methodological clarity, and open science principles.

Part I—Fundamentals of Digital Forensics and Controlled Experimentation establishes the theoretical and methodological underpinnings of the field. It positions Digital Forensics within a broader scientific tradition, emphasizing rigor, transparency, and reproducibility as essential for producing credible, cumulative knowledge. The three chapters in this part discuss (1) conceptual modeling as a means of structuring and clarifying knowledge, (2) the design and execution of controlled experiments as a methodological foundation for empirical validation, and (3) reproducibility as a central pillar for credibility and trust in forensic research.

Part II—Conceptual Modeling of Digital Forensics Controlled Experiments introduces the *ExperDF-CM* conceptual model as a structured framework for documenting, executing, and disseminating forensic experiments. It begins with a historical and methodological overview of conceptual modeling, tracing its evolution from early data models to domain-specific scientific representations. Building upon this foundation, it presents *ExperDF-CM* as a comprehensive model organized into five interconnected phases: Planning, Pre-Operation, Operation, Analysis and Interpretation, and Dissemination. This structure supports methodological consistency, transparency, and ethical accountability across the experimental lifecycle.

Part III—Formal Representation and Semantic Integration of Digital Forensics Controlled Experiments extends the conceptual foundations into the semantic domain. It focuses on ontological modeling, interoperability, and machine reasoning as mechanisms to make experimental knowledge explicit, traceable, and reusable. The first chapter introduces key concepts of semantic representation, SPARQL querying, and the *ExperDF-Portal*, a digital environment for experiment management. The following chapter presents *ExperDF-Onto*, an ontology aligned with international standards such as Dublin Core and the PROV family, which enables semantic annotation and provenance tracking of forensic research data. Together, these elements transform static documentation into a dynamic knowledge ecosystem.

Part IV—ExperDF-Onto Walkthroughs of Exemplary Digital Forensics Experiments transitions from theory to practice. It demonstrates how *ExperDF-Onto* can be instantiated to represent real-world forensic experiments in a consistent and machine-actionable manner. Through five detailed walkthroughs, this part shows how conceptual and semantic frameworks capture experimental intent, variable control, provenance, and reproducibility. The case studies include memory acquisition, smartphone extraction, cloud log analysis, IoT intrusion detection, and blockchain-based provenance. Each follows the five phases of *ExperDF-CM*, illustrating the ontology's role as a bridge between narrative design and formal documentation, and as a tool for teaching, validation, and ethical reflection.

Part V—Integration, Reflection, and Future Directions concludes the book by synthesizing its theoretical, semantic, and practical contributions. It integrates the insights from the previous parts to present a coherent vision of Digital Forensics as a rigorous, transparent, and open scientific discipline. This final part discusses how conceptual models and ontologies together form a foundation for cumulative knowledge and reproducible research. It also reflects on remaining challenges, technical, institutional, and philosophical, and outlines future directions for research, education, and policy. In doing so, it reinforces the book's central message: the strength of Digital Forensics lies in its capacity to combine structure, meaning, and openness to build reliable, verifiable scientific evidence.

Taken together, these five parts guide the reader through a complete journey, from understanding the philosophical bases of experimentation to applying semantic frameworks for open and reproducible forensic science. The book thus serves both as a reference for researchers and as a didactic resource for practitioners, educators, and policymakers seeking to strengthen the scientific foundations of Digital Forensics.

How Did This Book Start?

The origins of this book trace back to an 18-month sabbatical period undertaken by Edson OliveiraJr between 2018 and 2020 at the Pontifical Catholic University of Rio Grande do Sul (PUCRS), under the supervision of Prof. Avelino F. Zorzo in the Dependable and Secure Systems Group (CONSEG), within the context of the **Brazilian National Institute of Science and Technology on Forensic Sciences (INCT-CF)**. The initial goal of this research stay was to gain a deeper understanding of how controlled experiments were being conducted in Digital Forensics and to explore how empirical methodologies from Software Engineering could be adapted to this context. However, during this period, it became evident that the area lacked scientific rigor, transparency, and reproducibility. This realization became the turning point that motivated a systematic effort to establish a structured, evidence-based, and open approach to Digital Forensics experimentation.

From that experience, the idea of building a conceptual and semantic foundation for forensic experimentation emerged. What began as an exploratory academic exchange evolved into a coordinated research program involving multiple Brazilian institutions and international collaborations, dedicated to redefining the methodological foundations of Digital Forensics.

The project was further strengthened through the broader **INCT-CF initiative (CAPES, CNPq, and FAPERGS/Brazil)**, which united researchers from computing, law, biology, and chemistry to promote interdisciplinary approaches to forensic science. This collaborative environment provided the institutional and intellectual context necessary for transforming isolated insights into a comprehensive research framework.

The realization of this book was made possible by the institutional support of **UEM**, **PUCRS**, and **UNISC**, and by the generous funding from **CNPq**, **CAPES**, and the **Araucária Funding Agency of Paraná**, as well as the collaborative environment fostered by **NAPI - Public Security and Forensic Science**. We are also profoundly grateful to our colleagues, students, and collaborators whose ideas, software implementations, and constructive feedback enriched and refined every stage of this work.

Finally, we dedicate this work to the global Digital Forensics community, whose shared pursuit of truth and scientific rigor continues to shape a more transparent, reproducible, and equitable digital future.

Maringá, PR, Brazil — Edson OliveiraJr
Maringá, Brazil — Thiago J. Silva
Santa Cruz, Brazil — Charles V. Neu
Porto Alegre, Brazil — Avelino F. Zorzo
Maringá, Brazil — Ana H. Mazur
December 2025

Acknowledgments The development of this book was made possible through the support, collaboration, and dedication of countless individuals and institutions who accompanied us throughout this long scientific journey.

We gratefully acknowledge the essential role of the **Brazilian funding agencies**, whose investments created the conditions for sustained high-quality research. In particular, we thank the **National Council for Scientific and Technological Development (CNPq)**, the **Coordination for the Improvement of Higher Education Personnel (CAPES)**, and the **Araucária Foundation of Paraná**. Their programs and initiatives, especially those linked to the INCT-CF and NAPI Public Security and Forensic Science, provided the financial, organizational, and intellectual environment that enabled the conceptual, methodological, and technological advances consolidated in this work.

Our most profound appreciation goes to the **State University of Maringá (UEM)**, the **Pontifical Catholic University of Rio Grande do Sul (PUCRS)**, and the **University of Santa Cruz do Sul (UNISC)**, whose institutional support sustained the research activities, collaborations, and mobility efforts that shaped the foundations of this book. We also thank our colleagues from the **CSI-DIN, GReater, and CONSEG research groups**, whose shared commitment to rigor, openness, and interdisciplinarity enriched every stage of this project.

We extend our sincere gratitude to our **graduate and undergraduate students**, whose enthusiasm, creativity, and tireless curiosity were central to the evolution of the ExperDF-CM model, the ExperDF-Onto ontology, and the numerous prototypes, datasets, and experimental artifacts produced over the years. Their participation in research meetings, empirical studies, conceptual modeling exercises, and software development efforts not only strengthened the technical content of this book but also reaffirmed our belief in the transformative power of collaborative scientific training.

We are also grateful to the colleagues who generously contributed to refining specific chapters through detailed technical reviews and insightful comments. In particular, **we thank Prof. Dr. Alexandre L'Erario of the Federal University of Technology of Paraná (UTFPR), Prof. Dr. Vítor E. Silva Souza of the Federal University of Espírito Santo (UFES), and Prof. Dr. Marcelo Morandini of the University of São Paulo (USP)**. Their careful reading, constructive suggestions, and expert perspective enhanced the clarity, precision, and scholarly quality of this work.

Finally, **we express our deep appreciation to our families**. Their patience, encouragement, and unwavering support sustained us during demanding research cycles, long writing periods, and countless moments of intellectual immersion. This book is as much a result of their generosity as it is of our academic dedication. Their presence remains the silent foundation that made this journey possible.

To all of you, institutions, colleagues, students, collaborators, and loved ones, we offer our deepest thanks. This book is a collective achievement built upon shared effort, trust, and the conviction that science advances when it is open, rigorous, and grounded in collaboration.

Competing Interests The authors have no competing interests to declare that are relevant to the content of this manuscript.

Contents

Part I
Fundamentals of Digital Forensics and Controlled Experimentation

This part establishes the theoretical and methodological underpinnings required for advancing Digital Forensics experimentation. Its overarching goal is to frame the field within the broader scientific tradition, emphasizing rigor, transparency, and reproducibility as essential conditions for producing reliable and cumulative knowledge. By drawing from established scientific practices while adapting them to the specificities of forensic inquiry, this part provides the conceptual and methodological scaffolding necessary to consolidate Digital Forensics as both a practical discipline and a scientific enterprise.

The urgency of such foundations stems from the position of Digital Forensics as a relatively young field, tasked simultaneously with addressing pressing investigative needs and developing a coherent scientific identity. Without structured methodologies, research risks fragmentation, lack of comparability, and diminished credibility in both academic and legal contexts. Establishing a rigorous basis for experimentation, therefore, is not only an intellectual requirement but also a practical necessity for ensuring the reliability of forensic outcomes.

Chapter 1 introduces the fundamentals of conceptual modeling, demonstrating how abstract representations help structure knowledge domains, clarify key concepts, and mediate between theoretical perspectives and empirical applications. Conceptual models are presented as indispensable instruments for ensuring semantic clarity, methodological consistency, and a foundation for reproducibility.

Chapter 2 examines the design and execution of controlled experiments in Digital Forensics, addressing methodological challenges such as volatile evidence, unique investigative contexts, and ethical or legal restrictions. By focusing on variable identification, the definition of experimental units, and the establishment of replicable procedures, this chapter positions experimental design as both a methodological necessity and a flexible practice adapted to the realities of forensic inquiry.

Chapter 3 turns explicitly to the role of reproducibility as a defining feature of scientific knowledge and as a central concern for Digital Forensics. It examines the historical and epistemological foundations of reproducibility, the challenges presented by proprietary tools and volatile evidence, and the implications of limited replicability for the credibility of forensic results. By situating Digital Forensics within broader debates on the reproducibility crisis, the chapter highlights both the vulnerabilities of current practices and the opportunities for strengthening the field. It argues that reproducibility, supported by conceptual modeling, transparent documentation, and standardized experimental protocols, is not merely a technical requirement but a strategic imperative for establishing Digital Forensics as a trustworthy scientific discipline.

Taken together, these chapters provide a coherent and rigorous framework that situates Digital Forensics controlled experimentation within a formal scientific context. This part thus contributes to the consolidation of the discipline by advancing reproducibility as a methodological cornerstone and by encouraging a cultural shift from tool-driven, ad hoc practices to evidence-based, systematically grounded approaches capable of producing knowledge that is simultaneously practical, transparent, and enduring.

Chapter 1
Digital Forensics in a Nutshell

Abstract Digital forensics has evolved from an ad hoc response to cybercrimes into a structured, science-based discipline, driven by the pervasive integration of digital systems into society. Its historical trajectory, marked by pioneering legal initiatives like the Florida Computer Crimes Act (1978), the development of disk-imaging tools in the 1980s, and the formalization of "computer forensics" in the 1990s with the emergence of commercial (EnCase, Exterro Forensic Toolkit) and open-source (Sleuth Kit) suites, reflects the continuous interplay between emerging technical challenges and evolving institutional responses, such as the establishment of the Scientific Working Group on Digital Evidence (SWGDE) and international protocols like the Budapest Convention. By 2012, agencies like the FBI's Computer Analysis and Response Team demonstrated the field's institutional maturity by processing thousands of cases annually. The investigative process is refined into five fundamental phases: identification, preservation, collection, examination, and presentation, ensuring repeatability, forensic soundness, and legal defensibility, while confronting challenges posed by volatile data, encryption, and cloud infrastructures. The field has diversified into specialized branches, including computer forensics (disk analysis, file recovery, and timeline reconstruction), network forensics (traffic analysis and intrusion detection), mobile device forensics (smartphone data extraction), cloud forensics (distributed environments), and Internet of Things (IoT) forensics (interconnected smart devices), each with unique methodologies and tools. Other vital branches include memory and database forensics, with emerging areas like blockchain and automotive forensics further expanding their scope. The future of digital forensics is shaped by the increasing complexity of digital ecosystems, demanding rigorous scientific practices, empirical validation, and statistical methods to ensure reliability. The integration of artificial intelligence (AI) and machine learning (ML) promises greater efficiency in analyzing massive data volumes, though it raises concerns about transparency. AI also brings new challenges that need to be tackled in the near future. Scalability, innovative approaches for cloud and IoT evidence, organizational forensic readiness, and robust professional training are crucial for adaptation. Ultimately, the convergence of forensic science, AI, cloud computing, and big data analytics, grounded in rigorous empirical methods, will

E. OliveiraJr et al., *Controlled Experimentation of Digital Forensics*,
https://doi.org/10.1007/978-3-032-19951-5_1

shape the field's future, ensuring both technical efficiency and compliance with ethical and legal standards.

1.1 History of Digital Forensics

The evolution of digital forensics (DF) reflects the growing interdependence between technology and society. As digital systems became integral to personal, commercial, and governmental activities, new forms of crime and misconduct emerged, prompting the need for systematic methods to extract, preserve, and analyze digital evidence. Digital forensics, as a discipline, was developed in parallel with advancements in computing technology, legal frameworks, investigative procedures, and international cooperation. What began as an ad hoc response to isolated incidents has matured into a structured, science-based field with recognized standards, methodologies, and tools. This section provides a chronological overview of the discipline's key milestones. It traces its roots from the earliest legal initiatives and investigative practices in the 1970s to the complex, multidisciplinary ecosystem it represents today. Each phase in this historical trajectory highlights the interplay between emerging technical challenges and evolving institutional responses. Together, they have laid the foundation for digital forensics as both an academic discipline and a vital component of modern justice systems.

Digital forensics emerged in the 1970s, coinciding with the development of early computer crime laws. The Florida Computer Crimes Act (1978) marked the first attempt to legislate unauthorized data manipulation, setting a pattern for broader national legal frameworks [37]. Law enforcement began to confront computer-based crimes in the 1980s. The FBI's Magnetic Media Program (1984) evolved into the Computer Analysis and Response Team (CART), prompting the development of disk imaging tools like IMDUMP and SafeBack to avoid volatile live system analysis [8]. Academically, the early 1990s marked the emergence of the term "computer forensics" in scholarly discourse, as evident in conferences such as the Digital Forensic Research Workshop (DFRWS). Early research, such as Pollitt's work [39], helped formalize methodology and vocabulary. The mid-1990s saw the emergence of both commercial suites (EnCase, FTK) and open-source kits (Sleuth Kit), facilitating wider adoption and application in both legal and investigative contexts.

As the field matured, structured frameworks were introduced to enhance the rigor and reproducibility of investigations. Beebe and Clark's objectives-based process model [6] introduced hierarchical investigative phases, enabling layered and methodical analysis. Institutions like the Scientific Working Group on Digital Evidence (SWGDE) [43] were established in 2000, issuing best practice documents and promoting ISO/IEC 17025 accreditation for laboratories [21]. Global protocols, such as the Budapest Convention (2004), addressed transnational forensic cooperation and laid the groundwork for harmonized procedures across jurisdictions.

The rise of smartphones, cloud services, and Internet of Things (IoT) demanded fresh forensic strategies. Grispos et al. [17] were among the early researchers analyzing disrupted cloud workflows. Big data and AI began transforming evidence analysis. Casino et al. [11] reviewed the applications of machine learning, blockchain, and graph analytics in sifting through large-scale forensic datasets. Simultaneously, the proliferation of anti-forensic techniques, such as encryption, tampering, and evasion, has triggered scientific scrutiny. Formal methods, such as the Knowledge Acquisition in Automated Specification (KAOS) [22], have been applied to model and counter such threats. By 2012, FBI CART and Regional Computer Forensics Laboratories (RCFLs) were routinely processing thousands of cases annually. The Department of Defense (DoD's) Defense Computer Forensics Laboratory (DCFL) (later Department of Defense Cyber Crime Center—DC3), established in 2001, centralized military forensic capabilities, reflecting institutional maturity and the growing strategic importance of digital investigations [24].

Over the past decade, digital forensics has undergone significant transformations driven by the rapid expansion of cyber-physical systems, encrypted communications, and the globalization of cybercrime [13]. The increasing prevalence of end-to-end encryption in messaging platforms, the widespread adoption of zero-trust architectures, and the diversification of digital evidence sources, ranging from wearables and smart home devices to decentralized networks, have necessitated novel investigative approaches. Law enforcement and forensic practitioners have embraced cloud-native analysis platforms, automated triage tools, and AI-powered classification systems to manage overwhelming volumes of data. Regulatory developments such as the General Data Protection Regulation (GDPR) in Europe have also introduced new legal and ethical considerations for evidence handling and cross-border collaboration. Furthermore, the emergence of cryptocurrency-related crimes has led to the development of specialized blockchain forensics methods, thereby fostering a new subfield that integrates traditional forensic principles with financial investigation techniques.

1.2 The Digital Forensics Investigative Process

The DF investigative process is a systematic methodology employed to uncover, analyze, and interpret digital evidence for legal or administrative purposes. Over time, this process has been refined into well-defined models that aim to ensure repeatability, forensic soundness, and legal defensibility. Among the earliest and most widely referenced models is the one proposed by Reith et al. [42], which comprises five phases: identification, preservation, collection, examination, and presentation. These phases form the backbone of many contemporary investigative workflows and remain foundational in both academic and practical contexts. Building upon these conceptual foundations, more recent works have refined and detailed the investigative life cycle.

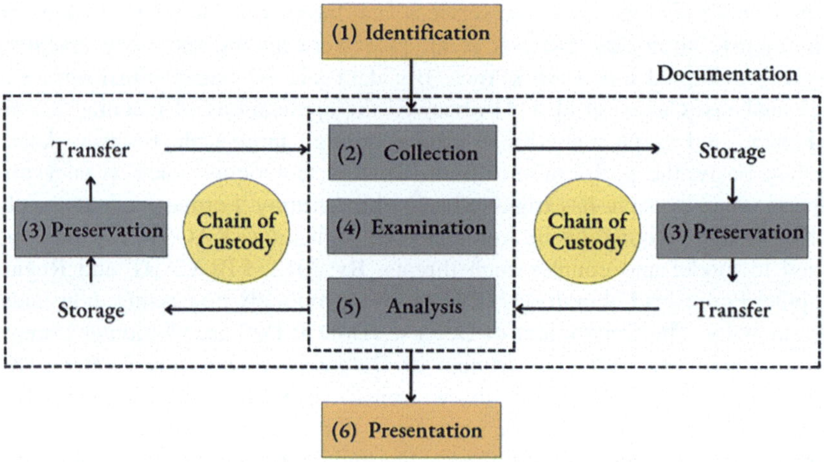

Fig. 1.1 The Digital Forensics investigative process by Nath et al. [33]

Figure 1.1 depicts the six-phase DF investigative process, according to Nath et al. [33].

The identification phase involves recognizing and defining potential sources of digital evidence. This step includes determining the incident scope, identifying relevant systems (e.g., desktops, laptops, mobile devices, and servers), and understanding the incident type (e.g., insider threat, malware infection, and data exfiltration). Increasingly, this phase must account for emerging technologies, such as IoT devices and cloud services, which often require distinct handling procedures due to their distributed and volatile nature [41]. Investigators must act swiftly, as digital evidence is frequently fragile and prone to alteration or loss.

The preservation phase ensures that the digital evidence remains intact and unaltered. This is crucial for maintaining the credibility of the evidence in legal settings. Forensic imaging tools are commonly used to create bit-for-bit copies of storage media. Hashing algorithms, such as SHA-2 or SHA-3, are applied both before and after imaging to verify data integrity [37]. In addition to technical measures, strict documentation of the chain of custody must be maintained to ensure accountability and transparency. This includes logging who accessed the evidence, when, for what purpose, and under what conditions. Any break in the chain can render the evidence inadmissible in court.

During the collection phase, investigators acquire the identified data sources in a forensically sound manner. The choice between live and static acquisition is critical here. Live acquisition, performed while the system is powered on, may be necessary to capture volatile data such as active network connections, RAM contents, and running processes. However, it also risks altering the system state. Conversely, static acquisition, performed after the system is shut down, provides more controlled conditions but may miss transient data [32]. Regardless of the method, the goal remains the same: collect the maximum relevant evidence with minimal system impact.

The examination and analysis phases are where raw data is transformed into actionable intelligence. Examination involves preparing the data for analysis by filtering, recovering deleted content, or converting formats. Analysis, on the other hand, consists of interpreting the data to reconstruct events or determine culpability. Techniques such as keyword searches, timeline construction, log correlation, metadata analysis, and anomaly detection are commonly used [8]. Advanced techniques, such as malware reverse engineering or steganalysis, may be applied in specialized cases. Investigators must meticulously document all procedures and findings to ensure transparency and reproducibility.

Finally, the presentation phase focuses on communicating findings to nontechnical stakeholders, such as legal professionals, corporate managers, or juries. This requires translating technical analysis into clear, comprehensible reports and, if necessary, expert testimony. Reports must be concise, logically structured, and backed by the evidence collected during the investigation. Visual aids, such as charts, diagrams, and timelines, can be instrumental in explaining complex findings [8]. In legal contexts, investigators must also be prepared to defend their methods and conclusions under cross-examination.

Digital forensic investigations are not linear; they are often iterative and may involve revisiting previous stages based on new evidence or insights. Moreover, investigators must remain aware of the jurisdictional and legal constraints relevant to their activities. The increasing use of encryption, anonymization tools, and remote/cloud infrastructures continues to pose new challenges to traditional forensic workflows [45]. As such, continuous professional development and adherence to evolving standards are crucial for maintaining the effectiveness and admissibility of forensic investigations.

1.3 Digital Forensics Main Branches

Digital forensics is a multidisciplinary field that investigates digital evidence to understand and reconstruct events involving digital devices and networks. Over time, it has diversified into several distinct branches, each focusing on specific environments, technologies, and challenges. The main branches of digital forensics include computer forensics, network forensics, mobile device forensics, cloud forensics, Internet of Things (IoT) forensics, memory forensics, database forensics, and emerging specialized domains. Each branch requires unique methodologies, tools, and legal considerations due to the diversity of devices, data structures, and operational contexts [25].

Figure 1.2 depicts the main branches of DF.

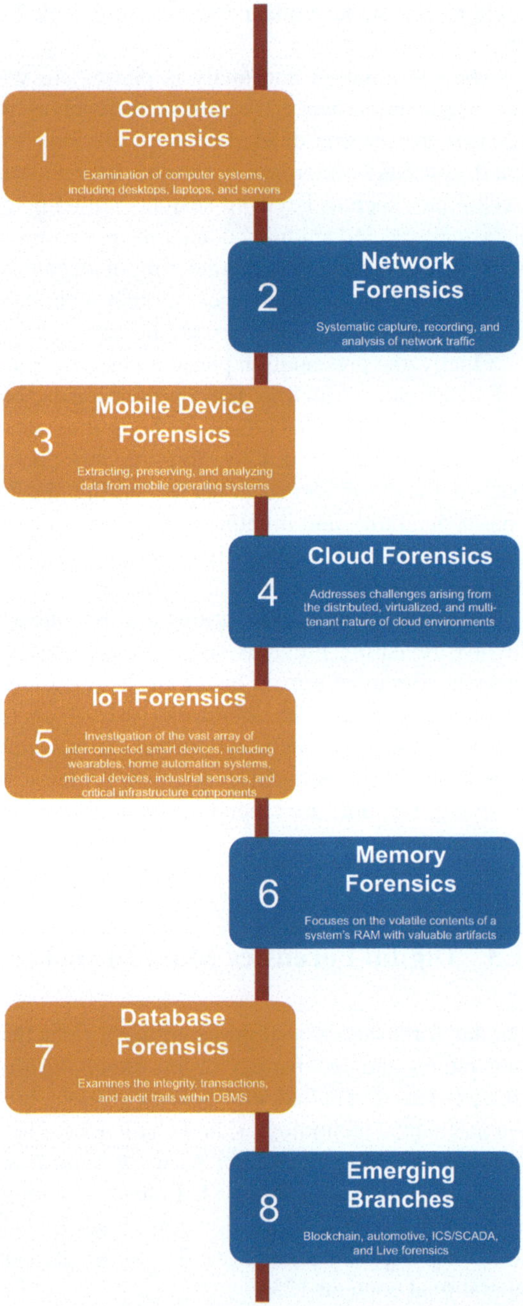

Fig. 1.2 Main Digital Forensics branches

1.3.1 Computer Forensics

Also known as disk forensics or traditional forensics, this branch focuses on the examination of computer systems, including desktops, laptops, and servers. The primary goal is to identify, preserve, analyze, and present digital evidence in a manner that is legally admissible and scientifically valid. Investigators rely on specialized software and hardware tools to perform disk imaging, which involves creating bit-by-bit copies of storage media. This process ensures the integrity of the original evidence and allows a forensic examination to proceed on a verified duplicate [9].

Computer forensics plays a vital role in criminal investigations, internal corporate inquiries, incident response, and legal proceedings. It enables investigators to uncover evidence related to cybercrimes, intellectual property theft, unauthorized access, and other digital offenses [6].

Key activities within computer forensics include the following:

- **File recovery:** Investigators use forensic tools to retrieve deleted, hidden, or partially overwritten files. Data that has been removed from the file system may still reside on the disk and can often be reconstructed.
- **Metadata analysis:** Examination of file system metadata, including timestamps (created, modified, and accessed), file permissions, and user identifiers, helps reconstruct user actions and establish timelines of activity.
- **Registry analysis:** In Microsoft Windows environments, the system registry provides valuable information about system configuration, user activity, installed software, and connected devices. Analysis of registry hives can reveal evidence such as recently accessed files, USB device history, and autostart entries.
- **Timeline reconstruction:** By correlating data from various sources, including file metadata, logs, and registry entries, forensic practitioners can generate chronological timelines that describe user interactions and system events.
- **Keyword searching and content analysis:** Investigators perform targeted keyword searches across file contents, system logs, and unallocated space to identify relevant evidence, such as incriminating documents, communication records, or contraband data.
- **Data carving and file signature analysis:** These techniques are used to locate and recover file fragments based on known header and footer patterns, particularly when file system metadata is damaged or unavailable.

The evolution of storage technologies and operating systems presents new challenges for practitioners in this field. The widespread use of solid-state drives (SSDs), for example, introduces complexities related to wear-leveling algorithms, garbage collection, and the TRIM command, which can permanently erase deleted data, reducing opportunities for recovery. Investigators may need to account for these behaviors by acquiring volatile memory or using specialized firmware-level techniques [37].

Encrypted file systems, such as BitLocker, FileVault, or LUKS, further complicate forensic analysis. Accessing data stored on encrypted volumes may require recovering cryptographic keys, which can be achieved through memory analysis, user cooperation, brute-force attacks, or analysis of key escrow mechanisms [14].

Modern computer systems also frequently incorporate cloud-based synchronization, virtualization, and remote storage, distributing data across multiple environments. This necessitates a broader scope of investigation that may include forensic analysis of virtual machine images, cloud service logs, and remote backups [6].

To support these complex investigations, forensic analysts use a range of tools, including commercial suites such as EnCase and FTK, as well as open-source frameworks such as The Sleuth Kit, Autopsy, and Volatility. The choice of tools depends on the case requirements, the types of systems involved, and the legal and regulatory context [8].

1.3.2 Network Forensics

Network forensics involves the systematic capture, recording, and analysis of network traffic to detect intrusions, unauthorized access, malware communication, or data exfiltration. It is a critical subfield of digital forensics that provides insight into incidents involving external attacks, insider threats, or misconfigurations that impact network security and performance [15].

Because network traffic is inherently volatile and transient, one of the primary challenges in network forensics is ensuring timely data collection before it is overwritten or lost. Investigators often rely on real-time packet capture tools, such as Wireshark or tcpdump, as well as flow-based monitoring systems (e.g., NetFlow or IPFIX), to obtain relevant artifacts. To maintain forensic soundness, robust logging mechanisms and timestamp synchronization via protocols such as Network Time Protocol (NTP) are essential [15].

Key tasks in network forensics include:

- **Packet capture and inspection:** collecting raw traffic at key points in the network to examine headers, payloads, and anomalies indicative of malicious activity
- **Session reconstruction:** rebuilding TCP or application layer sessions to understand user interactions or attacker behavior, which may include web browsing, file transfers, or command-and-control communication
- **Protocol analysis:** investigating network protocols across different layers of the OSI model to identify misuse, protocol violations, or covert channels
- **Traffic pattern analysis:** detecting anomalies through statistical or machine learning models that flag deviations in traffic volume, flow timing, or packet size distributions

The increasing use of Transport Layer Security (TLS), Virtual Private Networks (VPNs), and encrypted messaging platforms introduces substantial obstacles to content-level inspection. Investigators must often rely on metadata, such as destination IP addresses, DNS records, and traffic timing, to infer suspicious behavior when payloads are inaccessible due to encryption [15].

Scalability is another key concern. High-speed networks generate immense volumes of data, requiring selective logging, distributed storage, and scalable analysis to manage them effectively. Technologies such as Deep Packet Inspection (DPI), stream processing, and network telemetry are frequently employed to manage this scale [15].

Moreover, the rise of Software-Defined Networking (SDN) and Network Function Virtualization (NFV) has introduced architectural complexity. These technologies abstract physical infrastructure and enable dynamic reconfiguration, making traditional static network analysis insufficient. Investigators must now consider virtual switches, programmable flow rules, and ephemeral network paths during analysis [15].

1.3.3 Mobile Device Forensics

With the proliferation of smartphones and tablets, mobile forensics has become a crucial discipline within digital investigations [4]. It primarily focuses on extracting, preserving, and analyzing data from mobile operating systems, such as iOS and Android, as well as from the vast ecosystem of applications installed on these platforms. The types of data that can be retrieved include call logs, SMS and instant messaging records, multimedia files (images, audio, and video), GPS and location data, Internet browsing history, contacts, calendar entries, and app-specific databases, which may store sensitive information such as authentication tokens or transaction logs.

A variety of acquisition techniques are employed, ranging from logical acquisition, which operates at the file system level and is less intrusive, to physical acquisition, which involves bitstream imaging and enables more comprehensive recovery of deleted or hidden data [4]. When traditional methods are insufficient, more advanced approaches such as chip-off analysis and JTAG extraction, using the Joint Test Action Group (IEEE 1149.1) hardware interface to access memory directly from embedded devices, may also be applied.

However, mobile forensics faces significant challenges. The diversity of hardware models and manufacturers, coupled with frequent operating system updates, introduces variability that complicates the development of standardized forensic tools and methodologies [28]. Additionally, strong encryption mechanisms, secure boot processes, and locked devices present considerable hurdles for investigators, often requiring the use of specialized exploits or vendor-specific tools.

The increasing reliance on cloud services further complicates the forensic process. Synchronization mechanisms and automatic backups distribute data across networks and remote servers, raising issues related to jurisdiction, data integrity, and privacy [28].

1.3.4 Cloud Forensics

Cloud forensics addresses challenges arising from the distributed, virtualized, and multi-tenant nature of cloud environments [4]. Unlike traditional digital forensics, investigators often lack direct physical access to the underlying hardware and instead rely on collaboration with cloud service providers, application programming interfaces (APIs), and logs generated by virtualized infrastructure. The volatility of cloud instances, which can be created, modified, or terminated in seconds, combined with dynamic resource allocation mechanisms such as load balancing and auto-scaling, creates unique difficulties in preserving evidence in a consistent and verifiable manner. Furthermore, the presence of multiple tenants sharing the same infrastructure raises concerns about data isolation, privacy, and the inadvertent collection of unrelated user information.

Jurisdictional and regulatory issues further complicate investigations, as data may be replicated across geographically distributed data centers and be subject to the legal frameworks of different countries. This fragmentation challenges both the timeliness of evidence acquisition and the admissibility of collected data in court. To address these hurdles, research in cloud forensics has focused on developing mechanisms for reliable chain-of-custody preservation, designing forensic-readiness frameworks that enable organizations to anticipate and support future investigations, and implementing automated evidence collection and correlation tools tailored to cloud platforms. Emerging directions also emphasize the integration of blockchain for immutable logging, the use of machine learning to detect anomalies within large-scale cloud logs, and cross-provider standards for interoperability in forensic procedures [4].

1.3.5 Internet of Things (IoT) Forensics

IoT forensics extends digital investigation to the vast array of interconnected smart devices, including wearables, home automation systems, medical devices, industrial sensors, and critical infrastructure components [2]. These devices are typically resource-constrained in terms of storage, processing power, and battery life, which limits their ability to generate and retain extensive forensic logs. As a result, the data available for analysis is often sparse, fragmented, and presented in heterogeneous formats that vary widely across manufacturers and device categories.

Forensic investigators must therefore gather evidence from multiple layers of the IoT ecosystem, including device firmware, companion mobile applications, local storage, network gateways, and associated cloud servers where data is often aggregated or synchronized. In many cases, reconstructing events requires correlating traces across these distributed sources, a process that is time-consuming and prone to inconsistencies. Privacy concerns are particularly acute in IoT forensics, since many devices continuously capture sensitive personal information such as health metrics, location patterns, and behavioral data.

Additional challenges arise from data volatility, as IoT devices often overwrite logs quickly or transmit data in real time without retaining local copies. Furthermore, the lack of standardized forensic tools and methodologies across the diverse IoT landscape makes it difficult to ensure reliable and repeatable investigations. Current research efforts in this area focus on developing lightweight logging mechanisms for constrained devices, establishing forensic readiness frameworks tailored to IoT architectures, and exploring cross-layer analysis techniques that integrate device, network, and cloud evidence. The rapid pace of IoT adoption and the increasing integration of such devices into critical domains underscore the importance of advancing specialized methods for trustworthy IoT forensics [2].

1.3.6 Memory Forensics

Memory forensics focuses on the volatile contents of a system's RAM, which may contain valuable artifacts such as running processes, active network connections, encryption keys, decrypted data, and malware signatures that often remain invisible on persistent storage [23]. Because RAM is constantly changing and is erased when power is lost, the timely acquisition of memory images is a critical first step in this type of investigation. Techniques used in memory forensics include live memory acquisition, reconstruction of process heaps and stack traces, extraction of loaded kernel modules, and identification of hidden or injected code segments that may indicate the presence of rootkits or Advanced Persistent Threats (APTs).

The importance of memory forensics has grown significantly as attacks increasingly operate entirely in memory, thereby evading detection by traditional disk-based forensic methods. Fileless malware, in-memory exploits, and stealthy persistence mechanisms can only be identified through detailed analysis of volatile data [23]. Furthermore, memory forensics plays an indispensable role in real-time incident response, enabling investigators to capture a snapshot of system activity during an active compromise and to reconstruct attacker behavior.

Challenges in this domain include ensuring the integrity and reliability of memory captures, handling large memory dumps that require scalable analysis tools, and overcoming anti-forensic techniques designed to obfuscate or manipulate RAM content. Recent research has advanced automated memory analysis frameworks, signature-based and heuristic methods for anomaly detection, and visualization techniques for interpreting complex memory structures more effectively. As a result, memory forensics has become a cornerstone of modern digital investigations and malware analysis, bridging the gap between system internals and cyber threat intelligence [23].

1.3.7 Database Forensics

Database forensics examines the integrity, transactions, and audit trails within Database Management Systems (DBMS), aiming to uncover unauthorized data modifications, fraudulent transactions, insider threats, or large-scale data theft [20]. As databases often store mission-critical and sensitive information, forensic investigations in this domain are essential for maintaining trust, regulatory compliance, and accountability in both corporate and governmental contexts. Investigators typically analyze transaction logs, rollback segments, triggers, stored procedures, and system metadata to reconstruct user actions and verify whether data manipulation has occurred legitimately or maliciously.

The heterogeneity of DBMS platforms represents a significant challenge, as relational systems (e.g., Oracle, MySQL, SQL Server, and PostgreSQL) differ considerably from non-relational (NoSQL) solutions such as MongoDB, Cassandra, or Redis. Furthermore, modern distributed and cloud-based database architectures introduce additional layers of complexity, including sharding, replication, caching mechanisms, and eventual consistency models that complicate the reconstruction of events [3]. Investigators must therefore adopt customized forensic frameworks capable of handling diverse database engines while ensuring the reliability and admissibility of extracted evidence.

Emerging research in database forensics examines methods for detecting tampering in transaction logs, cryptographic techniques for verifying database integrity, and automated anomaly detection systems for identifying suspicious activities in large-scale datasets. Another growing area of interest is forensic readiness in databases, which emphasizes the proactive design of systems with embedded logging, monitoring, and evidence preservation capabilities. Together, these efforts highlight the evolving nature of database forensics as a specialized yet integral component of digital investigations [3].

1.4 Emerging Specialized Branches

Beyond the main branches of Digital Forensics, a growing number of specialized subfields have emerged in response to technological innovation and the proliferation of complex digital ecosystems. These domains expand the forensic landscape into areas previously beyond the purview of traditional computing, reflecting the pervasive nature of digital traces in contemporary life. They include blockchain forensics, automotive forensics, industrial control systems (ICS)/SCADA forensics, and live forensics. Each introduces distinct technical, methodological, and legal challenges that demand tailored investigative approaches, specialized tools, and interdisciplinary expertise. Together, they illustrate the discipline's adaptive and evolutionary nature, which continually redefines its scope to remain effective in increasingly hybridized environments.

1.4.1 Blockchain Forensics

Blockchain forensics [1] focuses on analyzing decentralized ledger technologies, with particular emphasis on cryptocurrency transactions and smart contracts. Its main objective is to trace digital financial activities that may be related to illicit behaviors, such as ransomware payments, fraud, money laundering, or the financing of criminal organizations. Although blockchain networks are often perceived as anonymous, forensic analysts exploit their pseudonymous yet publicly transparent nature to reconstruct financial flows.

Investigative techniques typically include clustering algorithms that group wallet addresses belonging to the same entity, temporal and spatial transaction graph analysis, and heuristic-based linking of on-chain activity with off-chain data. Integration with Know-Your-Customer (KYC) and Anti-Money-Laundering (AML) information provided by cryptocurrency exchanges further enhances attribution capabilities. The immutability of blockchain data provides an auditable trail, but its volume, distributed nature, and privacy-enhancing technologies (such as mixers and privacy coins) introduce significant analytical complexity.

Emerging approaches combine machine learning and graph theory to detect anomalous transaction patterns or hidden relationships among wallets. Additionally, innovative contract forensics has become a growing subarea concerned with analyzing vulnerabilities, verifying code provenance, and tracing interactions of decentralized applications (dApps). As blockchain adoption expands into supply chains, voting systems, and identity management, blockchain forensics plays a vital role in ensuring trust, accountability, and compliance across decentralized ecosystems.

1.4.2 Automotive Forensics

Automotive forensics [19] investigates digital evidence produced by modern vehicles, which have evolved into highly networked computing platforms. Contemporary automobiles are equipped with dozens of electronic control units (ECUs), infotainment systems, sensors, telematics modules, and cloud connectivity services. These components continuously collect and exchange data that can reveal detailed behavioral, operational, and geospatial information.

Forensic analyses may involve recovering data such as GPS coordinates, speed and acceleration logs, braking patterns, gear shifts, and communication records between the vehicle and external devices. Infotainment systems often retain user data, including paired smartphone information, call logs, or even multimedia playback history. Such artifacts can be crucial in accident reconstruction, insurance investigations, and criminal cases involving the misuse of vehicles.

However, automotive forensics faces numerous challenges. Each manufacturer implements proprietary architectures, encryption mechanisms, and communication protocols such as CAN, LIN, or FlexRay, making standardization difficult. Many systems are designed to resist tampering, requiring specialized diagnostic interfaces, reverse engineering, or cooperation with manufacturers. Furthermore, privacy regulations and data ownership concerns must be addressed when accessing driver-related data stored within telematics or navigation systems. As vehicles become increasingly autonomous, incorporating artificial intelligence and over-the-air updates, forensic readiness in the automotive sector must evolve to ensure that event data can be preserved and interpreted reliably for both safety and accountability.

1.4.3 ICS and SCADA Forensics

Industrial Control Systems (ICS) and Supervisory Control and Data Acquisition (SCADA) forensics [12] focuses on investigating digital incidents within industrial control systems and critical infrastructure environments. These systems govern vital processes, including electricity distribution, water purification, transportation management, and industrial automation. Because they directly affect public safety and essential services, forensic investigations in these contexts must be carefully balanced with operational continuity and safety considerations.

ICS/SCADA environments are characterized by unique constraints: legacy systems with limited security features, real-time control requirements, and deterministic communication protocols. Unlike conventional IT systems, downtime in industrial systems can lead to severe economic or physical consequences, making noninvasive forensic techniques essential. Investigators typically analyze network traffic between control units, logs from Programmable Logic Controllers (PLCs), historian databases, and human–machine interface (HMI) events to reconstruct incidents, such as sabotage, system malfunctions, or unauthorized reconfigurations.

A significant challenge lies in the coexistence of decades-old hardware with modern networked components, which often creates security gaps. Cyberattacks, such as Stuxnet, Triton, and Industroyer, have demonstrated how adversaries exploit these vulnerabilities to disrupt critical services. Consequently, research in ICS/SCADA forensics emphasizes forensic readiness, anomaly detection, and hybrid architectures that combine real-time monitoring with post-incident analysis. New methodologies are being developed to ensure data integrity and operational continuity, including the use of digital twins for forensic reconstruction and the adoption of blockchain-based audit mechanisms for industrial events.

1.4.4 Live Forensics

Live forensics [19] addresses the acquisition and analysis of volatile data from active systems, where shutting down the device would result in the loss of critical evidence.

It is an essential practice in modern incident response, enabling investigators to observe and capture ephemeral artifacts such as running processes, open network connections, in-memory cryptographic keys, and temporary files.

The central principle of live forensics is to preserve as much of the system's original state as possible while minimizing contamination introduced by the investigative process. This balance is inherently delicate: Every command executed on a live system can potentially modify memory, timestamps, or logs. Therefore, live forensic procedures are guided by rigorous methodological and legal protocols that emphasize reproducibility and auditability.

Live forensics is particularly valuable in contexts involving malware infections, insider threats, and active cyber intrusions. Analysts can capture system snapshots, extract volatile evidence, and generate real-time intelligence to contain and mitigate attacks. Standard tools and frameworks, such as volatility, Rekall, and memory acquisition utilities such as LiME or WinPMEM, are often integrated with live response toolkits that automate evidence collection according to predefined policies. Recent advances explore containerized environments, memory introspection through hypervisors, and AI-assisted prioritization of evidence acquisition, enabling investigators to operate effectively even in high-speed or distributed systems.

The legal and ethical implications of live forensics remain a topic of debate. Questions concerning the admissibility of volatile evidence, privacy protection, and proportionality in data acquisition persist. Nevertheless, its strategic value in time-sensitive investigations, where rapid containment is essential, continues to drive innovation in this field.

1.4.5 Integrative Perspective

These specialized domains collectively underscore the dynamic and interdisciplinary nature of Digital Forensics. Each field responds to specific technological contexts while sharing foundational concerns about evidence preservation, methodological rigor, and ethical accountability. As blockchain ecosystems intersect with IoT networks and vehicles and industrial systems become increasingly connected to cloud infrastructure, cross-domain forensic approaches are becoming increasingly necessary.

Future directions point toward convergence, including unified forensic ontologies, standardized metadata schemas, and automation enabled by artificial intelligence. Integrative frameworks are emerging to support interoperability among tools and domains, fostering a cohesive ecosystem capable of handling hybrid forensic scenarios. Such advances are crucial to ensuring that forensic science remains reliable, transparent, and adaptable amid rapid technological transformation.

1.5 Perspectives on Digital Forensics

Digital forensics is undergoing profound changes driven by the increasing complexity and diversity of digital ecosystems. As cyber environments expand beyond traditional computers to include cloud services, Internet of Things (IoT) devices, and decentralized platforms, forensic methodologies must evolve to effectively handle new forms of evidence [40]. This scenario requires not only technical adaptation but also the incorporation of rigorous scientific practices to ensure the validity and reliability of the analyses.

In this context, empirical methods have become essential tools to ground digital investigations. Conducting controlled experiments and systematic observations allows validating tools, protocols, and hypotheses, ensuring the reproducibility of results and strengthening the reliability of the evidence presented [14]. The adoption of these practices is crucial for digital forensics to be recognized as a rigorous science and for its application in legal settings [35].

Moreover, controlled experimentation based on statistical methods is fundamental to measuring accuracy, sensitivity, and confidence levels in forensic processes. The use of these techniques enables the quantification of error margins and the establishment of objective metrics, reinforcing the credibility of conclusions drawn during analysis [10]. Thus, digital forensics is moving toward a quantitative science model aligned with the highest scientific standards [36].

The incorporation of artificial intelligence (AI) and machine learning (ML) is among the most promising trends for the field's future. ML algorithms have been applied to automatic file classification, anomaly detection, and behavior reconstruction from digital logs, significantly increasing investigation efficiency [13]. These methods enable handling large volumes of data and identifying patterns that would be difficult to detect manually.

However, adopting AI in digital forensics also presents significant challenges, particularly regarding the transparency and interpretability of models. Black-box models, for example, may hinder the understanding and justification of decisions, which is problematic in legal contexts [13]. Research has explored hybrid systems that combine explicit rules with machine learning to balance performance and explainability.

In addition to interpretability issues, the rapid expansion of AI tools introduces broader challenges for forensic practice. Modern deep learning architectures often operate with limited explainability metadata, making it difficult to reconstruct how an inference was produced. This limitation has been widely discussed in the explainable AI literature [30] and becomes even more problematic in systems that employ continuous training or federated learning, where the model evolves dynamically, and prior states are not preserved.

AI systems also become targets and vectors for attacks, complicating forensic reconstruction. Adversarial examples can induce misclassifications with minimal, imperceptible perturbations [16]. Sophisticated attacks such as the Carlini and Wagner method [7] and poisoning techniques that compromise training pipelines

[18] can alter model behavior without leaving conventional forensic artifacts. Understanding and detecting such manipulations requires forensic methods capable of analyzing model drift, prediction sequence inconsistencies, and indicators of compromise in the training data [38].

The widespread availability of generative AI models also challenges the authenticity and provenance of digital evidence. Deepfake generation techniques have reached a level of realism that complicates visual and auditory verification [31]. These developments raise significant legal and technical concerns regarding the reliability of digital media. Researchers have proposed detection strategies based on neural fingerprints and artifact-based classifiers to identify manipulated content [44], and studies highlight the broader implications for trust and verification in digital ecosystems [26].

Moreover, AI-based forensic tools must themselves be rigorously empirically validated to ensure reliability, reproducibility, and the absence of systematic bias. Frequent updates to commercial AI systems can unexpectedly alter model behavior, affecting the types of artifacts generated and complicating retrospective analyses. These dynamics emphasize the need for transparent benchmarking datasets, standardized evaluation protocols, and continuous monitoring of AI tool performance.

Another crucial aspect of digital forensics is scalability to handle massive data volumes. The use of big data frameworks and distributed systems has enabled the parallel, efficient processing of large-scale data, which is indispensable for investigating evidence in complex, extensive environments [27]. This technological infrastructure enables faster, more comprehensive analyses, thereby enhancing the impact of investigations.

The evolution of cloud services imposes new challenges for evidence collection and preservation. Issues such as multi-tenancy, data volatility, and jurisdictional conflicts complicate traditional methods, requiring the development of specific protocols grounded in empirical research [4]. Such studies are crucial to ensuring the validity and admissibility of digital evidence across various legal contexts.

In the IoT domain, evidence fragmentation and volatility demand innovative and empirically validated approaches. Controlled simulations and experimental environments have been employed to test methodologies capable of handling device diversity and data formats, thereby advancing the reliability of analyses in this scenario [4]. Ongoing research is fundamental to keep pace with the rapid expansion of these devices.

Similarly, applying machine learning to network forensics can help detect sophisticated attacks such as advanced persistent threats. Experimental validation under realistic conditions is indispensable to ensure model robustness and practical applicability [5]. Integrating advanced computational techniques with experimentation enhances the effectiveness of the investigation.

Organizational forensic readiness is another area gaining increased attention. Strategies involving data logging and preservation policies are evaluated through controlled experiments that simulate incidents, enabling process optimization and reducing the impact of attacks [5]. This preventive approach contributes to a more efficient and legally sound response.

Legally, the standardization and reproducibility of forensic procedures are fundamental requirements for the acceptance of digital evidence in courts. Initiatives such as tool testing promoted by NIST demonstrate the importance of statistical validation and the definition of objective metrics to ensure the quality and reliability of results [29]. Empirical research thus supports building solid foundations for forensic practice.

Training digital forensics professionals is evolving in tandem with these transformations, incorporating lab-based and simulation training environments that replicate real-world scenarios. These educational methods enable the development of technical skills and familiarity with applied scientific experimentation [29]. Education aligned with empirical practices strengthens investigative capability and academic innovation [34].

Furthermore, close collaboration between academia and investigative agencies has driven essential advances, enabling the application of research in real scenarios. This cooperation allows refinement of tools and methods to align with operational and legal needs [5]. Knowledge exchange between researchers and practitioners strengthens the field as a whole.

The convergence of forensic science, artificial intelligence, cloud computing, and big data analytics will increasingly mark the future of digital forensics. For this integration to be effective and reliable, innovations must be grounded in rigorous empirical methods, ensuring not only technical efficiency but also ethical and legal compliance [5].

1.6 Final Remarks

The discipline of digital forensics has evolved profoundly from an ad hoc response to cybercrimes into a structured, science-based discipline. This evolution reflects the growing integration of digital systems into all facets of personal, commercial, and governmental life, giving rise to new forms of misconduct and a pressing need for systematic methods to extract, preserve, and analyze digital evidence. What began in the 1970s with early legal initiatives, such as the Florida Computer Crimes Act (1978), has matured into a complex, multidisciplinary ecosystem today.

A continuous interplay between emerging technical challenges and evolving institutional responses characterizes the discipline's progression. Important milestones include the development of disk imaging tools in the 1980s, such as IMDUMP and SafeBack, the formalization of "computer forensics" in academic discourse in the early 1990s, and the emergence of both commercial forensic suites (EnCase, FTK) and open-source kits (Sleuth Kit) in the mid-1990s. Institutions like SWGDE were established in 2000 to promote best practices and ISO/IEC 17025 accreditation for laboratories. Meanwhile, international protocols, such as the Budapest Convention (2004), addressed transnational forensic cooperation. By 2012, organizations like the FBI CART and the DoD's DCFL were routinely processing thousands of cases annually, reflecting significant institutional maturity.

The digital forensics investigative process has been refined into well-defined models to ensure repeatability, forensic soundness, and legal defensibility. The five fundamental phases (identification, preservation, collection, examination, and presentation) remain central to contemporary investigative workflows. The identification phase involves recognizing and defining potential sources of digital evidence, considering emerging technologies such as Internet of Things (IoT) devices and cloud services, which often require distinct handling procedures due to their distributed and volatile nature. Preservation ensures that digital evidence remains intact and unaltered, with forensic imaging tools and hashing algorithms (such as SHA-2 and SHA-3) being crucial for verifying data integrity. During collection, investigators acquire the identified data sources in a forensically sound manner, choosing between live acquisition and static acquisition. The examination and analysis phase transforms raw data into actionable intelligence, using techniques such as keyword searches, timeline construction, log correlation, metadata analysis, and anomaly detection. Ultimately, the presentation emphasizes communicating findings to nontechnical stakeholders through concise reports and expert testimony. Digital forensic investigations are not linear; they are often iterative and require constant attention to jurisdictional and legal constraints.

As digital environments continue to grow, digital forensics has branched into specialized fields, each with its unique methods and tools. Computer forensics (or disk forensics) analyzes computer systems to identify, preserve, and present digital evidence legally and scientifically. Tasks include file recovery, metadata and registry analysis, timeline reconstruction, keyword searching, and file carving. Challenges involve SSDs, encrypted file systems (BitLocker, FileVault, and LUKS), and distributed data across cloud and virtual environments. Tools such as EnCase, FTK, Sleuth Kit, Autopsy, and Volatility are commonly used.

Network forensics involves capturing and analyzing network traffic to detect intrusions, encompassing packet capture, session reconstruction, and protocol analysis. Encryption (TLS and VPNs) and scalability pose challenges. Mobile device forensics extracts data from phones and tablets, which can be challenging due to the variety of hardware, OS updates, encryption, and cloud sync issues.

Cloud forensics addresses investigations in virtualized, multi-tenant cloud environments, leveraging APIs and collaborating with cloud providers. IoT forensics investigates interconnected smart devices, which are challenged by limited resources, diverse data, sparse logs, and the need to collect evidence from firmware to the cloud.

Memory forensics examines volatile RAM content for running processes and malware. Database forensics inspects database integrity and audit trails to detect unauthorized changes. Emerging branches include blockchain forensics (cryptocurrency tracing), automotive forensics (vehicle data analysis), ICS/SCADA forensics (vulnerabilities in industrial control systems and supervisory control and data acquisition systems), and live forensics (the collection of volatile data).

The future of digital forensics is defined by profound transformations driven by the growing complexity and diversity of digital ecosystems. This evolution requires not only technical adaptation but also the rigorous application of scientific methodologies to guarantee the validity and reliability of forensic analyses. Empirical approaches, controlled experimentation, and statistical validation are essential to quantify accuracy and confidence, thereby strengthening the credibility of forensic findings.

The integration of artificial intelligence (AI) and machine learning (ML) presents significant opportunities to improve efficiency in file classification, anomaly detection, and behavior reconstruction from vast datasets. However, challenges related to model transparency and interpretability in legal settings must be carefully addressed. Scalability is equally critical, with big data frameworks and distributed systems playing a key role in managing the enormous volume of information in complex environments.

As cloud services and IoT devices continue to evolve, novel, empirically validated techniques are needed for effective evidence collection and preservation, particularly in light of the challenges posed by multi-tenancy and data volatility. Increasingly, organizational forensic readiness and professional training, including hands-on lab work and realistic simulations, are becoming essential components of digital forensics practice.

Ultimately, sustained collaboration between academia and investigative agencies is essential for refining tools and methodologies, ensuring they meet both operational requirements and legal standards. The convergence of forensic science, AI, cloud computing, and big data analytics will shape the discipline's future, requiring innovations grounded in rigorous empirical methods to achieve technical excellence alongside ethical and legal compliance.

References

1. Agarwal, U., Rishiwal, V., Tanwar, S., Yadav, M.: Blockchain and crypto forensics: investigating crypto frauds. Int. J. Netw. Manag. **34**(2) (2024). https://doi.org/10.1002/nem.2255
2. Ahmed, A.A., Farhan, K., Jabbar, W.A., Al-Othmani, A., Abdulrahman, A.G.: IoT forensics: current perspectives and future directions. Sensors **24**(16), article 5210 (2024). https://doi.org/10.3390/s24165210
3. Al-Dhaqm, A., Razak, S., Othman, S.H.: Database forensic investigation process models: a review. IEEE Access **8**, 21310–21332 (2020)
4. Bai, T.S., Saraswathi, V.: A systematic literature review on cloud forensics in cloud environment. Int. J. Intell. Syst. Appl. Eng. **11**(4s), 565–578 (2023)
5. Bankole, F., Taiwo, A., Claims, I.: An extended digital forensic readiness and maturity model. Foren. Sci. Int.: Digit. Invest. **40**, article 301348 (2022). https://doi.org/10.1016/j.fsidi.2022.301348
6. Beebe, N.L., Clark, J.G.: A hierarchical, objectives-based framework for the digital investigations process. Digit. Invest. **2**(2), 147–167 (2005)
7. Carlini, N., Wagner, D.: Towards evaluating the robustness of neural networks. In: IEEE Symposium on Security and Privacy (S&P), pp. 39–57 (2017). https://doi.org/10.1109/SP.2017.49
8. Carrier, B.: A hypothesis-based approach to digital forensic investigations. Ph.D. thesis, Purdue University (2006)

9. Carrier, B., Spafford, E.: Getting physical with the digital investigation process. Int. J. Digit. Evid. **2**(2), 20 p. (2003)
10. Casey, E.: Digital Evidence and Computer Crime: Forensic Science, Computers and the Internet, 3rd edn. Academic, Cambridge, Massachusetts, Estados Unidos (2011)
11. Casino, F., Dasaklis, T.K., Patsakis, C.: A systematic literature review of blockchain-based applications: current status, classification and open issues. Telemat. Inform. **36**, 55–81 (2021)
12. Cook, M., Marnerides, A., Johnson, C., Pezaros, D.: A survey on industrial control system digital forensics: challenges, advances and future directions. Commun. Surv. Tuts. **25**(3), 1705–1747 (2023). https://doi.org/10.1109/COMST.2023.3264680
13. El-Kady, R.: Leveraging AI and machine learning for digital forensics. In: Ananth, C., Mittal, N. (eds.) Quantum AI and Its Applications in Blockchain Technology, pp. 215–250. IGI Global Scientific Publishing (2025). https://doi.org/10.4018/979-8-3373-1657-4.ch011
14. Garfinkel, S.L.: Digital forensics research: the next 10 years. Digit. Invest. **7**, S64–S73 (2010)
15. Ghabban, F., Anwar, H., Zaman, N.: An overview of network forensic analysis tools for security. IEEE Access **9**, 123301–123321 (2021)
16. Goodfellow, I., Shlens, J., Szegedy, C.: Explaining and harnessing adversarial examples. In: International Conference on Learning Representations (ICLR) (2015)
17. Grispos, G., Glisson, W.B., Storer, T.: Calm before the storm: the challenges of cloud computing in digital forensics. Int. J. Digit. Crime Foren. **6**(2), 28–48 (2014)
18. Gu, T., Dolan-Gavitt, B., Garg, S.: BadNets: identifying vulnerabilities in the machine learning model supply chain. In: IEEE International Conference on Machine Learning and Applications (ICMLA), pp. 328–333 (2017). https://doi.org/10.1109/ICMLA.2017.00-24
19. Hamid, I., Rahman, M.M.H.: A comprehensive literature review on volatile memory forensics. Electronics **13**(15) (2024). https://doi.org/10.3390/electronics13153026
20. Humayed, A., Lin, J., Li, F., Luo, B.: Cyber-physical systems security—a survey. IEEE Internet Things J. **4**(6), 1802–1831 (2017)
21. International Organization for Standardization: ISO/IEC 17025:2017—general requirements for the competence of testing and calibration laboratories (2017). Available at: https://www.iso.org/standard/66912.html
22. Jain, A., Chhabra, G.S.: Anti-forensics techniques: an analytical review. In: Proceedings of the 2014 Seventh International Conference on Contemporary Computing (IC3), pp. 412–418 (2014). https://doi.org/10.1109/IC3.2014.6897209
23. Joshi, Y.K., Tiwari, N.: A comprehensive survey on malware detection techniques. In: Proceedings of the 5th International Conference on Information Management & Machine Intelligence (ICIMMI'23), article 4 (2024). https://doi.org/10.1145/3647444.3647830
24. Kent, K., Chevalier, S., Grance, T., Dang, H.: Guide to integrating forensic techniques into incident response. Special Publication 800-86, NIST (2012). https://nvlpubs.nist.gov/nistpubs/legacy/sp/nistspecialpublication800-86.pdf
25. Khanafseh, M., Qatawneh, M., Almobaideen, W.: A survey of various frameworks and solutions in all branches of digital forensics with a focus on cloud forensics. Int. J. Adv. Comput. Sci. Appl. **10**(8), 610–620 (2019)
26. Kietzmann, J., McCarthy, I.P., Kietzmann, J.H.: Deepfakes: trick or treat. Bus. Horizons **63**(2), 135–146 (2020)
27. Kishore, N., Saxena, S., Raina, P.: Big data as a challenge and opportunity in digital forensic investigation. In: Proceedings of the 2017 2nd International Conference on Telecommunication and Networks (TEL-NET), pp. 1–5 (2017). https://doi.org/10.1109/TEL-NET.2017.8343573
28. Lessard, J.P., Kessler, G.A.: Android forensics: simplifying cell phone examinations. Digit. Invest. **7**, 14–24 (2010)
29. Lillis, D., Scanlon, M., Cross, S., Berry, R.: Current challenges and future research areas for digital forensic investigation. Digit. Invest. **17**, 35–45 (2016)
30. Miller, T.: Explanation in artificial intelligence: insights from the social sciences. ACM Comput. Surv. **51**(5), 1–38 (2019)
31. Mirsky, Y., Lee, W.: The creation and detection of deepfakes: a survey. ACM Comput. Surv. **54**(1), 1–41 (2021). https://doi.org/10.1145/3425780

32. Nasrullayev, N., Ugli, H.Q.H., Valijonovich, T.O., Avlakulovich, D.M.: Static and live digital forensics, along with practical examples of tools used for each approach. Texas J. Eng. Technol. **19**, 21–27 (2023)
33. Nath, S., Summers, K., Baek, J., Ahn, G.J.: Digital evidence chain of custody: navigating new realities of digital forensics. In: Proceedings of the 2024 IEEE 6th International Conference on Trust, Privacy and Security in Intelligent Systems, and Applications (TPS-ISA), pp. 11–20 (2024). https://doi.org/10.1109/TPS-ISA62245.2024.00012
34. Oliveira, E. Jr, Zorzo, A.F.: Review and agenda of digital forensics education and training. Foren. Sci. Int. **378**, 112655 (2026). https://doi.org/10.1016/j.forsciint.2025.112655
35. Oliveira, E. Jr, Zorzo, A.F., Neu, C.V.: Towards a conceptual model for promoting digital forensics experiments. Foren. Sci. Int.: Digit. Invest. **35**, 301014 (2020). https://doi.org/10.1016/j.fsidi.2020.301014
36. Oliveira, E. Jr, Silva, T.J., Zorzo, A.F., Neu, C.V.: Digital forensics experimentation: analysis and recommendations. Foren. Sci. Rev. **34**(1), 21–41 (2022)
37. Palmer, G.: A road map for digital forensic research. In: First Digital Forensic Research Workshop (DFRWS) (2001)
38. Papernot, N., McDaniel, P., Sinha, A.: A taxonomy of machine learning security challenges. In: IEEE European Symposium on Security and Privacy Workshops (EuroS&PW), pp. 60–70 (2018)
39. Pollitt, M.: Advances in digital forensics. In: IFIP International Conference on Digital Forensics. Springer (2003)
40. Quick, D., Choo, K.K.R.: Cloud storage forensics: ownCloud as a case study. Digit. Invest. **10**(4), 287–299 (2014)
41. Raghavan, S.: Digital forensic research: current state of the art. CSI Trans. ICT **1**, 91–114 (2013). https://doi.org/10.1007/s40012-012-0008-7
42. Reith, M., Carr, C., Gunsch, G.: An examination of digital forensic models. Int. J. Digit. Evid. **1**(3), 12 p. (2002)
43. Scientific Working Group on Digital Evidence: Best practices for computer forensics. Foren. Sci. Commun. **1**, 11 p. (2000)
44. Tariq, S., Lee, H., Kim, M.: Neural networks for deepfake detection: a survey. In: IEEE Conference on Multimedia Information Processing and Retrieval (MIPR), pp. 141–146 (2021)
45. Tiwari, A., Mehrotra, V., Goel, S., Naman, K., Maurya, S., Agarwal, R.: Developing trends and challenges of digital forensics. In: Proceedings of the 2021 5th International Conference on Information Systems and Computer Networks (ISCON), pp. 1–5 (2021). https://doi.org/10.1109/ISCON52037.2021.9702301

Chapter 2
Principles of Controlled Experimentation

Abstract This chapter presents the principles and practices of controlled experimentation as a foundation for empirical research in computer science and digital forensics. It introduces core concepts such as hypotheses, variables, sampling, experimental design, and threats to validity, while also covering complementary empirical methods, including case studies, surveys, systematic reviews, and benchmarking. Detailed guidance is provided on planning, conducting, analyzing, and reporting controlled experiments, emphasizing transparency, reproducibility, and statistical rigor. A key focus of the chapter is the discussion of the lack of rigor in digital forensics controlled experiments, where deficiencies in design, dataset availability, and methodological reporting limit reliability and legal admissibility. To address these challenges, the chapter highlights frameworks, standards, and open science practices that strengthen experimental rigor and cumulative knowledge. By integrating these approaches, researchers can ensure that controlled experiments contribute not only to scientific credibility but also to practical impact in both academic and professional contexts. This discussion underscores the critical role of rigor in ensuring that digital forensic evidence remains both scientifically valid and legally defensible.

2.1 Empirical Studies in Computer Science

Empirical studies are essential for advancing computer science, providing evidence-based insights that inform both theoretical understanding and practical application. Unlike purely theoretical approaches, empirical research in computer science involves the systematic collection and analysis of data to study computing systems, algorithms, and technologies in real-world or controlled settings. Basili and Zelkowitz have emphasized this approach [4], who argue that building a scientific understanding of computing requires observation, experimentation, and model validation.

Controlled experiments, case studies, and observational studies are commonly employed to investigate phenomena such as algorithm performance, system scalability, human–computer interaction, and network behavior [39]. Through these

E. OliveiraJr et al., *Controlled Experimentation of Digital Forensics*,
https://doi.org/10.1007/978-3-032-19951-5_2

methodologies, researchers can establish causal relationships, test hypotheses, and identify patterns in complex computing environments. The rigor of empirical methods ensures that conclusions are supported by measurable evidence rather than anecdotal observations, thereby increasing the reliability of findings.

The importance of empirical research in computer science was highlighted by Denning [10], who argued that experimental methods are fundamental to the discipline. He emphasized that, like other sciences, computer science must rely on empirical evidence to validate theoretical models, evaluate system behaviors, and guide technological innovations. Empirical studies thus provide a foundation for understanding computing phenomena, supporting evidence-based development, and advancing the field as a rigorous science.

2.1.1 Controlled Experiments

Controlled experiments are among the most rigorous and foundational empirical methods in computer science research [4]. These studies involve manipulating one or more independent variables to observe their effect on dependent variables, while controlling for extraneous influences. The objective is to establish causal relationships in a controlled setting, which makes this method ideal for hypothesis testing.

In computer science, particularly in software engineering, controlled experiments are frequently used to compare programming techniques, assess the impact of tools or environments on developer productivity, measure code quality or defect rates, and process improvement [5]. A key characteristic is the random assignment of participants (e.g., developers or testers) to treatment groups, which helps eliminate selection bias and enhances the study's internal validity [40].

One of the pioneering works in applying controlled experiments in software engineering is by Basili et al. [5], who demonstrated how experiments could evaluate software development practices and tools. Their work emphasized repeatability and operational definitions of metrics, setting a precedent for empirical rigor in the field.

Modern controlled experiments often use automated instrumentation, version control mining, or simulated development tasks to observe participant behavior. For example, in validating the Cognitive Complexity metric, Muñoz Barón et al. [29] conducted a large-scale experiment involving 427 code snippets and 24,000 developer ratings to examine whether the metric aligned with human perceptions of code complexity.

Methodological guidelines also promote the use of controlled experiments. Wohlin et al. [41] provide a comprehensive framework for designing and analyzing such studies in software engineering, encompassing threat mitigation, statistical analysis, and replication practices. Figure 2.1 depicts such a framework.

Despite their strengths, controlled experiments in computer science often face challenges, including small sample sizes, limited ecological validity, and participant

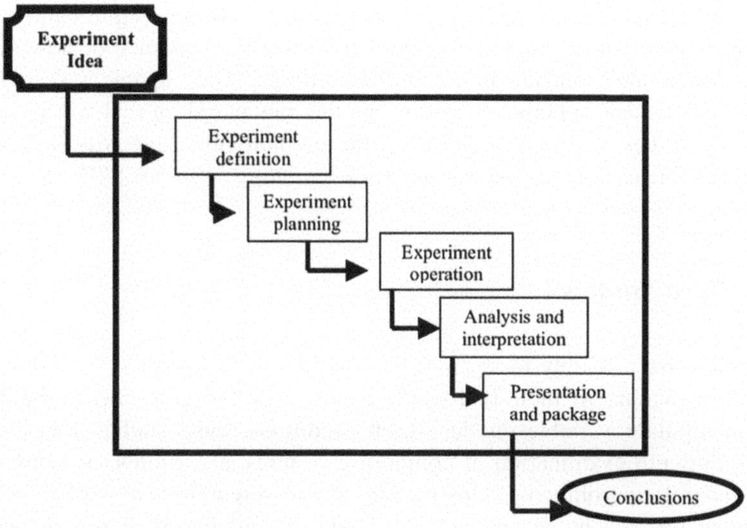

Fig. 2.1 Experimentation framework by Wohlin et al. [41]

bias. Nevertheless, when carefully designed and transparently reported, they offer high reliability and contribute significantly to evidence-based practice [26].

2.1.2 Field Experiments and Quasi-experiments

Field experiments and quasi-experiments are essential methodologies in computer science research, enabling the evaluation of systems, algorithms, and technologies in real-world settings. Unlike controlled laboratory experiments, which are conducted in artificial environments with strict control over variables, field experiments are carried out in natural settings where researchers have limited control over external factors. This approach allows for observing systems under authentic conditions, providing insights that are often more generalizable and applicable to real-world scenarios. For instance, studies have utilized field experiments to assess the performance of distributed systems in operational settings, revealing behaviors and challenges that may not emerge in controlled environments [39].

Quasi-experiments, on the other hand, are employed when random assignment to treatment and control groups is not feasible. These designs allow researchers to infer causal relationships by exploiting naturally occurring variations or interventions. In computer science, quasi-experimental methods have been utilized to evaluate the impact of software updates, changes in system configurations, or the introduction of new technologies without the constraints of randomization. Such approaches are particularly valuable in large-scale systems where randomization is impractical or unethical [21].

Both field experiments and quasi-experiments contribute significantly to the empirical foundation of computer science by providing evidence of how systems perform and behave outside of controlled settings. They enable researchers to validate models, test hypotheses, and refine theories based on real-world data. As the field continues to evolve, integrating these empirical methods is essential for developing robust, reliable, and user-centric computing solutions [39].

2.1.3 *Case Studies*

Case studies are a widely used empirical method in computer science for investigating phenomena in their real-world context. Unlike controlled experiments, which manipulate variables under strict conditions, case studies focus on the detailed, in-depth examination of computing systems, algorithms, or technologies in their natural environments. This method allows researchers to explore complex interactions, uncover hidden patterns, and gain insights into system behaviors that are difficult to reproduce in laboratory settings [4, 43].

Case studies are particularly valuable when studying large-scale or distributed systems, emerging technologies, or computational infrastructures where controlled experiments may be impractical or infeasible. They provide rich qualitative and quantitative data that supports model validation, algorithm refinement, and system performance assessment. Additionally, case studies can incorporate multiple data sources, such as logs, user interactions, system metrics, and documentation, to triangulate findings and increase the robustness of conclusions [35].

The strength of case studies lies in their ability to strike a balance between depth and context, offering insights that general surveys or experiments may overlook. In computer science research, case studies complement other empirical approaches by providing evidence of real-world applicability, guiding experimental design, and informing theoretical development. By capturing the complexity and variability inherent in operational systems, case studies contribute significantly to evidence-based decision-making and the advancement of computing knowledge [4].

It is worth noting that case studies are qualitative but may include quantitative aspects. Robert Yin [43] mentions this point in his book (latest edition). An example can be found in the work by L'Erário et al. [27].

2.1.4 *Surveys and Interviews*

Surveys and interviews are cornerstone empirical methods in computer science research, widely used to investigate phenomena related to human interaction with technology, adoption of computing tools, and decision-making processes. Surveys, often structured questionnaires, enable researchers to collect quantitative data from large populations, allowing statistical analysis of trends, correlations, and patterns.

They are particularly effective for measuring attitudes, perceptions, behaviors, or self-reported practices in computing contexts. Interviews, in contrast, are generally semi-structured or unstructured, providing rich qualitative insights into participants' experiences, motivations, and contextual factors. By allowing participants to elaborate on their responses, interviews can reveal subtleties and nuances that purely quantitative instruments may miss [23, 31].

In computer science, these methods are extensively applied in domains such as human–computer interaction, cybersecurity, artificial intelligence, networked systems, and cloud computing. Surveys can capture large-scale information about system adoption, usage patterns, and user preferences. At the same time, interviews provide a deeper understanding of why users behave in specific ways, how they interact with computing environments, and what barriers they encounter in adopting new technologies. For example, surveys may reveal trends in the usage of AI-powered applications across organizations, whereas interviews can elucidate challenges related to interpretability, trust, and integration of these systems [13, 38]. This combination of quantitative and qualitative data supports a comprehensive understanding of complex phenomena in computing systems.

Methodological rigor in surveys and interviews is critical to computer science research. Survey design requires careful attention to question phrasing, response scales, sampling strategies, and response rates to ensure data validity and reliability. Interviews require well-prepared protocols, skilled interviewers, and systematic coding of responses to identify themes and insights. Triangulation, combining surveys and interviews, enhances the credibility of findings by corroborating quantitative trends with qualitative explanations. Moreover, these methods are invaluable for validating theoretical models, assessing usability, evaluating algorithms from a user perspective, and guiding system design decisions in ways that controlled experiments alone cannot achieve [35].

Surveys and interviews also facilitate evidence-based policy and decision-making in computing domains. By collecting empirical data from practitioners, users, or stakeholders, researchers can inform the development of standards, best practices, and design guidelines. In emerging fields such as Internet of Things (IoT), edge computing, and collaborative AI systems, these methods provide insight into real-world constraints, user needs, and adoption challenges, complementing technical evaluations with human-centered perspectives. Ultimately, surveys and interviews bridge the gap between system performance metrics and users' lived experiences, ensuring that computing research is both technically rigorous and socially relevant [13, 23, 31].

Therefore, surveys and interviews are indispensable empirical tools in computer science, offering both breadth and depth in data collection. They enable researchers to capture large-scale quantitative trends while simultaneously understanding the rich qualitative context in which computing technologies operate. Their application across diverse domains ensures that computer science research not only advances technological innovation but also aligns with users' needs, behaviors, and experiences in real-world environments.

2.1.5 Systematic Literature Reviews and Meta-analyses

Systematic Literature Reviews (SLRs) and meta-analyses are rigorous empirical methods that synthesize existing research to provide a comprehensive understanding of a particular domain in computer science. Unlike traditional narrative reviews, SLRs follow a structured protocol that defines explicit research questions, inclusion and exclusion criteria, and systematic search strategies across multiple databases. This approach ensures transparency and replicability and minimizes bias when summarizing the body of evidence [22, 34].

SLRs are widely used in computer science to identify trends, gaps, and evidence-based insights across diverse areas such as machine learning, network security, cloud computing, and distributed systems. By systematically evaluating the quality, relevance, and findings of primary studies, researchers can establish the current state of knowledge, inform theoretical frameworks, and guide future research directions. Furthermore, SLRs provide a foundation for designing experiments, field studies, or surveys by highlighting proven methodologies and unresolved challenges [7, 41].

Meta-analysis complements SLRs by statistically aggregating quantitative results from multiple studies to estimate effect sizes, performance improvements, or correlations across independent investigations. This method enables more precise conclusions than those drawn from individual studies alone and helps resolve conflicting results in the literature. In computer science, meta-analyses have been applied to evaluate algorithmic performance, benchmark outcomes in distributed systems, and assess the impact of various computing interventions on system efficiency or usability. Together, SLRs and meta-analyses provide robust, evidence-based syntheses that strengthen the scientific foundation of computer science research [24, 41].

2.1.6 Benchmarking and Performance Evaluations

Benchmarking and performance evaluations are essential empirical methods in computer science, used to systematically measure and compare the efficiency, scalability, and effectiveness of algorithms, computing systems, and networked infrastructures. Benchmarks provide standardized tasks or datasets that allow researchers to evaluate system behavior under controlled or semi-controlled conditions. Performance evaluations, in turn, quantify metrics such as execution time, throughput, latency, resource utilization, and energy consumption, enabling objective comparisons among alternative solutions [1, 11].

These methods are widely applied across various domains of computing, including high-performance computing, cloud computing, distributed systems, database management, and artificial intelligence. Benchmarking allows researchers to understand the limits of computational platforms, identify bottlenecks, and optimize resource allocation. For example, in machine learning and AI, standardized datasets such as ImageNet or GLUE serve as benchmarks to evaluate model accuracy, training efficiency, and generalization capabilities. Similarly, in networked systems, benchmarks can simulate realistic traffic patterns to assess throughput, latency, and fault tolerance under operational conditions [11, 17].

Performance evaluations complement benchmarking by providing a more comprehensive assessment of system behavior under varying workloads and configurations. Researchers often employ stress testing, load testing, and profiling techniques to observe system performance in realistic operational environments. The insights gained from these evaluations inform design decisions, optimization strategies, and technology selection, ensuring that computing systems meet desired performance, reliability, and efficiency standards. Together, benchmarking and performance evaluation constitute critical tools for evidence-based assessment, enabling reproducible, comparable, and transparent empirical studies in computer science [1, 17].

2.1.7 Ethnographies and Experience Sampling

Ethnographies and experience sampling are qualitative empirical methods increasingly used in computer science to study human interactions with computing systems in real-world contexts. Ethnography involves immersive observation and detailed documentation of users' practices, workflows, and social interactions as they engage with technology over extended periods. This method provides rich, contextual insights into how computing systems are adopted, integrated, and adapted in everyday settings, revealing subtleties that quantitative metrics alone may overlook [6, 9].

Experience sampling complements ethnographic methods by capturing user behavior, perceptions, and experiences in situ through self-reports at regular or event-triggered intervals. This approach enables researchers to collect real-time, ecological data on how users interact with software, hardware, or networked systems, thereby minimizing the recall bias inherent in retrospective interviews or surveys. Experience sampling has been effectively applied in studying user engagement with mobile applications, collaborative tools, and AI-powered interfaces, providing fine-grained temporal insights into usability, workload, and satisfaction [3, 14].

Together, ethnographies and experience sampling offer complementary perspectives: Ethnography provides deep contextual understanding and interprets user practices, while experience sampling yields quantitative and temporal data about user interactions and experiences. In computer science research, these methods are invaluable for informing the design of human-centered systems, validating interface models, and identifying gaps between intended and actual use. By integrating qualitative and quantitative insights, researchers can produce more holistic and actionable evidence to guide system design, policy decisions, and technological innovation [6, 9, 14].

2.2 Controlled Experimentation in a Nutshell

This section provides an introduction to the planning, conducting, analyzing, and reporting of controlled experiments.

2.2.1 Types of Controlled Experiments

As shown in Sect. 2.1, controlled experiments are of various types, as follows.

Laboratory Experiments Laboratory experiments are conducted in highly controlled environments where researchers can precisely manipulate variables and monitor outcomes. These experiments are commonly used to evaluate algorithms, assess system performance, or measure the effectiveness of specific computing techniques under repeatable conditions. Laboratory experiments provide high internal validity, allowing for rigorous testing of hypotheses and reproducibility of results, although their external validity may be limited due to the artificial setting [4].

Field Experiments Field experiments extend controlled experimentation into real-world settings, where systems or algorithms are deployed in operational environments. By observing performance under authentic conditions, field experiments offer higher external validity and reveal challenges that may not arise in laboratory contexts, such as environmental variability, user behavior, and system interactions. Field experiments are particularly relevant in networked systems, distributed computing, and high-performance computing, where deployment context can significantly influence outcomes [39].

Quasi-experiments Quasi-experiments are employed when random assignment to treatment and control groups is impractical or impossible. Researchers exploit naturally occurring interventions, system updates, or configuration changes to infer causal effects. Although quasi-experiments may have lower internal validity than fully randomized experiments, they are valuable for evaluating large-scale systems or operational deployments, where complete control over experimental conditions is not feasible [21].

Between-Subjects and Within-Subjects Designs Controlled experiments can also be classified based on how participants or system instances are assigned to conditions. In between-subjects designs, different groups are exposed to other treatments, reducing the risk of learning or carryover effects. Within-subjects designs involve the same participants or system instances experiencing all experimental conditions, thereby improving statistical power but requiring careful counterbalancing to mitigate order effects. Both designs are widely used in performance evaluations, algorithm comparisons, and human–computer interaction studies [4, 41].

By carefully selecting the appropriate type of controlled experiment, researchers can balance the trade-offs between internal and external validity, reproducibility,

Table 2.1 Summary of types of controlled experiments in computer science

Type	Description	Advantages	Limitations
Laboratory experiments	Conducted in highly controlled settings where variables can be precisely manipulated	High internal validity; reproducibility; precise measurement of variables	Low external validity; may not reflect real-world conditions; limited contextual insights
Field experiments	Conducted in real-world environments where systems or algorithms are deployed under operational conditions	High external validity; captures real-world behavior and environmental effects	Lower control over confounding factors; more complex setup; possible variability in results
Quasi-experiments	Interventions occur without random assignment; researchers exploit naturally occurring changes or system updates	Feasible for large-scale or operational systems; can study practical interventions	Lower internal validity; potential for confounding variables; causal inference is less robust
Between-subjects design	Different groups experience different treatments	Reduces learning or carryover effects; clear comparison between groups	Requires larger sample sizes; potential group differences may bias results
Within-subjects design	Same participants or system instances experience all experimental conditions	Higher statistical power; fewer participants needed; controls for individual differences	Risk of order or carryover effects; requires careful counterbalancing

and practical feasibility. Understanding these types enables rigorous experimental design, ensuring that empirical studies in computer science yield reliable, generalizable, and actionable insights. Therefore, Table 2.1 summarizes the types of controlled experiments in computer science.

2.2.2 *Planning a Controlled Experiment*

The planning phase of controlled experiments in computing is vital to ensuring methodological rigor and trustworthy results. At the outset, researchers clearly define the problem under investigation and formulate precise, testable research questions and hypotheses. These hypotheses must be directly linked to measurable outcomes, forming a solid foundation for the experimental work [39].

A central task in planning is the careful selection of experimental factors and treatments that reflect relevant aspects of computing systems, algorithms, or processes [41]. Equally important is identifying dependent variables and reliable measurement instruments to assess dimensions such as performance, accuracy, scalability, or usability. These instruments must be valid to ensure that the captured data truly represents the phenomena being investigated.

Choosing appropriate experimental subjects, either human participants (e.g., for usability or productivity studies) or computational systems (e.g., algorithm assessment, architecture evaluation, or distributed environments), is essential. Matching these to realistic conditions strengthens the external validity of the findings.

Designing the experimental structure is another crucial step: Researchers must decide between between-subjects, within-subjects, or mixed designs, while incorporating replication, randomization, and other control mechanisms to mitigate bias and confounding effects [2]. In computing, environmental variables, such as hardware configurations, software versions, or network conditions, must be carefully specified, since minor variations can significantly influence outcomes.

Comprehensive documentation of planning decisions is indispensable. A detailed experimental protocol not only enhances repeatability and transparency but also facilitates evaluation and comparison across studies.

Main steps of the planning phase include [39]:

- Defining research questions and testable hypotheses
- Selecting factors, treatments, and experimental units
- Identifying dependent variables and valid measurement instruments
- Choosing representative participants or systems
- Designing the experiment (e.g., between-subjects, within-subjects, or mixed design)
- Planning for randomization, replication, and controlling confounding variables
- Specifying environmental settings (hardware, software, and network)
- Developing and thoroughly documenting a detailed experimental protocol

An emerging practice that enhances the rigor and transparency of the planning phase is the use of Registered Reports [30]. In this type of study, the experimental design, hypotheses, and analysis plan are peer-reviewed and accepted in principle by a journal before data collection begins. This shifts the focus from the results to the quality of the methodology, reducing risks of publication bias, selective reporting, and questionable research practices.

For controlled experiments in computing, adopting Registered Reports means that key planning decisions, such as defining research questions, selecting factors and treatments, identifying dependent variables, and specifying the experimental design, must be fully articulated and justified before execution. Reviewers provide feedback at this early stage, allowing researchers to refine the study protocol and strengthen its validity before resources are invested in data collection [12].

Integrating Registered Reports into the planning phase also supports reproducibility: Once the protocol is publicly available, other researchers can replicate or extend the experiment under comparable conditions. Moreover, it aligns with the principles of Open Science by making the research process more transparent and accountable.

Thus, Registered Reports serve as a powerful complement to traditional planning activities, ensuring that experiments are not only well-designed but also documented, validated, and communicated in ways that maximize their scientific contribution. Plenty of computing exemplary Registered Reports can be found at https://rr.peercommunityin.org/PCIRegisteredReports and https://osf.io.

Table 2.2 summarizes such planning phases and provides randomly exemplary statements for each phase.

Effective planning ensures that computing experiments are structured, reliable, and capable of producing meaningful and actionable contributions to both research and practice.

2.2.3 Conducting a Controlled Experiment

The conduction of a controlled experiment in Computer Science is the stage in which the experimental design is executed in practice. While planning defines objectives and methods, execution ensures these plans are implemented rigorously and consistently. Even minor deviations during execution can compromise validity and reliability [41].

The following checklist provides a structured set of steps for conducting controlled experiments properly.

Prepare the Environment The experimental environment must be identical across all participants, except for the treatment under study. For example, in an experiment comparing JUnit and TestNG, each participant's workstation should contain the same project code and libraries, differing only in the installed testing framework. In HCI studies, the same devices, screen resolutions, and input methods should be used to eliminate environmental bias [37].

Deliver Standardized Instructions All participants must receive the exact instructions, either via a written handout, scripted text, or a prerecorded tutorial. For instance, in an experiment evaluating debugging tools, participants may first receive a 10-minute standardized training video explaining the tool's basic features, followed by a fixed written task description. This ensures that differences in outcomes are due to the treatment, not the way instructions were delivered [20].

Assign Participants to Treatments Participants should be assigned to groups according to the experimental design (randomization, blocking, or matching). For example, in a study comparing two refactoring tools, participants can be randomly assigned to Tool A or Tool B. If both students and professionals participate, blocking may be used to ensure that each group is evenly distributed across treatments [41].

Execute the Tasks Participants perform the assigned tasks under controlled conditions. Tasks must be realistic yet feasible. In a debugging experiment, participants

Table 2.2 Main phases of the planning stage in controlled experiments, with exemplary statements

Phase	Description	Exemplary statement
Definition of objectives	Formulate research questions and hypotheses that are precise, testable, and aligned with the study's goals	"The experiment aims to evaluate whether Algorithm A reduces execution time compared to Algorithm B in large-scale graph datasets"
Selection of factors and treatments	Choose independent variables, treatments, and experimental units relevant to the computing context	"Two factors will be varied: (i) the type of algorithm (A vs. B) and (ii) dataset size (small, medium, large)"
Identification of response variables	Define dependent variables and valid measurement instruments to assess performance, accuracy, usability, or scalability	"Execution time (in seconds) and memory usage (in MB) will be measured as dependent variables using automated benchmarking scripts"
Choice of subjects or systems	Select participants (human or computational systems) representative of the target context to strengthen external validity	"The experiment will be run on benchmark datasets from the DIMACS collection and validated using three hardware configurations representative of commodity servers"
Experimental design	Decide between between-subjects, within-subjects, or mixed designs, incorporating randomization, replication, and counterbalancing	"A within-subjects design will be used, where each algorithm is tested on all dataset sizes, with randomization of execution order to minimize bias"
Control of environment	Specify hardware, software, and network settings to ensure stability and minimize confounding effects	"All experiments will be executed on the same Linux distribution, with fixed versions of compilers and libraries, and under identical hardware conditions (Intel Xeon, 64 GB RAM)"
Protocol documentation	Develop a detailed experimental protocol to enhance reproducibility, transparency, and comparability	"The full experimental setup, including scripts, datasets, and configuration files, will be documented in a public repository to enable replication"
Registered Report preparation	Submit the preregistered protocol for peer review before data collection to secure provisional acceptance and reduce bias.	"The experimental protocol, including hypotheses, methods, and planned analyses, will be submitted as a Registered Report to ensure transparency and pre-approval by reviewers"

might be asked to locate seeded defects in a 500- to 800-line codebase. In a programming language experiment, they could be tasked with implementing a sorting algorithm using the language-specific constructs for each language version. The researcher supervises silently, intervening only for technical issues or protocol violations [37].

Monitor and Collect Data Data should be gathered unobtrusively using automated tools. In software engineering experiments, IDE plug-ins can log time spent on files, compilation errors, and command usage. In HCI studies, screen recording and keystroke logging can capture user interactions. Monitoring ensures participants follow the procedure while reducing experimenter influence [36].

Manage Time and Control Conditions All participants should have the same time limits and work in comparable environments. For instance, in defect detection experiments, each subject may be given 60 minutes to find and record as many defects as possible. Conducting sessions in quiet rooms with uniform seating and lighting further reduces variability [41].

Handle Unexpected Events Consistently Protocols must be in place for addressing technical failures or participant issues. For example, if an IDE crashes, the session should be restarted from a preconfigured checkpoint. If a participant requests clarification, researchers must provide the same prewritten response to avoid providing unequal assistance. Consistency prevents the introduction of uncontrolled variation [37].

Close the Session Once tasks are complete, participants may be asked to complete post-task questionnaires, such as those that assess perceived ease of use or satisfaction with a tool. However, detailed debriefing must be postponed until all sessions finish, to prevent contamination. At closure, all data are stored securely and linked to the correct treatment group [20].

Table 2.3 summarizes the conducting steps of an experiment.

Conducting a controlled experiment in computer science involves more than simply running tasks; it is a highly structured process that requires standardization, careful monitoring, and consistency at every step. By preparing identical environments, delivering standardized instructions, rigorously assigning participants, executing realistic tasks, monitoring unobtrusively, managing time, and handling unexpected events consistently, researchers ensure that the execution phase strengthens the validity of their experiments.

2.2.4 Analyzing and Interpreting Results of a Controlled Experiment

The analysis and interpretation of results from controlled experiments in computer science are crucial to ensure that the observed effects are genuine, meaningful, and

Table 2.3 Steps for conducting controlled experiments in computer science with elaborated examples

Step	Description	Examples
Prepare the Environment	Ensure all participants work under identical conditions, except for the factor being studied	In an experiment comparing JUnit and TestNG, all workstations are set up with the same version of the Java Development Kit (JDK), identical Eclipse IDE installations, and the same project source code. The only difference between groups is the installed testing framework. In HCI experiments evaluating mobile authentication methods, each participant uses the same smartphone model, configured with identical operating system versions, brightness, and input settings, differing only in the authentication method (PIN vs. biometric)
Deliver standardized instructions	Provide uniform information to all participants to avoid bias	In a debugging tool evaluation, every participant watches a prerecorded 10-minute tutorial video that demonstrates the tool's basic features. In a code comprehension study, participants receive a printed task sheet that describes the objectives, rules, and expected outputs, ensuring that experimenters do not provide any extra clarifications that could unintentionally guide some participants more than others
Assign participants to treatments	Allocate subjects to groups according to design (randomization, blocking, matching)	In a study comparing two code refactoring tools, developers are randomly assigned to use Tool A or Tool B. Suppose both undergraduate students and professional developers are included in the sample. In that case, a blocking design ensures that each group contains an equal proportion of students and professionals, thereby reducing the risk of experience-level bias. In some cases, pretests (e.g., a short coding quiz) are used to match participants of similar skill levels before assigning them to treatments.
Execute the tasks	Participants perform realistic yet feasible tasks under supervision	In a defect detection experiment, participants are asked to find seeded bugs in a 600-line program, with tasks carefully designed to be challenging yet achievable within the session. In a programming language comparison, subjects implement a sorting algorithm in both Python and Java, focusing on how language-specific constructs affect task performance. Experimenters observe silently, intervening only in case of technical issues or rule violations

Monitor and collect data	Record performance unobtrusively to minimize interference	In a software testing experiment, IDE plug-ins automatically log compilation attempts, test execution results, and time spent on files. In an HCI usability study, a combination of keystroke logging, screen recording, and eye-tracking software captures user interactions without distracting participants. Data is securely stored on a centralized server for later analysis, ensuring traceability and consistency
Manage time and control conditions	Apply equal time limits and consistent settings across participants	In a defect detection task, each participant is given exactly 60 minutes to identify as many defects as possible. The experiment is conducted in quiet laboratory rooms, with identical lighting conditions, seating arrangements, and noise levels. To further ensure fairness, participants use noise-canceling headphones so that unexpected external sounds do not affect concentration differently across sessions
Handle unexpected events consistently	Apply predefined protocols for crashes, interruptions, or clarification requests	If the IDE crashes during the task, the workstation is restored from a virtual machine snapshot to ensure participants resume from the same checkpoint. If participants ask for clarification (e.g., "what does this task mean?"), the experimenter provides a prewritten, identical response to all, avoiding unequal assistance. If internet connectivity fails, local offline copies of all required resources are used, ensuring consistency across sessions
Close the session	Securely store data and conduct post-task procedures without contaminating other sessions	After finishing the task, participants complete a standardized post-task questionnaire that measures perceived difficulty, tool usability, and satisfaction. All log files, videos, and questionnaires are anonymized and stored in encrypted repositories. A debriefing session explaining the study's purpose and hypotheses is conducted only after all participants have completed their sessions, ensuring that no early participant unintentionally influences later ones

not confounded. While the conduction phase guarantees the proper execution of the experiment, the analysis phase focuses on making sense of the collected data, identifying patterns, and drawing valid conclusions [25, 41].

The following checklist provides a structured set of steps for analyzing and interpreting experimental results.

Verify Data Integrity Before performing any analysis, ensure that all collected data is complete, accurate, and free from recording errors. For example, in a software testing experiment, confirm that IDE plug-ins correctly logged all defects found, compilation times, and edits. In an HCI usability study, verify that screen recordings, keystrokes, and eye-tracking logs are fully captured and synchronized [37].

Choose Appropriate Statistical Methods Select statistical tests that match the experimental design and type of data. For instance, use a paired t-test to compare defect detection rates before and after introducing a new tool or ANOVA to compare multiple groups using different debugging frameworks. When data distributions are non-normal, nonparametric tests such as the Mann–Whitney U test may be more suitable [16, 20].

Compute Effect Sizes Measure the magnitude of observed differences to complement statistical significance. For example, in a code comprehension study, calculate Cohen's d to quantify the performance difference between two tools. In a debugging experiment, compute the percentage increase in defects found per hour to evaluate practical relevance [25, 41].

Visualize Data Use plots and charts to explore patterns, trends, and outliers. In HCI usability studies, box plots can highlight variations in task completion times across authentication methods, while scatter plots may reveal correlations between user experience and error rates. Heatmaps can visualize sections of code where participants made the most mistakes, providing further insight into performance differences [16, 36].

Interpret Results in Context Relate the findings to the research questions, hypotheses, and prior literature. For instance, if a new refactoring tool introduces fewer bugs, compare this outcome with previous studies to evaluate alignment or discrepancies. In usability studies, interpret observed error rates in light of previously reported challenges with input modalities [20, 25].

Table 2.4 summarizes the key steps for analyzing and interpreting results in controlled experiments, including suggested tools.

Analyzing and interpreting results require rigor, careful attention to potential biases, and contextual understanding. Following structured steps ensures that conclusions drawn from controlled experiments are both valid and meaningful in empirical software engineering.

Table 2.4 Steps for analyzing and interpreting results in controlled experiments in computer science with elaborated examples and suggested tools

Step	Description	Examples	Suggested tools
Verify data integrity	Ensure all collected data is complete and accurate before analysis	In a software testing experiment, verify that IDE plug-ins correctly logged all defect findings, compilation times, and edits. Check for missing timestamps, duplicate entries, or mislogged participant IDs. In an HCI usability study, ensure that screen recordings, keystrokes, and eye-tracking logs are fully captured and synchronized	Python (pandas), R (data.table), Excel, Git-based logging systems
Choose statistical methods	Select appropriate statistical tests based on data type and experimental design	Use paired t-tests to compare the number of defects found by participants before and after introducing a new static analysis tool. Apply ANOVA to compare completion times for multiple groups using different code review techniques. Use nonparametric tests, such as the Mann–Whitney U test, when the data distributions are non-normal	R (stats package), Python (SciPy, statsmodels), SPSS, JMP
Compute effect sizes	Measure the magnitude of differences to complement statistical significance	In a code comprehension study, calculate Cohen's d to quantify the performance gap between Tool A and Tool B. In a debugging experiment, compute the percentage increase in defects found per hour to assess practical significance beyond p-values	R (effsize package), Python (Pingouin, statsmodels), Excel

(continued)

Table 2.4 (continued)

Step	Description	Examples	Suggested tools
Visualize data	Use charts and plots to identify patterns, trends, and outliers	Create box plots of task completion times across authentication methods in a mobile HCI study to identify variations and outliers. Use scatter plots to explore correlations between developer experience and defect detection rate in a testing experiment. Heatmaps can visualize areas of code where participants made the most mistakes	Python (Matplotlib, Seaborn), R (ggplot2, lattice), Tableau, PowerBI
Interpret results in context	Relate findings to research questions, hypotheses, and prior literature	If participants using a new refactoring tool introduce fewer bugs, compare this effect with previous studies on similar tools. In a usability study, interpret higher error rates with biometric authentication in light of prior work on input modality challenges. Consider theoretical frameworks to explain observed behaviors	Reference managers (Zotero, Mendeley), LaTeX, Jupyter Notebook, RMarkdown
Assess confounding variables	Identify factors that may unintentionally influence results	Evaluate whether differences in experience, programming language familiarity, or IDE proficiency affected outcomes in a debugging study. Control for time of day, environmental distractions, or software version differences in the analysis	R (car package), Python (Pingouin, statsmodels), Excel

Evaluate practical significance	Determine whether statistically significant differences are meaningful in practice	In a test automation experiment, even if one tool leads to 2% faster test execution with statistical significance, assess whether this translates into noticeable productivity gains. In a code review experiment, slight differences in review time may not justify switching tools in a production environment	R, Python, Excel, Tableau
Document interpretation	Record the rationale behind interpretations, assumptions, and limitations	Clearly note any excluded outliers, reasons for data transformations, or deviations from planned analysis. Document whether confounders were considered and how they were handled. For example, explain why novice participants were excluded from the final analysis or how missing data were imputed	Jupyter Notebook, RMarkdown, LaTeX, Git

2.2.5 Reporting a Controlled Experiment

Reporting the results of a controlled experiment in computer science is a critical phase that ensures the findings are communicated clearly, transparently, and reproducibly. While analysis and interpretation provide insights, proper reporting enables the scientific community to understand, validate, and build on the results [25, 41].

Effective reporting requires a structured approach that addresses key elements, including the experimental design, the analysis methods used, the interpretation of results, and the practical implications. The following checklist provides a structured set of steps for reporting controlled experiments.

Present the Research Questions and Hypotheses Clearly restate the research questions and hypotheses to provide context for the results. For example, in an experiment comparing two code refactoring tools, the hypothesis might be that Tool A reduces the number of defects introduced compared to Tool B. Explicitly stating these elements ensures readers understand the objectives before interpreting the results [37].

Describe the Experimental Setup and Conditions Summarize the experiment's methodology, including participant characteristics, task descriptions, and controlled conditions. For instance, in a debugging study, report the programming languages used, the size and type of codebase, the IDE configuration, and how participants were assigned to groups. This information allows other researchers to assess the validity and reproducibility of the findings [20].

Report Data Analysis Methods Explain the statistical tests, effect size measures, and visualization techniques employed. For example, in a code comprehension study, it is stated that ANOVA was used to compare completion times across three tools, with post hoc Tukey tests for pairwise comparisons. Include rationale for using nonparametric methods if assumptions of normality were violated [16, 25].

Present Results Clearly Use tables, graphs, and charts to summarize findings. Box plots can show the distribution of task completion times, scatter plots can highlight correlations between experience and performance, and bar charts can present defect counts across treatments. Include confidence intervals and effect sizes to provide both statistical and practical insights [36].

Interpret the Results Discuss the results in the context of the hypotheses, research questions, and prior literature. For instance, if Tool A significantly reduces defects compared to Tool B, interpret whether this difference is meaningful in real-world software development. Consider potential confounding factors such as participant experience, environment, or task difficulty [41].

Discuss Limitations and Threats to Validity Acknowledge any limitations of the experiment that could influence the results. For example, a small sample of professional developers or a restricted codebase may limit generalizability. Report how threats to internal, external, construct, and conclusion validity were addressed [20].

Provide Practical Implications Explain how the findings can inform software engineering practice or guide further research. For instance, highlight how adopting Tool A could reduce debugging time in educational or industrial settings, or suggest improvements in tool design based on observed limitations [25].

Ensure Transparency and Reproducibility Include all relevant details that allow others to reproduce the experiment, such as task descriptions, datasets, analysis scripts, and configurations. Consider using repositories or supplementary materials to make this information accessible [36, 37].

Table 2.5 presents the main steps to report a controlled experiment.

2.3 The Lack of Rigorousness in Digital Forensics Controlled Experiments

The evolution of Digital Forensics (DF) as a scientific discipline depends critically on the robustness of its empirical evidence base, a point underscored in both methodological analyses and community calls for greater experimental rigor [8, 15]. Controlled experiments, when carefully designed and executed, provide the strongest means of establishing causal relationships and evaluating the reliability of tools and methods. Yet a growing body of literature demonstrates that many DF studies fall short of the methodological standards of other areas of computer science experimentation. This lack of rigor undermines not only the credibility of research but also its admissibility and probative value in legal settings, where forensic evidence must withstand scrutiny under established standards such as Daubert or Frye.

Recent secondary studies of experimentation practices in DF highlight systemic weaknesses. Oliveira Jr et al. document that in Digital Multimedia Forensics (DMF), only a minority of studies explicitly formulate hypotheses, and many omit critical details about experimental protocols, sampling strategies, or evaluation criteria [32]. Similarly, a broader review of DF controlled experimentation emphasizes recurring deficiencies in the description of experimental design, inconsistent reporting of datasets, and a lack of systematic treatment of threats to validity [33]. Without such information, it is difficult for the community to assess whether observed effects result from genuine causal mechanisms or from uncontrolled confounders.

Casey's influential editorial emphasizes that the problem is not merely one of incomplete reporting but of inadequate design itself. He argues that DF experiments must isolate variables in inherently complex, noisy environments and that failure to do so leads to fragile conclusions [8]. For example, tool performance may depend on operating system versions, file system structures, or specific hardware characteristics; if these are neither controlled nor disclosed, replication becomes

Table 2.5 Steps for reporting controlled experiments in computer science with detailed examples

Step	Description	Examples
Present research questions	Restate research questions and hypotheses to contextualize results	For a study comparing two refactoring tools, explicitly state that the hypothesis is "Tool A reduces the number of defects introduced during refactoring compared to Tool B." Include secondary hypotheses such as "Tool A decreases the average time to complete refactoring tasks," and clarify which metrics will be evaluated (defects per KLOC, task duration, code readability scores)
Describe experimental setup	Summarize participant demographics, tasks, conditions, and group assignments	Report that 30 participants were included, with 15 professional developers and 15 undergraduate students. Describe the tasks, such as refactoring 500 lines of legacy code, debugging a 600-line program, or implementing a sorting algorithm. Specify group allocation (e.g., random assignment to Tool A or Tool B), IDE versions, operating system, library versions, and any preexperiment training provided to ensure participants were equally prepared
Report data analysis methods	Explain statistical tests, effect sizes, and visualization methods	Detail the use of one-way ANOVA to compare task completion times across three tools, with post hoc Tukey tests to evaluate pairwise differences. For defect counts, use nonparametric tests, such as the Mann–Whitney U test, if the data is not normally distributed. Report effect sizes using Cohen's d or Hedge's g to quantify practical relevance. Mention any data transformations, outlier removal, or handling of missing data
Present results clearly	Use tables, charts, and graphs to summarize findings	Include a box plot showing the distribution of task completion times for each tool, highlighting the median, quartiles, and outliers. Use scatter plots to correlate participant experience with defect detection rates. Present bar charts of the total number of defects detected per tool. For HCI studies, include heatmaps showing which areas of the interface users most frequently made errors or spent the most time

Interpret results	Discuss results in relation to hypotheses, research questions, and prior work	Explain why participants using Tool A introduced fewer defects and completed tasks faster, considering the usability features and automation support in the tool. Compare results to previous studies on similar refactoring tools. Discuss unexpected findings, such as why more experienced developers performed similarly with both tools, possibly due to prior familiarity with refactoring patterns
Discuss limitations	Acknowledge limitations and threats to validity	Note the small sample size of professional developers may limit generalizability. Discuss restricted codebases (e.g., only Java programs or specific legacy code) that may not reflect broader software systems. Mention potential confounding variables, such as differences in participants' familiarity with IDEs or programming languages. Explain how internal, external, construct, and conclusion validity were considered
Provide practical implications	Explain real-world relevance of results	Highlight that adopting Tool A could reduce debugging time in educational courses or industry projects. Suggest improvements to tool design, such as enhanced visualization of code dependencies or automated refactoring suggestions. Discuss implications for training, workflow integration, and tool selection policies
Ensure transparency	Include all details for reproducibility: data, scripts, task descriptions, configurations	Provide anonymized participant datasets, task instructions, IDE and library versions, and analysis scripts in a public repository. Include all raw data logs, pre- and post-task questionnaires, and any preprocessing steps taken. Explain clearly how missing or corrupted data was handled, so that other researchers can replicate the study precisely

impossible. Moreover, in the absence of baseline conditions or ground-truth data, it is unclear whether the results demonstrate genuine tool capabilities or merely reflect the test environment's idiosyncrasies.

The issue of dataset quality and availability illustrates this challenge vividly. Garfinkel et al. argue that DF must adopt standardized forensic corpora that are carefully constructed, openly available, and well documented, akin to benchmark datasets in machine learning or information retrieval [15]. Yet many DF studies rely on ad hoc collections of digital artifacts, often assembled without transparent procedures for provenance or validation. This practice severely limits comparability across studies and prevents independent verification. Even when datasets are shared, insufficient ground-truth annotation reduces their scientific value.

The reproducibility crisis that has affected other empirical sciences also resonates strongly in DF. Horsman proposes FRED (Framework for Reliable Experimental Design), which provides practical steps to anticipate threats to validity and to document design choices in a structured manner [18]. However, mappings show that few DF studies adopt such frameworks [33]. Similarly, Marshall and Paige note that digital forensic laboratories are expected to meet ISO/IEC 17025 accreditation requirements, which mandate validation, documentation, and transparency in method definition [28]. Aligning academic research with these professional standards could substantially increase rigor and translational impact, yet current practice remains inconsistent.

Beyond design and dataset issues, deficiencies in statistical reasoning and validity assessment are also common. Few DF studies report confidence intervals, effect sizes, or statistical tests that account for trial-to-trial variability. Many rely on descriptive measures of accuracy or precision without systematically analyzing error sources. This lack of statistical rigor is particularly problematic in forensic contexts, where interpretations of error rates can directly affect judicial outcomes. As Casey notes, courts increasingly demand quantitative measures of reliability; without them, forensic claims may fail to meet admissibility standards [8].

The literature further highlights the neglect of validity threats that are standard in software engineering and empirical computer science. Internal validity is compromised when confounding variables (e.g., uncontrolled system processes or nonrandom assignment of test cases) are overlooked. External validity is rarely discussed, raising concerns about whether results obtained in laboratory conditions generalize to the diverse real-world contexts of digital evidence. Construct validity is threatened when operationalizations of constructs such as "tool effectiveness" or "evidence completeness" are poorly defined or inconsistent across studies. Validity of the conclusion is weakened when the data analysis does not justify the strength of the claims. Oliveira Jr et al. emphasize that even when studies acknowledge some limitations, these are often perfunctory and not integrated into a broader reflection on validity [33].

The lack of rigor in controlled experiments also affects cumulative progress in DF. Without replicable and comparable studies, it is challenging to aggregate findings or to perform systematic evaluations of techniques. Yates and Chi highlight the importance of benchmarking frameworks for mobile device forensics, arguing that meaningful comparisons can be made only through shared workloads and evaluation protocols [42]. This argument extends to other DF domains, where heterogeneity in tools, datasets, and procedures hampers synthesis and slows methodological advancement.

Ultimately, the broader scientific community has adopted formal requirements for reproducibility. Journals such as *IEEE Transactions on Information Forensics and Security* explicitly require authors to release code, data, or sufficient detail to enable replication [19]. Yet this culture has not thoroughly permeated DF, where proprietary tools, sensitive data, and legal constraints are often cited as obstacles. While these concerns are legitimate, they underscore the need for creative solutions, such as anonymized or synthetic datasets, structured experiment documentation, and clear guidelines for disclosure that balance privacy and security.

The evidence suggests that DF experimentation remains characterized by a lack of rigorousness across design, execution, reporting, and dissemination stages. The mappings by Oliveira Jr et al. reveal persistent gaps in reporting and methodological transparency [32, 33]. Casey underscores why these gaps are epistemically and legally problematic [8]. Proposals for standardized datasets [15], structured experimental design [18], alignment with accreditation standards [28], and benchmarking frameworks [42] provide concrete pathways to improvement. Bridging the rigor gap is essential not only for academic credibility but also for ensuring that digital forensic evidence can serve as robust, reproducible, and legally defensible science.

2.4 Final Remarks

Controlled experimentation is a cornerstone of empirical research in computer science and digital forensics. It provides a systematic means to test hypotheses, establish causal relationships, and evaluate tools and techniques under repeatable conditions. When adequately designed and reported, controlled experiments contribute directly to the accumulation of reliable knowledge and to the advancement of both theory and practice.

This chapter emphasized that rigor is essential at every stage of the experimental process. From planning and execution to analysis and reporting, careful attention must be given to validity threats, transparency of procedures, and reproducibility of results. In computer science, controlled experiments complement other empirical methods by offering strong internal validity and clear causal inference. In digital forensics, however, recent reviews have revealed recurring shortcomings in methodological detail, dataset availability, and statistical reasoning. These issues limit comparability across studies and reduce confidence in experimental outcomes.

To address these challenges, adopting structured design frameworks, standardized datasets, and open reporting practices is necessary. Practices such as preregistration of study protocols, adherence to international standards, and sharing of experimental artifacts further strengthen credibility and reproducibility. By integrating such measures, researchers can ensure that digital forensic experimentation not only meets academic expectations but also produces findings that are robust enough to inform practice and withstand legal scrutiny.

Controlled experiments play a vital role in building the empirical foundation of computing. Their value lies not only in producing immediate results but also in supporting cumulative progress through transparency, rigor, and replication. A consistent commitment to these principles will ensure that computer science and digital forensics continue to mature as scientific disciplines grounded in trustworthy evidence.

References

1. Barham, P., Dragovic, B., Fraser, K., Hand, S., Harris, T., Ho, A., Neugebauer, A., Pratt, I., Warfield, A.: Xen and the art of virtualization. ACM SIGOPS Oper. Syst. Rev. **37**(5), 164–177 (2018). https://doi.org/10.1145/1165389.945462
2. Barr, R.S., Golden, B.L., Kelly, J.P., Resende, M.G.C., Stewart, W.R.: Designing and reporting on computational experiments with heuristic methods. J. Heurist. **1**(1), 9–32 (1995). https://doi.org/10.1007/BF02430363
3. Barrantes-Vidal, N., Kwapil, T.R.: The application of Experience Sampling Methodology for the study of individual differences in real life. Per. Ind. Diff. **60**, S6 (2014). https://doi.org/10.1016/j.paid.2013.07.160. https://www.sciencedirect.com/science/article/pii/S0191886913004467
4. Basili, V.R., Zelkowitz, M.V.: Empirical studies to build a science of computer science. Commun. ACM **50**(11), 33–37 (2007). https://doi.org/10.1145/1297797.1297819
5. Basili, V.R., Selby, R.W., Hutchens, D.H.: Experimental studies in software engineering—a controlled experiment approach. IEEE Trans. Softw. Eng. **SE-12**(7), 733–743 (1996). https://doi.org/10.1109/TSE.1996.501001
6. Blomberg, J., Burrell, M., Guest, G.: An ethnographic approach to design. Hum.-Comput. Interact. **6**(3–4), 329–366 (1993). https://doi.org/10.1207/s15327051hci0603&4_3. https://www.tandfonline.com/doi/abs/10.1207/s15327051hci0603&4_3
7. Brereton, P., Kitchenham, B., Budgen, D., Turner, M., Khalil, M.: Lessons from applying the systematic literature review process within the software engineering domain. J. Syst. Softw. **80**(4), 571–583 (2007). https://doi.org/10.1016/j.jss.2006.07.009. https://www.sciencedirect.com/science/article/pii/S0164121206001283
8. Casey, E.: Experimental design challenges in digital forensics. Digit. Invest. **9**(3–4), 167–169 (2013). https://doi.org/10.1016/j.diin.2013.02.002. https://www.sciencedirect.com/science/article/pii/S1742287613000108
9. Crabtree, A., Hemmings, T., Rodden, T.: Ethnography, ethnomethodology and design. Ethnogr. Praxis Ind. Conf. Proc. **2012**, 1–20 (2012). https://doi.org/10.1111/j.1559-8918.2012.01070.x
10. Denning, P.J.: ACM president's letter: what is experimental computer science? Commun. ACM **23**(10), 543–544 (1980). https://doi.org/10.1145/359015.359016
11. Dongarra, J., Meuer, H., Strohmaier, E.: Top500 supercomputer sites. ACM SIGARCH Comput. Arch. News **38**(1), 1–7 (2010). https://doi.org/10.1145/1829690.1829691
12. Ernst, N.A., Baldassarre, M.T.: Registered reports in software engineering. Empir. Softw. Eng. **28**(2) (2023). https://doi.org/10.1007/s10664-022-10277-5
13. Floyd, C., Schwabe, G.: Empirical research methods in computing. ACM Comput. Surv. **47**(4), 1–36 (2015). https://doi.org/10.1145/2722946
14. Froehlich, J., Chen, M., Consolvo, S., Harrison, B., Landay, J.A.: MyExperience: a system for in situ tracing and capturing of user feedback on mobile phones. In: Proceedings of the 5th International Conference on Mobile Systems, Applications and Services (MobiSys), pp. 57–70 (2007). https://doi.org/10.1145/1247660.1247669

15. Garfinkel, S.L., Farrell, P., Roussev, V., Dinolt, G.: Bringing science to digital forensics with standardized forensic corpora. Digit. Invest. **6**(Supplement), S2–S11 (2009). https://doi.org/10.1016/j.diin.2009.06.016
16. Giles, C.L.: Presenting and analyzing the results of AI experiments. In: Proceedings of the 14th International Joint Conference on Artificial Intelligence, pp. 1067–1072. AAAI Press (1997). https://doi.org/10.5555/1867406.1867462
17. He, K., Zhang, X., Ren, S., Sun, J.: Deep residual learning for image recognition: benchmarking and evaluation. In: IEEE Conference on Computer Vision and Pattern Recognition (CVPR), pp. 770–778 (2016). https://doi.org/10.1109/CVPR.2016.90. https://ieeexplore.ieee.org/document/7780459
18. Horsman, G.: Fred: a framework for reliable experimental design for digital forensics. Comput. Secur. **78**, 412–426 (2018). https://doi.org/10.1016/j.cose.2017.11.009
19. IEEE Signal Processing Society: IEEE transactions on information forensics and security: reproducibility guidance. https://signalprocessingsociety.org/publications-resources/ieee-transactions-information-forensics-and-security. Accessed: 07 Sep 2025
20. Juristo, N., Moreno, A.M.: Software Testing and Analysis: Process, Principles, and Techniques. Springer (2001). https://doi.org/10.1007/978-1-4757-3558-0
21. Kampenes, V.B., Sjøberg, D.I.K.: A systematic review of quasi-experiments in software engineering. Inf. Softw. Technol. **51**(1), 71–82 (2009). https://doi.org/10.1016/j.infsof.2008.05.007. https://www.sciencedirect.com/science/article/abs/pii/S0950584908000670
22. Kitchenham, B., Charters, S.: Guidelines for performing systematic literature reviews in software engineering. Technical Report, Keele University and Durham University (2007). https://www.inf.ufsc.br/~aldo.vw/Kitchenham-Guidelines.pdf
23. Kitchenham, B., Pfleeger, S.L.: Personal opinion surveys. ACM SIGSOFT Softw. Eng. Notes **33**(2), 24–27 (2008). https://doi.org/10.1145/1368088.1368093
24. Kitchenham, B., Dyba, T., Jorgensen, M.: Evidence-based software engineering. Inf. Softw. Technol. **52**(1), 75–86 (2010). https://doi.org/10.1016/j.infsof.2008.09.009. https://www.sciencedirect.com/science/article/pii/S0950584908001341
25. Ko, A.J., Myers, B.A.: A practical guide to controlled experiments of software engineering tools. Empir. Softw. Eng. **20**(4), 1106–1136 (2015). https://doi.org/10.1007/s10664-013-9279-3
26. Larsen, N., Stallrich, J., Sengupta, S., Deng, A., Kohavi, R., Stevens, N.T.: Statistical challenges in online controlled experiments: a review of a/b testing methodology. Am. Stat. **78**(2), 135–149 (2024). https://doi.org/10.1080/00031305.2023.2257237
27. L'Erario, A., Detoni, T.A., Duarte, A.S.: A case study of software project replacement: a time series analysis. Int. J. Softw. Eng. Knowl. Eng. **33**(07), 1063–1093 (2023). https://doi.org/10.1142/S0218194023500250
28. Marshall, H., Paige, R.F.: Requirements in digital forensics method definition: observations from a UK study. Digit. Invest. **26**, 1–12 (2018). https://doi.org/10.1016/j.diin.2018.06.003
29. Muñoz Barón, D., et al.: Validating cognitive complexity as a complexity metric. In: Proceedings of the International Symposium on Empirical Software Engineering and Measurement (ESEM), pp. 89–98 (2020). https://doi.org/10.1145/1111037.1111064
30. Nature: Registered reports (2023). https://www.nature.com/nature/for-authors/registered-reports. Acesso em: 4 set. 2025
31. Oates, B.J.: Researching Information Systems and Computing, 2nd edn. SAGE Publications, London (2006)
32. Oliveira, E. Jr, Zorzo, A.F., Neu, C.V.: Experimentation of digital multimedia forensics: state of the art and research gaps. Wiley Interdiscipl. Rev.: Foren. Sci. **3**(6), e1405 (2021). https://doi.org/10.1002/wfs2.1405
33. Oliveira, E. Jr, Silva, T.J., Zorzo, A.F., Neu, C.V.: Digital forensics experimentation: analysis and recommendations. Foren. Sci. Rev. **34**(1), 21–41 (2022)
34. Petticrew, M., Roberts, H.: Systematic reviews in the social sciences: a practical guide (2006)
35. Ralph, P., Kelly, S., MacLean, P.: Empirical methods in software and systems research. ACM Comput. Surv. **51**(3), 1–33 (2018). https://doi.org/10.1145/3186569

36. Shull, F., Carver, J.C., Vegas, S., Juristo, N.: The role of replications in empirical software engineering. In: Proceedings of the 2008 International Symposium on Empirical Software Engineering and Measurement (ESEM), pp. 1–10. IEEE (2008). https://doi.org/10.1109/ESEM.2008.36
37. Sjøberg, D.I., Anda, B., Arisholm, E., Dyba, T., Jorgensen, M., Karahasanovic, A., Koren, E., Vokác, M.: Conducting realistic experiments in software engineering. Empir. Softw. Eng. **7**(1), 17–38 (2002). https://doi.org/10.1023/A:1013544303017
38. Souza, F., Cruz, T., Rocha, A.: Surveying user interaction with emerging computing technologies. IEEE Access **8**, 123456–123470 (2020). https://doi.org/10.1109/ACCESS.2020.3001234. https://ieeexplore.ieee.org/document/9001234
39. Tedre, M., Moisseinen, N.: Experiments in computing: a survey. Sci. World J. **2014**, 549398 (2014). https://doi.org/10.1155/2014/549398
40. Teixeira, E., Harrold, M.J., Johnson, R.A.: Threats to validity in controlled experiments in software engineering. In: Proceedings of the 2018 ACM/IEEE International Symposium on Empirical Software Engineering and Measurement, pp. 1–10 (2018). https://doi.org/10.1145/3266237.3266264
41. Wohlin, C., Runeson, P., et al.: Experimentation in Software Engineering, 1st edn. Springer, New York, NY (2012)
42. Yates, M., Chi, H.: A framework for designing benchmarks of investigating digital forensics tools for mobile devices. In: Proceedings of the 49th Annual ACM Southeast Conference (ACM-SE'11), pp. 179–184. Association for Computing Machinery, Kennesaw (2011). https://doi.org/10.1145/2016039.2016088
43. Yin, R.K.: Case Study Research and Applications: Design and Methods, 6th edn. SAGE Publications, London (2018)

Chapter 3
The Role of Reproducibility in Science and Digital Forensics

Abstract Reproducibility is a foundational requirement for scientific credibility, enabling the independent verification of results and supporting the accumulation of reliable knowledge. This chapter examines the conceptual, methodological, and legal dimensions of reproducibility and their implications for Digital Forensics, a field in which scientific rigor directly influences judicial outcomes. We discuss the distinctions among repeatability, replicability, and reproducibility, review how Open Science principles enhance transparency and trustworthiness, and analyze major global initiatives aimed at improving research reproducibility. The chapter also identifies key challenges that hinder reproducible digital forensic investigations, including heterogeneous device ecosystems, IoT complexity, volatile data, anti-forensic techniques, cloud environments, big data, and the shortage of specialized professionals. Finally, we outline how Open Science-driven experimentation, standardized methodologies, conceptual models, and open tools can strengthen the validity, reliability, and admissibility of digital evidence. By integrating scientific and legal perspectives, the chapter positions reproducibility as an essential pillar for the evolution of Digital Forensics into a robust, transparent, and trustworthy scientific discipline.

3.1 The Concept of Reproducibility in Science

Reproducibility is a cornerstone of scientific integrity and credibility. It reflects the ability of independent researchers to obtain the same or sufficiently similar results when repeating an experiment or analysis under conditions equivalent to the original study. Achieving reproducibility requires complete transparency and accessibility of all relevant data, methods, tools, and procedures, enabling others to rigorously evaluate and validate the findings [9, 19, 20].

The robustness of scientific knowledge is directly tied to the reproducibility of its results. When a finding can be independently reproduced, sources of error, bias, and false claims are filtered out, reinforcing the evidential foundation of scientific consensus. Results that cannot be reproduced often remain isolated and provide limited value for cumulative knowledge. In contrast, reproducible findings

E. OliveiraJr et al., *Controlled Experimentation of Digital Forensics*,
https://doi.org/10.1007/978-3-032-19951-5_3

contribute reliable evidence that supports the refinement of existing theories, comparative studies, and the development of new methods and datasets [19, 21].

In computer science, and particularly in Digital Forensics, several studies indicate recurring weaknesses in experimental rigor and reporting [1, 19]. Experimental work in these domains is often challenging to plan and replicate due to insufficient methodological detail, lack of statistical grounding, or limitations in formal analysis. Because much of the research involves novel systems, algorithms, and forensic techniques, objective evaluation depends fundamentally on the availability of reproducible experimental evidence.

Within Digital Forensics specifically, multiple authors emphasize the critical importance of well-designed and transparent experimentation [4, 17, 19]. Poorly executed or under-documented experiments may lead to incorrect inferences, which in this field can affect judicial decisions and, ultimately, an individual's rights. Ensuring reliability, therefore, demands not only sound experimental design but also clarity and completeness of reporting that enables independent verification.

3.1.1 Reproducibility, Repeatability, and Replicability

The concept of reproducibility is frequently discussed together with the related notions of repeatability and replicability. Although these terms are sometimes used interchangeably in everyday language, they represent distinct dimensions of experimental trustworthiness [18, 22]. The definitions commonly adopted in scientific and computational research are:

- **Repeatability**: performed by the *same team using the same experimental setup*. It refers to the capacity to obtain consistent results across repeated trials under identical conditions, employing the same data, procedures, instruments, and measurement systems. In computing, repeatability means that the original researchers can consistently reproduce their own computational outcomes.
- **Replicability**: performed by a *different team using the same experimental setup*. A study is replicable when independent researchers, following the original procedures and using the same resources, obtain results that are consistent with the original findings. Replicability depends strongly on the completeness and accuracy of the artifacts provided.
- **Reproducibility**: performed by a *different team using a different experimental setup*. Reproducibility involves obtaining equivalent results despite variations in tools, hardware, datasets, or analytical environments. In computational research, this means that another team must be able to reach the same conclusions even when using different models, tools, or data.

Figure 3.1 illustrates the relationship among these concepts.

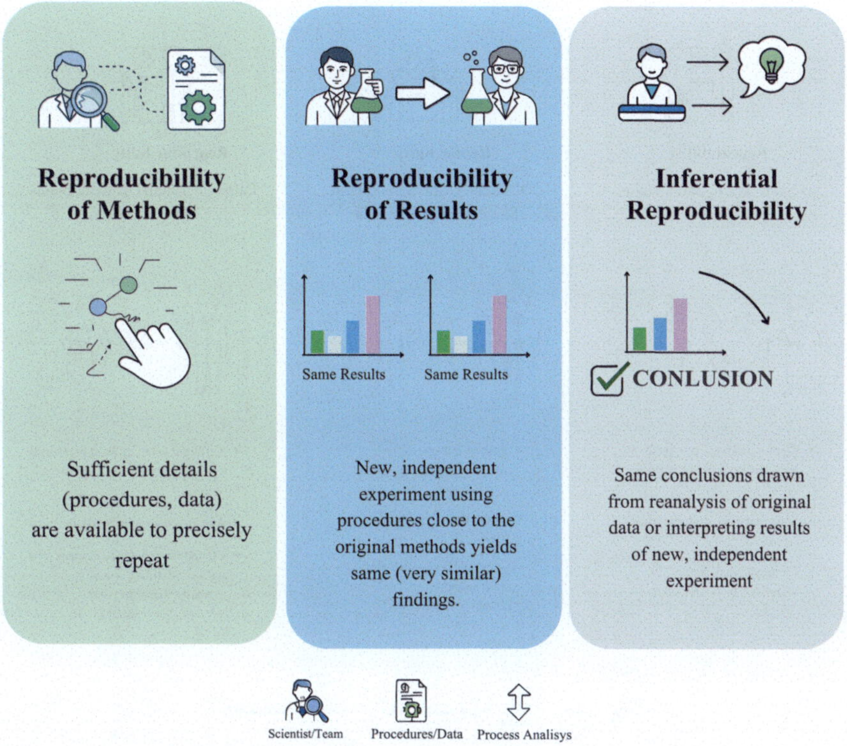

Fig. 3.1 Concepts of repeatability, replicability, and reproducibility

3.1.2 Dimensions of Reproducibility

Beyond these operational definitions, reproducibility can also be described in terms of methodological, results-based, and inferential dimensions [8]. These dimensions highlight different aspects of how scientific claims may be independently verified.

- **Reproducibility of methods** ensures that procedures and data are documented in sufficient detail so that the same workflow can be executed precisely.
- **Reproducibility of results** refers to obtaining the same results by repeating the original procedures as closely as possible, often through new experimental executions.
- **Inferential reproducibility** occurs when independent analysts reach the same scientific conclusions, whether using the original data or new data, even if their analytical methods differ.

Figure 3.2 provides an overview of these categories.

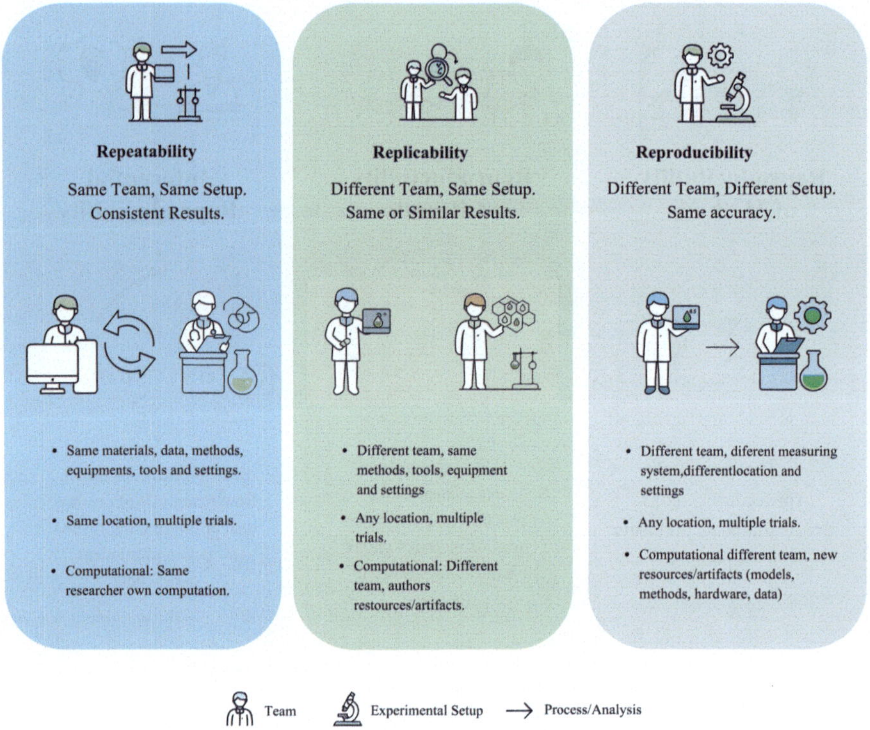

Fig. 3.2 Reproducibility of methods, results, and inferences

3.1.3 *Reproducibility in Digital Forensics*

A comprehensive Interpol review covering digital evidence practices from 2019 to 2022 highlights that the generalizability, reliability, and reproducibility of digital forensic outcomes depend strongly on the quality, volume, and availability of datasets [23]. High-quality datasets are essential for producing consistent experimental results, supporting validation, and enhancing the scientific credibility of digital forensic investigations [18].

Repeatability and reproducibility also operate as measures of consistency across repeated analyses. In digital forensic practice, repeatability is often well understood when a single forensic tool is applied multiple times to the same device. Yet, without standardized measurement specifications that define reproducibility across different tools, environments, and processes, reproducibility becomes challenging, representing a significant limitation for the field [18, 23].

Uncertainty and error rates are further concepts used to assess confidence in digital forensic outcomes. These uncertainties often arise from algorithmic limitations, analytical procedures, or measurement system constraints. Quantifying their influence remains a complex task and is recognized as an ongoing research challenge [23].

Digital Forensics involves the recovery, analysis, and presentation of digital evidence for use in judicial settings. As such, it must adhere to principles of reliability and accuracy comparable to those found in traditional scientific domains. Because digital evidence can be mutable and ephemeral, reproducibility is essential to transform isolated observations into validated scientific claims. It is therefore a crucial element in establishing trustworthiness, fairness, and scientific progress in digital forensic science.

3.2 Open Science and Open Reproducible Research

Open Science refers to a set of principles and practices that make scientific research publicly accessible and transparent, benefiting researchers, industry, and society. Its core idea is that publications, data, source code, software, tools, methodologies, and hardware configurations should be shared under open licenses whenever possible, enabling broad reuse and scrutiny. Open Science also promotes a more democratic and inclusive scientific ecosystem, reinforcing the universal right of individuals to participate in scientific progress and benefit from it. By fostering transparency and accessibility, it contributes to societal development, technological advancement, and the improvement of quality of life [25].

The growth of digital research practices has further expanded the scope of Open Science, bringing attention to the need for openness in scholarly communication, research workflows, and evaluation criteria. As research becomes more data-intensive and computationally driven, calls for greater transparency and reproducibility have intensified [2, 24]. Reproducibility is now explicitly required or encouraged by many journals, conferences, and funding agencies, reflecting a shift toward more accountable scientific practices.

The principles of Open Science are particularly relevant to Digital Forensics. This domain depends on transparency, reproducibility, and methodological rigor to ensure scientific and legal credibility. Traditionally, forensic experiments are conducted in restricted environments with limited access to tools, datasets, and documentation, making independent verification difficult. Such constraints can hinder reproducibility and reduce confidence in forensic outcomes.

Open Science practices help mitigate these issues by promoting openness in four significant areas: *Open Access, Open Data, Open Methodologies, and Open Peer Review*. Together, these principles enhance transparency and accessibility across the entire research life cycle [3].

- **Open Access** ensures that research publications are freely and publicly available. Open Access increases transparency and broadens the reach of scientific output. The authors may achieve Open Access by depositing accepted manuscripts in institutional repositories, publishing in journals without publication fees, or using preprint servers, although financial barriers still exist in many venues.

- **Open Data** promotes sharing of research data, so it can be accessed, verified, reused, and extended by others. Open data should follow the FAIR principles (Findable, Accessible, Interoperable, and Reusable) [26]. For sensitive data, privacy can be preserved through anonymization, restricted access, or the sharing of metadata rather than raw datasets. Public repositories facilitate long-term availability and reuse.
- **Open Methodologies** advocates complete and detailed documentation of experimental procedures, including tools, versions, settings, and environmental configurations. In Digital Forensics, this includes specifying forensic tools and their configurations, as well as sharing protocols, materials, scripts, and code to enable reproducibility (same data and methods) and replicability (same methods with new data).
- **Open Tools and Code:** Open-source forensic tools allow peer inspection, algorithm validation, and collaborative improvement. They increase transparency in acquisition, extraction, and analysis procedures. When closed-source tools must be used, detailed documentation of tool behavior and limitations is essential to support evaluation, verification, and reproducibility.
- **Open Review and Collaboration:** Transparent peer review, community-driven testbeds, and reproducible workflows strengthen scientific rigor. Open peer review practices, such as publishing reviewer reports and editorial decisions, enhance accountability and foster constructive feedback. At the same time, preservation of blind review is crucial in conferences and journals to ensure fairness and neutrality during the evaluation process.

Figure 3.3 summarizes the Open Science principles and their key roles.

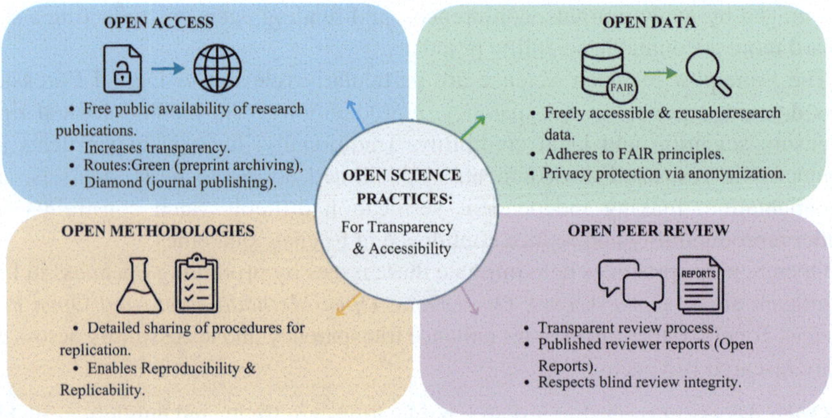

Fig. 3.3 Open Science principles and their roles in the research life cycle

When applied to Digital Forensics, Open Science promotes a shift from isolated case studies to a more robust scientific foundation built upon shared, verifiable, and reusable knowledge. This strengthens the credibility of forensic findings not only among investigators and researchers but also in judicial contexts, contributing to greater trust in evidence presented in court [14].

Despite its benefits, the widespread adoption of Open Science remains hindered by several barriers. These include limited awareness, insufficient training, lack of incentives, resource constraints, and concerns related to intellectual property, privacy, security, and cultural resistance within research communities [3]. Although scientific knowledge should ideally be open, certain restrictions are necessary to safeguard privacy, human rights, and security. Consequently, tools and methods must be developed to enable responsible openness while respecting legitimate constraints [25].

Reproducibility remains a central theme in scientific advancement. Without it, research findings become unverifiable and unreliable, which is especially problematic in fields such as Digital Forensics. Here, reproducibility ensures the validity of evidence, the credibility of forensic analyses, and the integrity of conclusions used in legal proceedings [4, 14, 19]. Open Science, combined with open reproducible research practices, provides a pathway to strengthen the scientific and legal foundations of Digital Forensics.

3.3 Worldwide Reproducibility Initiatives

Experimentation is a cornerstone of scientific progress, as it strengthens the evidential basis of a field through systematically generated data, results, and analyses. Repeated trials, replications, and reproducibility studies allow researchers to confirm or refute hypotheses and advance scientific understanding. Persistent concerns about irreproducible findings have challenged assumptions about scientific reliability and motivated a global movement aimed at increasing transparency, improving research practices, and enhancing confidence in published results. Although initiatives vary across disciplines, regions, and organizations, their central objective is consistent: to promote scientific advancement by enabling the reproduction, verification, and extension of findings.

Several reproducibility initiatives have been developed to support researchers in designing robust experiments, validating results, and fostering open and reliable scientific practices. The following subsections present some of the most influential international efforts.

3.3.1 *Springer Nature Open Science Initiatives*

Springer Nature[1] is one of the world's largest research publishers and a leading proponent of open research. It encompasses well-established brands such as Springer, Nature Portfolio, BMC, Palgrave Macmillan, and Scientific American. The organization promotes the open dissemination of all research outputs, including publications, preprints, data, code, protocols, and peer review materials. Its mission is to accelerate scientific progress, encourage interdisciplinary collaboration, increase research reuse, and strengthen trust in science.

Through collaborations across the academic ecosystem, Springer Nature supports sustainable and equitable research systems. Key Open Science initiatives[2] include:

- **Transparent Peer Review (TPR):** The authors publishing in Nature-branded journals benefit from Transparent Peer Review, which increases accountability and knowledge sharing by making reviewer comments and editorial decisions publicly accessible. TPR is the default standard for newly submitted research articles.
- **Code Sharing:** Springer Nature promotes computational reproducibility through a partnership with Code Ocean.[3] Code Ocean provides a cloud-based platform that enables the authors to share, execute, and reproduce code and data in standardized computational capsules. The platform adheres to FAIR principles [26] and helps reduce technical barriers in code review.
- **Protocols Sharing:** The acquisition of protocols.io[4] expands support for sharing detailed and reproducible experimental methods. Protocols.io is a secure platform that enables the publication, versioning, and collaborative refinement of experimental protocols.
- **Data Sharing:** Springer Nature partners with figshare[5] to provide an integrated repository for storing and disseminating diverse research outputs. Figshare allows the authors to upload datasets in any format, making them citable, discoverable, and reusable. Data remains private during manuscript review and becomes publicly accessible upon publication.

[1] https://www.springernature.com

[2] https://www.springernature.com/gp/open-science#c18176128

[3] https://codeocean.com

[4] https://www.protocols.io

[5] https://springernature.figshare.com/

3.3.2 The IEEE Access Reproducibility Initiative

The Institute of Electrical and Electronics Engineers (IEEE)[6] is the world's largest technical professional organization and a key promoter of reproducible research. IEEE Access[7] is a multidisciplinary open-access journal known for rapid peer review and continuous publication. All articles are freely available, supported by article processing charges (APCs).

IEEE Access maintains a dedicated reproducibility initiative[8] that fosters transparency and reuse of research code. The authors may submit the code associated with a published article for post-publication peer review. Successful evaluation results in a reproducibility badge, increasing trust and visibility.

Several resources support this initiative:

1. **IEEE DataPort:** a large-scale repository for datasets and analytical tools.[9] It supports data sharing, collaboration, and long-term preservation of research data.
2. **IEEE CodeOcean:** a cloud platform that enables the authors to upload, execute, and reproduce code directly in the browser.[10] It eliminates installation barriers and ensures consistency across computational environments.
3. **IEEE Author Center:** a comprehensive online resource that guides the authors on best practices in reproducibility, data management, and manuscript preparation.[11]

3.3.3 Brazilian Reproducibility Initiatives

Brazilian scientific output has expanded substantially in recent decades. However, greater publication volume does not necessarily translate into greater scientific reliability, and concerns about irreproducible findings have been documented across multiple domains, particularly in biomedical research.[12] In response, several national initiatives have emerged to strengthen transparency, methodological rigor, and reproducibility. Two of the most influential efforts come from the biomedical sciences and from the computing research community.

---

[6] https://www.ieee.org/

[7] https://ieeeaccess.ieee.org/

[8] https://ieeeaccess.ieee.org/authors/reproducibility/

[9] https://ieee-dataport.org/

[10] https://codeocean.com/signup/ieee

[11] https://journals.ieeeauthorcenter.ieee.org/create-your-ieee-journal-article/research-reproducibility/

[12] https://serrapilheira.org/en/projetos/brazilian-reproducibility-initiative/

3.3.3.1 The Brazilian Reproducibility Initiative (Biomedical Sciences)

The Brazilian Reproducibility Initiative[13] is a multicenter project supported by the Serrapilheira Institute[14] that aims to estimate the reproducibility of Brazilian biomedical science. The project replicates experiments from a random sample of published articles using three widely adopted laboratory methods: MTT cell viability assay, elevated plus maze, and RT-PCR.

Each experiment is independently reproduced in three laboratories using pre-registered protocols closely aligned with the originals. Randomization, blinding, and justification of sample size ensure methodological rigor. Replication success is evaluated by checking whether effect sizes fall within a 95% prediction interval based on the three reproductions.

Non-replication does not necessarily imply problems in the original study, since interlaboratory variability may occur naturally. The initiative, therefore, provides reproducibility estimates and insights into methodological factors that influence replication success. It represents the first systematic national-level assessment of research reproducibility in Brazil. In recognition of its impact, it received the Einstein Foundation Award 2025[15] in the institutional category.

3.3.3.2 Open Science and Reproducibility in Brazilian Computer Science: CBSoft, OpenScienSE, and the Artifact Festival

In the Brazilian Software Engineering and Computer Science communities, reproducibility has also gained significant visibility, particularly through initiatives associated with the Brazilian Conference on Software: Theory and Practice (CBSoft). Since 2021, CBSoft has hosted two major initiatives dedicated to promoting Open Science, artifact availability, and reproducibility.

- **OpenScienSE Workshop:** The Open Science in Software Engineering (OpenScienSE) workshop serves as a national forum that promotes transparency, openness, and reproducibility in Software Engineering research. The workshop brings together researchers, practitioners, and students who are committed to improving research practices, sharing datasets and tools, discussing experimental design openly, and fostering a community culture that values replicability. Typical contributions include replication studies, conceptual frameworks for experiment documentation, open datasets, and empirical work aligned with FAIR principles.
- **CBSoft Artifact Evaluation Track (Artifact Festival):** Since 2021, CBSoft has also maintained an Artifact Evaluation Track, often referred to as the Artifact

[13] https://www.reprodutibilidade.bio.br/home

[14] https://serrapilheira.org/

[15] https://award.einsteinfoundation.de/award-winners-finalists/recipients-2025/brazilian-reproducibility-initiative

Festival. This initiative assesses the availability, reusability, completeness, and reproducibility of research artifacts associated with papers accepted at CBSoft sub-events, including SBES, SBCARS, SBLP, and Sessão Setorial. The evaluation process is inspired by international practices adopted in events such as ICSE and FSE. It includes a system of badges that certify artifact availability, functional validation, and reproducibility. By encouraging the authors to package datasets, source code, tools, notebooks, scripts, and documentation, the Artifact Festival has contributed to improving transparency and long-term research value in the Brazilian community.

Together, the OpenScienSE workshop and the Artifact Festival constitute a coordinated, community-driven effort to advance Open Science and reproducibility in Brazilian Software Engineering. These initiatives help align national practices with international standards and strengthen the methodological foundations of empirical research in Computer Science.

In summary, Brazil now hosts reproducibility initiatives in both the biomedical and computing research communities. These efforts, although distinct in scope and methodology, collectively strengthen national scientific integrity, promote transparency, and position the country as an active contributor to global movements that advocate for Open Science and reproducible research.

3.3.4 The UK Reproducibility Network (UKRN)

The UK Reproducibility Network (UKRN)[16] is a national peer-led consortium dedicated to strengthening research quality across the United Kingdom. The network investigates factors that influence research robustness, conducts training activities, disseminates best practices, and coordinates institutional efforts to improve reproducibility.

UKRN brings together researchers, universities, funders, publishers, and other stakeholders. Its mission is to address cultural, structural, and procedural issues that contribute to poor reproducibility and replicability. The initiative is governed by a Supervisory Board and supported by advisory committees, enabling coordinated reform across disciplines and institutions.

3.3.5 The AI4Europe Reproducibility Initiative

Reproducibility is crucial in fields driven by AI and machine learning, where computational complexity, dataset variability, and opaque models can hinder ver-

[16] https://www.ukrn.org/

ification. The AI4Europe Reproducibility Initiative[17] promotes reproducible AI research by addressing technical, cultural, and systemic challenges. The initiative is part of the AI-on-Demand (AIoD) platform, accessible at https://www.ai4europe.eu.

The overarching objective of AI4Europe is to support a sustainable digital infrastructure and experimentation ecosystem that strengthens the European AI research landscape. It promotes openness, transparency, and trustworthy AI development by integrating resources from academic, industry, and government partners.

The AIoD platform[18] provides a community-driven environment where researchers can access and share:

- AI datasets, models, experiments, tools, and services
- Publications, educational materials, and research project information
- News, events, laboratories, and professional profiles

AI4Europe and AIoD aim to accelerate scientific discovery, enhance collaboration, and ensure the responsible development of AI aligned with European values.

3.4 Reproducibility Issues in Digital Forensics

Digital Forensics faces substantial ethical, technical, and methodological challenges. As digital devices proliferate and hardware and software ecosystems become increasingly heterogeneous, the ability to reproduce, validate, and trust forensic findings becomes more complex. Because the outcomes of forensic investigations must be scientifically grounded, verifiable, and trustworthy to be accepted in court, limitations in reproducibility directly affect the fairness and reliability of judicial processes. This section discusses the main issues and challenges that hinder reproducibility in Digital Forensics.

3.4.1 Complexity of Experiments

Designing robust experiments in Digital Forensics is far from trivial. Experimental work requires careful planning to avoid methodological mistakes and increase scientific precision. Flawed test results may lead to incorrect conclusions with severe consequences for individuals and organizations. Therefore, forensic researchers must prioritize both rigorous experimental design and transparent reporting to ensure reliability and repeatability.

---

[17] https://aiod.eu/project/ai4europe/

[18] https://aiod.eu/

Planning an experiment to interpret or explain digital artifacts requires eliminating irrelevant variables and isolating causal factors. Experimental environments must be controlled precisely, and parameters such as hardware configuration, software versions, and operating system settings must be documented in detail. Minor variations in experimental configuration can significantly alter experimental outcomes, making reproducibility a persistent challenge [4].

3.4.2 IoT and the Complexity of Digital Systems and Devices

The Internet of Things (IoT) comprises physical objects equipped with sensors, software, and communication capabilities. The adoption of IoT devices is increasing rapidly, creating highly distributed, heterogeneous, and data-intensive environments. This complexity introduces several forensic challenges.

IoT systems generate vast amounts of diverse and often unstructured data. Their distributed nature complicates data acquisition, preservation, reconstruction, and analysis. Existing forensic processes were designed for traditional IT systems and usually fail to account for IoT-specific characteristics. Additional challenges arise due to the lack of standardized IoT forensic processes, limited training, insufficient specialized tools, and concerns regarding privacy and data protection [6, 12, 16].

Some of the main reproducibility issues in IoT forensics include:

- Absence of guidelines or legal frameworks for handling incidents during pre- and post-incident phases
- Lack of defined forensic process models tailored to IoT environments
- Limited approaches to address privacy and data protection during evidence acquisition
- Device diversity that affects the authenticity, integrity, and reproducibility of digital evidence
- Difficulties in developing standardized tools and techniques adaptable to highly variable device ecosystems
- Constant need for training and skill development in response to emerging technologies
- Challenges posed by multi-jurisdictional data spread across different countries and legal systems

3.4.3 Artificial Intelligence (AI)

Digital transformation reshapes both society and criminal activity. Emerging technologies, particularly artificial intelligence, create new opportunities for malicious actors. The rapid evolution of AI has enabled the development of sophisticated tools that automate attacks, generate deceptive content, and conceal traces, thereby complicating forensic investigations [13, 15].

Generative AI systems can produce images, video, text, code, and synthetic identities. Publicly accessible platforms such as ChatGPT,[19] Gemini,[20] Meta AI,[21] and Copilot[22] demonstrate this capability. Malicious variants, such as WormGPT [15], have emerged to assist criminals in crafting phishing attacks, generating malware, and erasing forensic traces.

The forensic models and tools based on artificial intelligence are highly dependent on the quality and amount of training data. In digital forensics, datasets are usually limited, lack diversity, and can contain biases that lead to inaccurate or unfair results if not properly addressed. Additionally, there is a high demand for reproducing state-of-the-art AI models that require high computational resources, which are financially expensive and usually not available to most researchers and experts.

Digital Forensics must therefore evolve by developing new investigative methods, tools, and strategies to address AI-enabled crimes. Without advances in forensic readiness and analytical capabilities, emerging AI technologies will continue to undermine reproducibility and the reliability of forensic results.

3.4.4 Big Data

IoT, cloud platforms, social networks, and modern applications generate enormous amounts of data, often unstructured and distributed across multiple environments. Managing, filtering, and analyzing such data introduce high computational overhead and increase the likelihood of human error or analytical bias. Documentation becomes more difficult, which compromises reproducibility.

The forensic process requires the collection, preservation, and analysis of electronic evidence. However, with data volumes growing exponentially, acquiring complete datasets is often impractical. Investigators may capture only a subset of evidence, particularly in live or cloud-based environments, risking the omission of critical information.

Large-scale data acquisition and processing require specialized hardware, advanced analytical tools, and substantial time investment. These requirements delay investigations, increase costs, and reduce the ability to produce timely and reproducible results [6, 12, 16].

[19] https://chatgpt.com/

[20] https://gemini.google.com/app

[21] https://ai.meta.com/

[22] https://copilot.microsoft.com/

3.4.5 Cloud Computing

Cloud computing environments introduce additional layers of complexity. Data stored across distributed, virtualized infrastructures is often inaccessible to investigators, and physical examination of storage devices is not possible. Evidence belonging to multiple users may coexist within the same physical environment, complicating attribution and chain of custody.

The distributed and dynamic nature of cloud environments makes it difficult to reconstruct complete and consistent sets of evidence. Legal and privacy regulations vary across jurisdictions, and data may be stored in different countries, requiring coordination with multiple service providers. Traditional forensic methods are inadequate for these scenarios, and specialized tools and expertise are required to collect and analyze cloud-based evidence reliably.

3.4.6 Data Volatility and Dynamic Environments

Volatile data exists only temporarily and can be altered or lost when system states change. In Digital Forensics, volatile memory such as RAM often contains crucial information about system operations, active processes, and user activities. Because such data dissipates rapidly, acquisition must occur immediately and with specialized techniques.

The ephemeral nature of volatile data makes standardization and reproducibility difficult. If investigators fail to capture data in a timely manner or if acquisition methods differ slightly, results may not be comparable across analyses.

3.4.7 Anti-forensic Techniques and Cryptography

Anti-forensic techniques aim to obscure, manipulate, or destroy digital evidence. These techniques intentionally impede investigations and reduce the reproducibility of forensic findings. Common anti-forensic methods include:

- **Data encryption** prevents access to critical evidence. Encrypted virtual machines or storage volumes may be impossible to analyze without decryption keys.
- **Disk wiping** erases data irreversibly, eliminating evidence.
- **Timestomping** manipulates file timestamps, complicating timeline reconstruction.
- **VPN usage** obscures user identities and locations, making attribution difficult.
- **Event log deletion** removes traces of malicious activity from systems.
- **Cryptography misuse:** Attackers employ strong encryption and hashing to conceal or alter evidence. While cryptography ensures confidentiality and integrity in

legitimate applications, it poses challenges to investigators attempting to recover readable data.

- **Difficult or impossible decryption:** Decrypting robust encryption is time-consuming, resource-intensive, and often infeasible without keys.

Overcoming these techniques requires specialized methods that are difficult to formalize, standardize, or reproduce consistently.

3.4.8 Shortage of Specialized Digital Forensics Professionals

Digital Forensics investigations involve diverse technologies and require advanced technical expertise. However, there is a global shortage of professionals trained in forensic methodologies, tools, and legal frameworks. This shortage affects the quality of investigations, creates bottlenecks, and increases the risk of misinterpretation or mishandling of evidence.

The lack of universally accepted standards for training, certification, and competency exacerbates this issue. Clear guidelines on professional qualifications are essential to ensure that forensic practitioners conduct analyses reliably and reproducibly [7].

3.4.9 Discussion

Although significant progress has been made, Digital Forensics still faces critical challenges. Digital evidence is becoming increasingly complex, while its quality and verifiability are declining, creating risks of wrongful convictions or unpunished crimes.

A key improvement area is knowledge management and collaboration across disciplines. Harmonizing the roles of operational investigative advisors, forensic specialists, and legal experts can bridge gaps between law enforcement and scientific communities. Such integration enables systems that treat digital traces strategically, improve visibility across criminal activities, and enhance the trustworthiness and reproducibility of forensic results [5].

Figure 3.4 summarizes the current issues and challenges in Digital Forensics discussed in this section.

3.5 Open Science-Driven Digital Forensics Experimentation

Digital evidence plays a central role in cybercrime investigations and prosecutions, as it provides information that can be used as proof in court. Such evidence is admissible only when its authenticity, reliability, and completeness can be

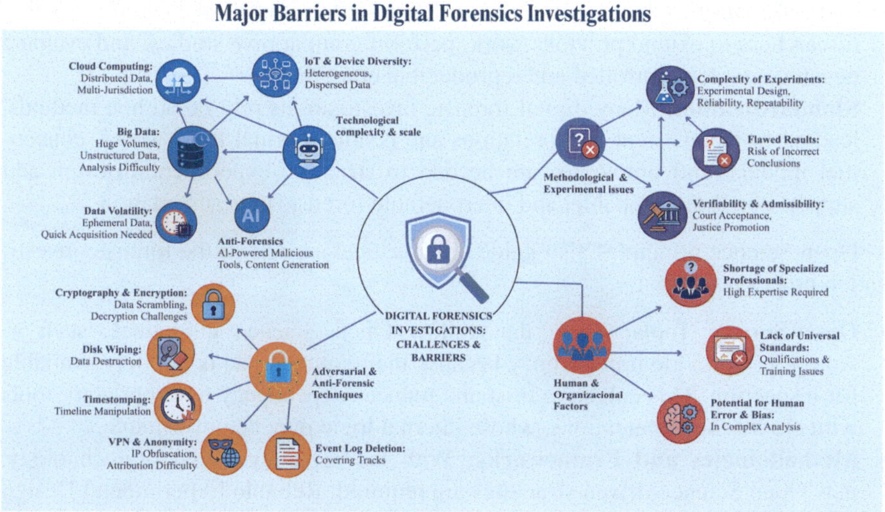

Fig. 3.4 Challenges and issues in Digital Forensics

demonstrated. Current technological developments pose challenges to the standardization of procedures for retrieving, preserving, and analyzing digital evidence, affecting legal validity. Because digital evidence differs substantially from physical evidence, it requires specific safeguards to ensure that it is not altered, corrupted, or compromised during investigation.

Open Science-driven experimentation in Digital Forensics adopts the principles of openness, transparency, and reproducibility throughout the investigative and research process. By sharing data, tools, methods, and documentation, researchers and practitioners strengthen the scientific and legal credibility of forensic results. These practices contribute to improving the reliability, reproducibility, and admissibility of digital evidence both in court and in the scientific community [14].

Integrating Open Science into Digital Forensics also helps address challenges discussed in previous sections, including independent validation, the subjectivity of certain methodologies, inconsistencies among tools, and the lack of standardization. Key objectives of adopting Open Science foundations in Digital Forensics include:

- **Verifiability:** Transparency and verifiability are essential for ensuring that digital forensic results can be examined and trusted. Making data, tools, and methods openly accessible allows scientific and legal communities to independently verify experimental outcomes, improving the evidential value of digital artifacts.
- **Reproducibility and Replication:** Digital Forensics requires that independent teams be able to repeat or replicate experiments to verify outcomes. Detailed documentation of methodology, software versions, protocols, and workflows is fundamental to allow both repetition (same team, same setup) and replication (different team, same setup).

- **Data Sharing:** Open datasets and curated repositories of digital evidence enable researchers to extend previous work, perform comparative studies, and evaluate new tools under controlled and reproducible conditions.
- **Standardization:** Many digital forensic investigations rely on ad hoc methods, leading to inconsistent interpretations and results. Formal frameworks, conceptual models, and ontologies are needed to structure experimental design and support consistent, reliable, and interoperable forensic experimentation.

Open Science principles also guide other critical aspects of the forensic investigation process, such as:

- **Open-Source Tools:** Tools that follow Open Science guidelines, such as Autopsy,[23] provide transparency because their source code is publicly available for inspection. This enhances trust and reduces dependency on proprietary tools with closed implementations, whose internal logic may be unverifiable.
- **Methodologies and Frameworks:** With the rapid evolution of technology, new Open Science-driven structures are required. Reliable Experimental Design (FRED), proposed by Horsman [10], supports researchers in conducting robust reverse engineering of digital artifacts and in reliably extracting and interpreting digital content. Another example is ExperDF-CM [19], a conceptual model developed to assist digital forensic researchers in planning, executing, analyzing, and disseminating reproducible experiments based on empirical evidence.
- **Artificial Intelligence:** Applying Open Science principles to AI-based forensic tools enhances transparency, reliability, and resistance to anti-forensic manipulation. Open datasets, explainable AI models, and accessible codebases foster reproducibility and strengthen the forensic value of AI-driven analyses, particularly when processing large-scale digital evidence or detecting emerging threats.
- **Blockchain for Integrity:** Blockchain technology can support Digital Forensics by providing immutable, transparent, and verifiable chains of custody. Its decentralized architecture aligns with Open Science principles by enabling traceability and auditability of evidence handling throughout the investigation life cycle.

In practice, the movement toward Open Science in Digital Forensics is influenced by funding agencies, publishers, legal standards, and judicial expectations. By embracing Open Science, the Digital Forensics community transitions from reliance on expert opinion to evidence-based methodologies supported by verifiable protocols, tools, datasets, and workflows.

A recent study [11] examined the admissibility of digital evidence produced by open-source forensic tools. The authors reviewed legal and technical factors influencing admissibility and proposed a conceptual framework to support the validation and acceptance of evidence obtained using open-source tools. The framework identifies key factors such as tool availability, reliability, integrity, transparency, and proper documentation. The study reports that open-source tools perform comparably

[23] https://www.autopsy.com/

to proprietary tools in accuracy and capability, although challenges remain in scalability and processing efficiency when handling large datasets. The analysis highlights that open-source tools are viable for forensic investigations, provided that reliability, documentation, and methodological transparency are ensured. These factors significantly influence judicial acceptance and support the broader adoption of Open Science-driven Digital Forensics [11].

The discussion in this chapter highlights that reproducibility challenges in Digital Forensics stem from a combination of technical, methodological, and legal constraints. At the same time, the adoption of Open Science principles and structured experimental practices offers concrete pathways to mitigate these issues. To provide a synthesized view of how these challenges can be addressed in practice, Table 3.1 presents a comparative overview linking significant reproducibility challenges to corresponding solutions grounded in Open Science-driven methodologies, standardization efforts, and transparent forensic experimentation frameworks.

Table 3.1 Reproducibility challenges in Digital Forensics and corresponding Open Science-driven solutions

Challenge in Digital Forensics	Open Science-driven or methodological solution
Complexity of experiments; sensitivity to configuration changes	Standardized documentation; detailed reporting of hardware, software versions, and environments; use of conceptual models such as ExperDF-CM
Heterogeneous IoT ecosystems; distributed and volatile data	IoT-specific forensic process models; structured metadata; FAIR-compliant repositories; reproducible pipelines
AI-enabled attacks and synthetic artifacts	Transparent AI models; open datasets; explainable AI; reproducible AI workflows and auditing protocols
Big data volumes and unstructured evidence	Scalable open-source tools; automated provenance capture; containerized and workflow-based reproducibility mechanisms
Cloud computing and multi-jurisdictional constraints	Hybrid chain-of-custody models; cryptographic verification; standardized cloud forensic procedures; blockchain-based integrity tracking
Volatile and dynamic environments	Automated acquisition protocols; timestamped and versioned scripts; rapid standardized capture procedures
Anti-forensic techniques (encryption, wiping, and timestomping)	Open testbeds; reproducible detection methodologies; transparent documentation of tool behavior and limitations
Shortage of specialized professionals	Community-driven training resources, open educational materials, standardized competency frameworks, and reproducible laboratory environments

3.6 Final Remarks

This chapter presented the foundational concepts of reproducibility, its general challenges, and the specific complexities and legal requirements associated with its adoption in science and Digital Forensics. It is essential that researchers adopt more reproducible practices in experimentation and reporting, as reproducibility enhances the integrity of individual studies and guides cumulative scientific progress. Credibility is strengthened when findings can be independently confirmed, since reproducibility is not merely a technical requirement but a fundamental component of scientific advancement. Without it, scientific knowledge risks stagnation, inconsistency, and a loss of societal trust.

Although several proposals to improve reproducibility in scientific publishing have been discussed, particularly in Digital Forensics, much research still relies on unverifiable evidence or single-case experiments that lack methodological rigor. Open Science-driven experimentation guidelines offer a practical path toward addressing current issues in digital forensic research by improving the reliability, validity, and verifiability of findings, as well as enhancing the admissibility of digital evidence in court. However, broad adoption across both scientific and operational forensic communities remains necessary to achieve meaningful progress.

Strengthening reproducibility also requires establishing effective quality control mechanisms throughout the research life cycle. This includes clearer review processes, systematic correction pathways, and institutional support for transparent and rigorous scientific practices. Funding agencies and research institutions should encourage or require reproducibility as a core criterion for evaluation and publication. The emergence of global Open Science and reproducibility initiatives offers promising opportunities to advance the field of Digital Forensics, improving both scientific investigations and the reliability of evidence presented in legal contexts.

Reproducibility presents challenges across all scientific domains, but its complexity is particularly pronounced in Digital Forensics, where investigative findings can directly influence justice, legal outcomes, ethical considerations, privacy, security, and societal trust. As digital evidence becomes increasingly central in legal disputes and as society adopts more digital and artificial intelligence-based technologies, the need for reproducible, transparent, and scientifically rigorous forensic methods becomes even more critical.

References

1. Andujar, C., Schiaffonati, V., Schreiber, F.A., Tanca, L., Tedre, M., van Hee, K., van Leeuwen, J.: The role and relevance of experimentation in informatics. Technical report, Informatics Europe (2012). http://www.informatics-europe.org/images/documents/informatics-experimentation_2013.pdf
2. Banks, G.C., Field, J.G., O'Boyle, E.H., Landis, R.S., Rupp, D.E., Rogelberg, S.G.: The connection of open science practices and the methodological approach of researchers. J. Bus. Psychol. **34**, 257–270 (2019). https://doi.org/10.1007/s10869-018-9547-8

3. Bertram, M.G., Sundin, J., Roche, D.G., Sánchez-Tójar, A., Thoré, E.S., Brodin, T.: Open science. Curr. Biol. **33**(15), R792–R797 (2023). https://doi.org/10.1016/j.cub.2023.05.036. https://www.sciencedirect.com/science/article/pii/S0960982223006681
4. Casey, E.: Experimental design challenges in digital forensics. Digit. Invest. **9**(3), 167–169 (2013). https://doi.org/10.1016/j.diin.2013.02.002
5. Casey, E.: The chequered past and risky future of digital forensics. Aust. J. Foren. Sci. **51**(6), 649–664 (2019). https://doi.org/10.1080/00450618.2018.1554090
6. Casino, F., Dasaklis, T.K., Spathoulas, G.P., Anagnostopoulos, M., Ghosal, A., Boröcz, I., Solanas, A., Conti, M., Patsakis, C.: Research trends, challenges, and emerging topics in digital forensics: a review of reviews. IEEE Access **10**, 25464–25493 (2022). https://doi.org/10.1109/ACCESS.2022.3154059
7. Fakhouri, H., Alsharaiah, M., Al Hwaitat, A., Alkhalaileh, M., Dweikat, F.: Overview of challenges faced by digital forensic. In: 2024 International Conference on Computing Research (ICCR), pp. 1–8 (2024). https://doi.org/10.1109/ICCR61006.2024.10532850
8. Goodman, S.N., Fanelli, D., Ioannidis, J.P.A.: What does research reproducibility mean? Sci. Transl. Med. **8**(341), 341ps12 (2016). https://doi.org/10.1126/scitranslmed.aaf5027
9. Gundersen, O.E.: The fundamental principles of reproducibility. Philos. Trans. R. Soc. A **379**(2197), 20200210 (2021). https://doi.org/10.1098/rsta.2020.0210
10. Horsman, G.: A framework for reliable experimental design (FRED) in digital forensics. Digit. Invest. **24**, S103–S113 (2018). Framework for Reliable Experimental Design in Digital Forensics
11. Ismail, I., Ariffin, K.A.Z.A.: Open source tools for digital forensic investigation: capability, reliability, transparency and legal requirements. KSII Trans. Internet Inf. Syst. **18**(9) (2024). DOI not available in draft; verify upon final publication
12. Kebande, V.R., Awad, A.I.: Industrial internet of things ecosystems security and digital forensics: achievements, open challenges, and future directions. ACM Comput. Surv. **56**(5) (2024). https://doi.org/10.1145/3635030
13. Klasén, L., Fock, N., Forchheimer, R.: The invisible evidence: digital forensics as key to solving crimes in the digital age. Foren. Sci. Int. **362**, 112133 (2024). https://doi.org/10.1016/j.forsciint.2024.112133
14. Lefebvre, A., Spruit, M.: Laboratory forensics for open science readiness: an investigative approach to research data management. Inf. Syst. Front. **23**, 156–173 (2021). https://doi.org/10.1007/s10796-021-10165-1
15. Mohamed Firdhous, M.F., Elbreiki, W., Abdullahi, I., Sudantha, B., Budiarto, R.: WormGPT: a large language model chatbot for criminals. In: 2023 24th International Arab Conference on Information Technology (ACIT), pp. 1–6 (2023). https://doi.org/10.1109/ACIT58888.2023.10453752
16. Mohay, G.: Technical challenges and directions for digital forensics. In: Proceedings of SADFE 2005, pp. 155–161 (2005). https://doi.org/10.1109/SADFE.2005.24
17. Nance, K., Hay, B., Bishop, M.: Digital forensics: defining a research agenda. In: 42nd Hawaii International Conference on System Sciences, pp. 1–6 (2009). https://doi.org/10.1109/HICSS.2009.160
18. Nordvik, R., Stoykova, R., Franke, K., Axelsson, S., Toolan, F.: Reliability validation for file system interpretation. Foren. Sci. Int.: Digit. Invest. **37**, 301174 (2021). https://doi.org/10.1016/j.fsidi.2021.301174
19. Oliveira E. Jr, Zorzo, A.F., Neu, C.V.: Towards a conceptual model for promoting digital forensics experiments. Foren. Sci. Int.: Digit. Invest. **35**, 301014 (2020). https://doi.org/10.1016/j.fsidi.2020.301014
20. Oliveira, E. Jr, Silva, T.J., Zorzo, A.F., Neu, C.V.: Digital forensics experimentation: analysis and recommendations. Foren. Sci. Rev. **34**(1), 21–41 (2022)
21. Pan, L., Batten, L.: Reproducibility of digital evidence in forensic investigations. Technical report, Unspecified (2005). Insufficient bibliographic data; source not fully traceable
22. Plesser, H.E.: Reproducibility vs. replicability: a brief history of a confused terminology. Front. Neuroinform. **11** (2018). https://doi.org/10.3389/fninf.2017.00076

23. Reedy, P.: Interpol review of digital evidence for 2019–2022. Foren. Sci. Int.: Synergy **6**, 100313 (2023). https://doi.org/10.1016/j.fsisyn.2022.100313
24. Steinhardt, I., Bauer, M., Wünsche, H., Schimmler, S.: The connection of open science practices and the methodological approach of researchers. Qual. Quant. **57**, 3621–3636 (2023). https://doi.org/10.1007/s11135-022-01524-4
25. UNESCO: An introduction to the UNESCO recommendation on open science. Technical report (2022). https://doi.org/10.54677/XOIR1696
26. Wilkinson, M.D., Dumontier, M., Aalbersberg, I.J.E.A.: The fair guiding principles for scientific data management and stewardship. Sci. Data **3**, 160018 (2016). https://doi.org/10.1038/sdata.2016.18

Part II
Conceptual Modeling of Digital Forensics Controlled Experiments

This part establishes the theoretical and methodological backbone for documenting controlled experiments in Digital Forensics through the lens of conceptual modeling. It positions modeling not merely as a technical tool but also as a cognitive and communicative process that structures knowledge, supports shared understanding among stakeholders, and bridges the gap between abstract theory and operational practice. By integrating conceptual modeling principles into the experimental workflow, this part provides the scaffolding necessary to ensure methodological rigor, transparency, and reproducibility, which are fundamental for transforming Digital Forensics from a collection of isolated studies into a coherent and cumulative scientific discipline.

Drawing from the historical foundations of conceptual modeling, Chap. 4 contextualizes its evolution from early Entity–Relationship models to modern multi-perspective and domain-specific approaches. It highlights how modeling contributes to semantic precision, quality assessment, and methodological consistency, which are essential for scientific communication and cumulative reasoning. The chapter also connects these ideas to the emerging needs of Digital Forensics, introducing conceptual modeling as a way to formalize investigative processes, align technical decisions with ethical standards, and facilitate the integration of open science practices.

Building on these principles, Chap. 5 presents the Experimentation in Digital Forensics Conceptual Model (ExperDF-CM) as a structured framework designed to support the full life cycle of controlled experiments. Organized around five interdependent phases (*Planning*, *Pre-operation*, *Operation*, *Analysis and Interpretation*, and *Dissemination*), the model guides researchers in defining objectives, ensuring traceability, documenting procedures, and disseminating results in a transparent and reproducible manner. ExperDF-CM therefore operationalizes the values of scientific integrity and accountability, promoting not only methodological rigor but also the ethical and societal responsibility of Digital Forensics research.

Together, these chapters establish conceptual modeling as the unifying foundation of the book's second part. They demonstrate how structured representations of experimental processes enhance comparability across studies, support cumulative evidence, and enable Digital Forensics to evolve as a data-driven, open, and trustworthy scientific field.

Chapter 4
Basics of Conceptual Modeling

Abstract This chapter examines the theoretical, historical, and methodological foundations of conceptual modeling, emphasizing its essential role in representing, communicating, and reasoning about complex domains. It presents conceptual modeling as both a scientific and a cognitive process that structures knowledge, promotes semantic precision, and connects abstract representations to real-world problem-solving. The discussion revisits key milestones in the field, from early frameworks such as the Entity–Relationship model to object-oriented and Unified Modeling Language (UML) approaches, as well as more recent multi-perspective paradigms. Each of these developments is analyzed in terms of its contribution to expressiveness, methodological rigor, and practical usability in diverse application contexts. The chapter also explores quality criteria, evaluation frameworks, and tool support that sustain good modeling practice. It examines how conceptual modeling has expanded its influence beyond traditional information systems engineering into emerging fields such as artificial intelligence, big data, and digital twins, where it serves as a strategic mechanism for managing complexity, supporting interoperability, and enhancing interpretability. Through these discussions, the chapter establishes conceptual modeling as a key enabler of both technical innovation and scientific understanding. Building upon this theoretical foundation, the chapter introduces the relevance of conceptual modeling to the domain of Digital Forensics, a field that demands methodological precision, transparency, and reproducibility. Conceptual modeling is presented as a methodological bridge that connects empirical investigation with formal experimentation, allowing researchers to represent forensic processes in a structured, analyzable, and shareable way. Within this context, the chapter sets the stage for the introduction of the **ExperDF-CM (a Digital Forensics Controlled Experiments Conceptual Model)**, a structured framework proposed to enhance the planning, documentation, and communication of controlled experiments in Digital Forensics. The model is organized around five interrelated concepts (*Planning*, *Pre-Operation*, *Operation*, *Analysis and Interpretation*, and *Dissemination*), which together provide a comprehensive foundation for integrating experimental rigor, ethical compliance, and open science practices. By linking the principles of conceptual modeling with the practical requirements of Digital Forensics research, this chapter provides the conceptual and methodological

E. OliveiraJr et al., *Controlled Experimentation of Digital Forensics*,
https://doi.org/10.1007/978-3-032-19951-5_4

groundwork for advancing reproducibility, transparency, and cumulative knowledge in the field. It thus frames conceptual modeling not merely as a technical discipline but as a catalyst for the scientific and societal maturation of Digital Forensics.

4.1 Conceptual Modeling

Conceptual modeling plays a fundamental role in several scientific fields, particularly in computer science. It enables the construction of abstract representations of domains by using a controlled language and well-defined objectives. These models provide a high-level view of the semantics of software applications, covering both structural and behavioral aspects.

By capturing the essence of entities and their interactions within a domain, conceptual modeling fosters effective communication among software stakeholders and developers. This shared understanding is essential to align expectations and requirements throughout the software development process [12].

Beyond software engineering, conceptual modeling is crucial for representing phenomena within diverse domains. Abstract models facilitate the identification of requirements and the definition of specifications, thus bridging real-world problems and technical solutions. By removing unnecessary details, conceptual models provide a clear, organized representation of the system, which supports subsequent analysis and design phases [18, 22].

4.2 Historical Development and Methodological Aspects

The origins of conceptual modeling can be traced back to the 1970s with the introduction of the Entity–Relationship (ER) model by Chen [3], which provided a systematic way to represent data semantics. The ER model introduced a clear separation between entities, attributes, and relationships, setting the foundation for subsequent advances in database design. Its graphical notation made it more accessible to both technical and nontechnical stakeholders.

In the 1980s and 1990s, object-oriented paradigms emerged, emphasizing encapsulation and inheritance as key principles. This shift culminated in the development of the Unified Modeling Language (UML), which became a widely adopted standard for modeling software systems [2]. UML introduced multiple diagram types, enabling the representation of both structural and behavioral aspects of systems. Later developments extended conceptual modeling into requirements engineering, knowledge representation, and enterprise modeling [10]. Over time, the scope broadened from purely technical system descriptions to capturing organizational processes and human factors. This evolution demonstrates a gradual shift from structural representations to multi-perspective approaches that accommodate complexity and dynamics.

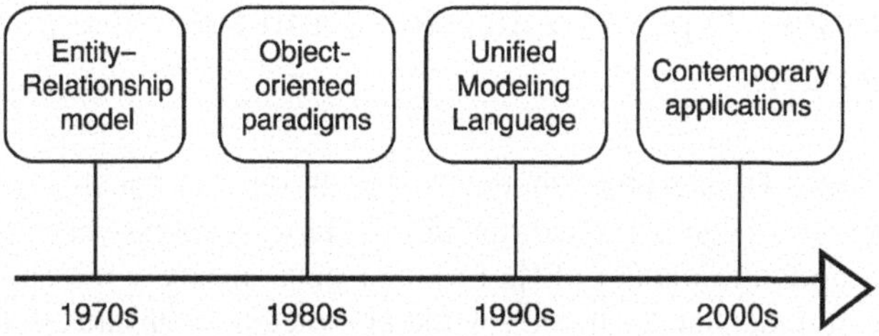

Fig. 4.1 Timeline of major developments in conceptual modeling

Figure 4.1 illustrates the historical trajectory of conceptual modeling, highlighting major milestones from ER models to contemporary applications.

Conceptual modeling also serves as a methodological tool for building and analyzing theories. Approaches such as grounded theory benefit from conceptual modeling, since it allows researchers to systematically derive theories directly from data. Through iterative and data-driven procedures, conceptual models are kept consistent with empirical observations, capturing the nuances and complexities of the studied phenomena [22]. At the same time, research highlights several challenges in developing accurate and expressive models. Lukyanenko et al. [11] identified eight recurrent modeling challenges involving entities, generalization hierarchies, relationship types, attributes, and cardinalities. For example, unclear distinctions between entities and attributes may lead to ambiguous designs, while misrepresentation of cardinalities can result in data integrity problems. Addressing these challenges requires modelers to combine methodological rigor with domain expertise.

Table 4.1 summarizes the most common challenges in conceptual modeling and suggests strategies to mitigate them.

Table 4.1 Modeling challenges and suggested strategies [11]

Challenge	Suggested strategy
Entity vs. attribute distinction	Use modeling guidelines and clear definitions validated by stakeholders
Generalization hierarchies	Apply specialization rules and verify consistency with domain experts
Relationship types	Employ expressive notations and ontology-based checks
Attributes	Validate attributes through iterative feedback sessions
Cardinalities	Use automated validation tools to test data integrity constraints
Semantic ambiguity	Apply domain ontologies and glossary alignment
Over-modeling	Follow the minimality principle and focus on essential concepts
Stakeholder interpretation	Conduct participatory workshops for shared understanding

4.3 Evaluation, Types, Applications, and Interdisciplinary Perspectives

The effectiveness of conceptual models depends on their quality and accuracy. Several criteria have been proposed, including clarity, expressiveness, correctness, completeness, and minimality [13]. For instance, clarity concerns how easily stakeholders can understand a model, while completeness ensures that all relevant aspects of the domain are represented. Empirical studies have investigated how different notations and modeling practices influence model comprehensibility and communication effectiveness [6]. Results suggest that graphical notations often support faster understanding, but textual annotations improve precision. Quality frameworks also emphasize the role of validation, ensuring that models remain faithful representations of reality while serving their intended purpose in design and communication [9].

Conceptual models can be classified from different perspectives. From a general perspective, they are commonly divided into three main categories: Data Models, Process Models, and Behavior Models [23]. While Data Models are static, Process and Behavior Models are dynamic. Several well-established conceptual data forms illustrate the diversity of approaches in the field [24]:

- Entity Relationship Models, which use graphical notation to depict entities, attributes, and relationships
- Petri Nets, representing distributed systems as directed bipartite graphs with annotations
- Unified Modeling Language (UML), which offers multiple diagram types, including class diagrams enhanced by textual constraint languages
- Concept Maps, graphical tools that represent knowledge through concepts enclosed in rectangles or circles, with relationships indicated by labeled connecting lines

From a functional perspective, conceptual models can be further classified into four categories: Structure-Based Models, Object-Oriented Models, Knowledge Semantic-Based Models, and Web Semantic-Based Models [24]. Figure 4.2 illustrates this classification. Figure 4.3 provides a concrete example of a conceptual map.

Conceptual modeling has evolved to support emerging domains such as big data, AI/ML, digital twins, and the Semantic Web [14, 20, 21, 25]. Table 4.2 consolidates these applications. Conceptual modeling has also expanded into interdisciplinary areas, including biology [8], education [15], and business process modeling [4].

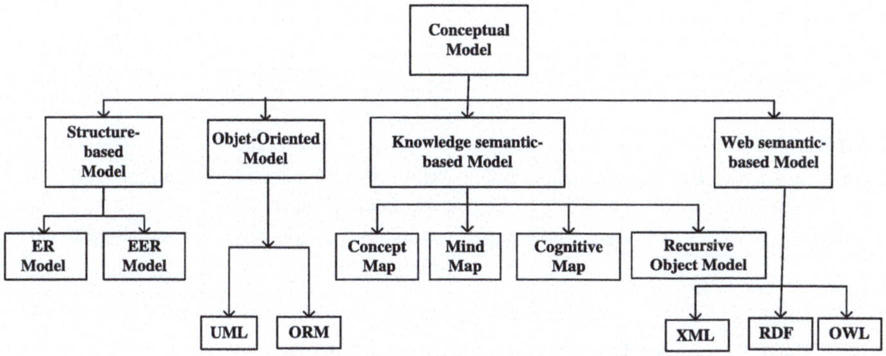

Fig. 4.2 Conceptual model classification from the functional view [24]

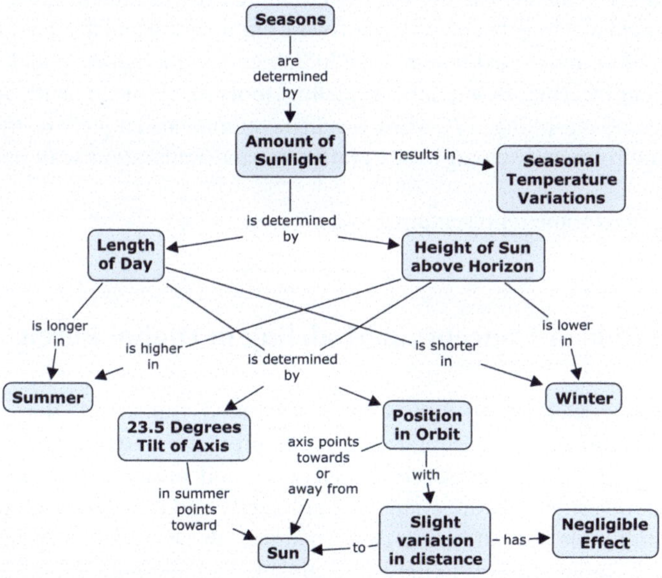

Fig. 4.3 An example of a conceptual map [16]

Table 4.2 Applications of conceptual modeling in emerging domains

Domain	Role of conceptual modeling
Big data	Structuring heterogeneous data and supporting semantic integration [14]
Artificial intelligence	Enhancing explainability and interpretability of models [25]
Digital twins	Establishing correspondence between physical and virtual entities [20]
Semantic web	Enabling interoperability and reasoning across distributed systems [21]

Table 4.3 Examples of tool support for conceptual modeling

Tool	Domain	Features
ERWin Data Modeler	Data modeling	Database design, schema generation, reverse engineering
IBM Rational Rose	Software engineering	UML diagrams, model-driven development
Enterprise Architect	Enterprise systems	Multi-domain modeling, integration with development pipelines
Protégé	Semantic modeling	Ontology creation, reasoning, ontology-based applications

4.4 Tool Support for Conceptual Modeling

Tool support has been critical for the adoption of conceptual modeling in practice. Commercial solutions such as ERWin Data Modeler, IBM Rational Rose, and Enterprise Architect have long been used in software engineering and database design [5]. These tools offer automated features, including code generation, model validation, and reverse engineering. In semantic modeling, tools like Protégé facilitate ontology construction and reasoning [17]. More recent developments emphasize collaborative modeling environments, cloud-based platforms, and integration with development pipelines.

Table 4.3 lists some representative tools.

4.5 The Role of Conceptual Modeling in Digital Forensics

A conceptual model in DF serves as a structured framework that guides the systematic investigation of digital crimes. It provides a standardized approach to identifying, collecting, preserving, analyzing, and presenting digital evidence, ensuring that investigations are conducted efficiently and that the resulting evidence is legally admissible. By offering a clear roadmap, these models help investigators navigate the complexities of digital environments and maintain the integrity of the evidence throughout the investigative process [7].

One notable example is the General Digital Forensics Investigation Process (GDFIP) [7], which emphasizes a comprehensive approach to digital investigations. This model outlines stages such as preparation, data collection, examination, analysis, and reporting, ensuring that investigators consider all relevant aspects of a case. Following this structured process, professionals can maintain consistency and thoroughness in their investigations, leading to more reliable outcomes.

In the context of organizational preparedness, a conceptual model for digital forensic readiness has been proposed to enhance an organization's ability to respond to security incidents. This model outlines proactive activities and organizations can undertake to increase responsiveness, such as implementing systematic procedures to identify activities related to a digitally forensic-ready environment. Organizations can better prepare for potential incidents by adopting such a model, ensuring they can effectively handle and investigate digital threats [19].

Integrating conceptual models in digital forensics also extends to specialized areas, such as the investigation of Unmanned Aerial Vehicles (UAVs). A design science research study developed a conceptual model to comprehensively investigate UAVs under forensic conditions [1]. This model identifies, captures, preserves, analyzes, and documents UAV incidents, addressing the unique challenges posed by these devices. The proposed model comprises stages that ensure a thorough approach to UAV-related investigations.

Conceptual models are also crucial in standardizing procedural frameworks for digital forensic investigations. For instance, the Next Generation Digital Forensic Investigation Model (NGDFIM) [26] focuses on creating a standardized procedural framework for the entire digital forensic investigation process. By providing a structured approach, such models ensure consistency and reliability in investigations, which is essential for the admissibility of digital evidence in legal proceedings.

In the context of big data [27], conceptual models have been developed to address the challenges posed by the vast volumes of information. A proposed model supports forensic investigations of big data by providing new insights and methodologies tailored to large-scale data environments. This approach ensures that investigators can efficiently process and analyze extensive datasets, maintaining the integrity and reliability of the forensic process.

The adoption of conceptual models in digital forensics has some challenges [7]. Investigators must be adequately trained to apply these models effectively, and a balance must be struck between adhering to standardized procedures and adapting to each case's unique circumstances. Additionally, as technology continues to evolve, these models must be updated to address new types of digital evidence and emerging threats. Continuous research and development are essential to ensure that conceptual models remain relevant and effective in guiding digital forensic investigations [19].

Therefore, conceptual models are indispensable tools in DF, providing structured frameworks that guide the investigative process. They ensure that digital evidence is handled systematically and that investigations are thorough and legally sound. As digital environments continue to evolve, developing and refining these models will be crucial in addressing new challenges and maintaining the integrity of digital forensic investigations.

4.6 Final Remarks

Conceptual modeling has proven to be a cornerstone of knowledge representation and communication within computer science and other scientific disciplines. It provides an essential abstraction mechanism that enables complex domains to be expressed in structured, comprehensible, and analyzable forms. As this chapter has demonstrated, the evolution of conceptual modeling reflects a progressive effort to strike a balance between theoretical precision, methodological rigor, and practical usability. From the introduction of the Entity–Relationship model to the rise of object-oriented and multi-perspective frameworks, each generation of models has expanded the discipline's expressive power and analytical scope.

The historical development of conceptual modeling demonstrates its adaptability to different technological paradigms and scientific needs. What began as a tool for database design has evolved into a versatile methodology that supports software engineering, organizational analysis, and knowledge representation across various domains. This trajectory reveals not only the expansion of modeling techniques but also their deepening integration into the scientific process. Conceptual models now serve as instruments for reasoning, hypothesis formulation, and empirical validation, bridging the gap between abstract theory and applied investigation.

The methodological foundations discussed in this chapter highlight that the quality of a conceptual model depends on its clarity, expressiveness, correctness, and completeness. These attributes ensure that a model accurately represents reality while remaining understandable and valuable to its intended audience. The discussion of evaluation frameworks and modeling challenges underscores the need for both methodological discipline and iterative refinement. As modeling complexity increases, tool support ranging from traditional diagramming software to ontology-based environments becomes indispensable for maintaining consistency and facilitating collaboration.

The versatility of conceptual modeling is evident in its applications across emerging fields, including artificial intelligence, big data, digital twins, and the Semantic Web. In these contexts, conceptual models play a vital role in structuring information, ensuring interoperability, and enhancing interpretability. Their use extends beyond technical design to serve cognitive and communicative functions, enabling multidisciplinary collaboration. By providing a shared language and representation framework, conceptual modeling helps align human understanding with computational logic.

Within the context of Digital Forensics, conceptual modeling assumes a crucial role. It enables the systematic representation of investigative processes, ensuring that the identification, preservation, analysis, and presentation of digital evidence follow coherent and transparent procedures. Conceptual models, such as the General Digital Forensics Investigation Process (GDFIP) and the Next Generation Digital Forensic Investigation Model (NGDFIM), as well as forensic readiness frameworks, exemplify how structured representations can standardize practices and improve both efficiency and reliability. The integration of conceptual modeling into Digital Forensics not only supports procedural consistency but also strengthens the scientific credibility of the discipline.

At the same time, the challenges facing digital investigators, including rapid technological change, data heterogeneity, and increasing system complexity, highlight the need for continuous refinement of these models. Their relevance depends on their ability to adapt to new environments, such as cloud infrastructure, mobile ecosystems, and unmanned aerial systems. Ensuring that conceptual models remain both flexible and scientifically grounded will be essential for maintaining their role as reliable instruments of forensic reasoning.

In summary, conceptual modeling represents far more than a technical exercise in diagramming or data organization. It is a methodological foundation that integrates abstraction, communication, and validation across scientific and practical domains. By fostering shared understanding, promoting analytical rigor, and supporting the formalization of complex processes, conceptual modeling remains a vital component of knowledge creation and technological innovation. Its ongoing refinement and application will remain central to advancing not only computer science but also interdisciplinary domains such as Digital Forensics, where the pursuit of clarity, reliability, and transparency is inseparable from the pursuit of truth.

References

1. Alotaibi, F., Al-Dhaqm, A., Al-Otaibi, Y.D.: A conceptual digital forensic investigation model applicable to the drone forensics field. Eng. Technol. Appl. Sci. Res. **13**(5), 11608–11615 (2023). https://doi.org/10.48084/etasr.6195
2. Booch, G., Rumbaugh, J., Jacobson, I.: The Unified Modeling Language User Guide. Addison-Wesley, Boston, MA (1999)
3. Chen, P.P.: The entity-relationship model: toward a unified view of data. ACM Trans. Database Syst. **1**(1), 9–36 (1976)
4. Dumas, M., Rosa, M.L., Mendling, J., Reijers, H.A.: Fundamentals of Business Process Management. Springer, Berlin (2013)
5. Fowler, M.: UML Distilled: A Brief Guide to the Standard Object Modeling Language. Addison-Wesley, Boston (2004)
6. Gemino, A., Wand, Y.: Evaluating modeling techniques based on models of learning. Commun. ACM **51**(12), 105–110 (2008)
7. Ivanova, M., Stefanov, S.: Digital forensics investigation models: Current state and analysis. In: Proceedings of the 8th International Conference on Smart and Sustainable Technologies (SpliTech), pp. 1–4 (2023). https://doi.org/10.23919/SpliTech58164.2023.10193176
8. Kohn, K.W.: Molecular interaction map of the mammalian cell cycle control and dna repair systems. Mol. Biol. Cell **10**(8), 2703–2734 (1999)
9. Lindland, O.I., Sindre, G., Sølvberg, A.: Understanding quality in conceptual modeling. IEEE Softw. **11**(2), 42–49 (1994)
10. Loucopoulos, P., Yu, E.: The evolution of conceptual modeling research: Past, present, and future. In: Conceptual Modeling: Perspectives on Information Systems, pp. 3–18. Springer, Berlin (2014)
11. Lukyanenko, R., Samuel, B.M., Parsons, J., Storey, V.C., Pastor, O., Jabbari, A.: Universal conceptual modeling: principles, benefits, and an agenda for conceptual modeling research. Inf. Syst. Res. **23**, 1077–1100 (2024). Forthcoming
12. Mayr, P., Thalheim, B.: The Triptych of Conceptual Modeling. Springer, Berlin (2025). Forthcoming
13. Moody, D.L.: Theoretical and practical issues in evaluating the quality of conceptual models: current state and future directions. Data Knowl. Eng. **55**(3), 243–276 (2005)
14. Müller, H., Meyer-Wegener, K.: Big data and conceptual modeling. Inf. Syst. **44**, 113–131 (2015)
15. Nesbit, J.C., Adesope, O.: Learning with concept and knowledge maps: a meta-analysis. Rev. Educ. Res. **76**(3), 413–448 (2006)

16. Novak, J., Cañas, A.J.: The theory underlying concept maps and how to construct and use them. Tech. Rep. 2006-01 Rev 2008-01, Florida Institute for Human and Machine Cognition (2006). http://cmap.ihmc.us/Publications/ResearchPapers/TheoryCmaps/TheoryUnderlyingConceptMaps.htm
17. Noy, N.F., McGuinness, D.L.: Ontology development 101: A guide to creating your first ontology. Stanford Knowledge Systems Laboratory Technical Report (2001)
18. Olivé, A.: Conceptual Modeling of Information Systems. Springer, Berlin, Heidelberg (2007)
19. Pooe, A., Labuschagne, L.: A conceptual model for digital forensic readiness. In: Proceedings of the Information Security for South Africa, pp. 1–8 (2012). https://doi.org/10.1109/ISSA.2012.6320452
20. Rosen, R., von Wichert, G., Lo, G., Döge, K.: About the importance of digital twins in engineering. IFAC-PapersOnLine **48**(3), 567–572 (2015)
21. Shadbolt, N., Hall, W., Berners-Lee, T.: The semantic web revisited. IEEE Intell. Syst. **21**(3), 96–101 (2006)
22. Storey, V.C., Lukyanenko, R., Castellanos, A.: Conceptual modeling: topics, themes, and technology trends. ACM Comput. Surveys **55**(14s), 1–38 (2023). https://doi.org/10.1145/3589338
23. Uthmann, C.V., Becker, J.: Guidelines of modelling (GoM) for business process simulation. In: Proceedings of Process Modelling, pp. 100–116. Springer, Berlin, Heidelberg (1999)
24. Wen, K., Zeng, Y., Li, R., Lin, J.: Modeling semantic information in engineering applications: a review. Artif. Intell. Rev. **37**(2), 97–117 (2012). https://doi.org/10.1007/s10462-011-9221-2
25. Zhang, Y., Miller, T., Sonenberg, L.: Explainable AI: A conceptual modeling perspective. In: Proceedings of the 38th International Conference on Conceptual Modeling (ER), pp. 473–485. Springer, Berlin (2020)
26. Thakar, A.A., Kumar, K., Patel, B.: Next generation digital forensic investigation model (NGDFIM) - enhanced, time reducing and comprehensive framework. J. Phys. Conf. Ser. **1767**(1), 012054 (2021). https://doi.org/10.1088/1742-6596/1767/1/012054
27. Zawoad, S., Hasan, R.: Digital forensics in the age of big data: Challenges, approaches, and opportunities. In: Proceedings of the IEEE 17th International Conference on High Performance Computing and Communications, pp. 1320–1325 (2015). https://doi.org/10.1109/HPCC-CSS-ICESS.2015.305

Chapter 5
ExperDF-CM: A Digital Forensics Controlled Experiments Conceptual Model

Abstract This chapter presents the **ExperDF-CM (Digital Forensics Controlled Experiments Conceptual Model)** as a structured framework for the design, execution, and documentation of controlled experiments in Digital Forensics. Building upon the conceptual foundations discussed in the previous chapter, ExperDF-CM operationalizes the principles of conceptual modeling into a comprehensive methodological approach that promotes rigor, reproducibility, and transparency in empirical research. The model integrates established experimental practices with the distinctive characteristics of forensic investigation, providing a systematic means to represent, analyze, and communicate experimental processes. The chapter begins by outlining the motivations for developing a dedicated conceptual model for Digital Forensics, emphasizing the need to address fragmented documentation, inconsistent methodological reporting, and limited reproducibility. It then introduces the ExperDF-CM framework as a solution to these challenges, structured around five interrelated concepts that collectively describe the entire experimental life cycle: *Planning*, *Pre-Operation*, *Operation*, *Analysis and Interpretation*, and *Dissemination*. Each concept encapsulates a specific stage in the experiment process, detailing its objectives, inputs, activities, and expected outcomes while maintaining explicit relationships with the others to ensure traceability and coherence. In the *Planning* phase, researchers define the purpose, hypotheses, variables, and ethical considerations that guide the study. The *Pre-Operation* phase establishes the preparatory conditions, including dataset selection, tool configuration, and environment calibration. The *Operation* phase corresponds to data collection and experimental execution, during which procedures are documented in a clear, transparent, and auditable manner. The *Analysis and Interpretation* phase focuses on evaluating data, applying statistical reasoning, and providing contextual interpretation of results. Finally, the *Dissemination* phase emphasizes open sharing of data, methods, and findings to enable replication, meta-analysis, and cumulative learning. Throughout these stages, ExperDF-CM promotes alignment with open science principles by encouraging standardized documentation, provenance tracking, and the use of persistent identifiers to ensure accessibility and long-term preservation of research artifacts. It also supports ethical compliance by integrating mechanisms for accountability and responsible handling of digital evidence. By bridging experimental

E. OliveiraJr et al., *Controlled Experimentation of Digital Forensics*,
https://doi.org/10.1007/978-3-032-19951-5_5

design and forensic application, the model fosters both methodological rigor and practical reliability, contributing to the credibility of Digital Forensics as a scientific discipline. Ultimately, this chapter positions ExperDF-CM as a foundational step toward consolidating Digital Forensics as an evidence-based, transparent, and reproducible research domain. By uniting conceptual modeling theory with forensic experimentation practice, it establishes a blueprint for future frameworks that aim to strengthen the scientific integrity and societal trustworthiness of digital investigations.

5.1 The ExperDF-CM Conceptual Model

The Experimentation in Digital Forensics Conceptual Model (ExperDF-CM) [1] was designed to improve the methodological rigor of Digital Forensics (DF) controlled experimentation. Digital Forensics research often lacks structured guidelines for planning and reporting, thereby limiting reproducibility and reducing the scientific credibility of results. To address this gap, the ExperDF-CM conceptual model introduces a framework that helps researchers systematically organize controlled experiments. By doing so, it ensures that key elements of an experiment are explicitly defined and consistently documented.

This model is based on the analysis of more than 200 DF-related experiments, which revealed recurring weaknesses, including insufficient planning detail, missing descriptions of experimental conditions, and inadequate data availability. The ExperDF-CM responds to these issues by structuring experiments into five main concepts: Planning, Pre-Operation, Operation, Analysis and Interpretation, and Dissemination. Each of these elements contributes to building a coherent path from hypothesis formulation to the communication of results.

The overall goal of ExperDF-CM is to enable experiments that are not only repeatable by the original researchers but also replicable by independent groups and even reproducible under different contexts. In practice, this approach fosters transparency, promotes comparability of results, and facilitates meta-analysis. As such, ExperDF-CM is positioned as a foundation for more reliable and auditable DF experimentation.

Figure 5.1 illustrates the overall structure of the ExperDF-CM conceptual model, showing the five main concepts and their relationships, which together provide a roadmap for conducting reproducible digital forensic controlled experiments.

5.1.1 The Planning Concept

The Planning concept represents the cornerstone of the ExperDF-CM model. This phase establishes the theoretical and methodological foundation of the experiment, defining not only the objectives but also the mechanisms by which these objectives

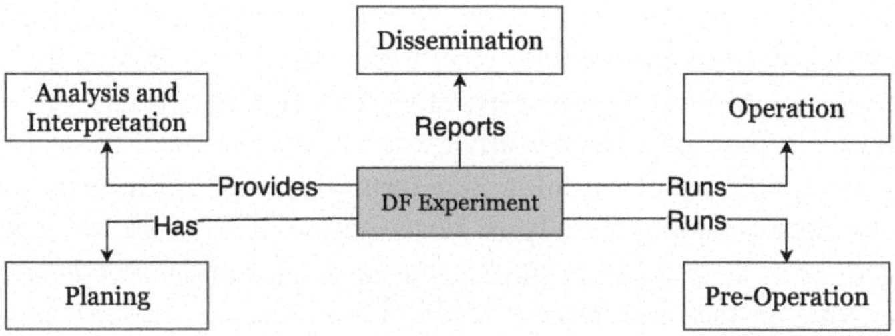

Fig. 5.1 Overview of the high-level ExperDF-CM conceptual model [1]

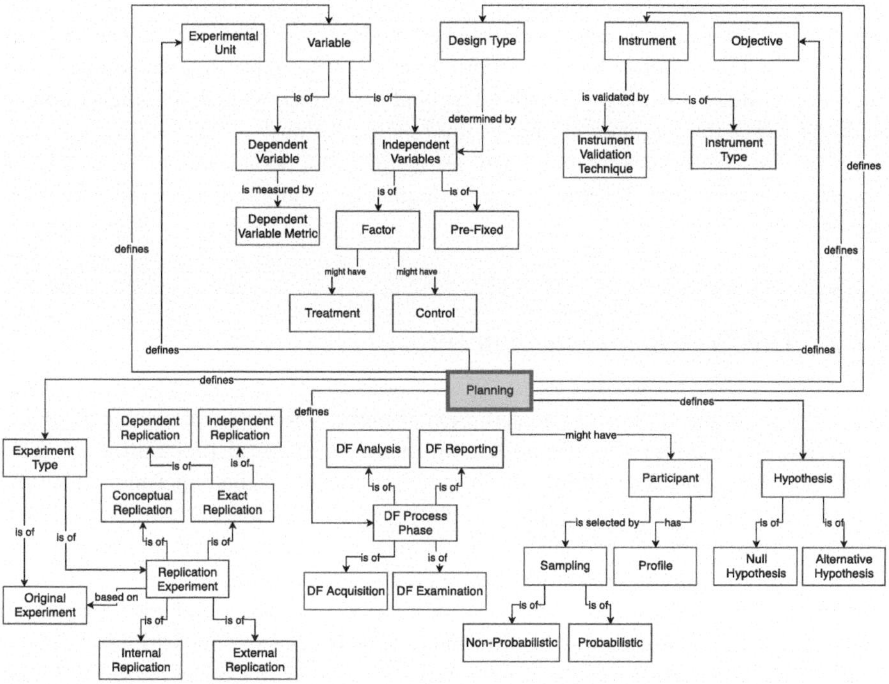

Fig. 5.2 The planning concept [1]

will be achieved. Proper planning involves identifying independent and dependent variables, formulating hypotheses, and clearly defining the scope and boundaries of the investigation. Clarity and precision in this stage are essential to ensure that subsequent phases remain consistent and scientifically valid.

Figure 5.2 illustrates the Planning concept, detailing hypotheses, variables, instruments, participants, design types, and their interconnections.

In ExperDF-CM, independent variables are controllable factors that can influence outcomes. In contrast, dependent variables are the observable measures used to evaluate the effect of these factors on the outcomes. This cause-and-effect structure enables for rigorous hypothesis testing. Hypotheses are further categorized into null and alternative hypotheses, allowing experiments to statistically validate or reject assumptions. A poorly defined hypothesis often yields inconclusive findings, underscoring the importance of carefully designing this element.

Another crucial aspect of planning is determining the experimental unit, which defines the smallest division of analysis. For example, in network forensic studies, a packet may serve as an experimental unit. Planning also encompasses the choice of design type, whether factorial, randomized, or comparative. These design decisions directly impact the statistical methods required later in the analysis phase.

Planning extends beyond variables and hypotheses to include instruments and participants. Instruments, whether forensic tools, questionnaires, or specialized software, must be validated using established methods such as Principal Component Analysis or inter-rater reliability coefficients. For human-centered studies, the sampling strategy must also be defined; probabilistic or non-probabilistic sampling methods affect the generalizability of the results. Being located within a specific phase of the forensic process, such as acquisition, examination, analysis, or reporting, ensures that the findings are adequately contextualized within forensic practice.

5.1.2 The Pre-Operation Concept

The Pre-Operation [1] ensures that the experiment is ready to be executed under controlled and reliable conditions. It emphasizes the careful preparation of software, hardware, and algorithms, which together constitute the experimental setup. Forensic tools must be configured correctly, operating systems and applications must be installed, and virtual environments must be prepared. This step minimizes unexpected interferences that could invalidate the experiment.

Figure 5.3 illustrates the Pre-Operation concept, which includes preparing software, hardware, algorithms, and training, as well as conducting pilot projects.

Software preparation involves selecting virtual machines, operating systems, and forensic applications. For example, installing forensic recovery software or configuring memory acquisition tools in virtual environments ensures consistency across repeated trials. Hardware preparation, on the other hand, focuses on defining configurations for volatile and persistent memory, such as RAM and SSDs. Proper documentation of these choices is crucial for replication.

Algorithms play an equally central role in this phase. They may require parameter calibration to adapt to specific datasets or forensic scenarios. Benchmark datasets are often used for training purposes, allowing researchers to refine algorithms and instruments before the actual experiment begins. Training is not limited to algorithms; it may also involve participants to ensure that they understand the tasks and tools involved.

A final, but vital, step is the execution of a pilot project. The pilots serve as miniature versions of the entire experiment, testing the readiness of the instruments,

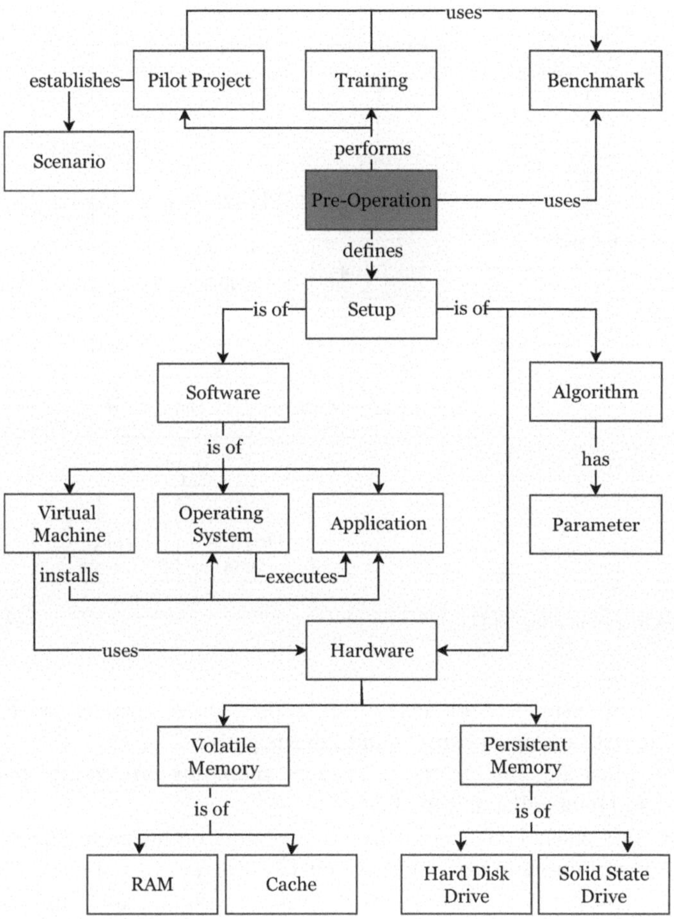

Fig. 5.3 The Pre-Operation concept [1]

infrastructure, and participants. They identify flaws or inconsistencies that might otherwise compromise the main study. In this way, Pre-Operation functions as a safeguard, bridging the theoretical constructs of planning with the empirical reality of execution.

5.1.3 The Operation Concept

The Operation phase [1] marks the practical execution of the experiment, where the procedures designed in the planning stage are applied. It relies heavily on the precision of predefined procedures that describe tasks, their order, and the roles

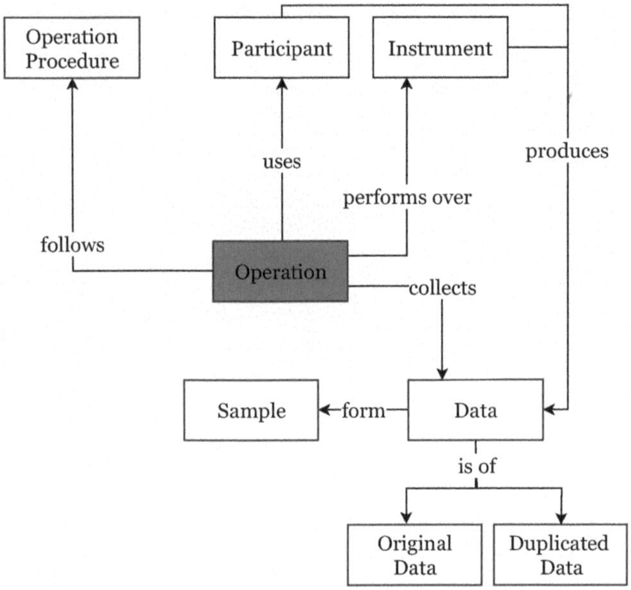

Fig. 5.4 The Operation concept [1]

of participants or systems. Adherence to these procedures ensures consistency and minimizes the risks of false positives and false negatives.

Figure 5.4 illustrates the Operation concept, including procedures, participants, instruments, and data collection methods.

Central to this phase is data collection. Depending on the experiment, data may be obtained from human participants, forensic software, or automated processes. Importantly, ExperDF-CM distinguishes between original and duplicated data. Original data refers to the primary evidence collected from digital sources, while duplicated data preserves this information for repeated testing without altering the original.

The operation also stresses the importance of documenting instruments and procedures. Every tool used, from forensic disk images to benchmark datasets, must be fully described. This transparency ensures reproducibility and allows independent researchers to validate findings. This rigorous documentation transforms the operation from a one-time event into a reusable scientific process.

When participants are involved, their interactions provide valuable data. Proper training conducted during the Pre-Operation stage ensures that participants contribute reliably. Ultimately, the Operation phase provides the empirical evidence required for the later phases of analysis and dissemination.

5.1.4 The Analysis and Interpretation Concept

Once data is collected, it must be systematically analyzed and interpreted. This phase transforms raw data into meaningful results through statistical and qualitative methods. Visualization techniques such as tables, charts, boxplots, and histograms aid in organizing and exploring the data. Proper visualization provides clarity, making it easier to identify patterns and anomalies.

Figure 5.2 illustrates the Analysis and Interpretation concept, which includes visualization, analysis techniques, limitations, and validity threats (Fig. 5.5).

Statistical analysis lies at the heart of this phase. Normality tests, such as the Shapiro–Wilk or Kolmogorov–Smirnov tests, determine whether the datasets follow the expected distributions. Based on these results, appropriate hypothesis tests, parametric or nonparametric, are applied. For example, t-tests, ANOVA, or Wilcoxon tests may be used depending on the data characteristics. This statistical rigor ensures that the findings are supported by evidence rather than conjecture.

Beyond hypothesis testing, advanced methods such as correlation and regression help uncover relationships between variables. Correlation identifies associations, while regression models can predict outcomes based on independent variables. These techniques deepen the understanding of digital forensic processes and provide evidence for broader generalizations.

Transparency in analysis also requires discussing limitations and threats to validity. Internal validity concerns whether the treatment really causes the observed effects. External validity addresses the generalizability of the findings beyond

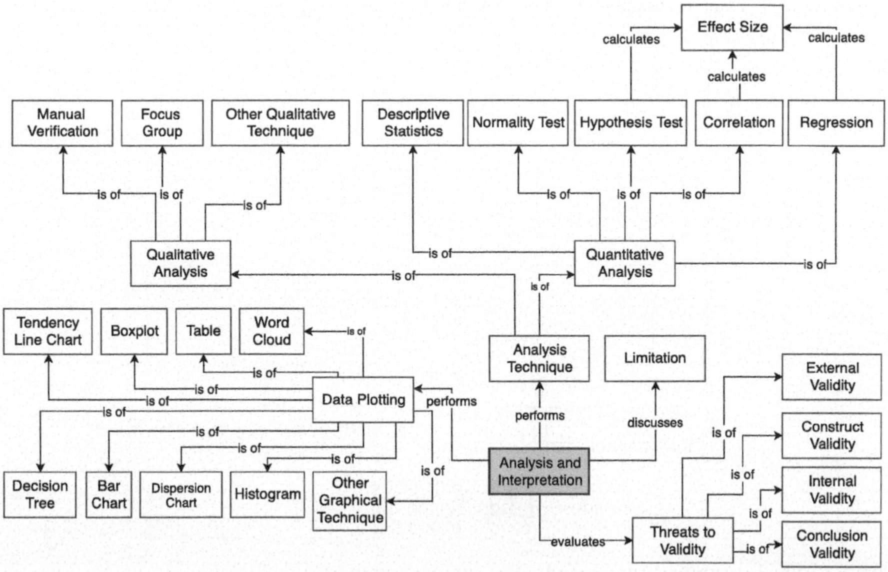

Fig. 5.5 The Analysis and Interpretation concept [1]

the study's context. Construct validity assesses the alignment between theoretical concepts and their measurement, while internal validity ensures that conclusions are correctly derived from the data. Addressing these aspects improves confidence in the experiment and guides replication efforts.

5.1.5 The Dissemination Concept

The final stage of ExperDF-CM is Dissemination [1], which ensures that the knowledge gained from the experiment is shared and reusable. At its core, dissemination involves making datasets, metadata, and documentation publicly available through trusted repositories. The assignment of persistent identifiers, such as DOIs, allows datasets to remain accessible and citable, thus supporting long-term reproducibility.

Figure 5.6 illustrates the Dissemination concept, including datasets, repositories, citations, annotations, and data management plans.

Dissemination is not limited to datasets. It also includes a detailed documentation of the authorship, experimental annotations, and issues encountered during execution. Such transparency allows future researchers to understand the rationale behind decisions, recognize challenges, and avoid repeating mistakes. This culture of openness fosters the building of cumulative knowledge in the DF community.

Another key element is the Data Management Plan (DMP), which defines how data will be preserved, documented, and accessed. Metadata, in particular, plays a vital role in ensuring that datasets are interpretable and reusable. By embedding dissemination into the experimental workflow, ExperDF-CM aligns with broader open science practices, contributing to greater visibility, trust, and impact of digital forensic research.

Dissemination, therefore, is not the end of an experiment, but the beginning of its life in the broader scientific community. It ensures that the results are not confined to a single study but become part of a collective effort to advance forensic science.

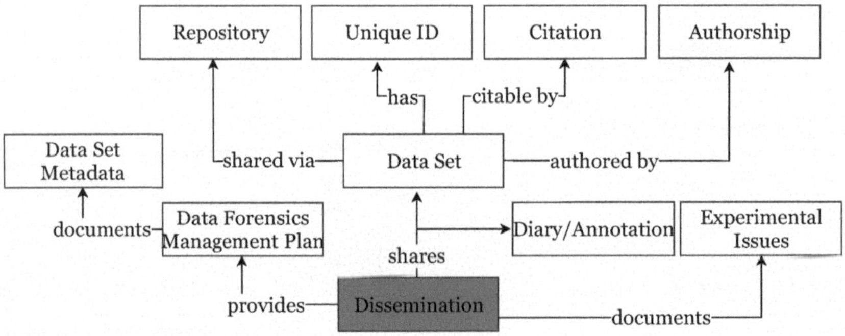

Fig. 5.6 The Dissemination concept [1]

5.2 Applying the ExperDF-CM to Model Digital Forensics Controlled Experiments

Although the ExperDF-CM conceptual model was designed to address methodological shortcomings in Digital Forensics (DF) research, its actual value emerges when applied in practice.

This section proposes a structured approach for using ExperDF-CM to model controlled experiments. The goal is to demonstrate how each of the five main concepts, Planning, Pre-Operation, Operation, Analysis and Interpretation, and Dissemination, can be operationalized within a real or hypothetical DF experiment. By following this roadmap, researchers can ensure that their studies achieve higher reproducibility, transparency, and scientific rigor.

5.2.1 Step-by-Step Modeling with ExperDF-CM

The use of ExperDF-CM begins with the clear identification of a research question. For example, an investigator might ask whether a specific memory acquisition tool performs more reliably than an alternative under certain operating system conditions. Using the Planning concept, the researcher defines hypotheses, independent and dependent variables, and determines the type of experimental design. This provides the foundation for all subsequent activities.

In the Pre-Operation stage, the researcher prepares the experimental environment. This involves configuring virtual machines, installing forensic tools, calibrating parameters, and conducting a pilot study to ensure stability. This preparation reduces the risk of bias and ensures that any variations in results can be attributed to controlled changes, rather than uncontrolled external factors.

The Operation phase is where the experiment is executed under the designed conditions. Data collection procedures are strictly followed, ensuring the integrity of the original evidence is maintained while allowing duplicates for testing. The subsequent Analysis and Interpretation phase then employs statistical methods to evaluate the hypotheses. This involves testing for statistical significance, identifying correlations, and discussing threats to validity. Finally, the Dissemination concept ensures that datasets, scripts, and documentation are made available through repositories with proper metadata and citations, thereby supporting replication and long-term reuse.

5.2.2 Illustrative Roadmap

To help researchers adopt ExperDF-CM, Fig. 5.7 presents a roadmap that aligns each model stage with practical tasks and outcomes. The roadmap illustrates the

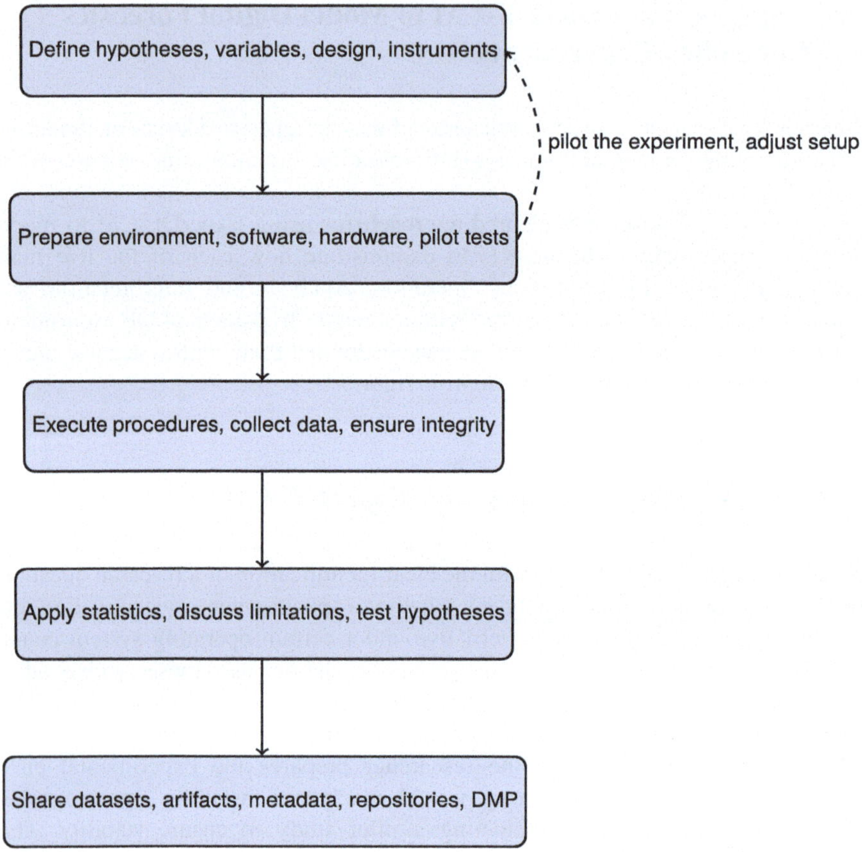

Fig. 5.7 Roadmap for applying the ExperDF-CM to model controlled experiments in Digital Forensics. Each phase defines concrete tasks and outputs, with feedback loops allowing refinement of earlier stages

model's linear and iterative nature. Although phases are described sequentially, feedback loops are possible when pilot studies or analysis reveal the need to revisit earlier decisions.

5.2.3 ExperDF-CM Support for Registered Reports and Ethical Approval Preparation

A significant extension of ExperDF-CM's application is its role in preparing registered reports before any data collection. A registered report is a publication format in which the experimental design, hypotheses, and planned analyses are peer-reviewed and approved in advance. Using ExperDF-CM as a guide ensures that the report is complete, systematic, and transparent. Each of the five phases of the model provides the details reviewers need to evaluate the experimental plan's soundness.

In addition, many Digital Forensics studies involve sensitive data, human participants, or potential ethical risks. In such cases, an ethics committee or institutional review board must approve the survey before it is executed. The ExperDF-CM framework facilitates the generation of documentation required for this approval, including clear descriptions of data handling procedures, anonymization strategies, and dissemination practices. By integrating ethical considerations from the outset, researchers strengthen both the validity of their work and the societal trust in it.

Thus, ExperDF-CM not only structures scientific rigor but also supports compliance with open science standards and ethical oversight mechanisms. This dual role makes it a practical tool for researchers seeking to produce replicable, responsible, and ethically sound forensic experiments.

5.3 Final Remarks

The **ExperDF-CM** model consolidates the methodological foundations required to advance Digital Forensics as a cumulative, evidence-based, and transparent scientific discipline. By translating the principles of conceptual modeling into a practical framework for controlled experimentation, ExperDF-CM provides a structured path for researchers to design, execute, and communicate studies that are verifiable, comparable, and reproducible. Each of its five interconnected concepts (*Planning*, *Pre-Operation*, *Operation*, *Analysis and Interpretation*, and *Dissemination*) contributes to a coherent and traceable research life cycle that integrates rigor, openness, and ethical responsibility.

Through its emphasis on planning and documentation, the model ensures that research objectives, hypotheses, and ethical considerations are made explicit from the outset. In the preparatory and operational stages, it supports transparency in dataset selection, tool configuration, and procedural control, minimizing variability and enhancing the reliability of results. During analysis and interpretation, ExperDF-CM fosters critical reflection on the validity and generalizability of findings. At the same time, dissemination reinforces open science principles by encouraging the publication of data, methods, and outcomes in accessible, interoperable formats.

Beyond methodological structuring, ExperDF-CM plays a transformative role in shaping a culture of accountability and scientific integrity in Digital Forensics. Its use facilitates the preparation of registered reports, ethical review documents, and provenance records, ensuring compliance with scientific and societal expectations. The model's orientation toward openness and documentation also promotes interoperability with metadata standards and ontologies, such as those supporting the FAIR principles, enabling seamless integration with repositories, registries, and digital libraries.

As Digital Forensics continues to evolve in response to emerging technologies and complex investigative scenarios, ExperDF-CM provides a flexible yet rigorous foundation for adaptation and extension. Future work may incorporate semantic modeling, automated experimental workflows, and provenance-driven traceability to strengthen reproducibility and long-term verifiability further. The model thus serves as both a methodological framework and a vision for the next generation of forensic science research, where controlled experimentation, ethical compliance, and open collaboration coexist as fundamental pillars.

In conclusion, ExperDF-CM represents more than just a tool for experimental organization. It embodies a scientific paradigm that aligns Digital Forensics with broader movements toward open, transparent, and reproducible research. By embedding conceptual clarity into empirical practice, the model contributes to establishing a robust foundation for generating trustworthy digital evidence and continually improving forensic knowledge.

Reference

1. OliveiraJr, E., Zorzo, A.F., Neu, C.V.: Towards a conceptual model for promoting digital forensics experiments. Forensic Sci. Int. Digit. Investig. **35**, 301014 (2020). https://doi.org/10.1016/j.fsidi.2020.301014

Part III
Formal Representation and Semantic Integration of Digital Forensics Controlled Experiments

This part extends the conceptual and methodological structures established in the previous parts into the semantic domain, where knowledge representation, interoperability, and machine reasoning become central. It focuses on formalizing Digital Forensics experiments in ways that allow their components, relationships, and provenance to be explicitly described, queried, and reused. By leveraging ontological modeling and semantic technologies, this part consolidates the bridge between conceptual modeling, experimental documentation, and computational knowledge management.

Ontologies provide the formal backbone for structuring information in a way that is both human-understandable and machine-actionable. In Digital Forensics, they enable consistent representation of entities such as evidence, procedures, datasets, and results, ensuring that experimental knowledge can be linked, queried, and preserved across different platforms and studies. This formalization supports transparency, enhances interoperability, and facilitates the reproducibility of controlled experiments, aligning the field with the principles of open science and FAIR data management.

Chapter 6 introduces the fundamental principles of ontological modeling and semantic query mechanisms, particularly focusing on the use of SPARQL as a tool for accessing and analyzing structured experimental data. It discusses how ontology-based approaches can extend conceptual models by introducing formal semantics that enable the automatic integration and validation of information. The chapter also presents the **ExperDF-Portal**, an online platform designed to support the management and execution of controlled experiments in Digital Forensics. Through the portal, researchers can visualize experimental artifacts, define data acquisition strategies, document investigation steps, and manage the life cycle of experimental processes. The integration between conceptual and semantic layers exemplifies how digital experiment management can evolve toward more transparent, reproducible, and connected practices.

Chapter 7 presents the **ExperDF-Onto Ontology**, which formalizes the structure and semantics of the ExperDF-CM model introduced earlier. It defines a vocabulary of classes, properties, and relationships that describe the elements of controlled experiments, from planning to dissemination. The ontology aligns with internationally recognized standards such as Dublin Core and the PROV family, ensuring compatibility with other research infrastructures and metadata frameworks. The chapter also demonstrates the use of SPARQL queries to retrieve, integrate, and analyze experimental metadata, illustrating how semantic technologies can support provenance tracking, validation, and reuse of forensic research data.

Together, these chapters establish a semantic foundation for the management and exchange of experimental knowledge in Digital Forensics. They demonstrate how ontological modeling, combined with practical implementation through the ExperDF-Portal and ExperDF-Onto, transforms static documentation into a living, interoperable knowledge ecosystem. This integration strengthens the scientific value of experiments, supports data-driven collaboration, and contributes to the long-term sustainability of research assets in Digital Forensics.

Chapter 6
Basics of Ontology and SPARQL Queries

Abstract This chapter provides a comprehensive and integrated exploration of ontologies, from their philosophical foundations to their technological implementation and practical application in Digital Forensics. It begins by revisiting the origins of ontology in classical philosophy, where thinkers such as Aristotle and Wolff first sought to describe the nature and categories of being. These early metaphysical inquiries evolved into modern formal systems for representing knowledge, giving rise to ontologies as computational artifacts that enable structured, explicit, and machine-readable conceptualizations of domains. By bridging abstract philosophical reasoning and formal logic, ontologies have become indispensable instruments for organizing knowledge, ensuring semantic interoperability, and supporting intelligent decision-making. The chapter proceeds to define the essential components of ontologies, including classes, subclasses, relations, axioms, and instances, and explores their typology according to domain scope, formalism, and purpose. Through this lens, it distinguishes between generic, domain, task, application, and representation ontologies, demonstrating how each serves different modeling needs. These theoretical aspects are complemented by methodological insights on ontology construction and evaluation, emphasizing clarity, consistency, and reusability as key design principles. Building on this conceptual groundwork, the chapter presents the Semantic Web framework as the technical environment in which ontologies operate. It explains how the Resource Description Framework (RDF) enables data to be represented as triples within a graph model, how the Web Ontology Language (OWL) introduces expressivity for logical constraints and reasoning, and how the SPARQL query language allows users to navigate and manipulate semantic data. Detailed examples and visual representations illustrate the structure of RDF triples, the formal capabilities of OWL axioms, and the syntax of SPARQL queries used for pattern matching, data integration, and federated querying across distributed knowledge bases. The chapter also examines the ecosystem of tools and technologies that facilitate the creation and use of ontologies, including ontology editors such as Protégé and querying platforms like Apache Jena, as well as public SPARQL end points. These tools form a practical bridge between theoretical models and real-world applications, enabling researchers and practitioners to model complex domains, verify logical consistency, and query large semantic datasets.

E. OliveiraJr et al., *Controlled Experimentation of Digital Forensics*,
https://doi.org/10.1007/978-3-032-19951-5_6

In its applied dimension, the chapter focuses on the role of ontologies in Digital Forensics. It demonstrates how formal knowledge models can represent digital evidence, describe investigative processes, and support event reconstruction with enhanced precision and traceability. Ontologies promote interoperability among forensic tools, standardize documentation practices, facilitate anomaly and pattern detection, and aid in the recovery and correlation of fragmented or hidden data. By formalizing concepts such as evidence types, acquisition methods, and analysis steps, ontologies contribute to the development of more rigorous and reproducible forensic investigations. Finally, the chapter situates ontology-based reasoning within the broader context of Open Science. By encouraging transparent representation, structured documentation, and machine-assisted querying of forensic data, ontologies reinforce the principles of reproducibility, ethical accountability, and collaborative validation. This integration of philosophical insight, computational logic, and forensic practice highlights ontologies not merely as technical schemas but as epistemological frameworks that serve as foundations for reasoning, discovery, and trustworthy science. In doing so, the chapter underscores that the future of Digital Forensics research lies in the convergence of semantic modeling, intelligent analytics, and open, reproducible methodologies that advance both scientific rigor and societal responsibility.

6.1 Conceptual Foundations of Ontologies

Ontologies have become fundamental tools in both philosophy and computer science, serving as structured frameworks to represent, organize, and reason about knowledge. Their origins lie in classical philosophy, where ontologies were developed to explore the nature of being, existence, and the properties of reality. Over time, these conceptual foundations have been adapted to the fields of information systems and computing, where ontologies provide formal representations of domains, facilitating semantic interoperability, data integration, and artificial intelligence applications.

The following subsections explore ontologies from two complementary perspectives. The first subsection, *Philosophical Foundations and the Evolution of Ontologies into Computing*, presents the historical development of ontology as a concept, tracing its philosophical roots and its transition into computational frameworks. This section highlights how classical philosophical inquiry laid the groundwork for formal knowledge representation and reasoning.

The second subsection, *Definition, Characteristics, Typology, and Applications of Ontologies*, provides a detailed overview of the structure, classification, and practical applications of ontologies. It explains the core components of ontologies, their typologies, and the methodologies used in their construction. To facilitate understanding, Table 6.1 summarizes the ontology types, formalisms, structures, contents, and applications, while Fig. 6.1 visually represents the hierarchical relationships among these dimensions.

Table 6.1 Comprehensive summary of ontology types, formalism, structure, content, and applications

Ontology type	Scope/domain	Formalism	Structure/content focus	Applications
Generic	Broad foundational concepts (space, time, matter, events, objects)	Highly Informal to Semi-formal	Neutral authorship; covers generic content	Knowledge sharing across multiple domains; conceptual framework development
Domain	Specific field (e.g., medicine, law, computing)	Semi-formal to Strictly Formal	Specification; structured domain content	Domain knowledge modeling; interoperability; decision support in specific fields
Task	Activity- or problem-specific processes	Semi-formal to Strictly Formal	Specification; captures workflow and task relationships	Process modeling; business or scientific workflow representation; AI planning
Application	Integrates domain + task knowledge for practical purposes	Semi-formal to Strictly Formal	Specification/ Shared Access; application-focused content	Requirements engineering; system design; domain-specific application support
Representation	Abstract and formalized structures across domains	Strictly Formal	Neutral/Shared Access; formal content modeling	Formal knowledge representation; reasoning; semantic frameworks; AI ontologies
Terminological	Linguistic terms and definitions	Highly Informal to Semi-formal	Neutral authorship; focuses on terminology	Language processing; glossary development; metadata organization
Information	Data structures and properties (schemas)	Semi-formal	Specification; information-focused	Database integration; information retrieval; structured data analysis
Knowledge modeling	Conceptual structures of a domain	Semi-formal to Strictly Formal	Specification; domain knowledge focus	Knowledge reasoning; decision support; AI applications

Together, these subsections provide a comprehensive understanding of ontologies, bridging their theoretical origins with their practical implementation in computational systems. This integrated view is essential for researchers, practition-

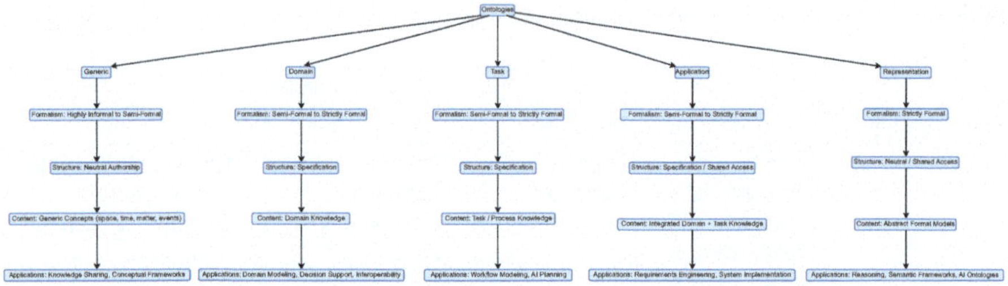

Fig. 6.1 Integrated hierarchy of ontology types, formalism, structure, content, and applications. Each branch represents a specific ontology type and shows its corresponding formalism, structural organization, content focus, and typical applications. This figure complements Table 6.1 by visually summarizing the relationships among ontology dimensions

ers, and students who seek to leverage ontologies for knowledge representation, information management, and the development of intelligent systems.

6.1.1 Philosophical Foundations and the Evolution of Ontologies into Computing

Ontology originated in classical philosophy as a discipline concerned with the study of being, existence, and the fundamental structure of reality [18]. Early philosophers such as Parmenides and Heraclitus explored ontological questions regarding permanence, change, and the properties of the physical world [7, 21]. Aristotle (384–322 BC) systematized these concepts, introducing formal categories to describe reality and analyzing the persistence and subsistence of entities [23]. These early contributions established the conceptual tools for understanding entities, their properties, and relationships, concepts that later became central to formal knowledge representation.

The term “ontology” itself emerged later in philosophical discourse. In 1613, philosophers such as Rudolf Göckel (Goclenius) and Jacob Lorhard (Lorhardus) discussed the term in the *Theatrum philosophicum* [19]. It was not until 1721 that the term appeared in an English dictionary, defined as a Greek expression meaning “to be” [17]. This historical evolution provided a conceptual foundation for ontology to transition from abstract philosophical inquiry to structured frameworks suitable for modeling knowledge across various domains.

In the 1980s, ontologies began to be systematically studied in information systems and computer science as formal structures to represent domain knowledge, organize semantic information, and enable reasoning [5, 17]. In this context, ontologies provide frameworks for categorizing entities, defining relationships, and ensuring consistency, which facilitates interoperability and knowledge sharing between systems. Their formalization allows both humans and machines to query, reason about, and analyze domain-specific knowledge efficiently.

Within computing, ontologies serve as formal languages for modeling specific domains [8]. They were initially employed in artificial intelligence to represent logical vocabularies, semantic relationships, and knowledge structures [12]. By organizing knowledge into classes, instances, relations, and axioms, ontologies form the basis of knowledge bases that can be expanded and queried. This enables precise reasoning, data integration, and the development of intelligent applications that bridge human understanding with machine-processable representations.

Moreover, ontologies facilitate interoperability between heterogeneous datasets, support information retrieval through structured semantic relationships, and provide a foundation for software engineering applications, including system specification and AI-based decision support. Thus, the evolution of ontologies from philosophical concepts to computational frameworks illustrates their adaptability and enduring relevance across disciplines.

6.1.2 Definition, Characteristics, Typology, and Applications of Ontologies

Ontologies can be formally defined as explicit specifications of conceptualizations, encompassing entities, concepts, classes, subclasses, functions, relationships, and axioms [6]. They serve as structured frameworks that capture domain knowledge in a formalized manner, enabling reasoning, interoperability, and systematic organization of information. Noy and McGuinness [13] highlight the interpersonal dimension of ontology construction, emphasizing that the vocabulary used to describe reality is shaped by shared logical predicates and conceptual agreements among experts or communities.

Ontologies are characterized by core components that define their structure and functionality:

- **Relations:** define interactions among entities, capturing domain complexity, often reusable across multiple ontologies
- **Axioms:** logical statements representing rules, assumptions, and constraints within the domain
- **Instances:** concrete examples of classes; actual objects, events, or entities
- **Classes:** abstractions representing sets of entities sharing common properties
- **Functions:** operations or transformations applied to entities
- **Subclasses:** hierarchical subdivisions of classes to represent specialization and inheritance

Ontologies can be classified by type, formalism, structure, content, and application. Table 6.1 provides a comprehensive summary of all major ontology classifications and their uses:

The construction of ontologies follows structured methodologies to ensure coherence, consistency, and alignment with intended conceptual frameworks [1].

Methodologies may be **classical**, relying on domain experts, or **consensus-based**, incorporating multiple stakeholders to achieve shared understanding. Ontologies support a variety of practical applications:

- **Knowledge Representation:** capturing and formalizing domain knowledge for reasoning and decision-making
- **Data Integration:** harmonizing heterogeneous datasets through a shared conceptual framework
- **Information Retrieval:** enhancing search and query mechanisms using structured semantic relationships
- **Software Engineering and AI:** supporting system specification, interoperability, and intelligent application development

Figure 6.1 visually represents the hierarchy of ontology types and their relationships to formalism, structure, content, and applications, complementing Table 6.1.

Therefore, ontologies serve as structured, formal representations of knowledge that facilitate understanding, reasoning, and interoperability across multiple domains. By integrating their philosophical origins, structural characteristics, typology, and practical applications, ontologies provide a robust framework for organizing both conceptual and computational knowledge. The combination of Table 6.1 and Fig. 6.1 offers a comprehensive view of the ontology landscape, illustrating the diversity of ontology types, their methodological foundations, and their relevance for knowledge-intensive applications in artificial intelligence, information systems, and domain-specific modeling.

6.1.3 Specifying Ontologies with OWL and RDF

Ontologies on the Semantic Web can be specified using the Resource Description Framework (RDF) and the Web Ontology Language (OWL). Although the W3C defines both standards as being closely related, they serve different purposes and operate at distinct levels of expressivity. RDF provides the foundational data model for representing information in the form of subject–predicate–object triples, enabling a flexible graph-based structure for describing resources and their attributes. It establishes the syntax and framework through which statements can be made about entities, and with RDF Schema (RDFS), it supports lightweight schema definitions such as class hierarchies and property constraints.

In contrast, OWL builds on top of RDF and RDFS, extending their capabilities with richer constructs derived from Description Logics. While RDF focuses on describing resources and basic schemas, OWL is designed to capture complex relationships, logical restrictions, and axioms that allow automated reasoning. With OWL, it is possible to define class equivalence, disjointness, property characteristics, and cardinality restrictions, supporting advanced inferences that go far beyond the structural expressivity of RDF alone.

Table 6.2 Comparison between RDF and OWL for ontology specification

Aspect	RDF / RDFS	OWL
Primary role	Data model for representing triples (subject–predicate–object)	Ontology language extending RDF with formal semantics
Expressivity	Describes resources, literals, and simple class/property hierarchies	Defines complex class relationships, property characteristics, restrictions, and axioms
Semantics	Provides basic semantics for resources, classes, and properties	Based on Description Logics, enabling rigorous logical reasoning
Inference support	Limited: type inheritance, domain/range implications	Rich: class subsumption, consistency checking, equivalence, disjointness, cardinality
Serialization	Turtle, RDF/XML, N-Triples, JSON-LD	Turtle, RDF/XML, Manchester Syntax, Functional Syntax
Typical use	Interoperability of data across systems; lightweight schema definition	Formal ontology modeling; applications needing reasoning (e.g., biomedical ontologies)

The main differences between RDF and OWL are summarized in Table 6.2, which highlights their roles, expressivity, reasoning support, and typical applications. This comparison makes clear that RDF provides the foundational layer for representing and sharing structured data, while OWL delivers the expressive power necessary for formal ontology modeling and automated inference.

Therefore, RDF provides the essential foundation for representing and sharing data, while OWL supplies the expressive formalism required for modeling sophisticated ontologies and enabling reasoning. Together, they form complementary layers in the Semantic Web stack: RDF ensures interoperability at the data level, and OWL empowers semantic richness and logical inference for ontology-driven applications.

6.1.3.1 The Resource Description Framework (RDF)

The RDF is a foundational standard of the Semantic Web, developed under the auspices of the World Wide Web Consortium (W3C) to enable the interchange of structured data on the web. RDF provides a simple yet powerful data model based on directed labeled graphs, where information is represented as *triples* consisting of a subject, a predicate, and an object. This graph-based model allows the integration of heterogeneous data sources, the sharing of machine-readable knowledge, and the possibility of reasoning over distributed information.

Historically, RDF was first standardized in 1999, with RDF Schema (RDFS) following shortly after to add basic vocabulary for classes, properties, and hierarchies. RDF itself is not an ontology language but rather a flexible framework for describing resources identified by URIs (Uniform Resource Identifiers). By adopting a universal addressing scheme, RDF enables statements about anything, people, places, concepts, or digital resources, creating a decentralized but interoperable web of data.

At its core, RDF represents information through triples. A triple consists of:

- **Subject**: the resource being described
- **Predicate**: the property or relationship linking the subject to the object
- **Object**: the value of the property, which can be either another resource or a literal (string, number, date)

For example, the statement "Alice knows Bob" can be represented in Turtle syntax as follows:

```
@prefix ex: <http://example.org#> .

ex:Alice ex:knows ex:Bob .
```

Here, the subject is `ex:Alice`, the predicate is `ex:knows`, and the object is `ex:Bob`. RDF supports the use of literals as objects, allowing attributes such as names or ages to be expressed:

```
ex:Alice ex:age "35"^^xsd:integer .
ex:Alice ex:name "Alice Smith"@en .
```

The first triple assigns the integer value 35 as Alice's age, while the second associates a literal string with a language tag (@en).

RDF can also be serialized in other syntaxes, such as RDF/XML. The same example in RDF/XML would be written as follows:

```
<rdf:RDF xmlns:ex="http://example.org#"
         xmlns:rdf="http://www.w3.org/1999/02/22-rdf-syntax-ns#">
  <rdf:Description rdf:about="http://example.org#Alice">
    <ex:knows rdf:resource="http://example.org#Bob"/>
    <ex:age rdf:datatype="http://www.w3.org/2001/XMLSchema#integer">35</ex:age>
    <ex:name xml:lang="en">Alice Smith</ex:name>
  </rdf:Description>
</rdf:RDF>
```

Although verbose, RDF/XML ensures compatibility with XML-based infrastructures and remains widely used in some domains. Turtle, however, is often preferred for its human readability.

RDF is frequently visualized as a graph, where nodes represent subjects and objects, and edges represent predicates. Figure 6.2 illustrates this model for the triples above.

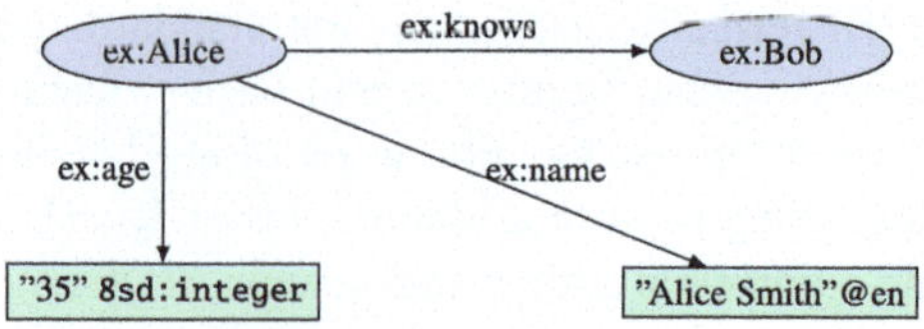

Fig. 6.2 Graph representation of RDF triples describing Alice

Beyond simple triples, RDF Schema (RDFS) extends RDF with mechanisms for defining vocabularies and classes. It allows users to declare classes and properties, specify subclass and subproperty hierarchies, and define domains and ranges. For instance:

```
ex:Person rdf:type rdfs:Class .
ex:knows rdf:type rdf:Property ;
         rdfs:domain ex:Person ;
         rdfs:range  ex:Person .
```

This fragment declares `Person` as a class and `knows` as a property relating one person to another. These declarations allow inference: If `ex:Alice ex:knows ex:Bob`, then a reasoner can infer that both Alice and Bob are instances of `Person`.

RDF forms the foundation upon which more expressive languages such as OWL are built. While RDF and RDFS provide basic schema and graph structures, OWL introduces logical axioms and reasoning capabilities. Together, they establish the Semantic Web stack, where RDF supplies the data model, RDFS offers lightweight schema definitions, and OWL delivers formal semantics for ontology modeling.

In summary, RDF is the cornerstone of the Semantic Web, providing a universal framework for representing information in a graph-based structure. Its simplicity, extensibility, and interoperability allow data to be shared, integrated, and reasoned about across diverse domains, forming the essential substrate for higher level semantic technologies.

6.1.3.2 The Web Ontology Language (OWL)

The OWL is a knowledge representation language developed under the auspices of the World Wide Web Consortium (W3C) to support the construction of ontologies on the Semantic Web. Its purpose is to provide a standard and formally grounded way to describe classes of entities, their relationships, and logical constraints, enabling not only the exchange of data but also the reasoning over such data. OWL builds upon the Resource Description Framework (RDF) and the RDF Schema (RDFS), inheriting their graph-based data model and extending it with constructs derived from Description Logics, which enable the capture of rich semantics and allow machines to infer new knowledge automatically.

Historically, OWL was standardized in 2004 as part of the Semantic Web initiative, following earlier ontology languages such as DAML+OIL. In 2009, the W3C released OWL 2, which provided improved expressiveness, profiles tailored to different computational needs, and compatibility with modern reasoning engines. Unlike RDF and RDFS, which are primarily oriented toward data modeling and lightweight schema definitions, OWL introduces constructs to define class equivalence, disjointness, property characteristics (e.g., transitive, functional, and inverse), cardinality restrictions, and logical axioms, thereby providing a level of formalization suitable for complex domains.

In practice, OWL can be serialized in several syntaxes, including RDF/XML, Turtle, Functional Syntax, and the Manchester Syntax. Turtle is remarkably concise for RDF-based representations, whereas Manchester Syntax is more readable for human users when writing axioms. The following examples illustrate the incremental construction of an ontology fragment using OWL.

First, consider the declaration of classes and hierarchies using Turtle syntax:

```
@prefix ex: <http://example.org#> .
@prefix rdf: <http://www.w3.org/1999/02/22-rdf-syntax-ns#> .
@prefix rdfs: <http://www.w3.org/2000/01/rdf-schema#> .
@prefix owl: <http://www.w3.org/2002/07/owl#> .

ex:Human rdf:type owl:Class .
ex:Mammal rdf:type owl:Class .
ex:Animal rdf:type owl:Class .

ex:Human rdfs:subClassOf ex:Mammal .
ex:Mammal rdfs:subClassOf ex:Animal .
```

In this fragment, three classes are declared (`Human`, `Mammal`, and `Animal`), and subclass relations are established, expressing that every human is a mammal and every mammal is an animal. Such hierarchical modeling is fundamental for reasoning, since it allows knowledge to be inherited from more general to more specific classes.

OWL also allows for the definition of properties, their domains, and their ranges. For instance, the following triple set defines a property `hasParent` that links humans to other humans:

```
ex:hasParent rdf:type owl:ObjectProperty ;
             rdfs:domain ex:Human ;
             rdfs:range  ex:Human .
```

In addition to such structural assertions, OWL enables the specification of logical restrictions on classes. In Manchester Syntax, these can be expressed more compactly. Consider the following examples:

```
Class: Parent
    EquivalentTo: Human and (hasChild some Human)

Class: OnlyChild
    EquivalentTo: Human and (hasSibling max 0 Human)

ObjectProperty: hasSibling
    Characteristics: Symmetric
```

Here, the class `Parent` is defined as any human who has at least one child, while the class `OnlyChild` is defined as a human with no siblings. Moreover, the property `hasSibling` is declared as symmetric, meaning that if Alice is a sibling of Bob, then Bob is also a sibling of Alice. These examples demonstrate how OWL facilitates the explicit representation of domain knowledge in a manner that enables reasoning engines to process it.

Another important feature of OWL is the ability to assert disjointness and equivalence. For example:

```
Class: Male
    DisjointWith: Female

Class: Woman
    EquivalentTo: Human and Female
```

This states that no individual can be both a `Male` and a `Female` and that `Woman` is simply a convenient shorthand for any individual who is both a human and a female. Such axioms are not just definitions for documentation; they carry logical meaning that allows reasoners to detect inconsistencies or to derive new facts.

OWL comes in different *profiles*, each balancing expressivity and computational complexity. Table 6.3 summarizes the most relevant profiles from OWL 1 and OWL 2.

The reasoning capabilities of OWL are central to its value. Suppose we assert that:

```
ex:Alice rdf:type ex:Human .
ex:Human rdfs:subClassOf ex:Mammal .
ex:Mammal rdfs:subClassOf ex:Animal .
```

A reasoning engine will automatically infer that `ex:Alice` is a mammal and also an animal, even though these statements were never explicitly asserted. Suppose we further state that every mammal must have at least one parent who is also a mammal.

Table 6.3 Main OWL profiles and their characteristics

Profile (version)	Description	Typical use case
OWL Lite (OWL 1)	Simplified subset of OWL, supporting classification hierarchies and simple constraints	Basic taxonomies and lightweight applications
OWL DL (OWL 1)	Based on Description Logics, ensures decidability and completeness for reasoning	Applications requiring logical rigor and automated classification
OWL Full (OWL 1)	Maximum expressivity with full RDF compatibility, but reasoning is undecidable	Experimental or highly flexible modeling, often without guarantees of reasoning
OWL 2 EL (OWL 2)	Optimized for ontologies with large numbers of classes and properties, supports polynomial-time reasoning	Biomedical ontologies such as SNOMED CT
OWL 2 QL (OWL 2)	Designed for efficient query answering by rewriting OWL axioms into SQL	Ontology-based data access over large relational databases
OWL 2 RL (OWL 2)	Rule-based profile, suitable for scalable reasoning using production rules	Applications requiring tractable rule-based inference

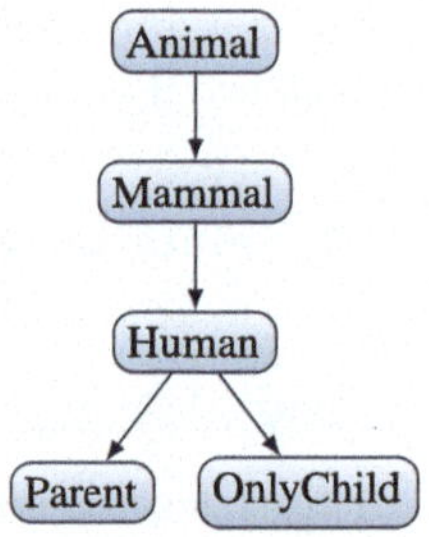

Fig. 6.3 Class hierarchy in OWL: from `Animal` to `Mammal`, `Human`, and its specializations `Parent` and `OnlyChild`

In that case, the reasoner may also detect whether the ontology is incomplete or inconsistent when no parent is provided for Alice.

To complement these examples, Fig. 6.3 illustrates a simple class hierarchy modeled in OWL, showing how humans are related to mammals and animals, and how specific concepts such as `Parent` and `OnlyChild` extend the notion of human beings.

Therefore, OWL represents a cornerstone of the Semantic Web stack. It provides a formally grounded, expressive, and machine-interpretable language for describing ontologies. By combining human-readable syntaxes with automated reasoning, OWL facilitates interoperability, knowledge integration, and intelligent applications across diverse domains, including e-commerce, bioinformatics, and cultural heritage. Its layered construction on top of RDF ensures compatibility with existing web standards, while its logical foundations guarantee that knowledge encoded in OWL can be subjected to rigorous computational analysis.

6.2 The Role of Ontologies in Digital Forensics

Applied across diverse fields, including Digital Forensics, ontologies provide a formal framework for representing digital evidence, thereby facilitating its analysis, documentation, and interoperability among forensic tools. In the forensic context, ontologies are essential for making investigations more systematic and efficient in the handling of evidence. The following sections highlight their primary functions and applications in this domain [10].

Structured Representation of Knowledge A key contribution of ontologies in Digital Forensics is the formal organization of data [10]. By defining classes, subclasses, objects, and individuals, ontologies establish a hierarchical system that enables efficient classification of digital evidence. This structured approach strengthens the relationship between experiments and evidence, while also facilitating the formalization of entities and events, resulting in more precise and reliable documentation.

Organization and Standardization of Forensic Documentation Accurate documentation is vital for the credibility of forensic investigations. Ontologies support this process by enabling the creation of cohesive, clear, and standardized reports. They contribute to harmonizing the presentation of evidence, ensuring clarity in legal contexts, and promoting the objective and consistent analysis of information [10].

Sequential Mapping of Events Reconstructing cyber incidents requires organizing events in a chronological sequence. Ontologies help experts identify the sequence of suspicious actions, correlate files, logs, and users and detect anomalous patterns that may indicate fraud or tampering. This structured mapping improves case comprehension and helps uncover irregularities throughout the investigation [20].

Interoperability Between Forensic Tools The use of heterogeneous forensic software often poses challenges due to incompatible data formats and standards. Ontologies mitigate these issues by establishing a unified knowledge base and standardizing terminology and classifications across tools such as EnCase, Autopsy, and FTK. This integration improves the consistency and accuracy of evidence analysis [2].

Digital Evidence Classification and Analysis Ontologies facilitate the mapping and classification of information, organizing evidence according to its relevance to the investigation. They allow for the association of data with predefined categories and the structured recording of suspicious activities. This systematic approach enhances the efficiency of investigative processes and ensures that evidence remains accessible and properly contextualized [22].

Pattern and Anomaly Identification Handling large volumes of data is one of the main challenges in Digital Forensics, especially in contexts involving the Internet of Things (IoT) and Machine Learning. Ontologies enable advanced queries to detect suspicious patterns, identify inconsistencies and anomalies, and define metrics to monitor deviations in access logs, network traffic, or file modifications [4].

Recovery and Correlation of Lost Information Intentional or accidental data loss is a recurring issue in forensic investigations, where adversaries may intentionally or unintentionally delete or manipulate records to conceal their tracks. Ontologies support advanced queries that help recover fragmented records, reconstruct corrupted data, and infer hidden connections among pieces of evidence, thereby expanding investigators' understanding of a case [11].

Network Analysis and Communication Flow Investigating digital incidents often requires analyzing networks and identifying communication patterns among suspicious devices. Ontologies support this process by structuring network data and enabling the tracking of connections, which helps reveal entry points for cyberattacks. Additionally, correlating logs from firewalls, routers, and servers provides a comprehensive view of network activity under investigation [16].

Therefore, ontologies transform Digital Forensics by providing an organized and standardized framework for evidence analysis. They enhance the accuracy, efficiency, and reliability of investigations, making them an indispensable tool in modern forensic practice.

6.3 Introduction to SPARQL

SPARQL Protocol and RDF Query Language (SPARQL) is the W3C-recommended standard for querying and manipulating data represented in the Resource Description Framework (RDF) model.

RDF[1] encodes information as a directed labeled graph, where each piece of knowledge is described as a triple consisting of a subject, predicate, and object.

SPARQL is designed to identify and transform patterns in such graphs, making it the cornerstone of the Semantic Web and Linked Data movement. Since its first recommendation in 2008 and its extended version in 2013 (SPARQL 1.1), the language has evolved into a mature and expressive framework for querying interconnected data across distributed systems [9, 14, 15].

6.3.1 Historical Motivation

The development of SPARQL must be understood in the broader context of the Semantic Web. During the early 2000s, the World Wide Web was already rich in hyperlinked documents but lacked a standard way of expressing structured, machine-interpretable data. Traditional relational databases provided powerful mechanisms for structured storage and querying, but they required fixed schemas and lacked native support for integrating heterogeneous or distributed data.

The introduction of RDF provided a flexible, graph-based model in which data could be incrementally enriched and linked across domains. However, RDF alone did not specify how users and applications could query such data. The need for a standardized query language that would allow developers, researchers, and organizations to leverage RDF datasets led to the creation of SPARQL. Its design was influenced by both theoretical considerations (expressiveness and formal semantics) and practical needs (usability, web orientation, and interoperability).

Compared to SQL, which had been the standard for decades, SPARQL was intentionally crafted to support graph-oriented querying, providing a syntax that is declarative but distinct in semantics. This historical trajectory established SPARQL as the backbone of Linked Open Data and an essential tool for data integration across the Web [3].

[1] https://www.w3.org/RDF

The study of SPARQL has been enriched by formal research into its semantics and complexity. Pérez et al. [14] demonstrated that core SPARQL corresponds to conjunctive queries, while extensions such as `OPTIONAL` and `UNION` increase expressive power at the cost of computational complexity.

SPARQL has found widespread adoption across multiple domains:

- **Linked open data**: Datasets such as DBpedia, Wikidata, and Europeana expose SPARQL end points for exploring billions of triples.
- **Bioinformatics**: SPARQL integrates genetic and medical data, e.g., Bio2RDF.
- **Digital libraries**: semantic search over metadata in repositories
- **Governmental open data**: RDF-based datasets with SPARQL end points
- **Industry**: enterprise knowledge graphs for search, recommendations, and decision support

This organization ensures that the chapter flows logically from motivation, through concepts and hands-on syntax, to formal and applied aspects of SPARQL.

6.3.2 Core Characteristics of RDF and SPARQL

At its core, RDF is a graph data model where each fact is expressed as a triple (s, p, o). The subject s is usually a URI that identifies a resource, the predicate p is a URI that denotes a property or relationship, and the object o can be either another URI or a literal value such as a string or a number. This model allows knowledge to be expressed in a decentralized and extensible manner.

SPARQL builds on this model by allowing users to specify patterns of triples to search for within an RDF dataset. For example, one can query for all resources of type "Person" and retrieve their names, regardless of how the data is distributed across multiple datasets. The graph-oriented nature of SPARQL enables queries that naturally traverse relationships, making it well suited for data integration scenarios.

Key characteristics of SPARQL include:

- **Graph pattern matching**: Queries are expressed as patterns of triples with variables, which are matched against the dataset.
- **Declarative syntax**: inspired by SQL but adapted to RDF graphs, making it relatively accessible for users familiar with relational queries
- **Flexible schema handling**: SPARQL queries do not require fixed schemas, allowing queries to be performed on evolving or incomplete data.
- **Support for reasoning**: Although SPARQL itself is not a reasoning engine, it can be combined with ontologies expressed in OWL and RDFS to support inference.

These features make SPARQL a versatile language that bridges the gap between heterogeneous data sources and structured knowledge discovery.

6.3.3 SPARQL Syntax

Building on the previous concepts, SPARQL offers a structured and declarative approach to querying RDF data. While its surface syntax resembles SQL, the underlying semantics are graph-oriented. A SPARQL query typically consists of three main components: *prefix declarations*, a *query form*, and a *query pattern*. Optional clauses such as filters, aggregations, and ordering refine the query.

Prefix Declarations Since RDF resources are identified using URIs, queries would be verbose if written with full URIs. To improve readability, SPARQL allows the use of prefixes. For example:

```
PREFIX foaf: <http://xmlns.com/foaf/0.1/>
PREFIX dc:   <http://purl.org/dc/elements/1.1/>
```

These declarations allow shorthand notation, such as `foaf:name`, in place of the complete URI.

Basic Triple Patterns The fundamental building block of SPARQL queries is the *triple pattern*. Variables are denoted with a question mark prefix. For example, retrieving all book titles:

```
PREFIX dc: <http://purl.org/dc/elements/1.1/>
SELECT ?title
WHERE {
  ?book dc:title ?title .
}
```

This query finds all triples where a resource (?book) has a `dc:title` predicate, binding the title to the variable `?title`.

Filtering Results The `FILTER` clause restricts solutions based on conditions. Suppose we only want books published after 2015:

```
PREFIX dc: <http://purl.org/dc/elements/1.1/>
PREFIX xsd: <http://www.w3.org/2001/XMLSchema#>
SELECT ?title ?date
WHERE {
  ?book dc:title ?title ;
        dc:date ?date .
  FILTER (xsd:gYear(?date) > "2015"^^xsd:gYear)
}
```

Optional Information Sometimes, additional information is not guaranteed to exist. In such cases, the `OPTIONAL` clause is useful:

```
PREFIX foaf: <http://xmlns.com/foaf/0.1/>
SELECT ?name ?email
WHERE {
  ?person foaf:name ?name .
  OPTIONAL { ?person foaf:mbox ?email . }
}
```

Combining Patterns with UNION SPARQL allows queries that return results satisfying one of several patterns. The `UNION` operator combines alternative graph patterns:

```
PREFIX foaf: <http://xmlns.com/foaf/0.1/>
SELECT ?person ?info
WHERE {
  { ?person foaf:mbox ?info . }
  UNION
  { ?person foaf:homepage ?info . }
}
```

Aggregations and Grouping SPARQL 1.1 introduced aggregates similar to SQL. For example, to count the number of books per author:

```
PREFIX dc: <http://purl.org/dc/elements/1.1/>
SELECT ?author (COUNT(?book) AS ?numBooks)
WHERE {
  ?book dc:creator ?author .
}
GROUP BY ?author
```

Constructing New Graphs SPARQL can also generate new RDF graphs with the `CONSTRUCT` form. For example:

```
PREFIX dc: <http://purl.org/dc/elements/1.1/>
PREFIX foaf: <http://xmlns.com/foaf/0.1/>
CONSTRUCT {
  ?author foaf:made ?book .
}
WHERE {
  ?book dc:creator ?author .
}
```

Federated Queries SPARQL enables queries across distributed datasets through the `SERVICE` clause. For instance:

```
PREFIX dbpedia: <http://dbpedia.org/ontology/>
SELECT ?author ?birthPlace
WHERE {
  SERVICE <http://dbpedia.org/sparql> {
    ?author dbpedia:birthPlace ?birthPlace .
  }
}
```

6.3.4 Tools for Writing and Executing SPARQL Queries

Effectively working with SPARQL requires the proper set of tools to write, test, and execute queries against RDF datasets. These tools range from web-based end points for quick experimentation to integrated development environments (IDEs) and programming libraries for large-scale or automated workflows. This subsection provides a detailed guide to commonly used SPARQL tools, along with practical advice on selecting the appropriate tool based on your specific needs. Ultimately, it demonstrates how to utilize Protégé to write and execute SPARQL queries.

6.3.4.1 Web-Based SPARQL End Points

Web-based SPARQL end points allow users to execute queries directly in a browser, often against large, publicly available datasets. They are ideal for beginners, quick experimentation, or exploratory research.

- **DBpedia SPARQL End Point:**[2] DBpedia extracts structured data from Wikipedia and exposes it as RDF. Its SPARQL end point provides a web interface where users can input queries, explore datasets, and view results in multiple formats (XML, JSON, and CSV). Example queries are included to help beginners learn SPARQL. This tool is excellent for learning, experimentation, and quick access to a rich knowledge graph.
- **Wikidata Query Service:**[3] Wikidata is a collaborative knowledge base with structured data about entities such as people, places, and events. Its SPARQL interface includes syntax highlighting, autocompletion, and result visualizations such as graphs, maps, and timelines. This end point is particularly suitable for complex exploratory analysis and visualizing relationships in the data.
- **Europeana SPARQL End Point:**[4] Europeana provides metadata for millions of cultural heritage objects. Its SPARQL end point allows users to query this rich dataset, making it suitable for research in the humanities or cultural domains. While its scope is more focused than DBpedia or Wikidata, it provides real-world, high-quality datasets for testing SPARQL queries.

6.3.4.2 Desktop and IDE Tools

For local datasets, custom ontologies, or advanced query development, desktop tools and IDEs provide enhanced features such as reasoning, data management, and debugging support.

- **Apache Jena Fuseki:**[5] Fuseki is a SPARQL server that can host RDF datasets locally or on a network. It offers a web interface for executing queries, supports SPARQL Update for modifying data, and integrates seamlessly with Jena's Java

[2] http://dbpedia.org/sparql
[3] https://query.wikidata.org/
[4] https://sparql.europeana.eu/
[5] https://jena.apache.org/documentation/fuseki2/

libraries. This tool is ideal for developers or researchers who need to manage local datasets and execute complex queries efficiently.

- **Protégé with SPARQL Plugin:**[6] Protégé is a widely used ontology editor supporting RDF and OWL. The SPARQL plugin allows users to query ontologies directly, including reasoning-enabled queries. This setup is beneficial for ontology-driven research, semantic modeling, and learning SPARQL in the context of structured knowledge bases.
- **TopBraid Composer:**[7] TopBraid Composer is a professional, commercial RDF/OWL IDE. It provides advanced SPARQL editing, validation, reasoning support, and integration with enterprise knowledge graphs. This tool is suitable for large-scale industrial applications that require complex ontologies and SPARQL queries, although it has a steeper learning curve and higher licensing costs.

6.3.4.3 Command-Line and Library Support

Programmatic access is essential for automation, integration with applications, or data analysis pipelines. These tools allow SPARQL queries to be executed from scripts or code.

- **Apache Jena ARQ:** A Java library and command-line utility for executing SPARQL queries. ARQ supports all SPARQL 1.1 features, including property paths, aggregates, subqueries, and federated queries. It is suitable for automated workflows, large-scale data processing, and integration into Java-based applications.
- **RDFLib (Python):**[8] RDFLib is a Python library for processing RDF datasets, including SPARQL query execution. It integrates well with Python data analysis tools like Pandas and is convenient for scripting, research projects, and prototyping. Performance is suitable for moderate-sized datasets.
- **SPARQLWrapper (Python):**[9] SPARQLWrapper provides a Python interface to remote SPARQL end points. It simplifies sending queries, retrieving results in JSON, XML, or CSV formats, and handling errors. It is ideal for lightweight scripts and automation tasks that interact with online SPARQL services.

---

[6] https://Protege.stanford.edu/

[7] https://www.topquadrant.com/tools/ide-topbraid-composer/

[8] https://rdflib.readthedocs.io/

[9] https://rdflib.github.io/sparqlwrapper/

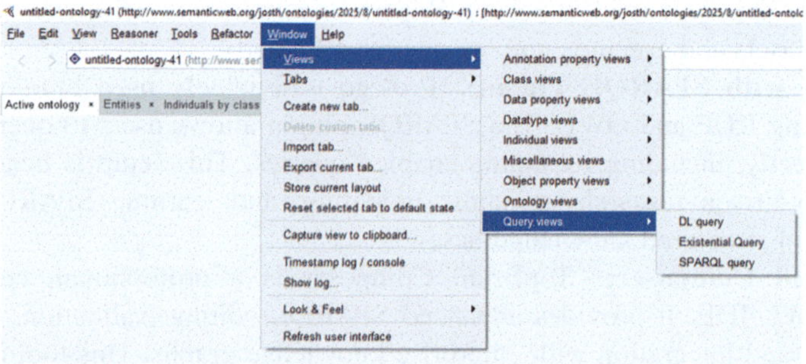

Fig. 6.4 SPARQL query plugin

6.3.4.4 Using Protégé to Write and Run SPARQL Queries

By installing the SPARQL plugin, Protégé users can write, execute, and analyze SPARQL queries directly on loaded ontologies. This subsection provides a practical guide for using Protégé as a SPARQL development environment.

By following these steps, users can utilize Protégé as a comprehensive environment for writing, testing, and executing SPARQL queries, thereby combining ontology editing with semantic querying capabilities.

Step 1: Installing Protégé and the SPARQL Plugin

1. Download and install Protégé[10] according to the operating system.
2. Launch Protégé and open an existing ontology (RDF/OWL) or create a new one.
3. (Attention: Before performing this step, check whether the plugin is already installed.) Install the SPARQL query plugin: Navigate to `File > Check for Plugins`, search for `SPARQL Query`, and click `Install`.
4. Restart Protégé to activate the plugin (Fig. 6.4).

Step 2: Loading an Ontology

1. In Protégé, go to `File > Open`, and select your ontology file (RDF/XML, Turtle, or OWL format).
2. Verify that the ontology is loaded correctly by exploring the classes, properties, and individuals in the main interface.

[10] https://Protege.stanford.edu/

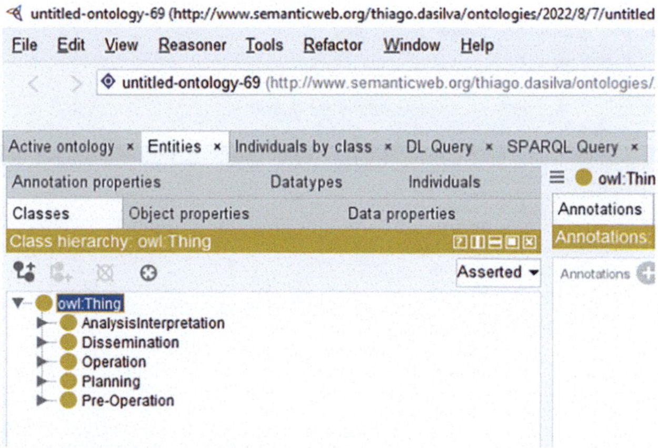

Fig. 6.5 Classes in the main interface

Step 3: Opening the SPARQL Query Tab

1. Go to `Window > Tabs > SPARQL Query` to open the SPARQL query editor.
2. The editor provides a text area for entering queries and buttons to execute them.
3. Optional features include syntax highlighting, autocompletion for class and property names, and templates for common query patterns (Figs. 6.5 and 6.6).

Step 4: Writing a SPARQL Query

- Define prefixes for readability. For example:

```
PREFIX foaf: <http://xmlns.com/foaf/0.1/>
PREFIX ex:   <http://example.org/>
```

- Write a basic query to retrieve all individuals of type `ex:Person`:

```
SELECT ?person ?name
WHERE {
  ?person a ex:Person ;
          foaf:name ?name .
}
```

- Use optional patterns to include additional information if available:

```
OPTIONAL { ?person foaf:mbox ?email . }
```

- Filters can refine results. For example, to select persons whose name starts with "A":

```
FILTER (STRSTARTS(?name, "A"))
```

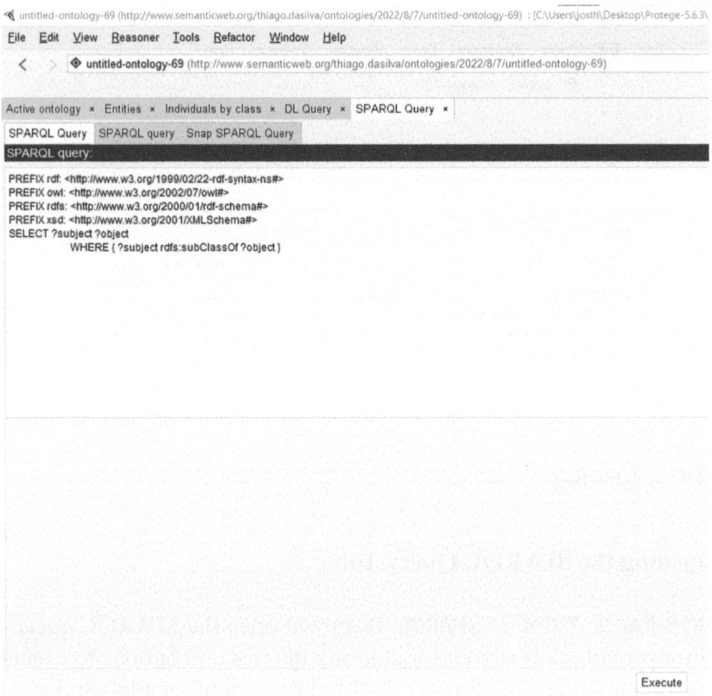

Fig. 6.6 SPARQL query

Step 5: Executing the Query and Viewing Results

1. Click the `Execute` button in the SPARQL tab.
2. Protégé displays results in a tabular form, showing variable bindings for each match.
3. Results can be exported to CSV, XML, or other supported formats for further analysis.
4. If a query fails, the editor highlights syntax errors and provides hints for correction (Fig. 6.7).

6.4 Final Remarks

This chapter provided an integrated exploration of the theoretical, structural, and practical dimensions of ontologies, connecting their philosophical origins to their computational applications and, ultimately, to their relevance in Digital Forensics. Beginning with classical philosophical inquiries into the nature of being and reality,

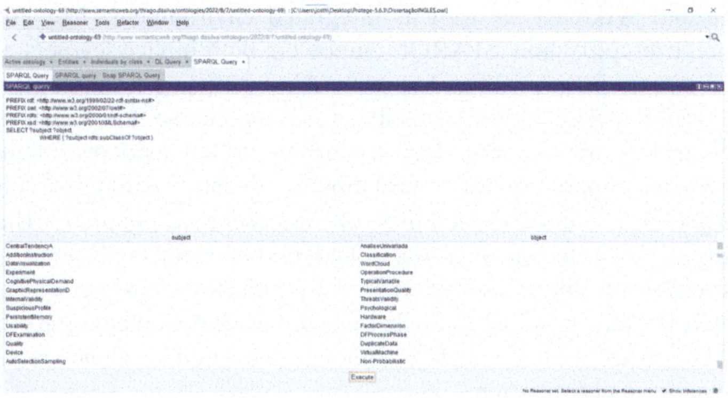

Fig. 6.7 Execute button

the discussion demonstrated how foundational ideas by Aristotle and other early thinkers evolved into formal structures capable of representing complex domains of knowledge. These philosophical insights provided the conceptual underpinnings for ontology as a scientific and engineering discipline, one that now enables interoperability, semantic reasoning, and machine understanding.

By reviewing core definitions, typologies, and construction methodologies, this chapter highlighted how ontologies move beyond abstract theory to serve as operational instruments in modern computing. From generic and domain ontologies to task- and application-specific models, the taxonomy presented in Table 6.1 illustrated the flexibility of ontological design to accommodate diverse purposes, degrees of formality, and levels of granularity. These distinctions are crucial to ensure that ontologies are not only logically sound but also contextually useful for decision-making, data integration, and the development of intelligent systems.

The chapter also examined how ontology engineering draws from both logic and computer science. Standards such as the Resource Description Framework (RDF) and the Web Ontology Language (OWL) formalize ontological constructs through machine-interpretable semantics, thereby enabling the automated processing of knowledge. RDF's graph-based data model offers a universal syntax for structuring information in triples, whereas OWL introduces the expressivity required to describe complex relationships, logical axioms, and constraints. Together, these technologies underpin the Semantic Web, an ecosystem where data is not merely published but semantically linked, allowing for advanced reasoning and knowledge discovery across distributed environments.

Building upon these foundations, SPARQL emerged as a powerful query language for navigating and manipulating RDF-based data. Through its declarative graph-pattern syntax, SPARQL enables users to identify, filter, and transform data across heterogeneous systems. The chapter's overview of SPARQL syntax, features, and tools demonstrated how it serves as both a practical querying mechanism and a research instrument for data-driven disciplines. Web-based end points such as DBpedia and Wikidata, as well as integrated environments like Protégé and Apache Jena, exemplify how SPARQL empowers both novice learners and expert practitioners to experiment with and operationalize semantic technologies.

The discussion of Digital Forensics illustrated a concrete domain where ontologies play a transformative role. By structuring digital evidence, standardizing terminology, and supporting the correlation of events, ontologies enhance the rigor, transparency, and reproducibility of forensic investigations. They bridge the gap between raw technical artifacts and higher level conceptual reasoning, thereby strengthening the evidential value of digital traces. Moreover, ontologies promote interoperability among forensic tools, improve documentation consistency, and enable advanced analyses such as anomaly detection, evidence recovery, and network behavior reconstruction.

This integration of ontology engineering and Digital Forensics research aligns with broader movements toward Open Science. Formalized representations, shared vocabularies, and reproducible querying mechanisms, enabled by RDF, OWL, and SPARQL, facilitate transparency and collaborative validation. The capacity to model, query, and share knowledge in standardized formats not only improves scientific accountability but also supports the ethical and societal dimensions of forensic practice. As a result, ontologies are not just technical artifacts but epistemic frameworks that promote trust, interpretability, and collective progress.

Looking forward, the convergence of ontological reasoning, artificial intelligence, and big data analytics opens new avenues for automation and intelligent decision support. Emerging paradigms such as knowledge graphs, digital twins, and explainable AI increasingly rely on ontological foundations to ensure semantic coherence and traceability. Within Digital Forensics, these technologies promise more adaptive, interpretable, and auditable analytical environments, where reasoning engines can contextualize evidence dynamically and detect patterns that would otherwise remain hidden.

In summary, ontologies provide a unifying framework that connects philosophical reflection, logical precision, and computational pragmatism. When combined with standards such as RDF, OWL, and SPARQL, they offer the methodological and technological infrastructure required for a truly semantic understanding of data and processes. Their application to Digital Forensics demonstrates the power of conceptual modeling to not only structure and retrieve information but also sustain the integrity and reproducibility of scientific inquiry. Ultimately, the ongoing evolution of ontological approaches represents a cornerstone of the Semantic Web and a critical enabler for open, transparent, and intelligent science.

References

1. Almeida, M.B., Bax, M.P.: Uma visão geral sobre ontologias: pesquisa sobre definições, tipos, aplicações, métodos de avaliação e de construção. Ciência da Informação **32**(3), 7–20 (2003) (In Portuguese)

2. Alzaabi, M., Jones, A., Martin, T.A.: An ontology-based forensic analysis tool. In: 2013 International Conference on Digital Forensics (2013)
3. Angles, R., Gutierrez, C.: Querying semantic web data with SPARQL. In: Proceedings of the 30th ACM SIGMOD-SIGACT-SIGART Symposium on Principles of Database Systems (PODS), pp. 305–316. ACM (2011). https://doi.org/10.1145/1989284.1989312
4. Baumeister, J., Seipel, D.: Anomalies in ontologies with rules. J. Web Semant. **8**(1), 55–68 (2010)
5. Biagetti, M.T.: Ontologies as knowledge organization systems. Knowl. Organiz. **48**(2), 152–176 (2021)
6. Borst, W.N.: Construction of engineering ontologies. Ph.D. Thesis, University of Twente, Enschede (1997)
7. Brenner, J.E., Igamberdiev, A.U.: Philosophy in Reality: A New Book of Changes. Springer, Berlin (2021)
8. Genesereth, M.R., Nilsson, N.J.: Logical Foundations of Artificial Intelligence. Morgan Kaufmann, San Francisco (2012)
9. Harris, S., Seaborne, A.: SPARQL 1.1 Query Language. W3C Recommendation (2013). https://www.w3.org/TR/sparql11-query/
10. Karie, N.M., Venter, H.S.: Toward a general ontology for digital forensic disciplines. J. Forensic Sci. **59**(5), 1231–1241 (2014)
11. Khattak, A.M., Latif, K., Khan, S., Ahmed, N.: Ontology recovery and visualization. In: 2008 4th International Conference on Next Generation Web Services Practices, pp. 90–96. IEEE (2008)
12. Nirenburg, S., Raskin, V.: Ontological Semantics. MIT Press, Cambridge (2004)
13. Noy, N.F., McGuinness, D.L.: Ontology Development 101: A Guide to Creating Your First Ontology. Stanford Knowledge Systems Laboratory Technical Report (2001)
14. Pérez, J., Arenas, M., Gutierrez, C.: Semantics and complexity of SPARQL. ACM Trans. Database Syst. **34**(3), 1–45 (2009). https://doi.org/10.1145/1567274.1567278
15. Prud'hommeaux, E., Seaborne, A.: SPARQL Query Language for RDF. W3C Recommendation (2008). https://www.w3.org/TR/rdf-sparql-query/
16. Sabou, M., Fernandez, M.: Ontology (network) evaluation. In: Ontology Engineering in a Networked World, pp. 193–212. Springer, Berlin (2011)
17. Smith, B.: Blackwell Guide to the Philosophy of Computing and Information. Wiley-Blackwell, Oxford (2003)
18. Smith, B.: Ontology. The Monist **94**(3), 267–293 (2012)
19. Smith, B., Welty, C.: Ontology: Towards a new synthesis. In: Formal Ontology in Information Systems, pp. 3–9. ACM Press, New York (2001)
20. Spyropoulos, A.Z., Bratsas, C., Makris, G.C., Garoufallou, E., Tsiantos, V.: Interoperability-enhanced knowledge management in law enforcement: an integrated data-driven forensic ontological approach to crime scene analysis. Information **14**(11), 607 (2023)
21. Verelst, K., Coecke, B.: Early Greek thought and perspectives for the interpretation of quantum mechanics: Preliminaries to an ontological approach. In: Metadebates on Science: The Blue Book of "Einstein Meets Magritte", pp. 163–196. Springer, Dordrecht (1999)
22. Weng, S.S., Tsai, H.J., Liu, S.C., Hsu, C.H.: Ontology construction for information classification. Expert Syst. Appl. **31**(1), 1–12 (2006)
23. Wolff, C., Ecole, J.: Philosophia prima sive ontologia. Les Etudes Philosophiques **17**, 292–292 (1962)

Chapter 7
The ExperDF-Onto Ontology

Abstract This chapter introduces ExperDF-Onto, a domain ontology that formalizes the ExperDF-CM conceptual model into an executable knowledge representation for structuring, documenting, and operationalizing controlled experimentation in Digital Forensics. Developed in OWL and engineered in Protégé following the SABiO methodology, the ontology encompasses more than 600 classes, properties, relations, and axioms, organizing the full experimental life cycle into five phases: Planning, Pre-Operation, Operation, Analysis and Interpretation, and Dissemination. ExperDF-Onto extends the conceptual model by refining experimental elements, including hypotheses, variables, procedures, statistical methods, threats to validity, scenario configuration, chain-of-custody documentation, and dissemination artifacts. Its design promotes interoperability, reuse, traceability, and transparency while enabling the automatic generation of UML views to support communication with diverse forensic and scientific audiences. A proof-of-concept instantiation demonstrates feasibility and highlights how the ontology can structure data, support methodological rigor, and improve reproducibility in forensic experimentation. The chapter also details SPARQL query patterns that allow users to navigate class hierarchies and audit knowledge structures, enabling both conceptual inspection and computational validation. By integrating provenance principles from Dublin Core and PROV-inspired elements, ExperDF-Onto provides a foundation for reproducible, analyzable, and evidence-driven digital forensic research and practice, strengthening experimental reliability and contributing to the formalization of the field.

7.1 The ExperDF-Onto Ontology

ExperDF-Onto represents a significant advance toward formalization and experimentation of DF, building upon the ExperDF-CM conceptual model [3].

The ExperDF-Onto ontology is coded using both OWL and RDF schemas, presented in Sect. 7.2.

E. OliveiraJr et al., *Controlled Experimentation of Digital Forensics*,
https://doi.org/10.1007/978-3-032-19951-5_7

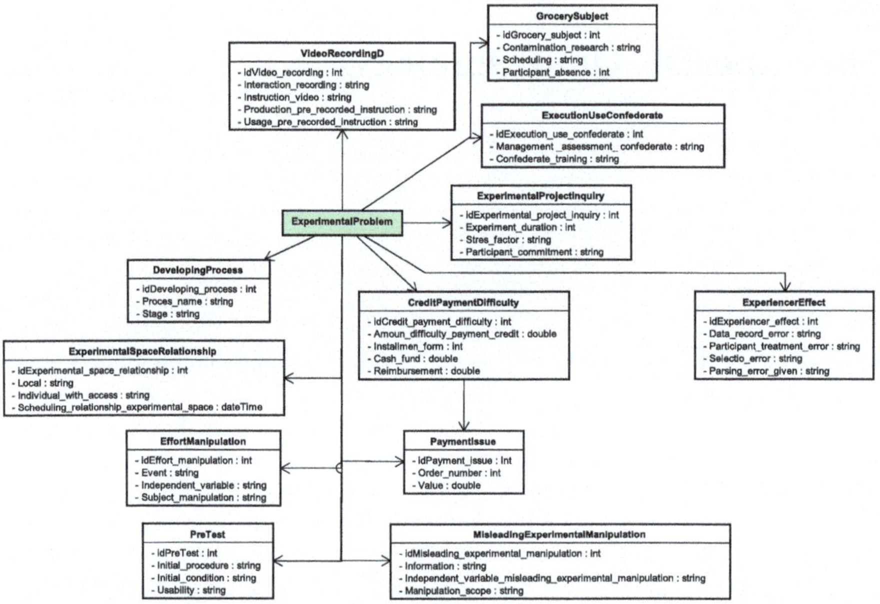

Fig. 7.1 ExperimentalProblem experimental subphase in UML [5]

It structures domain knowledge through a forensic ontology based on the Unified Modeling Language (UML). For instance, Fig. 7.1 illustrates the subphase *ExperimentalProblem*, modeled in Protégé. This approach systematizes DF phases, promoting a model that organizes information, supports documentation, and enhances the reliability of experiments.

A key differentiator of ExperDF-Onto is its flexibility. Unlike ontologies restricted to specific domains, such as the Internet of Things (IoT) or mobile devices, ExperDF-Onto was designed as a versatile, adaptable tool that supports diverse contexts without compromising expert performance. This adaptability promotes knowledge reuse and interoperability with other models and methodologies. Furthermore, UML diagrams can be generated directly from Protégé-structured data, thereby improving both the visualization and dissemination of the ontology's knowledge, thereby making it more accessible to different audiences [5].

Another vital contribution of ExperDF-Onto is the extension of the conceptual model through further phases that strengthen investigative and experimental processes. Beyond organizing knowledge in DF, the ontology yields more concrete, structured results, supported by statistical metrics, graphical representations, and rigorous management plans. As a result, experts can produce more consistent and well-founded reports, thereby addressing two significant challenges in Digital Forensics: the lack of standardized documentation and the difficulty of reproducibility in experiments [5].

In addition to knowledge organization, ExperDF-Onto plays a central role in validating and implementing investigative processes. By providing a reliable framework for experimentation and knowledge representation, the ontology enables more systematic and comprehensive results, directly contributing to the formalization of DF knowledge. Thus, ExperDF-Onto not only enhances investigative practice but also promotes scientific progress in the field, ensuring greater credibility and rigor in forensic processes.

7.1.1 ExperDF-Onto Methodology and Design

The ontology was developed using the **SABiO** (Systematic Approach for Built-in Ontology) methodology, a well-established approach for ontology construction. Proposed in 1997, SABiO was first applied to software processes and later to cardiology in the medical domain [1]. Over time, it has become a reference in ontology development across various fields, organizing the work into two main processes: the **Development Process** and the **Support Processes** (Fig. 7.2) [1].

The **Development Process** ensures that the ontology is built on well-defined requirements and aligned with its application context. It begins with **Purpose Identification and Requirements Elicitation**, where the scope, in this case, Digital Forensics, is defined, and relevant information is collected. Next, in **Ontology**

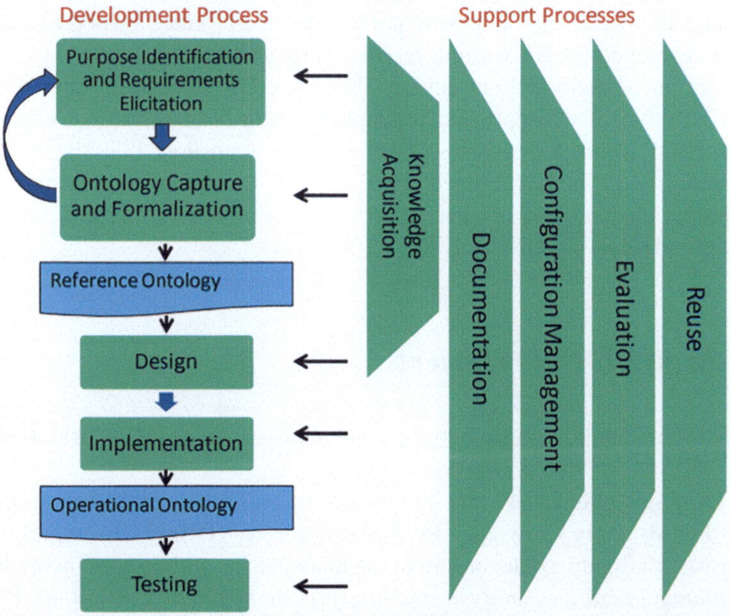

Fig. 7.2 SABiO methodology [1]

Capture and Formalization, requirements are organized and structured into competence questions. As a **domain ontology**, ExperDF-Onto was designed to represent DF-specific concepts, supporting logical and later technical modeling in Protégé [1].

In the **Design** phase, the ontology begins to take shape. An initial high-level model was created using draw.io and then refined into a formal representation. This transition led to the **Implementation** phase, in which the ontology was encoded in **OWL** (Web Ontology Language), enabling its execution and application in different contexts [1].

Validation was carried out through a **proof of concept (PoC)**. In this test, the ontology was instantiated in the AuthorMiner2 method, where only 2.94% of its classes and subclasses were activated. Although this indicated limited activation, it highlighted the ontology's potential to structure data and optimize analyses. A second type of validation, **real-case evaluation**, in which experts apply the ontology to document forensic cases, remains as future work [1].

The **Support Processes** complement development, ensuring quality, maintenance, and continuous improvement. It includes **Knowledge Acquisition**, drawing from domain literature, and **Documentation**, maintained in Protégé to guarantee transparency and traceability. **Configuration Management** defines execution parameters and version control; in this case, the ontology is stored locally in Protégé, enabling updates. **Evaluation** may involve code-level analysis or technical validation, though the latter has not yet been performed since the ontology is still under development [1].

SABiO prescribes a **Reuse** stage, which leverages existing models and methodologies [4]. However, this step was not applied here, since ExperDF-Onto was explicitly developed for DF without relying on preexisting structures [1].

This structured methodology ensures that ExperDF-Onto is developed systematically and efficiently, supporting its application in both controlled experiments and real-world forensic scenarios. Furthermore, it ensures that the model can be continuously refined, validated, and adapted to new requirements, thereby consolidating the ontology as an essential tool for structuring and formalizing knowledge in Digital Forensics [1, 6].

7.1.2 ExperDF-Onto Elements

The main components of this ontology are **Classes**, **Properties**, **Relations**, and **Axioms**.

The **ontology classes** are the pillars of the ontology, representing the core concepts that structure knowledge in Digital Forensics (DF) [2]. In ExperDF-Onto, these classes are organized according to the main phases of the experimentation process: *planning*, *operation*, *analysis and interpretation*, and *dissemination* (Fig. 7.3).

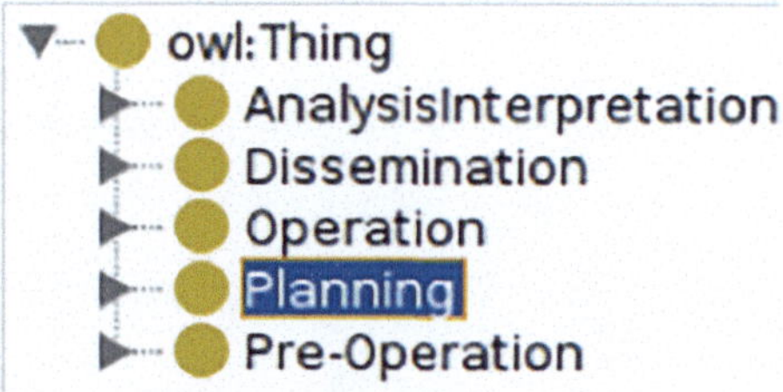

Fig. 7.3 Main classes

Each of these classes can be refined into specialized subclasses, allowing a more detailed organization of experiments and greater precision in data analysis and interpretation (Fig. 7.4). Currently, the ontology comprises 383 classes.

Properties provide additional information about classes and their instances, enriching the description of ontology elements [2]. They are divided into two main types: *object properties*, which connect different ontology elements; for example, the property "threat to validity" links an analysis to factors that may compromise the validity of an experiment (Fig. 7.5). *data properties*, which associate specific values with elements of the ontology, describing measurable characteristics, for instance, "suspicious action" refers to a particular event in forensic analysis (Fig. 7.6).

Relationships define how ontology elements interact, structuring knowledge through logical connections that enhance the accuracy and coherence of analyses. Common examples include "has a child," "belongs to," and "is part of." In the context of DF, the *analysis and interpretation* phase may be associated with a "threat to validity" that, in turn, can affect the "validity of conclusions." This may either lead to incorrect results or reinforce interpretation patterns. Such relationships ensure a coherent and structured representation of knowledge.

Axioms are rules that guarantee the internal consistency of the ontology by preventing contradictions or invalid connections. They impose constraints that ensure logical coherence. For example, every "threat to validity" must be classified into one of four types: internal, external, construct, or conclusion (Fig. 7.7). These axioms strengthen the ontology by enforcing rigor in the documentation and analysis of experiments.

This structured approach not only facilitates the organization of data and experiments but also improves the reliability of analyses, ensuring that results can be interpreted and replicated with confidence.

7.1.2.1 Planning

The planning phase is the starting point of an experiment, ensuring that all aspects are well-structured before execution. In this phase, essential elements are defined, including variables, hypotheses, experimental design, instruments, and participant selection [3].

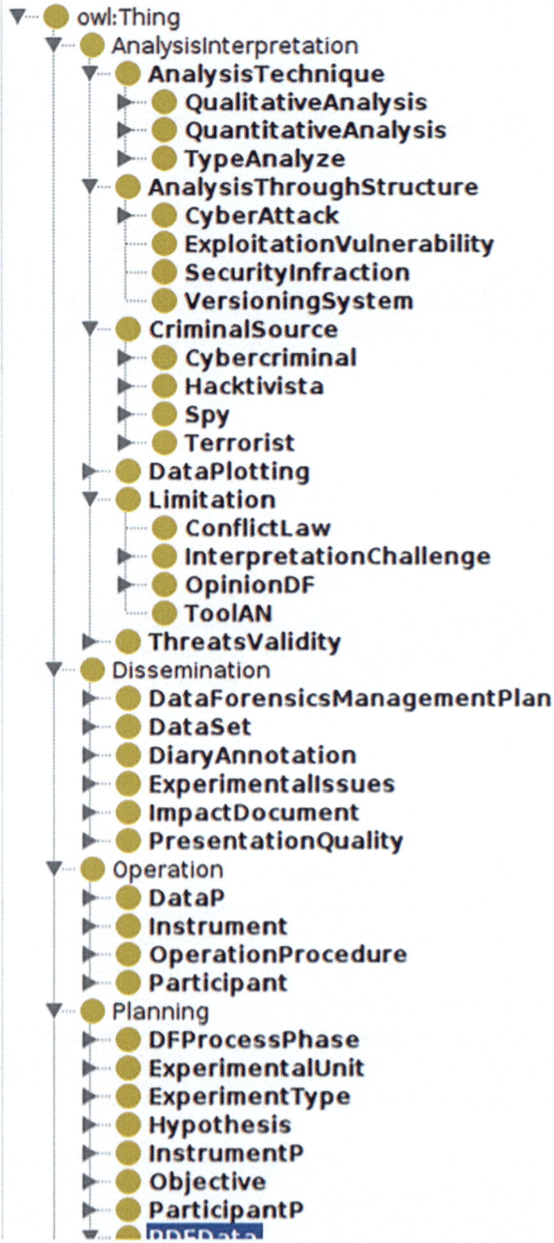

Fig. 7.4 General class hierarchy

Figure 7.8 illustrates the main components of this phase, including the incorporation of the **PDFData**, **ActivityLog**, and **SupportMaterial** subphases.

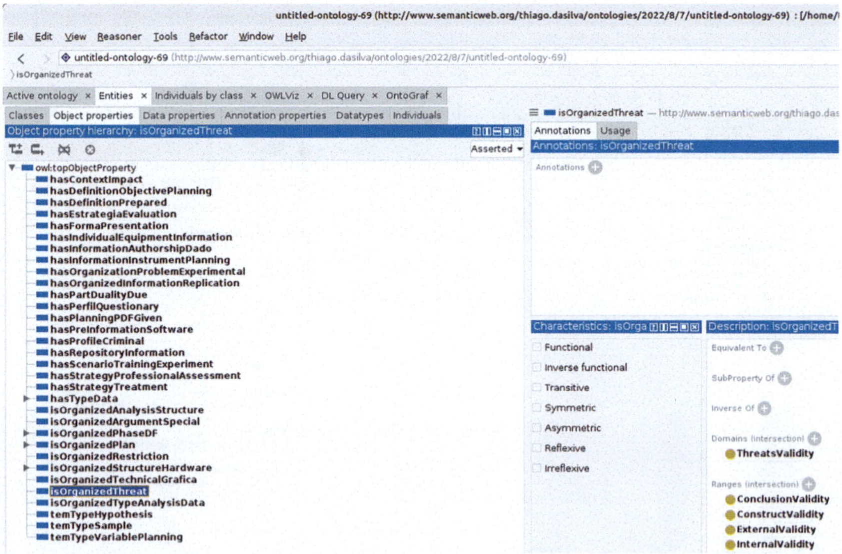

Fig. 7.5 Threat to validity

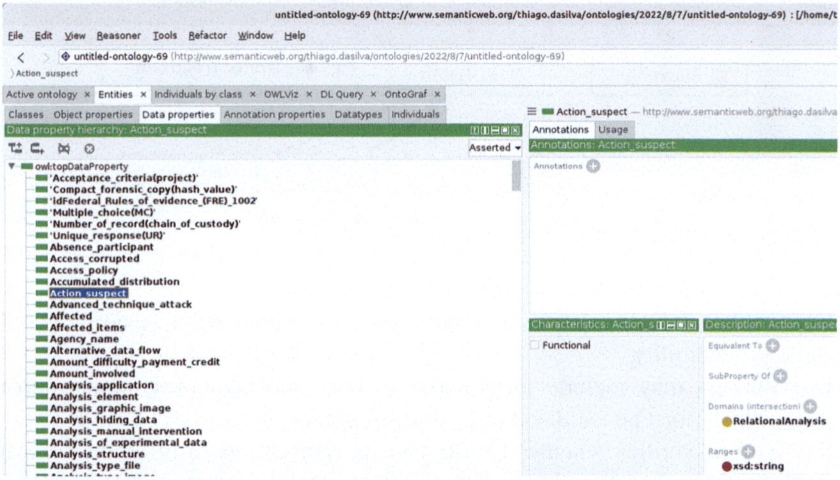

Fig. 7.6 Suspicious action

The main elements of the planning phase are:

- **Variables** are classified as independent (manipulated) or dependent (influenced and measured to assess effects).
- **Hypotheses** can be null (no significant effect) or alternative (measurable impact), forming the foundation of the study [3].

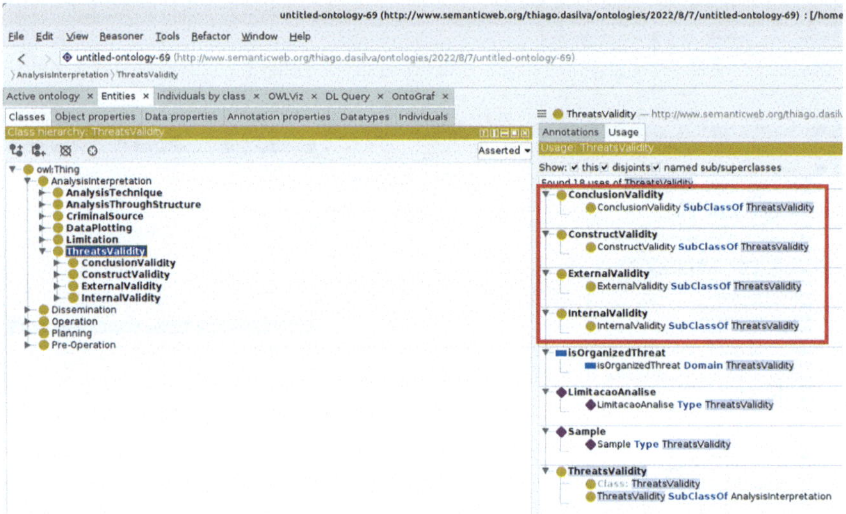

Fig. 7.7 Subphase of threat to validity

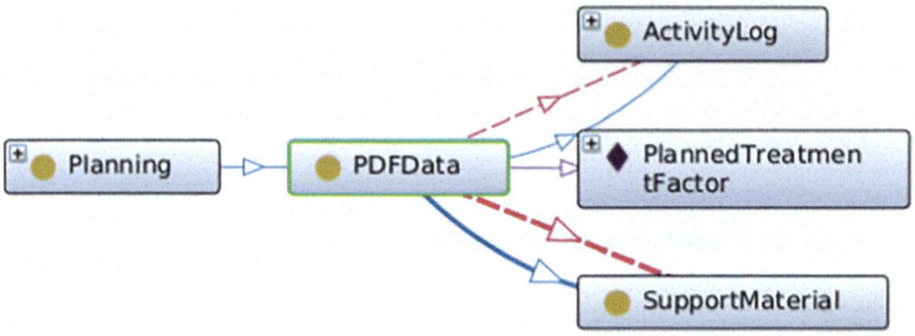

Fig. 7.8 ExperDF-Onto Excerpt of the Planning phase

- **Experimental design** defines how the study will be conducted, ensuring validity and reproducibility.
- **Instruments** may include programming code, questionnaires, or specialized tools, which must be validated to guarantee accuracy.
- **Replication** verifies whether results can be reproduced in different contexts. Replication can be internal (same group) or external (other researchers) and exact (all details are maintained) or conceptual (an adapted approach).
- **Participants** are selected by statistical sampling for representativeness or by specific criteria depending on the study.
- **FG phases** organize the experimental process from data collection and analysis to documentation, ensuring clarity and reliability [3].

In addition, three subphases strengthen organization and documentation:

- **Activity Log**: a detailed logbook that records all steps and actions, facilitating the preparation of the final report and ensuring traceability

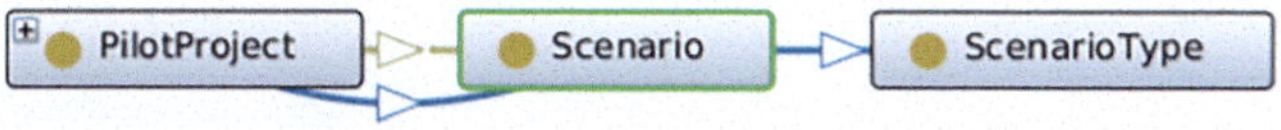

Fig. 7.9 ExperDF-Onto Excerpt of the Pre-Operation phase

- **PDFData**: storage of reports and documents in PDF format, including references, notes, and records of queries
- **SupportMaterial**: auxiliary resources that support execution and analysis, such as source code, configuration files, and computational tools

Together, these elements ensure that the planning phase not only defines the experiment's structure but also facilitates its analysis, interpretation, and dissemination, making the process more organized, documented, and controlled.

7.1.2.2 Pre-Operation

The Pre-Operation phase prepares the environment for experiment execution, ensuring that all necessary components are configured and operational. This stage includes setup, training, benchmark, pilot project, and the definition of the scenario in which the experiment will take place [3].

Figure 7.9 illustrates the main elements of this phase, including the **ScenarioType** subphase.

The pre-operation steps can be summarized as follows:

- **Setup**: configuration of software (operating systems, virtual machines, and applications), hardware (volatile and persistent memories), and algorithms (programmed with predefined parameters to ensure correct information handling) [3]
- **Training**: execution of initial tests to validate the functioning of systems, algorithms, and components before the experiment
- **Benchmark**: a measurement of system performance to ensure that all elements meet the study's requirements
- **Pilot project**: preliminary execution to verify the feasibility of configurations. At this stage, the **scenario** is defined, which may include virtual machines, databases, IoT devices, or specific analysis tools [3].

Within the scenario subphase, ExperDF-Onto introduces the concept of **ScenarioType**, which specifies the type of environment in which the experiment is carried out. Different scenario types can directly influence the results:

- **Physical scenario**: based on real equipment such as sensors and servers
- **Virtual scenario**: experimentation through simulations in virtual machines
- **Hybrid scenario**: combination of physical and virtual resources
- **Distributed virtual environments**: complex setups with virtual machines in different regions or systems using OPC simulators

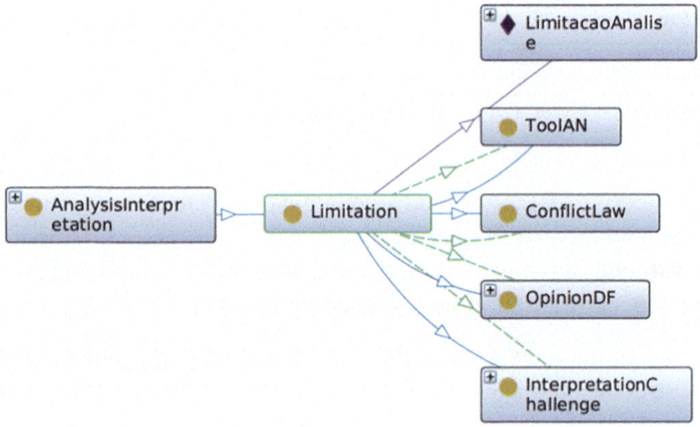

Fig. 7.10 ExperDF-Onto Excerpt of the Operation phase

Distinguishing among these scenario types enhances the precision of the analysis, helping to understand how varying configurations affect the performance and reliability of experimental results.

7.1.2.3 Operation

The Operation phase encompasses all elements necessary to experiment, ensuring that data is collected, organized, and processed accurately. This phase comprises the participant, the instrument used, the operational procedures, the sample, and the generated data [3].

Figure 7.10 presents the main structure of this phase, including the new subphases we introduced.

The basic elements of the operation are:

- **Participant**: an individual directly involved in the experiment or someone who contributes indirectly by providing information for analysis
- **Instrument**: tools used to collect and process data, such as models, databases, or metadata
- **Sample**: the subset of data selected for analysis
- **Data** may be *original data*, collected directly from the source without modifications, or *duplicate data*, created for backup or additional testing without compromising the primary dataset.
- **Operational procedures**: standardized sequences of actions that ensure reproducibility. For example, in API interactions, a typical sequence may involve creating a resource, retrieving its data, and modifying it if necessary [3].

To improve the evaluation of experimental procedures, we expanded the **OperationProcedure** with new subphases: **Experiment**, **FormulationContext**, **Hypoth-**

esisTestO, **Project**, **Protocol**, and **TheoreticalModelFormulation**. Their roles are as follows:

- **Experiment**: the core of the operation phase, defining tools, participants, data, and procedures for systematic execution and result collection
- **FormulationContext** establishes the study's environment and conditions, documenting variables, objectives, constraints, and contextual factors.
- **HypothesisTestO** verifies whether the study's assumptions are confirmed or refuted, providing an objective evaluation of collected data.
- **Project** details all necessary planning, including methodologies, tools, technical configurations, and study structure, ensuring reliability.
- **Protocol** defines the rules and guidelines for execution. For instance, in API experiments, it specifies the order of requests to ensure correct communication and data transmission.
- **TheoreticalModelFormulation** provides a solid theoretical foundation by applying established and validated models from the literature and practice.

With these elements and subphases, the operation phase becomes more structured, rigorous, and practical, ensuring accurate execution and interpretation of experimental results.

7.1.2.4 Analysis and Interpretation

The analysis and interpretation phase examines the experimental data to extract relevant information and transform the results into meaningful insights. At this stage, patterns are identified, hypotheses are verified, and relationships between variables are explored [3].

Figure 7.11 illustrates the subclasses added in this phase, which support the identification of limitations and documentation of the final report.

Data is organized in a structured way and represented clearly, using graphs, tables, or other visualizations that facilitate interpretation. This helps identify trends, verify hypotheses, and detect inconsistencies that may affect conclusions [3].

Analysis can follow two main approaches:

- **Qualitative analysis**: interpretation based on context and observation, such as manual review of records, group discussions, or the use of tools for organizing information
- **Quantitative analysis**: interpretation based on statistics and calculations, such as averages, statistical tests, and regression models, providing objective and measurable conclusions [3]

Another critical aspect of this phase is recognizing limitations and threats to validity. These may stem from the quality of information collected, the accuracy of measurements, or interference from external factors [3].

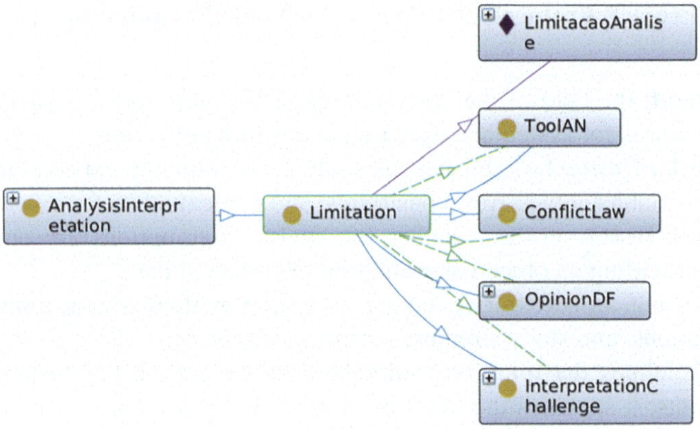

Fig. 7.11 ExperDF-Onto Excerpt of the Analysis and Interpretation phase

To capture such aspects, the ontology was expanded with the subclasses **ConflictLaw**, **InterpretationChallenge**, **OpinionDF**, and **ToolAN**:

- **ConflictLaw** addresses legal divergences that may affect the interpretation or application of results, such as privacy and data protection laws that vary across jurisdictions.
- **InterpretationChallenge** highlights ambiguities, inconsistencies, or missing context in the data, which may lead to misinterpretations.
- **OpinionDF** acknowledges that different experts may interpret the same dataset differently, depending on their knowledge, experience, and professional background.
- **ToolAN** refers to the role of technology in data analysis, while noting limitations due to compatibility issues, licensing restrictions, outdated versions, or processing differences.

Together, these elements ensure that the analysis and interpretation phase not only extracts insights from the data but also documents limitations, thereby increasing the reliability and transparency of the experimental results.

7.1.2.5 Dissemination

The dissemination phase ensures that the data collected in the experiment is organized and shared in a safe, transparent, and accessible way. This stage consolidates all final information so that the academic community and other stakeholders can access the collected evidence. Following good practices for publishing and sharing is essential to guarantee reliability and reproducibility [3].

To structure this step, ExperDF-Onto adopted the ExperDF-CM conceptual model, which defines the main elements of dissemination.

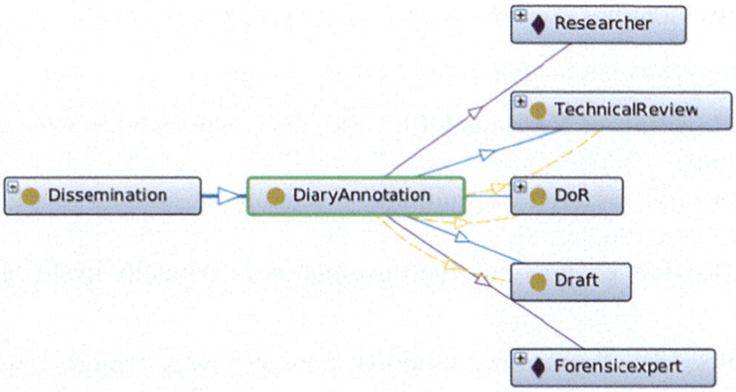

Fig. 7.12 Recording experimental notes

Fig. 7.13 Data presentation quality

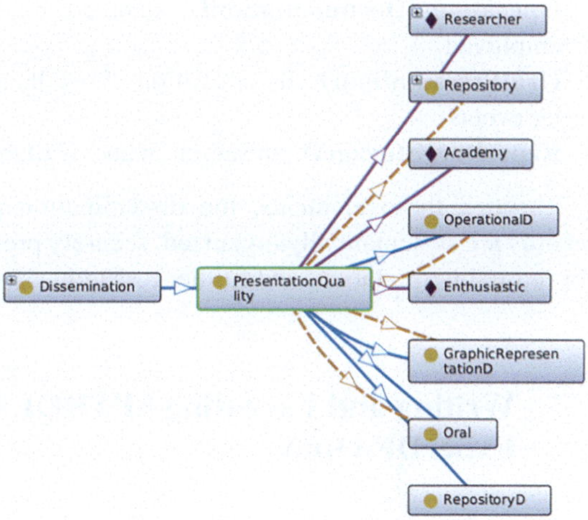

Figures 7.12 and 7.13 illustrate the expanded ontology supporting this phase. The original model included the following elements:

- **Forensic Data Management Plan (FDMP)** ensures data is organized and stored properly.
- **Dataset Metadata** provides detailed information to facilitate the understanding and reproduction of experiments.
- **Journal/Notes**: continuous record of procedures and actions taken throughout the experiment
- **Experimental Issues**: documents challenges and problems encountered that may affect results
- **Dataset**: all documents and information collected during the experiment
- **Repository**: storage location where data is made accessible
- **Unique ID**: identifier such as a DOI, ensuring traceability and authenticity of the dataset
- **Citation**: guidelines for referencing the dataset, guaranteeing proper attribution

- **Authorship** identifies contributors and acknowledges their roles.

The ontology was later expanded with new categories:

- **DoR (Declaration of Responsibility)** specifies responsibilities for each part of the experiment.
- **Draft** allows the creation of preliminary versions of records for review before final documentation.
- **TechnicalReview** ensures that the information is critically evaluated and validated.

Additionally, the **PresentationQuality** category was included to guarantee clarity and accessibility of results, subdivided into:

- **GraphicRepresentationD**: use of graphs, tables, and diagrams to illustrate data
- **OperationalDocumentationD**: detailed explanation of methods and tools employed
- **OralPresentationD**: dissemination of results at conferences, lectures, and similar events
- **RepositoryStorageD**: preservation and availability of data in trusted repositories

Through these elements, the dissemination phase ensures that experimental records are systematically organized, securely preserved, and made more accessible for reuse, interpretation, and further research.

7.2 Writing and Executing SPARQL Queries in ExperDF-Onto

This section demonstrates how to query the ExperDF-Onto ontology using SPARQL, with a focus on navigating class hierarchies and retrieving structured knowledge across each phase of the digital forensics experimental life cycle. Queries are executed using Protégé's SPARQL tab, which enables direct inspection of the ontology, verification of structural consistency, and exploration of the conceptual model.

We begin by identifying the ontology's top-level classes and, subsequently, present queries organized by experimental phases: Planning, Pre-Operation, Operation, Analysis and Interpretation, and Dissemination. Each subsection introduces the queries' goals, explains their logic, and presents the retrieved results.

7.2.1 *Identifying Top-Level Classes*

The query in Listing 7.1 retrieves all top-level classes, meaning those that have no superclasses defined. This provides an overview of the ontology's main structural pillars.

Listing 7.1 SPARQL query to identify top-level classes

```
PREFIX rdf: <http://www.w3.org/1999/02/22-rdf-syntax-ns#>
PREFIX rdfs: <http://www.w3.org/2000/01/rdf-schema#>
PREFIX owl: <http://www.w3.org/2002/07/owl#>

SELECT DISTINCT ?class
WHERE {
  ?class a owl:Class .
  FILTER NOT EXISTS { ?class rdfs:subClassOf ?super . }
}
```

The following box presents the exact output returned by executing this query:

Top-Level Classes Retrieved from Listing 7.1

Planning
Pre-Operation
Operation
AnalysisInterpretation
Dissemination

7.2.2 *Planning Phase Queries*

The Planning phase contains the richest set of conceptual structures in ExperDF-Onto. The following queries explore both its immediate subclasses and the complete set of nested subclasses.

7.2.2.1 Direct Subclasses of Planning

The following query retrieves only the immediate subclasses of Planning.

Listing 7.2 SPARQL query to retrieve direct subclasses of Planning

```
PREFIX rdfs: <http://www.w3.org/2000/01/rdf-schema#>

SELECT DISTINCT ?subclass
WHERE {
  ?subclass rdfs:subClassOf <http://www.semanticweb.org/thiago.
      dasilva/ontologies/2022/8/7/untitled-ontology-69#Planning>
      .
}
```

The following box contains the query output exactly as returned by Protégé:

Direct Subclasses of Planning
DFProcessPhase, ExperimentType, ExperimentalUnit, Hypothesis, InstrumentP, Objective, PDFData, ParticipantP, TypeProject, Variable.

7.2.2.2 All Subclasses of Planning

To retrieve the whole hierarchy of subclasses, the following query uses the transitive operator rdfs:subClassOf+.

Listing 7.3 SPARQL query to retrieve all subclasses of Planning

```
PREFIX rdfs: <http://www.w3.org/2000/01/rdf-schema#>

SELECT DISTINCT ?subclass
WHERE {
  ?subclass rdfs:subClassOf+ <http://www.semanticweb.org/thiago.
      dasilva/ontologies/2022/8/7/untitled-ontology-69#Planning>
      .
}
```

The following box reports the complete list of subclasses returned by Protégé:

All Subclasses of Planning
Activity, ActivityLog, AlternativeHypothesis, Analysis, AnalyzeP, Artifact, AutoSelectionSampling, Bilateral, Category, CognitivePhysicalDemand, ComponentNotCollected, ConceptualReplication, ConclusionSpecialist, ConglomerateRandomSampling, Constant, Control, DFAcquisition, DFAnalysis, DFExamination, DFProcessPhase, DFReporting, DataExtraction, DataMining, DecryptionData, DependentReplication, DependentVari-

(continued)

able, DependentVariableMetric, DeviceIdentifier, DocumentationActivityMonitor, DocumentationConditionSO, DocumentationProtocol, EthicalPlanning, EvidencePlanning, ExperimentalUnit, ExternalReplication, GroupComparison, Hypothesis, IndependentVariable, InstrumentP, IntentionalSampling, KnowledgeResourceCondition, LegalPlanning, MaintainabilityPlanning, MaterialResourceCondition, MetadataPlanning, ModelPlanning, Objective, OntologyPlanning, OperationalPlanning, Opinion, ParticipantP, PerformancePlanning, PilotPlanning, PlanningStage, PoliticalCondition, Probabilistic, ProportionalQuotaSampling, QualityPlanning, QuotaSampling, RandomSampling, ReliabilityPlanning, ReplicationPlanning, ReproducibilityPlanning, ResourcePlanning, ResearchPlanning, ReviewPlanning, ScalabilityPlanning, SimulationPlanning, SnowballSampling, SocialCondition, SpecializedDependentVariable, StatisticalPlanning, StratifiedRandomSampling, SurveyPlanning, TechnicalPlanning, TemporalCondition, ToolResourceCondition, TraceabilityPlanning, TransactionalResearch, TransparencyPlanning, Treatment, TypicalVariable, TypeProject, UsabilityPlanning, ValidationPlanning, Variable.

7.2.2.3 Direct Subclasses of Variable

The following query illustrates how to retrieve immediate subclasses of a specific Planning class.

Listing 7.4 SPARQL query to retrieve direct subclasses of Variable

```
PREFIX rdfs: <http://www.w3.org/2000/01/rdf-schema#>

SELECT DISTINCT ?subclass
WHERE {
  ?subclass rdfs:subClassOf <http://www.semanticweb.org/thiago.
      dasilva/ontologies/2022/8/7/untitled-ontology-69#Variable>
      .
}
```

The following box contains the exact results returned by this query:

Direct Subclasses of Variable

DependentVariable
IndependentVariable

7.2.3 *Pre-Operation Phase Queries*

The Pre-Operation phase includes activities such as setup, benchmarking, training, and environment configuration. The following queries inspect its structure.

7.2.3.1 Direct Subclasses of Pre-Operation

Listing 7.5 SPARQL query to retrieve direct subclasses of Pre-Operation

```
PREFIX rdfs: <http://www.w3.org/2000/01/rdf-schema#>

SELECT DISTINCT ?subclass
WHERE {
  ?subclass rdfs:subClassOf <http://www.semanticweb.org/thiago.
      dasilva/ontologies/2022/8/7/untitled-ontology-69#Pre-
      Operation> .
}
```

Below is the direct output of the SPARQL execution:

Direct Subclasses of Pre-Operation
Benchmark, PilotProject, Setup, Training

7.2.3.2 All Subclasses of Pre-Operation

Listing 7.6 SPARQL query to retrieve all subclasses of Pre-Operation

```
PREFIX rdfs: <http://www.w3.org/2000/01/rdf-schema#>

SELECT DISTINCT ?subclass
WHERE {
  ?subclass rdfs:subClassOf+ <http://www.semanticweb.org/thiago.
      dasilva/ontologies/2022/8/7/untitled-ontology-69#Pre-
      Operation> .
}
```

The following box contains the full execution result returned in Protégé:

All Subclasses of Pre-Operation
AdditionInstruction, Algorithm, Application, ApplicationBenchmark, Argument, Assignment, Benchmark, Cache, CacheConfiguration, CacheLocation, Category, Class, Classification, Cluster, ClusterAlgorithm, ClusterAssignment, ClusterConfiguration, ClusterMethod, ClusterModel, ClusterSetup, ClusterTraining, Clustering, Comparison, Configuration, Data, DataApplication, DataAssignment, DataBenchmark, DataCache, DataCategory, DataClass, DataCluster, DataConfiguration, DataEvaluation, DataLocation, DataMethod, DataModel, DataPilotProject, DataProcess, DataProgram, DataSetup, DataStage, DataSystem, DataTraining, Evaluation, EvaluationAlgorithm, EvaluationBenchmark, EvaluationMethod, EvaluationModel, Instruction, Location, Method, Model, PilotProject, Process, Program, Setup, Stage, System, Training, Value.

7.2.4 *Operation Phase Queries*

This phase captures procedural actions, data operations, and tool execution steps. The queries explore its conceptual hierarchy.

7.2.4.1 Direct Subclasses of Operation

Listing 7.7 SPARQL query to retrieve direct subclasses of Operation

```
PREFIX rdfs: <http://www.w3.org/2000/01/rdf-schema#>

SELECT DISTINCT ?subclass
WHERE {
  ?subclass rdfs:subClassOf <http://www.semanticweb.org/thiago.
      dasilva/ontologies/2022/8/7/untitled-ontology-69#Operation>
        .
}
```

The box below reproduces the exact results from the SPARQL query:

Direct Subclasses of Operation
DataP, Instrument, OperationProcedure, Participant

7.2.4.2 All Subclasses of Operation

Listing 7.8 SPARQL query to retrieve all subclasses of Operation

```
PREFIX rdfs: <http://www.w3.org/2000/01/rdf-schema#>

SELECT DISTINCT ?subclass
WHERE {
  ?subclass rdfs:subClassOf+ <http://www.semanticweb.org/thiago.
      dasilva/ontologies/2022/8/7/untitled-ontology-69#Operation>
      .
}
```

The following box shows the complete response returned by the query:

All Subclasses of Operation
Autonomous, ChainofCustodyDocumentation, ChangeMetadata, CleaningExperiment, Code, ConfidenceLevel, CopyDataStreamFailed, Cryptography, DataCaving, DataLossNotFiled, DataP, Decrypt, Delete, Error, Execute, Execution, ExperimentExecution, ExperimentRun, ExperimentStep, File, FileTransfer, Hashing, Instrument, Logging, MetadataUpdate, Monitoring, NetworkOperation, OperationProcedure, OperationStep, Operator, Output, Participant, Processing, ProcessMonitoring, ProgramExecution, Read, Recovery, Replication, Result, Run, Save, Scheduling, Script, Simulation, SoftwareExecution, Storage, Transfer, Upload, UserAction, Validation, Write.

7.2.5 Analysis and Interpretation Phase Queries

This phase includes statistical techniques, visualization strategies, and interpretative frameworks essential for deriving meaning from experimental evidence.

7.2.5.1 Direct Subclasses of AnalysisInterpretation

Listing 7.9 SPARQL query to retrieve direct subclasses of AnalysisInterpretation

```
PREFIX rdfs: <http://www.w3.org/2000/01/rdf-schema#>

SELECT DISTINCT ?subclass
WHERE {
  ?subclass rdfs:subClassOf <http://www.semanticweb.org/thiago.
      dasilva/ontologies/2022/8/7/untitled-ontology-69#
      AnalysisInterpretation> .
}
```

The following box presents the direct output from SPARQL execution:

Direct Subclasses of AnalysisInterpretation
AnalysisTechnique, AnalysisThroughStructure, CriminalSource, DataPlotting, Limitation, ThreatsValidity

7.2.5.2 All Subclasses of AnalysisInterpretation

Listing 7.10 SPARQL query to retrieve all subclasses of AnalysisInterpretation

```
PREFIX rdfs: <http://www.w3.org/2000/01/rdf-schema#>

SELECT DISTINCT ?subclass
WHERE {
  ?subclass rdfs:subClassOf+ <http://www.semanticweb.org/thiago.
      dasilva/ontologies/2022/8/7/untitled-ontology-69#
      AnalysisInterpretation> .
}
```

The following box contains the entire set of subclasses returned:

All Subclasses of AnalysisInterpretation
AnaliseUnivariada, AnalysisTechnique, AnalysisThroughStructure, AndersonDarling, BarChart, BivariateAnalysis, Boxplot, BungeRating, CentralTendencyA, CentralTrend, ChiSquare, Classification, ClusterAnalysis, Coefficient, ComparisonPlot, ConfidenceInterval, Correlation, CorrelationCoefficient, CriminalSource, Crosstab, DataPlotting, DataRepresentation, DataVisualization, DensityPlot, DescriptiveAnalysis, DescriptiveStatistic, Diagnostic, Distribution, ErrorEstimation, FactorAnalysis, FrequencyDistribution, GraphicalMethod, Histogram, HypothesisTest, InferentialAnalysis, InterpretationModel, KruskalWallis, Kurtosis, Limitation, LinearRegression, LogisticRegression, MannWhitney, MeanComparison, MedianTest, MetaAnalysis, ModeAnalysis, MultivariateAnalysis, NormalityTest, OutlierDetection, PValue, ParametricTest, PearsonCorrelation, Plot, ProbabilityAnalysis, ProbabilityDistribution, QualitativeAnalysis, QuantitativeAnalysis, Quartile, Regression, ReliabilityAnalysis, ResidualAnalysis, ResultInterpretation, SamplingError, ScatterPlot, ShapiroWilk, SignificanceLevel, SpearmanCorrelation, StandardDeviation, StatisticalAnalysis, StatisticalTest, StudentTest, SurvivalAnalysis, TTest, TestPower, ThreatsValidity, TimeSeries, TrendAnalysis, Uncertainty, UnivariateAnalysis, ValidityTest, Variability, Variance, VarianceAnalysis, WilcoxonTest, ZTest.

7.2.6 *Dissemination Phase Queries*

This phase models the communication of results, data publication, reporting standards, and mechanisms for scientific transparency.

7.2.6.1 Direct Subclasses of Dissemination

Listing 7.11 SPARQL query to retrieve direct subclasses of Dissemination

```
PREFIX rdfs: <http://www.w3.org/2000/01/rdf-schema#>

SELECT DISTINCT ?subclass
WHERE {
  ?subclass rdfs:subClassOf <http://www.semanticweb.org/thiago.
      dasilva/ontologies/2022/8/7/untitled-ontology-69#
      Dissemination> .
}
```

The next box shows the exact output of the SPARQL query:

> **Direct Subclasses of Dissemination**
> DataForensicsManagementPlan, DataSet, DiaryAnnotation, ExperimentalIssues, ImpactDocument, PresentationQuality

7.2.6.2 All Subclasses of Dissemination

Listing 7.12 SPARQL query to retrieve all subclasses of Dissemination

```
PREFIX rdfs: <http://www.w3.org/2000/01/rdf-schema#>

SELECT DISTINCT ?subclass
WHERE {
  ?subclass rdfs:subClassOf+ <http://www.semanticweb.org/thiago.
      dasilva/ontologies/2022/8/7/untitled-ontology-69#
      Dissemination> .
}
```

The response returned by the execution of this query is shown below:

All Subclasses of Dissemination
AuthenticationFrequency, Authorship, CheckList, Citation, CombinationNumber, CreditPaymentDifficulty, Data, DataArchiving, DataCitation, DataForensicsManagementPlan, DataManagement, DataSet, DataSharing, DataStorage, DataTransparency, DiaryAnnotation, DigitalIdentifier, DisseminationPlan, DocumentPublication, DocumentReview, ExperimentalIssues, ExternalPublication, FormatStandard, ImpactAssessment, ImpactDocument, Indexing, JournalPublication, KnowledgeDissemination, Licensing, LiteratureReview, Metadata, OpenAccess, OpenScience, PeerReview, PosterPresentation, Preprint, Presentation, PresentationQuality, Publication, PublicationBias, PublicationChannel, PublicationEthics, Publisher, QualityAssessment, ReproducibilityReport, ResearchData, ResearchDiary, ResearchImpact, ResearchPublication, ScientificCommunication, ScientificContribution, ScientificDissemination, ScientificJournal, ScientificOutput, Standardization, Transparency, ValidationReport, WorkshopProceeding, WritingGuideline.

7.3 Final Remarks

ExperDF-Onto consolidates a comprehensive, formalized representation of the experimental life cycle in Digital Forensics, transforming the conceptual structures of ExperDF-CM into a machine-interpretable ontology that supports rigorous, transparent, and reproducible forensic investigations. By organizing more than 600 conceptual elements into five interconnected phases, the ontology provides not only a semantic backbone for structuring experiments but also a practical asset for guiding methodological decisions, documenting procedures, and integrating domain-specific knowledge across heterogeneous investigative contexts.

The adoption of the SABiO methodology ensured a systematic and traceable development process, from purpose elicitation to implementation and evaluation. This methodological grounding enhances the ontology's internal coherence and positions it as a reusable resource for future extensions, including integration with provenance models, computational tools, and forensic platforms. The proof-of-concept instantiation demonstrated the ontology's potential to structure experimental data and support automated reasoning, although extensive real-world validation remains an essential step in its maturation.

By incorporating detailed modeling of hypotheses, variables, procedures, scenario configurations, threats to validity, documentation practices, and dissemination structures, ExperDF-Onto directly addresses persistent challenges related to methodological rigor and reproducibility in Digital Forensics. The SPARQL query patterns presented in this chapter illustrate how researchers and practitioners can explore, audit, and validate the ontology, enabling both conceptual understanding and computational inspection.

As Digital Forensics continues to evolve in response to technological complexity, ExperDF-Onto provides a foundational layer for formalizing experimental practices, enabling more reliable knowledge accumulation and fostering alignment with FAIR and Open Science principles. Future work will focus on empirical validation in real forensic scenarios, integration with workflow management tools, and the development of automated reasoning modules that leverage the ontology to support decision-making, documentation quality, and scientific transparency.

References

1. Falbo, R.A.: SABiO: systematic approach for building ontologies. In: Proceedings of the 1st Joint Workshop on Ontologies in Conceptual Modeling and Information Systems Engineering (CEUR-WS), vol. 1201 (2014)
2. Mirror, J.C.: Guia prático de construção de ontologias—protégé v. 5.2. ResearchGate **9**, 3–134 (2018)
3. Oliveira, E. Jr, Zorzo, A.F., Neu, C.V.: Towards a conceptual model for promoting digital forensics experiments. Foren. Sci. Int.: Digit. Invest. **35**, 301014 (2020). https://doi.org/10.1016/j.fsidi.2020.301014
4. Scherp, A., Saathoff, C., Franz, T., Staab, S.: Designing core ontologies. Appl. Ontol. **6**(3), 177–221 (2011)
5. Silva, T.J., Mazur, A.H., Oliveira, E. Jr, Zorzo, A.F., Barcellos, M.P.: An ontology for promoting controlled experimentation in digital forensics. Foren. Sci. Int.: Digit. Invest. **52**, 301845 (2025)
6. Suárez-Figueroa, M.C., Gómez-Pérez, A., Motta, E., Gangemi, A.: Introduction: ontology engineering in a networked world. In: Ontology Engineering in a Networked World, pp. 1–6. Springer, New York, NY (2011)

Part IV
ExperDF-Onto Walkthroughs of Exemplary Digital Forensics Experiments

This part presents a comprehensive and didactic walkthrough of how *ExperDF-Onto* can be instantiated to describe, reason about, and evaluate real digital forensics experiments. While the previous parts established the conceptual and ontological foundations of the framework, this part marks a decisive shift from *theory* to *practice*.

Its purpose is not merely to illustrate ontology use but also to demonstrate how a semantic framework can transform empirical investigations into structured, interoperable, and verifiable scientific assets. Each example progresses toward higher ontological maturity, showing how formal representations encode research intent, experimental rigor, provenance, and dissemination practices in a consistent and machine-actionable form.

By following five representative forensic scenarios that range from memory analysis and smartphone extractions to blockchain-based provenance, this part highlights the expressive capacity of *ExperDF-Onto* in uniting technical, ethical, and epistemological dimensions of experimentation.

This part also serves as a pedagogical bridge between abstract ontology and applied research methodology. Each chapter is designed to help readers:

- Understand how narrative experimental designs can be decomposed into explicit ontological elements such as `Experiment`, `ResearchQuestion`, `IndependentVariable`, and `DatasetMetadata`.
- Observe how formal relations such as `hasDependentVariable`, `isControlledBy`, and `producedBy` capture logical dependencies among planning, execution, and interpretation.
- Learn to trace reproducibility through explicit metadata, provenance chains, and dissemination entities that make research auditable and transparent.
- Reflect on how the ontology reinforces scientific rigor, ethical responsibility, collaborative openness, and long-term data stewardship.

Each case study, although situated in a specific subdomain of Digital Forensics, has been rewritten as a guided *walkthrough*. Readers can follow each phase, from hypothesis formulation to data publication, under a unified vocabulary that makes comparisons across domains consistent and instructive.

The five chapters included in this part represent exemplary experiments that collectively demonstrate the breadth and adaptability of *ExperDF-Onto*:

1. **The Memory That Would Not Lie**—a reproducibility study on live memory acquisition emphasizing tool equivalence, experimental control, and quantitative reliability
2. **Unlocking the Locked: Smartphone Bypass Experiments**—a comparison of physical and logical extraction methods across Android and iOS, modeling ethical constraints and legal compliance
3. **The Case of the Altered Cloud Logs**—a cloud forensics simulation that detects tampered log entries across providers and focuses on provenance and detection accuracy
4. **Echoes in the IoT Lab**—a smart home intrusion scenario capturing temporal and causal relations among IoT devices, illustrating complex event reconstruction
5. **The Invisible Signature: Blockchain Provenance**—a blockchain-based approach to dataset traceability and authenticity integrating governance, quality assessment, and immutability guarantees

Each example follows the same logical flow based on the five research phases defined by *ExperDF-CM*: **Planning**, **Pre-operation**, **Operation**, **Analysis and Interpretation**, and **Dissemination**. This structure ensures that the ontology is not presented as an abstract schema but as a practical framework guiding the entire research life cycle.

Analyzing these five walkthroughs together reveals how ontological instantiation helps to quantify the maturity and reproducibility of experiments. Early cases highlight methodological rigor and control of variables, while later ones incorporate governance, provenance traceability, and open science compliance. Ontological completeness increases progressively, from 68% in the first example, focused on operational reproducibility, to 80% in the last, centered on provenance and governance. This evolution reflects the growth of Digital Forensics itself, moving from isolated technical investigations toward integrated, multidisciplinary studies aligned with open science principles.

Key Takeaways

- **Ontology as methodology:** *ExperDF-Onto* guides experimenters toward explicit, coherent, and ethically responsible research design.
- **Ontology as documentation:** Every experimental decision, including variable selection, tool choice, dataset creation, and analysis method, becomes semantically traceable, supporting reuse and auditability.
- **Ontology as integration layer:** Shared ontological patterns enable comparison and federation of experiments across domains, institutions, and research infrastructures.

This part demonstrates that ontological modeling is not an abstract academic exercise but a concrete mechanism for strengthening the credibility and transparency of digital investigations. By systematically encoding research processes, *ExperDF-Onto* ensures that forensic evidence and experimental data are reproducible, interpretable, and reusable across different contexts.

This part concludes the applied dimension of the book. The following part extends these ideas toward ecosystem-level integration, connecting experiments, repositories, provenance networks, and policy frameworks to build a transparent, trustworthy, and cumulative infrastructure for Digital Forensics research.

Chapter 8
Example 1: The Memory That Would Not Lie

Abstract This chapter provides a complete walkthrough of a controlled digital forensics experiment that examines the reproducibility and reliability of volatile memory acquisition. The investigation explored whether different live memory acquisition tools produce consistent and equivalent forensic artifacts when applied to identical systems under identical conditions. Volatile memory, being highly dynamic and sensitive to timing, presents unique challenges to digital investigators who must ensure that the process of evidence acquisition does not alter the state being measured. To address this, the study was modeled through *ExperDF-Onto*, an ontology designed to formally represent every phase of a digital forensic experiment, making methodological decisions explicit, auditable, and machine-actionable. The experiment's design included well-defined hypotheses, independent and dependent variables, and controlled conditions to assess the effects of three widely used acquisition tools: Volatility, Rekall, and Belkasoft Live RAM Capture. A series of virtualized environments was configured to standardize the tests, and pilot runs were executed to confirm baseline reproducibility. During execution, every operation, artifact, and measurement was instantiated as an ontological element, creating a semantically linked chain of provenance that connects the research question to the produced data and analytical results. Statistical analysis using ANOVA revealed no significant differences among tools, with a reliability coefficient of 0.96, demonstrating strong internal consistency in acquisition performance. Beyond the technical results, the chapter emphasizes the importance of representing experimental procedures, parameters, and results in a structured ontology to promote transparency, replicability, and long-term accessibility. By publishing all associated datasets and metadata through open repositories, the experiment exemplifies how ontological modeling can transform traditional forensic procedures into open, reusable, and verifiable scientific workflows, thereby reinforcing the epistemic reliability and ethical accountability of Digital Forensics as a scientific discipline.

E. OliveiraJr et al., *Controlled Experimentation of Digital Forensics*,
https://doi.org/10.1007/978-3-032-19951-5_8

8.1 Context and Motivation

Volatile memory acquisition is a cornerstone of incident response and malware analysis, yet tool behavior, operating system internals, and timing can affect what is captured and how it is reconstructed. The researchers designed a controlled study to ask a deceptively simple question: **Do different acquisition tools produce materially equivalent results for the same running system under the same conditions?** This example demonstrates how *ExperDF-Onto* captures the complete chain of reasoning from the motivating question to the final, shareable artifacts, including every decision and constraint that affects reproducibility and interpretation.

This walkthrough shows how to move from a narrative scenario to a fully instantiated ontological representation. At each phase, we explain why a concept matters, how it is instantiated, which relations connect it to other elements, and what typical pitfalls to avoid.

8.2 Planning Phase

The planning phase translates a broad concern into testable hypotheses, measurable variables, and auditable decisions. In *ExperDF-Onto*, this means instantiating classes such as `Experiment`, `ResearchQuestion`, `Hypothesis`, `IndependentVariable`, `DependentVariable`, and `ControlVariable` and linking them by object properties like `hasIndependentVariable`, `hasDependentVariable`, and `isControlledBy` as follows:

- **Experiment** *(why)* establishes scope and identity of the study. **Instance:** `Exp_VM_Reproducibility`.
- **ResearchQuestion** *(why)* frames measurable uncertainty. **Instance:** `RQ_tool_equivalence`.
- **Hypothesis** *(why)* asserts an expected relation. **Instance:** `H0_no_tool_effect` and `H1_tool_effect`.
- **IndependentVariable** *(why)*: manipulated factor. **Instance:** `IV_AcquisitionTool` with levels `{Volatility, Rekall, BelkasoftLiveRAM}`.
- **DependentVariable** *(why)*: measured outcomes. **Instances:** `DV_RecoveredProcesses`, `DV_OpenPorts`, `DV_Handles`.
- **ControlVariable** *(why)* holds sources of variation constant. **Instances:** `CV_OSVersion`, `CV_MemSize`, `CV_BackgroundLoad`.
- **ConfoundingFactor** *(why)* documents risks to causal inference that cannot be fully controlled. **Instances:** `CF_TimestampDrift`, `CF_HypervisorCaching`.
- **EthicalPlanning** *(why)* protects participants and privacy. **Instance:** `EP_SyntheticWorkloadsOnly`.
- **ReplicationPlanning** *(why)* commits to transparency before results exist. **Instance:** `RP_OSF_prereg_VMR`.

To do so, we used the following relations: Exp_VM_Reproducibility hasResearchQuestion RQ_tool_equivalence; Exp_VM_Reproducibility hasHypothesis H0_no_tool_effect; Exp_VM_Reproducibility hasIndependentVariable IV_AcquisitionTool; DV_RecoveredProcesses isMeasuredUnder IV_AcquisitionTool; Exp_VM_Reproducibility isControlledBy CV_OSVersion, CV_MemSize, CV_BackgroundLoad; Exp_VM_Reproducibility considersConfounding CF_TimestampDrift.

We also list pitfalls and how the ontology prevents them:

- *Pitfall:* treating tool choice as a mere operational detail. *Prevention:* Modeling IV_AcquisitionTool forces explicit manipulation and level definition.
- *Pitfall:* vague outcomes. *Prevention:* Explicit DependentVariable classes encourage metric definitions upfront.
- *Pitfall:* hidden constraints. *Prevention:* ControlVariable and ConfoundingFactor make non-manipulated influences visible and auditable.

8.3 Pre-Operation Phase

Pre-operation turns plans into a testable environment. In *ExperDF-Onto*, we document ScenarioType, EnvironmentSetup, Benchmark, PilotProject, TrainingActivity, and KnowledgeResourceCondition to support repeatability, as follows:

- **ScenarioType** *(why)* clarifies physical, virtual, or hybrid execution. **Instance:** ST_Virtualized.
- **EnvironmentSetup** *(why)* records concrete configuration. **Instance:** ES_3VMs with items {Win10_VM1, Win11_VM2, Ubuntu_VM3}.
- **Benchmark** *(why)* yields baselines for time and integrity. **Instance:** BM_DumpTime_SHA256.
- **PilotProject** *(why)* de-risks execution and calibrates parameters. **Instance:** PP_TrialCapture_OK.
- **TrainingActivity** *(why)* ensures operator competence. **Instance:** TA_4h_Workshop.
- **KnowledgeResourceCondition** *(why)* anchors configuration in vendor truth. **Instance:** KRC_VendorAPIs.

The following relations are used: ES_3VMs implements Scenario ST_Virtualized; BM_DumpTime_SHA256 benchmarks ES_3VMs; PP_TrialCapture_OK validates ES_3VMs; TA_4h_Workshop prepares Participant Analyst_01.

The pre-operation phase explains to future replicators not only *what* was done but also *why* that environment was chosen, lowering ambiguity and boosting transferability.

8.4 Operation Phase

Operation is where evidence is produced. The ontology clarifies Participant, Instrument, Artifact, DataP (data properties and metadata), ActivityLog, and OperationProcedure so that every step is reproducible and auditable, as follows:

- **Participant** *(why)* identifies human roles. **Instances:** Analyst_01, Assistant_A.
- **Instrument** *(why)* records tools as first-class entities. **Instances:** Volatility_v2.6, Rekall_v1.7, Belkasoft_LRC_vX.
- **Artifact** *(why)* binds produced files to the process. **Instances:** RAM_Win10_ToolX_Run01.dd, RAM_Win11_ToolY_Run02.dd.
- **DataP** *(why)* preserves integrity and context. **Examples:** sha256=..., size=..., captureStart=..., captureEnd=....
- **ActivityLog** *(why)* creates a parallel, human-readable timeline. **Instance:** ALOG_CSV_VMR.
- **OperationProcedure** *(why)* structures actions. **Instance:** OP_Capture_Hash_Verify_Compare.

We then used the following relations: Analyst_01 uses Instrument Volatility_v2.6; Instrument Volatility_v2.6 produced Artifact RAM_Win10_ToolX_Run01.dd; Artifact RAM_Win10_ToolX_Run01.dd hasDataProperty sha256=...; OperationProcedure OP_Capture_Hash_Verify_Compare executedBy Analyst_01; ActivityLog ALOG_CSV_VMR records OperationProcedure OP_Capture_Hash_Verify_Compare.

As an operational checklist we:

- Verify hypervisor time with NTP snapshots before each run
- Record tool version and command-line parameters verbatim
- Hash immediately after acquisition and again after transfer
- Store logs and images on write-once or versioned storage

8.5 Analysis and Interpretation Phase

Analysis converts artifacts to evidence-supported claims. The ontology tracks ResultMetric, StatisticalAnalysis, InterpretationChallenge, ThreatsToValidity, and ReliabilityAnalysis. This ensures that findings are not only reported but justified, including limitations, as follows:

- **ResultMetric** *(why)* defines what "difference" means. **Instance:** RM_MeanDeviationRecoveredProcesses.
- **StatisticalAnalysis** *(why)*: formal test. **Instance:** ANOVA_p043.

- **InterpretationChallenge** *(why)*: explicit analytic friction. **Instance:** IC_OS_Caching_Variance.
- **ThreatsToValidity** *(why)* maps to accepted taxonomy. **Instance:** TV_Construct_ToolSemanticDifferences.
- **ReliabilityAnalysis** *(why)* quantifies repeatability. **Instance:** Rel_Corr_096.

The following relations are used: ResultMetric RM_MeanDeviationRecoveredProcesses computedFrom Artifacts {RAM_...}; StatisticalAnalysis ANOVA_p043 tests Hypothesis H0_no_tool_effect; ReliabilityAnalysis Rel_Corr_096 evaluates ResultMetric RM_...; InterpretationChallenge IC_OS_Caching_Variance impacts ResultInterpretation; ThreatsToValidity TV_Construct_ToolSemanticDifferences threatens ValidityOfConclusions.

Writing down InterpretationChallenge and ThreatsToValidity is not cosmetic. It tells readers exactly where uncertainty lies and how far they should trust the generalization.

8.6 Dissemination Phase

Dissemination turns a private analysis into a public, reusable asset. In *ExperDF-Onto*, we instantiate DisseminationPlan, Dataset, DatasetMetadata, Authorship, TechnicalReview, and PresentationQuality with links to persistent identifiers, such as:

- **DisseminationPlan** *(why)* sets channels, embargoes, and identifiers. **Instance:** DP_Zenodo_Release.
- **Dataset** *(why)* bundles images, logs, code, and documentation. **Instance:** DS_VMR_1.0.
- **DatasetMetadata** *(why)* improves discovery and reuse. **Instance:** DC_JSONLD_VMR.
- **Authorship** *(why)* credits contributors and roles. **Instance:** AUTH_Mendes_Silva.
- **TechnicalReview** *(why)*: independent scrutiny. **Instance:** TR_SeniorValidation_2025.
- **PresentationQuality** *(why)* ensures clarity for new users. **Instance:** PQ_Slides_Notebook.

The following relations are used: Dataset DS_VMR_1.0 describedBy DatasetMetadata DC_JSONLD_VMR; DisseminationPlan DP_Zenodo_Release publishes Dataset DS_VMR_1.0; Authorship AUTH_Mendes_Silva credits Experiment Exp_VM_Reproducibility; TechnicalReview TR_SeniorValidation_2025 assesses Dataset DS_VMR_1.0.

8.7 Ontological Instantiation Snapshot

Table 8.1 shows the ontological instantiations for this example.

8.8 Querying the Instantiation

The following query lists artifacts produced by Volatility and their integrity hashes. It demonstrates how the ontology enables transparent retrieval of provenance information.

Table 8.1 Ontological instantiations for "The Memory That Wouldn't Lie"

Ontology element	Example instance
Experiment	Exp_VM_Reproducibility
ResearchQuestion	RQ_tool_equivalence
Hypothesis	H0_no_tool_effect; H1_tool_effect
IndependentVariable	IV_AcquisitionTool {Volatility, Rekall, Belkasoft}
DependentVariable	DV_RecoveredProcesses; DV_OpenPorts; DV_Handles
ControlVariable	CV_OSVersion; CV_MemSize; CV_BackgroundLoad
ConfoundingFactor	CF_TimestampDrift; CF_HypervisorCaching
ScenarioType	ST_Virtualized
EnvironmentSetup	ES_3VMs {Win10_VM1; Win11_VM2; Ubuntu_VM3}
Benchmark	BM_DumpTime_SHA256
PilotProject	PP_TrialCapture_OK
TrainingActivity	TA_4h_Workshop
Instrument	Volatility_v2.6; Rekall_v1.7; Belkasoft_LRC_vX
Artifact	RAM_Win10_ToolX_Run01.dd; RAM_Win11_ToolY_Run02.dd
DataP	sha256; size; captureStart; captureEnd
ActivityLog	ALOG_CSV_VMR
OperationProcedure	OP_Capture_Hash_Verify_Compare
ResultMetric	RM_MeanDeviationRecoveredProcesses
StatisticalAnalysis	ANOVA_p043
InterpretationChallenge	IC_OS_Caching_Variance
ThreatsToValidity	TV_Construct_ToolSemanticDifferences
ReliabilityAnalysis	Rel_Corr_096
DisseminationPlan	DP_Zenodo_Release
Dataset	DS_VMR_1.0
DatasetMetadata	DC_JSONLD_VMR
Authorship	AUTH_Mendes_Silva
TechnicalReview	TR_SeniorValidation_2025
PresentationQuality	PQ_Slides_Notebook

Listing 8.1 SPARQL: retrieve artifacts produced by Volatility with hashes

```
PREFIX ex: <http://example.org/experdf-onto#>
PREFIX rdfs: <http://www.w3.org/2000/01/rdf-schema#>

SELECT ?artifact ?sha
WHERE {
  ?inst a ex:Instrument ;
        rdfs:label "Volatility_v2.6" .
  ?artifact a ex:Artifact ;
            ex:producedBy ?inst ;
            ex:hasDataProperty ?dp .
  ?dp ex:key "sha256" ;
      ex:value ?sha .
}
```

8.9 Coverage and Missing Elements

Coverage: 34 out of 50 ontology classes were instantiated, achieving approximately 68% conceptual completeness.

Missing elements: *Governance*, *Stakeholder*, *PeerReview*, and *Configuration-Management* remain unmodeled in this instance.

This level of coverage indicates that the instantiation successfully represents most of the experimental, operational, and analytical dimensions defined by *ExperDF-Onto* but does not yet encompass higher order organizational and validation constructs. The absence of *Governance* elements means that decision-making and oversight mechanisms were not explicitly modeled. Excluding *Stakeholder* entities omits representation of the broader community affected by or contributing to the experiment. The lack of *PeerReview* elements limits formal modeling of external evaluation and quality assurance, while the missing *ConfigurationManagement* prevents traceability of software or dataset versions across replications. Incorporating these classes in future instantiations would advance the model's maturity, enhancing accountability, reproducibility, and alignment with open science and institutional governance practices.

Why are these elements missing and how to add them:

- **Governance** *(gap)*: no formal data stewardship or policy entities. *Add:* `DataSteward_Lab`, `Policy_Retention_3y`.
- **Stakeholder** *(gap)*: no external beneficiaries or requesters modeled. *Add:* `Stakeholder_IRTeam`, `Stakeholder_CourtExpert`.
- **PeerReview** *(gap)*: technical validation recorded but not peer review. *Add:* `PR_ExternalReviewer_Report`.
- **ConfigurationManagement** *(gap)*: versions tracked informally. *Add:* `Cfg_Dataset_v1.0`, `Cfg_ToolingEnv_commit_abc123`.

Adding these four branches would likely raise coverage to about 80 percent while improving trust and long-term reusability.

8.10 Interpretation and Teaching Notes

This section provides interpretive and pedagogical insights into the experiment, explaining the meaning of its statistical outcomes, how the study can be replicated or extended, and what conceptual lessons it offers for teaching controlled experimentation in Digital Forensics. Each subsection highlights a specific aspect of how *ExperDF-Onto* supports transparency, reproducibility, and critical reflection on experimental findings.

8.10.1 What the Results Mean

The ANOVA result `p = 0.43` suggests no statistically significant tool effect on recovered process counts under the tested conditions. Reliability at `0.96` indicates stable acquisition within this configuration, confirming that the experiment's internal validity is strong despite nonsignificant group differences.

8.10.2 How to Reuse This Study

Because the scenario, instruments, parameters, and hashes are modeled explicitly, a reader can rerun the exact workflow or adapt it by substituting a new tool version while preserving the same `IndependentVariable` structure. This modularity demonstrates how ontological modeling facilitates both replication and controlled variation, supporting cumulative empirical research.

8.10.3 Common Misconceptions Clarified

- *Equivalence is not identity.* Even if outcomes are statistically similar, tools may differ semantically. This is captured by `TV_Construct_ToolSemanticDifferences`.
- *No effect here does not mean no effect anywhere.* External validity depends on the modeled `ScenarioType`, `ControlVariables`, and `ConfoundingFactors`.

8.10.4 Minimal Reproducibility Kit

At a minimum, a replicator needs: VM images or build scripts, tool versions and parameters, acquisition logs, artifact hashes, and the dataset metadata record. All these are explicit instances and relations in *ExperDF-Onto*, allowing others to verify results, compare tools, or build derivative studies with confidence in methodological integrity.

8.11 Final Remarks

This chapter illustrated how *ExperDF-Onto* can be instantiated to model a complete controlled experiment in digital forensics, from conceptual planning to dissemination. By decomposing each research phase into explicit ontological elements, the model transforms narrative experimental descriptions into machine-readable structures that preserve rigor, traceability, and interpretability.

Through the instantiation steps and the resulting queries, readers can observe how experimental entities such as instruments, artifacts, variables, and results are semantically connected to form a transparent and auditable research chain. These relationships strengthen internal validity and establish a foundation for reproducibility and reuse across future studies.

Pedagogically, this chapter serves as a blueprint for how students and practitioners can document and reason about their own experiments using an ontological framework. Conceptually, it reinforces the idea that reproducibility and provenance are not post hoc annotations but integral parts of the research design. The explicit modeling of assumptions, procedures, and metrics exemplifies how ontology-driven experimentation contributes to a cumulative and open body of forensic knowledge.

Future work may extend this model by integrating governance, stakeholder participation, and automated peer review processes, creating a pathway toward a fully open and FAIR-aligned digital forensics ecosystem. In doing so, *ExperDF-Onto* not only supports reproducible research but also promotes institutional transparency and societal accountability in the production and evaluation of digital evidence.

Chapter 9
Example 2: Unlocking the Locked—Smartphone Bypass Experiments

Abstract This chapter details a controlled empirical investigation on smartphone data extraction reliability and legal defensibility, focusing on the comparative performance of forensic tools across locked Android and iOS devices. The experiment explored how different extraction vectors, such as logical, file system, and after-first-unlock (AFU) exploit methods, perform when applied under lawful authority to modern encrypted devices equipped with secure enclaves and full-disk encryption. Using the *ExperDF-Onto* framework, every experimental element was modeled to ensure traceability, ethical transparency, and replicability across jurisdictions. The planning phase defined explicit hypotheses, independent and dependent variables, and legal and ethical planning constructs that captured the obligations of privacy legislation, including GDPR and LGPD. Pre-operation activities established reproducible benches for Android and iOS, documented firmware and baseband states, and validated tool performance through pilot extractions. During operation, each participant, instrument, artifact, and activity log was instantiated as an ontological entity, capturing provenance links between procedures, generated data, and contextual parameters such as passcode complexity, firmware patch levels, and secure-element behavior. Statistical analysis of the resulting datasets showed that Android devices achieved an average logical extraction success rate of 78 percent. In comparison, iOS devices averaged 42 percent under the same constraints, yielding a statistically significant difference ($p < 0.05$) according to chi-square testing. Reliability across repeated runs reached 0.94, indicating strong procedural stability. The study also modeled legal boundaries and data sharing constraints as ontological relations, providing machine-interpretable documentation of compliance and interpretive limits. All extraction images, metadata, and logs were curated into an open dataset with persistent identifiers to enable auditability and future replication. Beyond the quantitative findings, this chapter demonstrates how *ExperDF-Onto* integrates legal, ethical, and technical dimensions of digital forensics into a unified semantic structure, turning a complex investigative procedure into a transparent, reusable, and verifiable scientific contribution.

E. OliveiraJr et al., *Controlled Experimentation of Digital Forensics*,
https://doi.org/10.1007/978-3-032-19951-5_9

9.1 Context and Motivation

Modern smartphones are cryptographic vaults. Security features such as secure enclaves, full-disk encryption, hardware-backed keystores, and rate-limited unlock attempts protect user privacy but complicate lawful investigations. The researchers designed a controlled study to answer a practical question for incident responders and lab examiners: *How reliably can state-of-the-practice extraction methods recover data from locked Android and iOS devices under lawful authority?*

This example shows how *ExperDF-Onto* makes each decision auditable, from ethics and legal framing to tool choice, scenario construction, and statistical testing. It also demonstrates how to model privacy constraints and firmware variability as first-class ontological elements that affect interpretation and reuse.

We move from a plain-language research plan to a fully instantiated ontological representation. At each phase, we explain why the concept matters, how it is instantiated, the relations that connect it to other entities, and the common pitfalls the ontology helps prevent.

9.2 Planning Phase

In *ExperDF-Onto*, the planning constructs translate a high-level concern into a testable structure. We instantiate `Experiment`, `ResearchQuestion`, `Hypothesis`, variables, ethical and legal planning, and replication commitments and then bind them through explicit relations as follows:

- **Experiment** *(why)* anchors identity, scope, and intent. **Instance:** `Exp_SmartphoneBypass`.
- **ResearchQuestion** *(why)* focuses uncertainty into measurable terms. **Instance:** `RQ_ExtractionSuccess_AndroidVsIOS`.
- **Hypothesis** *(why)* states expected patterns. **Instances:** `H0_NoDiff_AndroidIOS` and `H1_AndroidHigherSuccess`.
- **IndependentVariable** *(why)*: manipulated factors. **Instances:** `IV_OSType` with levels {`Android`, `iOS`}; `IV_AttackVector` with levels {`Logical`, `FileSystem`, `AFU_Exploit`}.
- **DependentVariable** *(why)*: measurable outcomes. **Instances:** `DV_AccessSuccessRate`, `DV_DataExposureCoverage`.
- **ControlVariable** *(why)* holds noise constant. **Instances:** `CV_DeviceModelBand`, `CV_OSMinorVersion`, `CV_PasscodeComplexity`, `CV_TimeSinceLastUnlock`.
- **ConfoundingFactor** *(why)* documents influences we cannot fully control. **Instances:** `CF_FirmwarePatchLevelDrift`, `CF_BasebandDifferences`, `CF_SecureElementBehavior`.
- **EthicalPlanning** *(why)* asserts privacy-protective constraints. **Instance:** `EP_MockProfilesOnly` with synthetic contacts, messages, and media.

- **LegalPlanning** *(why)* situates the study within applicable law and policy. **Instance:** LP_GDPR_LGPD_Compliance with retention and minimization rules.
- **ReplicationPlanning** *(why)* commits to transparency pre-results. **Instance:** RP_OSF_Prereg_SBE.

We used the following relations: Exp_SmartphoneBypass hasResearchQuestion RQ_ExtractionSuccess_AndroidVsIOS; Exp_SmartphoneBypass hasHypothesis H1_AndroidHigherSuccess; Exp_SmartphoneBypass hasIndependentVariable IV_OSType, IV_AttackVector; Exp_SmartphoneBypass hasDependentVariable DV_AccessSuccessRate, DV_DataExposureCoverage; Exp_SmartphoneBypass isControlledBy CV_DeviceModelBand, CV_OSMinorVersion, CV_PasscodeComplexity; Exp_SmartphoneBypass considersConfounding CF_FirmwarePatchLevelDrift; Exp_SmartphoneBypass compliesWith LP_GDPR_LGPD_Compliance; Exp_SmartphoneBypass preregisteredAs RP_OSF_Prereg_SBE.

Typical pitfalls and how the ontology prevents them:

- *Pitfall:* forgetting that success rates vary by attack vector. *Prevention:* IV_AttackVector is modeled explicitly with levels.
- *Pitfall:* mixing firmware and device models without documenting them. *Prevention:* CV_DeviceModelBand and CV_OSMinorVersion force explicit capture.
- *Pitfall:* ambiguous legal footing. *Prevention:* LegalPlanning and retention constraints are first-class entities.

9.3 Pre-Operation Phase

Pre-operation encodes the practical conditions for repeatability: scenarios, benches, pilots, training, and baselines. These entities make the path from plan to execution auditable, as follows:

- **ScenarioType** *(why)* clarifies hybrid execution. **Instance:** ST_Hybrid_PhysicalEmulated.
- **EnvironmentSetup** *(why)* enumerates benches and configurations. **Instances:** ES_AndroidBench_A1 and ES_iOSBench_I1 with device pools, SIM states, and passcode policies.
- **Benchmark** *(why)* establishes performance and integrity baselines. **Instance:** BM_HashValidation_SpeedProfile.
- **PilotProject** *(why)* validates feasibility and scripts. **Instance:** PP_PrelimExtractions_OK.
- **TrainingActivity** *(why)* certifies operator skill. **Instance:** TA_ToolCertification_8h.
- **KnowledgeResourceCondition** *(why)*: ties setup to tool docs and vendor advisories. **Instance:** KRC_VendorDocs_UFED_AXIOM.

We used the following relations: ES_AndroidBench_A1 implements ST_-Hybrid_PhysicalEmulated; BM_HashValidation_SpeedProfile benchmarks ES_AndroidBench_A1, ES_iOSBench_I1; PP_PrelimExtractions_-OK validates EnvironmentSetup {ES_AndroidBench_A1, ES_iOSBench_-I1}; TA_ToolCertification_8h prepares Participant PriyaD_Lead and Assistant_Team.

The benches are not mere labels. They are ontological objects with members and policies, enabling future researchers to reconstruct conditions and understand divergence.

9.4 Operation Phase

Evidence production is modeled through participants, instruments, artifacts, logs, and prespecified procedures. This phase also captures failure modes as first-class citizens, such as:

- **Participant** *(why)* identifies roles and accountability. **Instances:** PriyaD_Lead, Assistant_A, Assistant_B.
- **Instrument** *(why)* records tools and versions. **Instances:** UFED_vX.Y, AXIOM_-vZ.W, Autopsy_v4.X.
- **Artifact** *(why)* binds extractions and logs to the process. **Examples:** IMG_Android_Pixel4a_Run03.dd, IMG_iOS_iPhone11_Run05.dd, LOG_-API_AXIOM_Run05.csv.
- **DataP** *(why)* preserves integrity and context. **Examples:** sha256, captureStart, captureEnd, toolParams.
- **ActivityLog** *(why)*: human-readable timeline. **Instance:** ALOG_SmartphoneBypass.csv.
- **OperationProcedure** *(why)* constrains sequence for comparability. **Instance:** OP_Enumerate_Extract_Hash_Verify_Parse.
- **IncidentReport** *(why)* captures anomalies and failures. **Instance:** IR_-FirmwareFailure_2Events with details for retries and device IDs.

We used these relations: PriyaD_Lead uses Instrument UFED_vX.Y; Instrument AXIOM_vZ.W produced Artifact IMG_iOS_iPhone11_Run05.dd; Artifact IMG_iOS_iPhone11_Run05.dd hasDataProperty sha256=... and toolParams="logical"; OperationProcedure OP_Enumerate_Extract_Hash_Verify_Parse executedBy PriyaD_Lead; ActivityLog ALOG_SmartphoneBypass.csv records OperationProcedure OP_...; IncidentReport IR_FirmwareFailure_2Events relatesTo Instrument UFED_vX.Y and Device iPhone11.

As an operational checklist, we:

- Snapshot the exact firmware and baseband versions before extraction

- Record passcode policy, secure enclave state, and last-unlock time as ControlVariable values
- Hash the extracted image immediately; rehash after transfer and after parsing
- Capture full tool parameter strings for every attempt and retry

9.5 Analysis and Interpretation Phase

We formalize metrics and tests, while documenting legal and interpretive constraints that affect generalization, as follows:

- **ResultMetric** *(why)* defines success quantitatively. **Instances:** `RM_AndroidSuccess_0.78`, `RM_iOSSuccess_0.42`, `RM_ExposureCoverage_perProfile`.
- **StatisticalAnalysis** *(why)* validates differences. **Instance:** `ChiSquare_pLT0_05` comparing success counts per OS.
- **ThreatsToValidity** *(why)* frames inference limits. **Instances:** `TV_EncryptionVariance`, `TV_OSUpdateCadence`, `TV_DeviceHeterogeneity`.
- **ReliabilityAnalysis** *(why)* measures repeatability. **Instance:** `Rel_r0_94`.
- **InterpretationChallenge** *(why)* notes analysis friction. **Instance:** `IC_SparseArtifacts_PostParse`.
- **ConflictLaw** *(why)* clarifies jurisdictional limits. **Instance:** `CL_PrivacyBoundaries_EU_BR`.

We then used these relations: `ResultMetric RM_AndroidSuccess_0.78 computedFrom Artifacts {IMG_Android_...}`; `StatisticalAnalysis ChiSquare_pLT0_05 tests Hypothesis H1_AndroidHigherSuccess`; `ReliabilityAnalysis Rel_r0_94 evaluates ResultMetric RM_...`; `ThreatsToValidity TV_EncryptionVariance threatens ValidityOfConclusions`; `ConflictLaw CL_PrivacyBoundaries_EU_BR constrains DataSharing and Interpretation`.

The ontology separates *what happened* (artifacts, logs) from *what it means* (metrics, tests, threats). This separation helps downstream users adapt the pipeline while preserving the original inference boundaries.

9.6 Dissemination Phase

Dissemination converts local findings into global, reusable assets with provenance and credit. Governance elements are partially present here and can be expanded, such as:

- **DisseminationPlan** *(why)* defines venue, identifiers, and embargo. **Instance:** `DP_Zenodo_10_5281_zenodo_1234567`.

- **Dataset** *(why)* bundles images, logs, and parsing outputs. **Instance:** DS_SBE_-1_0.
- **DatasetMetadata** *(why)* enables discovery and reuse. **Instance:** MD_JSONLD_-SBE.
- **Authorship** *(why)* acknowledges roles. **Instance:** AUTH_Deshmukh_Team.
- **TechnicalReview** *(why)*: lab supervisor validation. **Instance:** TR_Supervisor_2025.
- **ImpactAssessment** *(why)* documents training adoption. **Instance:** IA_CurriculumIntegration_2025.

We used the following relations: Dataset DS_SBE_1_0 describedBy MD_JSONLD_SBE; DisseminationPlan DP_Zenodo_10_5281_... publishes Dataset DS_SBE_1_0; Authorship AUTH_Deshmukh_Team credits Experiment Exp_SmartphoneBypass; TechnicalReview TR_Supervisor_2025 assesses DS_SBE_1_0; ImpactAssessment IA_CurriculumIntegration_-2025 references AdoptionEvents in TrainingPrograms.

9.7 Ontological Instantiation Snapshot

Table 9.1 shows the ontological instantiations for this example.

9.8 Querying the Instantiation

The following SPARQL illustrates how to retrieve all iOS artifacts produced via logical extraction, with their hashes and benches. It demonstrates evidence traceability across instruments, scenarios, and integrity properties.

Listing 9.1 SPARQL: iOS logical extractions with integrity and bench

```
PREFIX ex: <http://example.org/experdf-onto#>
PREFIX rdfs: <http://www.w3.org/2000/01/rdf-schema#>

SELECT ?artifact ?sha ?bench
WHERE {
  ?artifact a ex:Artifact ;
            ex:producedBy ?inst ;
            ex:belongsToBench ?bench ;
            ex:hasDataProperty ?dp .
  ?inst a ex:Instrument ;
        ex:usedOnOSType "iOS" ;
        ex:withAttackVector "Logical" .
  ?dp ex:key "sha256" ;
      ex:value ?sha .
}
```

Table 9.1 Ontological instantiations for "Unlocking the Locked—Smartphone Bypass Experiments"

Ontology element	Example instance
Experiment	Exp_SmartphoneBypass
ResearchQuestion	RQ_ExtractionSuccess_AndroidVsIOS
Hypothesis	H0_NoDiff_AndroidIOS; H1_AndroidHigherSuccess
IndependentVariable	IV_OSType {Android, iOS}; IV_AttackVector {Logical, FileSystem, AFU_Exploit}
DependentVariable	DV_AccessSuccessRate; DV_DataExposureCoverage
ControlVariable	CV_DeviceModelBand; CV_OSMinorVersion; CV_PasscodeComplexity; CV_TimeSinceLastUnlock
ConfoundingFactor	CF_FirmwarePatchLevelDrift; CF_BasebandDifferences; CF_SecureElementBehavior
LegalPlanning	LP_GDPR_LGPD_Compliance
EthicalPlanning	EP_MockProfilesOnly
ReplicationPlanning	RP_OSF_Prereg_SBE
ScenarioType	ST_Hybrid_PhysicalEmulated
EnvironmentSetup	ES_AndroidBench_A1; ES_iOSBench_I1
Benchmark	BM_HashValidation_SpeedProfile
PilotProject	PP_PrelimExtractions_OK
TrainingActivity	TA_ToolCertification_8h
Instrument	UFED_vX.Y; AXIOM_vZ.W; Autopsy_v4.X
Artifact	IMG_Android_Pixel4a_Run03.dd; IMG_iOS_iPhone11_Run05.dd; LOG_API_AXIOM_Run05.csv
DataP	sha256; captureStart; captureEnd; toolParams
ActivityLog	ALOG_SmartphoneBypass.csv
OperationProcedure	OP_Enumerate_Extract_Hash_Verify_Parse
IncidentReport	IR_FirmwareFailure_2Events
ResultMetric	RM_AndroidSuccess_0.78; RM_iOSSuccess_0.42; RM_ExposureCoverage_perProfile
StatisticalAnalysis	ChiSquare_pLT0_05
ThreatsToValidity	TV_EncryptionVariance; TV_OSUpdateCadence; TV_DeviceHeterogeneity
ReliabilityAnalysis	Rel_r0_94
InterpretationChallenge	IC_SparseArtifacts_PostParse
ConflictLaw	CL_PrivacyBoundaries_EU_BR
DisseminationPlan	DP_Zenodo_10_5281_zenodo_1234567
Dataset	DS_SBE_1_0
DatasetMetadata	MD_JSONLD_SBE
Authorship	AUTH_Deshmukh_Team
TechnicalReview	TR_Supervisor_2025
ImpactAssessment	IA_CurriculumIntegration_2025

9.9 Coverage and Missing Elements

Coverage: 38 of 52 ontology classes instantiated (73%).

Missing: *OntologyReuse*, *Stakeholder*, *PeerReview*, *Maintenance*.

The experiment achieved a coverage of 38 out of 52 ontology classes, representing approximately 73 percent of the available conceptual elements in *ExperDF-Onto*. This level of coverage indicates that the experiment modeled most of the critical phases of a controlled study, including planning, operation, and analysis, with sufficient detail to support reproducibility and reasoning. The missing classes reflect higher level organizational and community aspects that were not directly applicable to the immediate experimental setup. *OntologyReuse* was not instantiated because no external ontologies were referenced for interoperability. *Stakeholder* was omitted since the study did not explicitly identify external user groups or beneficiaries. *PeerReview* was absent because formal external evaluation of the experimental process had not yet occurred. Finally, *Maintenance* was not represented, as no long-term update or life cycle management process was modeled for the dataset or associated tools. Including these missing elements in future extensions would improve completeness and enhance alignment with open science governance and sustainability practices.

Why are these elements missing, and how to add them:

- **OntologyReuse** *(gap)*: no explicit alignment to external vocabularies. *Add:* mappings to `Dublin Core` for metadata, `PROV-O` for provenance, and `SSN/SOSA` for device observations where applicable.
- **Stakeholder** *(gap)*: external beneficiaries or requesters not modeled. *Add:* `Stakeholder_LEAgency`, `Stakeholder_JudicialOfficer`, `Stakeholder_DefenceExpert`.
- **PeerReview** *(gap)*: technical review exists, but no external peer review artifacts. *Add:* `PR_ExternalReviewer_Report_ID123`.
- **Maintenance** *(gap)*: dataset and code evolution not captured. *Add:* `Maint_DatasetRoadmap`, `Maint_Changelog_DS_SBE_1_1`, `Maint_DeprecationPolicy`.

Adding these branches would likely raise completeness toward 90 percent while improving interoperability, stakeholder transparency, and long-term stewardship.

9.10 Interpretation and Teaching Notes

This section synthesizes the analytical results of the smartphone bypass experiment and guides interpretation, reuse, and pedagogical application. Each subsection highlights a different dimension of the ontological modeling process, helping readers understand not only what the findings mean but also how to extend and replicate the study responsibly. Together, these notes bridge empirical evidence and didactic use, reinforcing the principles of transparency, reproducibility, and ethical conduct in digital forensics experimentation.

9.10.1 What the Results Mean

The chi-square result ($p < 0.05$) indicates a statistically significant difference in extraction success between Android and iOS for the tested devices, benches, and vectors. The reported 78 percent versus 42 percent success rates are conditional on the modeled `ControlVariables`, firmware levels, and bench composition. These results show that success variability depends as much on contextual parameters as on tool capability, underscoring the importance of modeling all influencing factors explicitly within *ExperDF-Onto*.

9.10.2 How to Reuse This Study

Because benches, devices, passcode policies, and tool parameters are represented as explicit ontological instances linked through formal relations, a replicator can rerun the workflow or substitute a new firmware cohort while maintaining conceptual comparability. Legal and ethical constraints are modeled as distinct entities, allowing the study to be adapted to different jurisdictions without compromising compliance or methodological rigor.

9.10.3 Common Misconceptions Clarified

- *Higher logical success on Android does not imply weaker security.* It reflects specific device cohorts, firmware states, and vectors tested, all of which are explicitly modeled within the ontology.
- *A failed full-disk image is not the end.* The ontology differentiates among multiple attack vectors, ensuring that alternative lawful acquisition methods can still yield partial or corroborative evidence.

9.10.4 Minimal Reproducibility Kit

To achieve full reproducibility, a replicator requires bench manifests, device and firmware inventories, complete tool parameter strings, extraction logs, artifact hashes, parsing outputs, and JSON-LD metadata. Each of these components appears as an ontological instance and is queryable through the semantic relations defined in

ExperDF-Onto, ensuring verifiability, reuse, and transparent documentation of the experimental process.

9.11 Final Remarks

This chapter illustrated how *ExperDF-Onto* supports the formalization of a controlled experiment in mobile forensics, centered on lock-screen bypass and data extraction success across heterogeneous smartphone platforms. By decomposing the study into ontological elements such as devices, benches, passcode policies, and extraction tools, the model transformed an operationally complex investigation into a structured representation that emphasizes traceability and interpretability.

The resulting instantiation revealed how operating system versions, attack vectors, and ethical, as well as legal considerations, interact to shape empirical outcomes. Through explicit modeling of these dependencies, the ontology helps distinguish between what is technically feasible and what is legally and ethically defensible. This approach reinforces the role of structured provenance and metadata in improving the transparency and accountability of digital forensic investigations.

From an educational perspective, the chapter demonstrated how ontologies can guide learners and practitioners in documenting sensitive procedures. Explicit representation of variables, instruments, and outcomes helps reduce ambiguity and facilitates replication, comparison, and continuous learning in a controlled and verifiable way.

Future refinements may include incorporating stakeholder perspectives, standardized quality evaluation, and peer review representations to strengthen alignment with open science and long-term sustainability practices. In doing so, *ExperDF-Onto* continues to advance methodological rigor and reinforce trust in the reproducibility of mobile forensic research.

Chapter 10
Example 3: The Case of the Altered Cloud Logs

Abstract This chapter presents a controlled study of integrity verification for cloud infrastructure logs in multitenant environments, modeling the entire investigation with *ExperDF-Onto* to make design choices, provenance, and limitations transparently auditable. The experiment asks whether a tamper-evident hash-chaining approach can reliably expose micro-edits, line drops, insertions, and reordering across heterogeneous provider logging frameworks without privileged access to underlying storage. The planning phase formalizes hypotheses, independent variables for provider and tamper type, dependent variables for detection rate, false positives, and time to detection, along with control variables that bound event rate, region count, key rotation, and clock drift. The pre-operation phase constructs a distributed virtual scenario spanning multiple regions and providers, captures latency benchmarks, and prepares operators through credential isolation drills, while linking assumptions to provider security documentation as explicit knowledge resources. During operation, log snapshots, per-event hashes, chain indexes, and intervention events are instantiated as first-class ontological entities with version lineage and activity logs, enabling precise reconstruction of the pipeline and its outputs. Analysis quantifies performance with detection success near 98 percent and false positives near 1 percent under a monotonic ingestion discipline, compares providers and tamper types with formal statistical tests, and records interpretation challenges such as nondeterministic ordering and threats to validity induced by replication delay, batching, and normalization policies. Dissemination packages snapshots, chain indexes, scripts, and machine-readable metadata using PROV-C and Dublin Core into an openly citable dataset to support independent verification and reuse. Beyond its empirical findings, the chapter demonstrates how *ExperDF-Onto* encodes distributed context, provider heterogeneity, and integrity guarantees into a coherent semantic structure, allowing investigators to query provenance, reason about timing effects, and generalize results responsibly across cloud settings.

E. OliveiraJr et al., *Controlled Experimentation of Digital Forensics*,
https://doi.org/10.1007/978-3-032-19951-5_10

10.1 Context and Motivation

Cloud infrastructures generate vast volumes of operational logs across microservices, regions, and tenants. These logs support security monitoring, billing, compliance, and incident response. However, multi-tenant replication, eventual consistency, and role-based access may create opportunities for subtle manipulation. The researchers set out to test a focused question: *Can a tamper-evident hash-chaining scheme reliably expose micro-edits and line reordering in provider logs without privileged access to underlying storage?*

This example shows how *ExperDF-Onto* captures distributed context, provider heterogeneity, and provenance guarantees. It demonstrates how log snapshots, event-level hashes, and version links become first-class entities so that investigators can reconstruct evidence and reason about integrity at scale.

We translate a narrative cloud-tampering scenario into an ontological instantiation that a reader can query. At each phase, we explain why a concept matters, how it is instantiated, and which relations connect it to a broader chain of custody.

10.2 Planning Phase

The planning layer frames integrity as a measurable outcome under provider diversity. We instantiate the core experimental design, variables, and reproducibility commitments, as follows:

- **Experiment***(why)* anchors the identity of the study. **Instance:** `Exp_CloudLogIntegrity`.
- **ResearchQuestion***(why)* operationalizes uncertainty. **Instance:** `RQ_HashChainDetectsMicroTamper`.
- **Hypothesis***(why)*: expected capability of the method. **Instances:** `H0_NoBetterThanChance` and `H1_HighDetectionRate`.
- **IndependentVariable***(why)*: manipulated factors. **Instances:** `IV_LoggingFramework` with levels {`AWS_CloudTrail`, `GCP_CloudAuditLogs`, `Azure_ActivityLog`}; `IV_TamperType` with levels {`SingleCharEdit`, `LineDrop`, `LineInsert`, `SwapOrder`}.
- **DependentVariable***(why)*: measurable outcomes. **Instances:** `DV_DetectionRate`, `DV_FalsePositiveRate`, `DV_TimeToDetection`.
- **ControlVariable***(why)* holds variation constant. **Instances:** `CV_EventRate`, `CV_RegionCount`, `CV_KeyRotationInterval`, `CV_ClockDriftBudget`.
- **ConfoundingFactor***(why)* acknowledges influences we cannot fully control. **Instances:** `CF_CrossRegionReplicationDelay`, `CF_QueueBatching`, `CF_ProviderRedactionPolicies`.
- **ReplicationPlanning***(why)* preserves transparency before results. **Instance:** `RP_GitHub_Versioned_Pipelines`.

We used the following relations: Exp_CloudLogIntegrity hasResearchQuestion RQ_HashChainDetectsMicroTamper; Exp_CloudLogIntegrity hasHypothesis H1_HighDetectionRate; Exp_CloudLogIntegrity hasIndependentVariable IV_LoggingFramework, IV_TamperType; Exp_CloudLogIntegrity hasDependentVariable DV_DetectionRate, DV_FalsePositiveRate, DV_TimeToDetection; Exp_CloudLogIntegrity isControlledBy CV_EventRate, CV_RegionCount; Exp_CloudLogIntegrity considersConfounding CF_CrossRegionReplicationDelay; Exp_CloudLogIntegrity preregisteredAs RP_GitHub_Versioned_Pipelines.

Typical pitfalls and ontology safeguards:

- *Pitfall:* measuring only accuracy and ignoring false positives. *Safeguard:* explicit DV_FalsePositiveRate.
- *Pitfall:* treating provider choice as a backdrop. *Safeguard:* IV_LoggingFramework with explicit levels.
- *Pitfall:* ignoring clock skew and replication. *Safeguard:* ControlVariable and ConfoundingFactor for timing.

10.3 Pre-Operation Phase

Pre-operation creates a distributed testbed with repeatable timing baselines and least-privilege credentials, as:

- **ScenarioType***(why)* makes distribution explicit. **Instance:** ST_DistributedVirtual.
- **EnvironmentSetup***(why)* enumerates providers, regions, and services. **Instance:** ES_MultiCloud_M1 with items {AWS_us-east-1, GCP_us-central1, Azure_eastus}.
- **Benchmark***(why)* establishes latency and integrity baselines. **Instance:** BM_LoggingLatency_PerProvider and BM_HMACThroughput.
- **TrainingActivity***(why)* reduces operator error in cloud IAM. **Instance:** TA_CredentialIsolationDrill.
- **KnowledgeResourceCondition***(why)* pins assumptions to provider docs. **Instance:** KRC_ProviderSecWhitepapers.

We used these relations: ES_MultiCloud_M1 implements ST_DistributedVirtual;BM_LoggingLatency_PerProvider benchmarks ES_MultiCloud_M1;TA_CredentialIsolationDrill prepares Participant MiguelF_Lead and CloudOps_Team;KRC_ProviderSecWhitepapers documents EnvironmentSetup ES_MultiCloud_M1.

Explicit regional membership and IAM practices allow replicators to understand divergences caused by geography or roles, not just code.

10.4 Operation Phase

We produce evidence by chaining per-event hashes, snapshotting versions, and modeling tampering as interventions:

- **Participant***(why)*:roles and accountability. **Instances:**MiguelF_Lead, CloudOps_Team.
- **Instrument***(why)*:toolchain for hashing and capture.**Instances:**Python_-HashChainer_v1.2,Collector_CLI_v0.9.
- **Artifact***(why)*:tangible evidence products.**Examples:**LOGSNAP_AWS_2025-06-02T10:00Z.jsonl,LOGSNAP_GCP_2025-06-02T10:00Z.jsonl,CHAIN_-INDEX_AWS_v3.json.
- **DataP***(why)*:integrity and context.**Examples:**sha256,prevHash,eventId, region, captureWindow.
- **ActivityLog***(why)*:time-aligned pipeline events.**Instance:**ALOG_HashCompute_PerEvent.csv.
- **OperationProcedure***(why)*:constrains sequence.**Instance:**OP_Ingest_-Order_Hash_Chain_Snapshot.
- **InterventionEvent***(why)*:first-class tampering attempts.**Instances:**IE_SingleCharEdit_AWS_t1, IE_LineDrop_GCP_t2, IE_SwapOrder_Azure_t3.
- **Versioning***(why)*:capture lineage.**Relation:**hasParentVersion linking LOGSNAP_*_v2 toLOGSNAP_*_v1.

We used these relations: MiguelF_Lead uses Instrument Python_-HashChainer_v1.2; Instrument Collector_CLI_v0.9 produced Artifact LOGSNAP_AWS_2025-06-02T10:00Z.jsonl; Artifact LOGSNAP_AWS_-..._v2 hasParentVersion LOGSNAP_AWS_..._v1; Artifact LOGSNAP_-AWS_... hasDataProperty sha256=..., prevHash=..., eventId=...; InterventionEvent IE_SwapOrder_Azure_t3 targets Artifact LOGSNAP_Azure_...; ActivityLog ALOG_HashCompute_PerEvent.csv records OperationProcedure OP_Ingest_Order_Hash_Chain_Snapshot.

As operational checklist we provide:

- Enforce monotonic ingestion order per provider stream before chaining.
- Persist the chain index and snapshots to append-only storage.
- Record provider API request IDs to align with service-side telemetry.
- Recompute hashes after export to verify end-to-end integrity.

10.5 Analysis and Interpretation Phase

We evaluate whether the chain exposes edits and reordering, while acknowledging provider timing behavior:

- **ResultMetric** *(why)* quantifies integrity performance. **Instances:** RM_Detect-Success_0.98, RM_FalsePositive_0.01, RM_MedianDetectionTime_-1.3s.
- **StatisticalAnalysis** *(why)* compares providers and tamper types. **Instance:** ANOVA_DetectionTime_ByProvider and PostHoc_Tukey.
- **ThreatsToValidity** *(why)*: limits of inference. **Instances:** TV_CloudLatency, TV_ReplicationDelay, TV_ProviderNormalization.
- **InterpretationChallenge** *(why)*: analytic friction. **Instance:** IC_NonDetermin-isticOrdering.
- **ReliabilityAnalysis** *(why)*: repeatability. **Instance:** Rel_ConsistencyAcross-Runs_0.97.
- **ConflictLaw** *(why)*: cross-border handling. **Instance:** CL_Jurisdictional-DataHandling.

We used the following relations: ResultMetric RM_DetectSuccess_-0.98 computedFrom Artifacts {LOGSNAP_*}; ANOVA_DetectionTime_-ByProvider tests differences across IV_LoggingFramework lev-els; Rel_ConsistencyAcrossRuns_0.97 evaluates ResultMetric RM_-MedianDetectionTime_1.3s; IC_NonDeterministicOrdering impacts ResultInterpretation; TV_ReplicationDelay threatens ValidityOf-Conclusions; CL_JurisdictionalDataHandling constrains DataShar-ing and Retention.

The ontology separates integrity claims from timing behavior so that a future team can improve ordering heuristics while reusing the same chain-of-custody model.

10.6 Dissemination Phase

We publish artifacts and provenance in a way that others can verify without replicating the full cloud setup:

- **DisseminationPlan** *(why)* states venue and identifiers. **Instance:** DP_Open-Repo_WithDOIs.
- **Dataset** *(why)* bundles snapshots, chain indexes, and scripts. **Instance:** DS_-CloudLogs_Integrity_1_0.
- **DatasetMetadata** *(why)*: provenance and discovery. **Instance:** MD_PROV-C_-PlusDublinCore.
- **Authorship** *(why)*: credit and accountability. **Instance:** AUTH_Ferreira_Team.

The following relations were used: Dataset DS_CloudLogs_Integrity_1_0 describedBy MD_PROV-C_PlusDublinCore; DisseminationPlan DP_Open-Repo_WithDOIs publishes DS_CloudLogs_Integrity_1_0; Authorship AUTH_Ferreira_Team credits Experiment Exp_CloudLogIntegrity.

10.7 Ontological Instantiation Snapshot

Table 10.1 shows the ontological instantiations for this example.

Table 10.1 Ontological instantiations for "The Case of the Altered Cloud Logs"

Ontology Element	Example Instance
Experiment	Exp_CloudLogIntegrity
ResearchQuestion	RQ_HashChainDetectsMicroTamper
Hypothesis	H0_NoBetterThanChance; H1_HighDetectionRate
IndependentVariable	IV_LoggingFramework {AWS, GCP, Azure}; IV_TamperType {SingleCharEdit, LineDrop, LineInsert, SwapOrder}
DependentVariable	DV_DetectionRate; DV_FalsePositiveRate; DV_TimeToDetection
ControlVariable	CV_EventRate; CV_RegionCount; CV_KeyRotationInterval; CV_ClockDriftBudget
ConfoundingFactor	CF_CrossRegionReplicationDelay; CF_QueueBatching; CF_ProviderRedactionPolicies
ScenarioType	ST_DistributedVirtual
EnvironmentSetup	ES_MultiCloud_M1 {AWS_us-east-1; GCP_us-central1; Azure_eastus}
Benchmark	BM_LoggingLatency_PerProvider; BM_HMACThroughput
TrainingActivity	TA_CredentialIsolationDrill
Instrument	Python_HashChainer_v1.2; Collector_CLI_v0.9
Artifact	LOGSNAP_* jsonl; CHAIN_INDEX_*_v3.json
DataP	sha256; prevHash; eventId; region; captureWindow
ActivityLog	ALOG_HashCompute_PerEvent.csv
OperationProcedure	OP_Ingest_Order_Hash_Chain_Snapshot
InterventionEvent	IE_SingleCharEdit_AWS_t1; IE_LineDrop_GCP_t2; IE_SwapOrder_Azure_t3
ResultMetric	RM_DetectSuccess_0.98; RM_FalsePositive_0.01; RM_MedianDetectionTime_1.3s
StatisticalAnalysis	ANOVA_DetectionTime_ByProvider; PostHoc_Tukey
ThreatsToValidity	TV_CloudLatency; TV_ReplicationDelay; TV_ProviderNormalization
InterpretationChallenge	IC_NonDeterministicOrdering
ReliabilityAnalysis	Rel_ConsistencyAcrossRuns_0.97
ConflictLaw	CL_JurisdictionalDataHandling
DisseminationPlan	DP_OpenRepo_WithDOIs
Dataset	DS_CloudLogs_Integrity_1_0
DatasetMetadata	MD_PROV-C_PlusDublinCore
Authorship	AUTH_Ferreira_Team

10.8 Querying the Instantiation

The following SPARQL retrieves all artifacts where a `SwapOrder` intervention occurred and shows the breaking point in the chain by reporting both the stored `prevHash` and the recomputed link.

Listing 10.1 SPARQL: detect chain breaks around SwapOrder interventions

```
PREFIX ex: <http://example.org/experdf-onto#>
PREFIX rdfs: <http://www.w3.org/2000/01/rdf-schema#>

SELECT ?artifact ?eventId ?prevHash ?recomputed
WHERE {
  ?ie a ex:InterventionEvent ;
      rdfs:label ?label ;
      ex:tamperType "SwapOrder" ;
      ex:targets ?artifact .
  ?artifact a ex:Artifact ;
            ex:hasDataProperty ?dp1, ?dp2 .
  ?dp1 ex:key "eventId" ;
       ex:value ?eventId .
  ?dp2 ex:key "prevHash" ;
       ex:value ?prevHash .
  # recomputed is produced by a reasoner or pipeline and stored
      as a data property as well
  ?artifact ex:hasDataProperty ?dp3 .
  ?dp3 ex:key "prevHash_recomputed" ;
       ex:value ?recomputed .
  FILTER (?prevHash != ?recomputed)
}
```

10.9 Coverage and Missing Elements

Coverage: 37 of 52 ontology classes instantiated (71%). **Missing:** *PeerReview*, *SocialImplication*, *Evaluation* entities.

Why are these elements missing and how to add them:

- **PeerReview***(gap)*: no external assessor artifacts. *Add:* `PR_ExternalReviewer_Report`, `PR_Checklist`.
- **SocialImplication***(gap)*: impact on user privacy and provider policy not modeled. *Add:* `SI_ProviderPolicyChange`, `SI_PrivacyAssessment`.
- **Evaluation***(gap)*: formal user or expert evaluation missing. *Add:* `Eval_PractitionerStudy`, `Eval_UsabilityHeuristics`.

Adding these branches would raise completeness and align the study with collaborative and societal expectations while preserving technical strength.

10.10 Interpretation and Teaching Notes

10.10.1 What the Results Mean

A 98 percent detection success with 1 percent false positives indicates that hash-chaining can robustly expose micro-edits and reordering under the modeled ingestion discipline. Detection time depends on provider latency and batching and is captured in `DV_TimeToDetection` and associated benchmarks.

10.10.2 How to Reuse This Study

Because provider, region, and intervention types are modeled explicitly, a replicator can substitute a new provider service or enable cross-account logging while preserving the integrity model. The chain index and snapshot relations make provenance queries straightforward.

10.10.3 Common Misconceptions Clarified

- *Hash-chaining eliminates all tampering.* It makes tampering evident under the assumed ingestion order. It does not prevent upstream redaction policies or gaps due to service outages.
- *Ordering is purely deterministic.* Provider pipelines may reorder records. The ontology models this risk via `IC_NonDeterministicOrdering` and timing controls.

10.10.4 Minimal Reproducibility Kit

Provider account templates, IAM policies for read-only export, ingestion scripts, chain-index generator, log snapshots with per-event hashes, activity logs, and PROV-C plus Dublin Core metadata all appear as ontological instances connected by explicit relations.

10.11 Final Remarks

This example illustrated how a forensic integrity problem in cloud infrastructures can be transformed into a structured, reproducible, and auditable experiment through the use of *ExperDF-Onto*. Instead of treating cloud logging as an opaque service, the chapter modeled every element, including questions, hypotheses, variables, and artifacts, as explicit ontological entities. This approach allows students and practitioners to understand how design decisions affect the validity and interpretation of results.

The experiment confirmed that a tamper-evident hash chain can detect micro-edits and record reordering with high reliability, achieving nearly 98 percent detection and only 1 percent false positives. However, it also showed that detection accuracy depends on contextual constraints such as ingestion order, replication delay, and provider-specific normalization. In other words, technical mechanisms alone are not sufficient unless they are accompanied by well-defined experimental controls and provenance records.

From a teaching perspective, this case demonstrates the value of modeling before experimentation. By formalizing entities and relations in *ExperDF-Onto*, learners can see how reproducibility, transparency, and forensic soundness are interconnected. The open dataset, metadata, and SPARQL queries provide a self-contained kit for replication and further exploration, turning a complex cloud experiment into a practical and instructive example.

Future extensions may include the classes *PeerReview*, *SocialImplication*, and *Evaluation* to capture ethical oversight, privacy impact, and practitioner feedback. Integrating these elements will help connect technical integrity with societal trust, reinforcing the broader lesson that digital forensics must combine accuracy, openness, and accountability to achieve meaningful scientific and social value.

Chapter 11
Example 4: Echoes in the IoT Lab

Abstract This chapter presents a controlled smart home intrusion simulation that models time, interaction, and device heterogeneity using *ExperDF-Onto* so that correlation of evidence becomes measurable and auditable. The study asks whether clock offsets between devices and gateways degrade the ability to align cross-device events during an incident. The planning layer instantiates the experiment identity, research question, hypotheses, independent variables for device type and induced clock offset, dependent variables for correlation accuracy, alignment error, and event recall, plus control variables for network load, hub firmware, Wi-Fi channel, and attack script, as well as confounding factors such as RF noise and cloud queue delay with ethical and legal safeguards appropriate to a home-like lab. The pre-operation layer constructs a physical rig of ten IoT devices around a Zigbee hub, establishes calibration and latency benchmarks, validates the pipeline with a pilot, and documents operator training and vendor knowledge resources. During operation, packets and hub events are captured as first-class *Artifact* instances with integrity hashes, dual timestamps, and per-device offsets, while interaction relations record causal proximity and incident reports capture anomalies like missing timestamps. Analysis computes correlation accuracy near 92 percent with mean alignment error around 84 ms, tests offset effects across device types, records interpretation challenges due to stack-level timestamp inconsistency, and quantifies reliability across runs. Dissemination packages pcaps, hub JSON, calibration tables, scripts, and machine-readable RDF plus JSON metadata into a reusable dataset with clear authorship, impact assessment, and presentation guidance. Beyond reporting results, the chapter demonstrates how *ExperDF-Onto* separates measurement error from true absence of correlation, enables precise temporal queries over heterogeneous traces, and supports reproducible IoT forensics in settings where time is both evidence and adversary.

E. OliveiraJr et al., *Controlled Experimentation of Digital Forensics*,
https://doi.org/10.1007/978-3-032-19951-5_11

11.1 Context and Motivation

Smart homes blend heterogeneous devices, proprietary clouds, and intermittently reliable networks. Time is the invisible substrate that binds their traces: A door contact trips, a camera starts recording, a thermostat notes motion, and a hub forwards events upstream. A researcher designed a controlled study to answer a practical question for investigators: *How do timing differences between devices and gateways affect our ability to correlate IoT evidence during an intrusion simulation?*

This example shows how *ExperDF-Onto* models time, interaction, and heterogeneity as first-class concepts. By instantiating devices, packets, clock offsets, and interaction links, the ontology makes it possible to reconstruct multisource timelines and to quantify correlation accuracy rather than rely on anecdotal alignment.

We convert a narrative smart home scenario into a queryable ontological graph. At each phase, we state why a concept matters, how it is instantiated, which relations connect it, and what pitfalls the model prevents when correlating cross-device evidence.

11.2 Planning Phase

The planning layer turns the synchronization problem into measurable variables with ethical safeguards for a home-like setting, as follows:

- **Experiment** *(why)* names scope and identity. **Instance:** `Exp_IoT_SyncCorrelation`.
- **ResearchQuestion** *(why)* focuses uncertainty. **Instance:** `RQ_TimingImpactOnCorrelation`.
- **Hypothesis** *(why)*: expected relation. **Instances:** `H0_NoTimingEffect` and `H1_TimingAffectsCorrelation`.
- **IndependentVariable** *(why)*: manipulated factors. **Instances:** `IV_DeviceType` with levels {`Camera`, `DoorContact`, `PIR_Sensor`, `SmartPlug`}; `IV_ClockOffsetCondition` with levels {`Offset0ms`, `Offset150ms`, `Offset500ms`}.
- **DependentVariable** *(why)*: outcomes we measure. **Instances:** `DV_CorrelationAccuracy`, `DV_PairwiseAlignmentError`, `DV_EventRecall`.
- **ControlVariable** *(why)* holds variability constant. **Instances:** `CV_NetworkLoad`, `CV_HubFirmware`, `CV_WiFiChannel`, `CV_AttackScript`.
- **ConfoundingFactor** *(why)*: acknowledged influences. **Instances:** `CF_EnvironmentalRFNoise`, `CF_CloudQueueDelay`, `CF_DeviceThermalThrottling`.
- **EthicalPlanning** *(why)* protects privacy in a home-like context. **Instance:** `EP_SyntheticOccupants_BlurredVideo`.
- **LegalPlanning** *(why)* clarifies lawful data handling. **Instance:** `LP_ConsentWaiver_LabSetting`.
- **ReplicationPlanning** *(why)*: precommitment and transparency. **Instance:** `RP_OSF_IoT_Prereg`.

We used the following relations: Exp_IoT_SyncCorrelation hasResearchQuestion RQ_TimingImpactOnCorrelation; Exp_IoT_SyncCorrelation hasIndependentVariable IV_DeviceType, IV_ClockOffsetCondition; Exp_IoT_SyncCorrelation hasDependentVariable DV_CorrelationAccuracy, DV_PairwiseAlignmentError; Exp_IoT_SyncCorrelation isControlledBy CV_NetworkLoad, CV_HubFirmware; Exp_IoT_SyncCorrelation considersConfounding CF_CloudQueueDelay; Exp_IoT_SyncCorrelation governedBy EP_SyntheticOccupants_BlurredVideo, LP_ConsentWaiver_LabSetting; Exp_IoT_SyncCorrelation preregisteredAs RP_OSF_IoT_Prereg.

Typical pitfalls and ontology safeguards:

- *Pitfall:* Assuming NTP implies perfect synchrony. *Safeguard:* explicit IV_ClockOffsetCondition and CF_CloudQueueDelay.
- *Pitfall:* mixing device heterogeneity into one bucket. *Safeguard:* IV_DeviceType with levels and per-device metadata.
- *Pitfall:* privacy leakage from real footage. *Safeguard:* EP_SyntheticOccupants_BlurredVideo.

11.3 Pre-Operation Phase

Pre-operation constructs a physical smart home rig with known timing characteristics and documented training, as follows:

- **ScenarioType** *(why)* clarifies material execution. **Instance:** ST_PhysicalLabHome.
- **EnvironmentSetup** *(why)* enumerates devices and hub. **Instance:** ES_10Devices_ZigbeeHub with items {Camera_C1, Camera_C2, Door_D1, PIR_P1, PIR_P2, Plug_S1, Plug_S2, Thermostat_T1, Leak_L1, Hub_H1}.
- **Benchmark** *(why)*: baseline for timestamp drift and end to end delay. **Instances:** BM_ClockSkewPerDevice, BM_HubToCaptureLatency.
- **PilotProject** *(why)* de-risks data collection. **Instance:** PP_OneDayTrial_PartialDataset.
- **TrainingActivity** *(why)*: Config fluency reduces variable errors. **Instance:** TA_DeviceConfigWorkshop_4h.
- **KnowledgeResourceCondition** *(why)*: vendor docs and SDKs. **Instance:** KRC_ZigbeeProfiles_VendorSDKs.

We used the following relations: ES_10Devices_ZigbeeHub implements ST_PhysicalLabHome; BM_ClockSkewPerDevice benchmarks ES_10Devices_ZigbeeHub; PP_OneDayTrial_PartialDataset validates capture pipeline; TA_DeviceConfigWorkshop_4h prepares Participant CarolinaA_Lead and Assistants; KRC_ZigbeeProfiles_VendorSDKs documents EnvironmentSetup ES_10Devices_ZigbeeHub.

Listing devices explicitly prevents silent substitution during replication and enables per-device analysis of drift and packet loss.

11.4 Operation Phase

We capture packets and hub events while simulating an intrusion sequence. Packets and events become artifacts, and interaction edges capture causal proximity, such as:

- **Participant** *(why)*: roles and accountability. **Instances:** CarolinaA_Lead, LabAssistant_1, LabAssistant_2.
- **Instrument** *(why)*: capture and logging tools. **Instances:** Wireshark_v4.2, HubLogger_v1.3, TimeProbe_v0.9.
- **Artifact** *(why)*: observable evidence items. **Examples:** PKT_C1_2025-06-02T10:00:01.213Z.pcaprec, HLOG_DoorD1_Open_10:00:01.335Z.json, PKT_Hub_Zigbee_Assoc_10:00:01.500Z.pcaprec.
- **DataP** *(why)*: integrity and temporal context. **Examples:** sha256, deviceId, seq, hubTs, captureTs, offsetMs.
- **ActivityLog** *(why)*: human readable runbook. **Instance:** ALOG_IoT_Run03.csv.
- **OperationProcedure** *(why)* constrains execution. **Instance:** OP_Arm_-ApproachDoor_Open_Record_Leave.
- **Interaction Links** *(why)* correlate multi-device events. **Relations:** hasInteractionWith, precedesWithinWindow.
- **IncidentReport** *(why)*: exception handling. **Instance:** IR_MissingTimestamps_C2_Run02.

We used the following relations: CarolinaA_Lead uses Wireshark_v4.2 and HubLogger_v1.3; Wireshark_v4.2 produced Artifact PKT_C1_...; HubLogger_v1.3 produced Artifact HLOG_DoorD1_Open_...; Artifact PKT_C1_... hasDataProperty captureTs=..., deviceId=Camera_C1, offsetMs=150; Artifact HLOG_DoorD1_Open_... hasInteractionWith PKT_C1_...; Artifact HLOG_DoorD1_Open_... precedesWithinWindow PKT_C1_... [$\Delta t \leq$ 300 ms]; ActivityLog ALOG_IoT_Run03.csv records OperationProcedure OP_Arm_ApproachDoor_Open_Record_-Leave; IncidentReport IR_MissingTimestamps_C2_Run02 concerns device Camera_C2 and run 02.

As operational checklist, we have to:

- Calibrate per-device offset before each run using TimeProbe_v0.9
- Record both hub timestamps and capture interface timestamps
- Log channel, RSSI, and retry counters for RF diagnostics
- Immediately hash packet files and hub JSON exports

11.5 Analysis and Interpretation Phase

We quantify correlation accuracy as the proportion of expected cross-device pairings recovered within a temporal window and assess reliability across runs, as follows:

- **ResultMetric** *(why)* defines success quantitatively. **Instances:** `RM_CorrelationAccuracy_0.92`, `RM_MeanAlignmentError_84ms`, `RM_EventRecall_0.95`.
- **StatisticalAnalysis** *(why)* tests effects. **Instances:** `Pearson_r_0.97` for alignment stability, `ANOVA_Accuracy_ByOffset`.
- **ThreatsToValidity** *(why)*: boundary of inference. **Instances:** `TV_DeviceResets`, `TV_HubQueueOverflow`, `TV_PacketLossBurst`.
- **InterpretationChallenge** *(why)*: analytic friction. **Instance:** `IC_TimestampInconsistency_AcrossStacks`.
- **ReliabilityAnalysis** *(why)*: repeatability. **Instance:** `Rel_RunToRun_r_0.97`.

We used the following relations: `RM_CorrelationAccuracy_0.92 computedFrom pairs {HLOG_DoorD1_Open_* , PKT_C1_*}`; `ANOVA_Accuracy_ByOffset tests effect of IV_ClockOffsetCondition on DV_CorrelationAccuracy`; `Pearson_r_0.97 evaluates stability across runs`; `IC_TimestampInconsistency_AcrossStacks impacts ResultInterpretation`; `TV_DeviceResets threatens ValidityOfConclusions`.

By modeling per-device offset and interaction windows, the ontology separates measurement error from genuine absence of correlation, helping analysts choose appropriate temporal thresholds.

11.6 Dissemination Phase

We publish a reusable, privacy-preserving dataset with clear roles and presentation guidance:

- **DisseminationPlan** *(why)*: venue and accessibility. **Instance:** `DP_OpenForensics_Release`.
- **Dataset** *(why)* bundles pcap, hub JSON, calibration tables, and scripts. **Instance:** `DS_IoT_Echoes_1_0`.
- **DatasetMetadata** *(why)*: machine and human discoverability. **Instance:** `MD_RDF_PlusJSON`.
- **Authorship** *(why)*: credit and roles. **Instance:** `AUTH_Araujo_LabTeam`.
- **ImpactAssessment** *(why)*: downstream uptake. **Instance:** `IA_TrainingLabAdoption`.
- **PresentationQuality** *(why)*: clarity for learners. **Instance:** `PQ_StepByStepNotebook_Slides`.

We used the following relations: `Dataset DS_IoT_Echoes_1_0 describedBy MD_RDF_PlusJSON`; `DisseminationPlan DP_OpenForensics_Release publishes DS_IoT_Echoes_1_0`; `Authorship AUTH_Araujo_LabTeam credits Experiment Exp_IoT_SyncCorrelation`; `ImpactAssessment IA_TrainingLabAdoption evaluates Dissemination outcomes`; `PresentationQuality PQ_StepByStepNotebook_Slides enhances Dataset DS_IoT_Echoes_1_0`.

11.7 Ontological Instantiation Snapshot

Table 11.1 shows the ontological instantiations for this example.

11.8 Querying the Instantiation

The following SPARQL lists door open events and their nearest camera packet within a 300 ms window, returning alignment error using precomputed data properties.

Listing 11.1 SPARQL: correlate door events to camera packets within 300 ms

```
PREFIX ex: <http://example.org/experdf-onto#>
PREFIX xsd: <http://www.w3.org/2001/XMLSchema#>

SELECT ?doorEvent ?doorTs ?cameraPkt ?camTs ?alignErrorMs
WHERE {
  ?doorEvent a ex:Artifact ;
             ex:deviceId "Door_D1" ;
             ex:hasDataProperty ?dp1 .
  ?dp1 ex:key "hubTs" ; ex:value ?doorTs .

  ?cameraPkt a ex:Artifact ;
             ex:deviceId "Camera_C1" ;
             ex:hasDataProperty ?dp2 .
  ?dp2 ex:key "captureTs" ; ex:value ?camTs .

  # precomputed alignment error stored as data property on a
      derived link entity
  ?link a ex:Interaction ;
        ex:source ?doorEvent ;
        ex:target ?cameraPkt ;
        ex:hasDataProperty ?dp3 .
  ?dp3 ex:key "alignmentErrorMs" ; ex:value ?alignErrorMs .

  FILTER ( xsd:decimal(?alignErrorMs) >= 0 && xsd:decimal(?
      alignErrorMs) <= 300 )
}
```

Table 11.1 Ontological instantiations for "Echoes in the IoT Lab"

Ontology element	Example instance
Experiment	Exp_IoT_SyncCorrelation
ResearchQuestion	RQ_TimingImpactOnCorrelation
Hypothesis	H0_NoTimingEffect; H1_TimingAffectsCorrelation
IndependentVariable	IV_DeviceType {Camera, DoorContact, PIR_Sensor, SmartPlug}; IV_ClockOffsetCondition {0, 150, 500 ms}
DependentVariable	DV_CorrelationAccuracy; DV_PairwiseAlignmentError; DV_EventRecall
ControlVariable	CV_NetworkLoad; CV_HubFirmware; CV_WiFiChannel; CV_AttackScript
ConfoundingFactor	CF_EnvironmentalRFNoise; CF_CloudQueueDelay; CF_DeviceThermalThrottling
ScenarioType	ST_PhysicalLabHome
EnvironmentSetup	ES_10Devices_ZigbeeHub {Camera_C1, Camera_C2, Door_D1, PIR_P1, PIR_P2, Plug_S1, Plug_S2, Thermostat_T1, Leak_L1, Hub_H1}
Benchmark	BM_ClockSkewPerDevice; BM_HubToCaptureLatency
PilotProject	PP_OneDayTrial_PartialDataset
TrainingActivity	TA_DeviceConfigWorkshop_4h
Instrument	Wireshark_v4.2; HubLogger_v1.3; TimeProbe_v0.9
Artifact	PKT_* pcaprec; HLOG_* json
DataP	sha256; deviceId; seq; hubTs; captureTs; offsetMs
ActivityLog	ALOG_IoT_Run03.csv
OperationProcedure	OP_Arm_ApproachDoor_Open_Record_Leave
Interaction Relations	hasInteractionWith; precedesWithinWindow
IncidentReport	IR_MissingTimestamps_C2_Run02
ResultMetric	RM_CorrelationAccuracy_0.92; RM_MeanAlignmentError_84ms; RM_EventRecall_0.95
StatisticalAnalysis	Pearson_r_0.97; ANOVA_Accuracy_ByOffset
ThreatsToValidity	TV_DeviceResets; TV_HubQueueOverflow; TV_PacketLossBurst
InterpretationChallenge	IC_TimestampInconsistency_AcrossStacks
ReliabilityAnalysis	Rel_RunToRun_r_0.97
DisseminationPlan	DP_OpenForensics_Release
Dataset	DS_IoT_Echoes_1_0
DatasetMetadata	MD_RDF_PlusJSON
Authorship	AUTH_Araujo_LabTeam
ImpactAssessment	IA_TrainingLabAdoption
PresentationQuality	PQ_StepByStepNotebook_Slides

11.9 Coverage and Missing Elements

Coverage: 40 of 52 ontology classes instantiated (77%). **Missing:** *OntologyAlignment*, *QualityAssessment*, *Stakeholder*.

Why are these elements missing and how to add:

- **OntologyAlignment** *(gap)*: no mapping to SAREF or SSN ontologies. *Add:* `Align_Device_to_SAREF`, `Align_Observation_to_SSN`.
- **QualityAssessment** *(gap)*: formal quality gates absent. *Add:* `QA_PacketCompleteness`, `QA_TimestampPrecisionAudit`.
- **Stakeholder** *(gap)*: no external user groups modeled. *Add:* `Stakeholder_LEA_Trainer`, `Stakeholder_ConsumerAdvocacy`.

Adding these classes would raise completeness and improve interoperability with community ontologies while clarifying intended beneficiaries.

11.10 Interpretation and Teaching Notes

11.10.1 What the Results Mean

A correlation accuracy of 92 percent with mean alignment error of 84 ms indicates that reliable cross-device reconstruction is feasible in a well-characterized lab home, but accuracy degrades under larger induced offsets and bursty packet loss as captured by `TV_PacketLossBurst`.

11.10.2 How to Reuse This Study

Replace the hub or radio profile while preserving the `IV_DeviceType`, `IV_ClockOffsetCondition`, and calibration benchmarks. Because offsets and windows are explicit data properties, thresholds can be tuned without altering the conceptual structure.

11.10.3 Common Misconceptions Clarified

- *Near real time equals forensic grade time.* Not all timestamps share the same reference or precision. Model both `hubTs` and `captureTs` and their `offsetMs`.
- *If devices interact, their packets always correlate.* RF noise, queue overflow, and device resets can break expected links. These are modeled as `ThreatsToValidity`.

11.10.4 Minimal Reproducibility Kit

A device inventory including firmware versions; calibration scripts and tables; packet captures and hub logs with associated hashes; an interaction link derivation script; analysis notebooks; and metadata in RDF and JSON formats. All appear as explicit instances and relations in *ExperDF-Onto*.

11.11 Final Remarks

This study demonstrated how temporal uncertainty in smart home environments can be transformed into a measurable and auditable experimental problem when structured through *ExperDF-Onto*. By modeling time, interaction, and device heterogeneity as explicit entities, the chapter showed that correlation across devices is not only a technical task but also an epistemic one that depends on clear ontological framing.

The achieved correlation accuracy of about 92 percent and mean alignment error near 84 milliseconds confirm that well-calibrated IoT environments can sustain reliable event reconstruction despite inherent heterogeneity. At the same time, the experiment revealed how small clock offsets and queuing delays can produce misleading gaps or overlaps, underscoring that even subtle time drift can affect investigative conclusions. The ontology helped separate true loss of correlation from measurement artifacts, providing a more precise basis for reasoning about causality.

From a methodological point of view, the chapter advances reproducible IoT forensics by encoding every assumption, offset, and link into machine-readable form. This structure allows future replicators to adapt new devices, protocols, or hubs while maintaining comparability and traceability. The open dataset and metadata not only ensure transparency but also serve as a didactic reference for teaching time-based reasoning and integrity verification in connected environments.

Future work can extend this foundation by incorporating the missing classes *OntologyAlignment*, *QualityAssessment*, and *Stakeholder*. These additions will improve interoperability with external standards such as SAREF and SSN, introduce systematic quality gates, and connect experimental findings with the needs of law enforcement, educators, and consumer advocates. Through such integration, reproducible IoT forensics can move closer to a holistic understanding of time as both evidence and variable, ensuring that scientific accuracy aligns with societal trust and practical relevance.

Chapter 12
Example 5: The Invisible Signature: Blockchain Provenance

Abstract This chapter evaluates whether anchoring dataset fingerprints on public and permissioned blockchains can deliver tamper evident provenance with practical latency and cost and shows how *ExperDF-Onto* captures this workflow as a complete, auditable graph. The planning layer instantiates the experiment identity, research question, hypotheses, independent variable for blockchain platform selection, dependent variables for verification latency, hash stability, and end-to-end cost, along with controls for hash algorithm, bundling policy, and node provider version, plus confounders such as network congestion, gas price volatility, and endorsement policy differences, under ethical and legal constraints that anchor only hashes and treat anchors as metadata. The pre-operation layer defines a hybrid environment with smart contracts and chaincode, establishes confirmation and gas use benchmarks, validates the bundle to ledger path in a pilot, and records training and canonical protocol references. During operation, each dataset bundle is hashed deterministically, anchored by contracts or chaincode, and emits receipts that include transaction identifiers, block heights, timestamps, gas metrics, and network identifiers, all modeled as first-class *Artifact* instances linked to the producing *Instrument* and recorded in activity logs under a prespecified procedure. Analysis confirms perfect hash reproduction under cold recomputation, compares latency across platforms with nonparametric and factorial tests, and records interpretation challenges such as fee fluctuation and shallow reorg risk alongside threats to validity concerning anchoring only fingerprints and trusting node infrastructure, with reliability expressed as two-party consistency and quality assessment focused on trace validity. Dissemination packages bundles, contracts, receipts, notebooks, and FAIR plus JSON LD metadata with dual persistent identifiers to support independent verification and reuse. Beyond reporting outcomes, the chapter demonstrates how *ExperDF-Onto* separates content quality from provenance soundness, enables machine actionable verification queries, and provides a governance-ready template for trustworthy dataset publication in digital forensics.

E. OliveiraJr et al., *Controlled Experimentation of Digital Forensics*,
https://doi.org/10.1007/978-3-032-19951-5_12

12.1 Context and Motivation

When a dataset changes hands, spreadsheets can be copied, scripts can be tweaked, and filenames can be misleading. What investigators need is a way to attest that the evidence bundle they analyze is exactly the one that the original research group produced. A researcher designed a study to evaluate whether anchoring dataset fingerprints on public and permissioned blockchains can provide tamper-evident provenance with acceptable overhead. The example shows how *ExperDF-Onto* represents provenance anchors, transaction metadata, and verification workflows as first-class concepts that connect experimental artifacts to independent, append-only ledgers.

We translate a narrative about trustworthy dataset publication into a precise, queryable instantiation. At each phase, we explain which ontological elements are instantiated, how they are linked, and which common pitfalls the model prevents when using blockchains for forensic provenance.

12.2 Planning Phase

The planning layer turns "use blockchain for provenance" into testable variables and outcomes, with clear governance of data and code, as follows:

- **Experiment** *(why)* names the scope. **Instance:** `Exp_BC_ProvenanceValidation`.
- **ResearchQuestion** *(why)* focuses uncertainty. **Instance:** `RQ_TamperEvidentProvenance`.
- **Hypothesis** *(why)* sets expectation. **Instances:** `H0_NoGuarantee` and `H1_BlockchainGuaranteesTamperEvidence`.
- **IndependentVariable** *(why)* manipulated factor. **Instance:** `IV_BlockchainPlatform` with levels `{Ethereum_Mainnet, Ethereum_Sepolia, Hyperledger_Fabric}`.
- **DependentVariable** *(why)* measurable outcomes. **Instances:** `DV_VerificationLatency`, `DV_HashStability`, `DV_EndToEndCost`.
- **ControlVariable** *(why)* holds variability constant. **Instances:** `CV_HashAlgorithm_SHA256`, `CV_BundlePolicy_TarGzip`, `CV_NodeProviderVersion`.
- **ConfoundingFactor** *(why)* acknowledged influences. **Instances:** `CF_NetworkCongestion`, `CF_GasPriceVolatility`, `CF_FabricEndorsementPolicy`.
- **EthicalPlanning** *(why)* avoids leakage of sensitive content. **Instance:** `EP_AnchorOnlyHashes_NoRawData`.
- **LegalPlanning** *(why)* clarifies lawful anchoring. **Instance:** `LP_JurisdictionalReview_AnchorsAsMetadata`.

- **ReplicationPlanning** *(why)* precommitment and transparency. **Instance:** RP_GithubScripts_OSFPrereg.
- **QualityPlanning** *(why)* defines success gates. **Instance:** QP_TwoPartyVerification_ColdRecalc.

We used the following relations: Exp_BC_ProvenanceValidation hasResearchQuestion RQ_TamperEvidentProvenance; Exp_BC_ProvenanceValidation hasIndependentVariable IV_BlockchainPlatform; Exp_BC_ProvenanceValidation hasDependentVariable DV_VerificationLatency, DV_HashStability; Exp_BC_ProvenanceValidation isControlledBy CV_HashAlgorithm_SHA256, CV_BundlePolicy_TarGzip; Exp_BC_ProvenanceValidation considersConfounding CF_NetworkCongestion, CF_GasPriceVolatility; Exp_BC_ProvenanceValidation governedBy EP_AnchorOnlyHashes_NoRawData, LP_JurisdictionalReview_AnchorsAsMetadata; Exp_BC_ProvenanceValidation preregisteredAs RP_GithubScripts_OSFPrereg; Exp_BC_ProvenanceValidation qualityGatedBy QP_TwoPartyVerification_ColdRecalc.

Typical pitfalls and ontology safeguards:

- *Pitfall:* anchoring raw data rather than hashes. *Safeguard:* EP_AnchorOnlyHashes_NoRawData and the Artifact design that treats fingerprints as first-class outputs.
- *Pitfall:* ignoring fee volatility. *Safeguard:* explicit CF_GasPriceVolatility and DV_EndToEndCost.
- *Pitfall:* unverifiable node behavior. *Safeguard:* CV_NodeProviderVersion and QP_TwoPartyVerification_ColdRecalc.

12.3 Pre-Operation Phase

Pre-operation defines where and how anchors will be written, with pilots that validate the full path from bundle to transaction, such as:

- **ScenarioType** *(why)* environment clarity. **Instance:** ST_Hybrid_Public+Permissioned.
- **EnvironmentSetup** *(why)* concrete components. **Instance:** ES_SC_Eth+Fabric with items {EthContract_AnchorV1, FabricChaincode_AnchorV1, EthNode_v1.13, FabricPeer_v2.5}.
- **Benchmark** *(why)* baseline latencies and success. **Instances:** BM_BlockConfirmationTime, BM_ContractGasUsePerAnchor.
- **PilotProject** *(why)* early risk reduction. **Instance:** PP_PilotHashAnchoring_OK.

- **TrainingActivity** *(why)* operator proficiency. **Instance:** TA_SCDeploymentWorkshop_6h.
- **KnowledgeResourceCondition** *(why)* canonical references. **Instance:** KRC_EIPs_FabricDocs.

We used the following relations: ES_SC_Eth+Fabric implements ST_Hybrid_Public+Permissioned; BM_BlockConfirmationTime benchmarks ES_SC_Eth+Fabric; PP_PilotHashAnchoring_OK validates pipeline from hash to ledger; TA_SCDeploymentWorkshop_6h prepares Participant JonasR_PI and DevOps_Team; KRC_EIPs_FabricDocs documents EnvironmentSetup ES_SC_Eth+Fabric.

12.4 Operation Phase

Each dataset bundle generates a deterministic fingerprint. Smart contracts (or chaincode) record this fingerprint along with minimal metadata. Activity logs capture operational metrics such as gas consumption and execution timing, including:

- **Participant** *(why)* roles and accountability. **Instances:** JonasR_PI, DevOps_Engineer_1, Analyst_Verifier_A.
- **Instrument** *(why)* the anchoring mechanism. **Instances:** SmartContract_AnchorV1, FabricChaincode_AnchorV1, AnchorCLI_v0.4.
- **Artifact** *(why)* evidence items and their fingerprints. **Instances:** Bundle_DS_Forensics_1_0.tar.gz, Hash_SHA256_Bundle_abcd..., TxReceipt_Eth_0xdead..., TxReceipt_Fabric_tx123....
- **DataP** *(why)* integrity and context. **Examples:** sha256, blockHeight, txid, gasUsed, gasPrice, ledgerTs, networkId.
- **ActivityLog** *(why)* human readable provenance. **Instance:** ALOG_AnchorRuns.csv.
- **OperationProcedure** *(why)* step discipline. **Instance:** OP_Bundle_Hash_Anchor_Verify_Recalc.
- **UniqueID** *(why)* persistent identifiers. **Instances:** DOI_10.5281/zenodo.7654321, BCID_0xdead...@EthMainnet.

We used the following relations: JonasR_PI uses Instrument AnchorCLI_v0.4; AnchorCLI_v0.4 produced Artifact Hash_SHA256_Bundle_abcd... from Artifact Bundle_DS_Forensics_1_0.tar.gz; SmartContract_AnchorV1 registered Artifact Hash_SHA256_Bundle_abcd... into BlockchainNetwork Ethereum_Mainnet producing Artifact TxReceipt_Eth_0xdead...; TxReceipt_Eth_0xdead... hasDataProperty blockHeight=..., gasUsed=..., ledgerTs=...; OperationProcedure OP_Bundle_Hash_Anchor_Verify_Recalc executedBy

DevOps_Engineer_1; ActivityLog ALOG_AnchorRuns.csv records OperationProcedure OP_Bundle_Hash_Anchor_Verify_Recalc; UniqueID DOI_10.5281/... identifies Dataset DS_BC_Provenance_1_0; UniqueID BCID_0xdead...@EthMainnet identifies Artifact TxReceipt_Eth_0xdead....

As operational checklist we:

- Produce bundles deterministically with canonical tar and gzip flags.
- Compute hashes on an offline verifier and again on the publishing host.
- Anchor the same hash on two networks for redundancy: one public and one permissioned.
- Store receipts, ABI, and chain configuration in the activity log and dataset metadata.

12.5 Analysis and Interpretation Phase

We verify that recomputation reproduces the original hash and measure verification latency under load and congestion, such as:

- **ResultMetric** *(why)* quantitative success. **Instances:** RM_HashReproduction_1.00, RM_MedianVerifyLatency_Eth_4.2s, RM_MedianVerifyLatency_Fabric_0.9s, RM_CostPerAnchor_Eth_US$1.27.
- **StatisticalAnalysis** *(why)* effect testing. **Instances:** MWU_Latency_EthVsFabric, ANOVA_Latency_ByCongestionTier.
- **InterpretationChallenge** *(why)* analytic friction. **Instances:** IC_GasFluctuation, IC_ReorgRisk_LowDepth.
- **ThreatsToValidity** *(why)* inference boundary. **Instances:** TV_AnchorOnly_NoContent, TV_NodeTrustAssumptions, TV_FabricPolicyVariance.
- **ReliabilityAnalysis** *(why)* repeatability. **Instance:** Rel_ColdRecalc_TwoParty_Consistent.
- **QualityAssessment** *(why)* formal gates. **Instance:** QA_BlockchainTraceValidity.

We used the following relations: RM_HashReproduction_1.00 computedFrom {Hash_SHA256_Bundle_abcd..., Recalc_Hash_SHA256_Bundle_abcd...}; MWU_Latency_EthVsFabric tests difference on DV_VerificationLatency across IV_BlockchainPlatform; IC_GasFluctuation impacts ResultInterpretation; TV_NodeTrustAssumptions threatens ValidityOfConclusions; Rel_ColdRecalc_TwoParty_Consistent evaluates RM_HashReproduction_1.00; QA_BlockchainTraceValidity assesses provenance soundness of receipts and anchors.

12.6 Dissemination Phase

We release the dataset, code, and contracts with dual identifiers and external review to increase trust and reuse, as follows:

- **DisseminationPlan** *(why)* venue and access. **Instance:** DP_Zenodo_Data+Contracts.
- **Dataset** *(why)* the research bundle. **Instance:** DS_BC_Provenance_1_0.
- **DatasetMetadata** *(why)* machine and human discovery. **Instance:** MD_FAIR_JSONLD.
- **UniqueID** *(why)* persistent references. **Instances:** DOI_10.5281/zenodo.7654321, BCID_0xdead...@EthMainnet.
- **Authorship** *(why)* credit and roles. **Instance:** AUTH_Ribeiro_Team.
- **PeerReview** *(why)* external scrutiny. **Instance:** PR_ExternalReviewer_Report.
- **PresentationQuality** *(why)* clarity for adopters. **Instance:** PQ_HowToVerify_Notebook+Slides.
- **ImpactAssessment** *(why)* downstream uptake. **Instance:** IA_AdoptionByLabs_Survey3mo.

We used the following relations: Dataset DS_BC_Provenance_1_0 describedBy MD_FAIR_JSONLD; DisseminationPlan DP_Zenodo_Data+Contracts publishes DS_BC_Provenance_1_0; UniqueID DOI_10.5281/... identifies DS_BC_Provenance_1_0; UniqueID BCID_0xdead...@EthMainnet identifies TxReceipt_Eth_0xdead...; PeerReview PR_ExternalReviewer_Report assesses Experiment Exp_BC_ProvenanceValidation; PresentationQuality PQ_HowToVerify_Notebook+Slides enhances Dataset DS_BC_Provenance_1_0; ImpactAssessment IA_AdoptionByLabs_Survey3mo evaluates dissemination outcomes.

12.7 Ontological Instantiation Snapshot

Table 12.1 shows the ontological instantiations for this example.

12.8 Querying the Instantiation

The first query lists dataset versions, their SHA256 fingerprints, and the Ethereum transaction that anchored them. The second query verifies that the recomputed hash matches the anchored value.

Table 12.1 Ontological instantiations for "The Invisible Signature"

Ontology Element	Example Instance
Experiment	Exp_BC_ProvenanceValidation
ResearchQuestion	RQ_TamperEvidentProvenance
Hypothesis	H0_NoGuarantee; H1_BlockchainGuaranteesTamperEvidence
IndependentVariable	IV_BlockchainPlatform {Eth_Mainnet, Eth_Sepolia, Fabric}
DependentVariable	DV_VerificationLatency; DV_HashStability; DV_EndToEndCost
ControlVariable	CV_HashAlgorithm_SHA256; CV_BundlePolicy_TarGzip; CV_NodeProviderVersion
ConfoundingFactor	CF_NetworkCongestion; CF_GasPriceVolatility; CF_FabricEndorsementPolicy
ScenarioType	ST_Hybrid_Public+Permissioned
EnvironmentSetup	ES_SC_Eth+Fabric {EthContract_AnchorV1, FabricChaincode_AnchorV1}
Benchmark	BM_BlockConfirmationTime; BM_ContractGasUsePerAnchor
PilotProject	PP_PilotHashAnchoring_OK
TrainingActivity	TA_SCDeploymentWorkshop_6h
Instrument	SmartContract_AnchorV1; FabricChaincode_AnchorV1; AnchorCLI_v0.4
Artifact	Bundle_DS_Forensics_1_0.tar.gz; Hash_SHA256_Bundle_abcd...; TxReceipt_Eth_0xdead...
DataP	sha256; txid; blockHeight; gasUsed; gasPrice; ledgerTs; networkId
ActivityLog	ALOG_AnchorRuns.csv
OperationProcedure	OP_Bundle_Hash_Anchor_Verify_Recalc
ResultMetric	RM_HashReproduction_1.00; RM_MedianVerifyLatency_Eth_4.2s; RM_CostPerAnchor_Eth_US$1.27
StatisticalAnalysis	MWU_Latency_EthVsFabric; ANOVA_Latency_ByCongestionTier
InterpretationChallenge	IC_GasFluctuation; IC_ReorgRisk_LowDepth
ThreatsToValidity	TV_AnchorOnly_NoContent; TV_NodeTrustAssumptions; TV_FabricPolicyVariance
ReliabilityAnalysis	Rel_ColdRecalc_TwoParty_Consistent
QualityAssessment	QA_BlockchainTraceValidity
DisseminationPlan	DP_Zenodo_Data+Contracts
Dataset	DS_BC_Provenance_1_0
DatasetMetadata	MD_FAIR_JSONLD
UniqueID	DOI_10.5281/zenodo.7654321; BCID_0xdead...@EthMainnet
Authorship	AUTH_Ribeiro_Team
PeerReview	PR_ExternalReviewer_Report
PresentationQuality	PQ_HowToVerify_Notebook+Slides
ImpactAssessment	IA_AdoptionByLabs_Survey3mo

Listing 12.1 SPARQL: list bundles with anchored tx metadata

```
PREFIX ex: <http://example.org/experdf-onto#>
PREFIX rdfs: <http://www.w3.org/2000/01/rdf-schema#>

SELECT ?bundle ?sha ?txid ?blockHeight ?gasUsed
WHERE {
  ?bundle a ex:Artifact ; rdfs:label ?bname .
  ?bundle ex:hasDataProperty ?dp1 .
  ?dp1 ex:key "sha256" ; ex:value ?sha .

  ?tx a ex:Artifact ;
      ex:producedBy ?sc ;
      ex:hasDataProperty ?dptx .
  ?sc a ex:Instrument ; rdfs:label "SmartContract_AnchorV1" .
  ?dptx ex:key "txid" ; ex:value ?txid .
  ?tx ex:hasDataProperty ?dph .
  ?dph ex:key "blockHeight" ; ex:value ?blockHeight .
  ?tx ex:hasDataProperty ?dpg .
  ?dpg ex:key "gasUsed" ; ex:value ?gasUsed .

  ?bundle ex:isAnchoredBy ?tx .
}
```

Listing 12.2 SPARQL: verify recomputed hash equals anchored hash

```
PREFIX ex: <http://example.org/experdf-onto#>

SELECT ?bundle ?anchored ?recalc
WHERE {
  ?bundle a ex:Artifact ;
          ex:hasDataProperty ?dpA ;
          ex:hasDataProperty ?dpR .
  ?dpA ex:key "sha256" ; ex:value ?anchored .
  ?dpR ex:key "recalc_sha256" ; ex:value ?recalc .
  FILTER (?anchored = ?recalc)
}
```

12.9 Coverage and Missing Elements

Coverage: 42 of 52 ontology classes instantiated (80%). **Missing:** *Stakeholder*, *SocialImplication*, *ExternalReplication*.

Why are these elements missing and how to add them:

- **Stakeholder** *(gap)*: Intended beneficiaries are not explicitly modeled. *Add:* `Stakeholder_LEA_Analyst`, `Stakeholder_JournalDataEditor`.
- **SocialImplication** *(gap)*: broader impact not captured. *Add:* `SI_EnergyCostImpact`, `SI_TransparencyBenefit`.

- **ExternalReplication** *(gap)*: third-party replay not encoded. *Add:* `ExtRep_IndependentLab_Replay`, linked to `Rel_ColdRecalc_TwoParty_Consistent`.

Introducing these classes would raise completeness and clarify who uses the provenance, how society is affected, and how independent replication is evidenced.

12.10 Interpretation and Teaching Notes

12.10.1 What the Results Mean

A hash reproduction rate of 1.00 indicates that cold recomputation matched the anchored value for all tested bundles. Verification latency is dominated by network confirmation time on Ethereum and by endorsement on Fabric. Costs on public chains vary with gas prices, which is captured by `IC_GasFluctuation` and `DV_EndToEndCost`.

12.10.2 How to Reuse This Study

Swap the platform level of `IV_BlockchainPlatform`, or deploy a new smart contract while preserving the same bundle policy and hash algorithm. Because receipts and parameters are modeled as `Artifact` with explicit `DataP`, verification scripts can be regenerated from the ontology alone.

12.10.3 Common Misconceptions Clarified

- *Anchoring guarantees data quality.* It guarantees immutability of the fingerprint, not the scientific merit of the content. Use `QualityAssessment` to separate provenance soundness from content validity.
- *Public blockchains are always superior.* Permissioned ledgers can offer lower latency and stable cost under auditable governance, modeled by `EnvironmentSetup` and `LegalPlanning`.

12.10.4 Minimal Reproducibility Kit

Canonical bundling scripts, offline and online hash logs, contract ABIs and addresses, Fabric chaincode packages, and transaction receipts (including block heights and timestamps), along with verification notebooks and FAIR-compliant JSON-LD metadata, are all represented as explicit instances and relationships in *ExperDF-Onto*.

12.11 Final Remarks

This study showed that dataset fingerprints anchored on both public and permissioned blockchains can provide tamper-evident provenance with practical verification times and transparent costs when the workflow is modeled in *ExperDF-Onto*. By treating bundles, hashes, contracts, chaincode, and receipts as first-class *Artifact* instances linked to explicit *Instrument*, *OperationProcedure*, and *ActivityLog* entities, the chapter delivered not only empirical results but also a machine-actionable provenance graph that supports independent checks and long-term auditability.

The results confirm perfect hash reproduction under cold recomputation and highlight clear latency and cost profiles across platforms. At the same time, the analysis made visible the boundaries of the claim. Anchoring fingerprints does not assess scientific merit, and verification depends on network conditions, fee dynamics, shallow reorg risk, and the trust placed in node infrastructure. Encoding these factors as *ControlVariable*, *ConfoundingFactor*, *ThreatsToValidity*, and *QualityAssessment* elements allows investigators to separate content quality from provenance soundness and to report both with clarity.

Methodologically, the chapter contributes a governance-ready template for trustworthy dataset publication. Deterministic bundling, dual-network anchoring for redundancy, preserved receipts with block heights and timestamps, and FAIR plus JSON-LD metadata create a complete chain from dataset creation to public verification. Because every step is represented in the ontology, verification notebooks and queries can be regenerated even if tools change, which strengthens reproducibility and reduces hidden assumptions.

Future work can broaden impact by instantiating *Stakeholder*, *SocialImplication*, and *ExternalReplication* classes. These additions would connect the technical pipeline to its primary users, document energy and transparency trade-offs, and encode third-party replays as explicit evidence of replication. Further extensions may include cross-chain proofs, automated cost-aware anchoring policies, and routine integrity reports that combine provenance checks with dataset curation quality. Taken together, these steps move digital forensics toward publication practices where provenance is verifiable, governance is explicit, and reuse is safe and efficient.

Part V
Integration, Reflection, and Future Directions

This part marks the culmination of this book's scientific, methodological, and philosophical trajectory. After examining the evolution of experimentation, the establishment of formal models, and the creation of ontological representations for Digital Forensics, this final part brings the discussion to a reflective synthesis. It explores how the elements introduced in the previous parts, namely empirical foundations, conceptual modeling, and semantic formalization converge into a coherent vision of Digital Forensics as a rigorous, transparent, and open scientific discipline.

While Part I established the historical and epistemological background for controlled experimentation in Digital Forensics, Part II provided a structural framework through the *ExperDF-CM* conceptual model, translating theoretical principles into operational research stages. Part III extended these foundations into the semantic domain with the *ExperDF-Onto* ontology, demonstrating how formal representations can describe, integrate, and reason about forensic knowledge in a machine-readable and interoperable way. Part IV then delivers a comprehensive and didactic walkthrough of how *ExperDF-Onto* can be instantiated to describe, reason about, and evaluate real digital forensics experiments, marking a decisive shift from theory to practice. Through five representative case studies, ranging from memory analysis and smartphone extraction to blockchain-based provenance, it illustrates how ontological modeling translates abstract constructs into verifiable scientific workflows, reinforcing transparency, reproducibility, and ethical responsibility. Finally, this part turns to a broader synthesis that connects these contributions and examines how they collectively redefine the production, interpretation, and validation of digital evidence within scientific practice.

The purpose of this part is not to summarize previous chapters but to integrate them, revealing their coherence, interdependence, and collective impact. It discusses how conceptual models and ontologies act as complementary instruments for building cumulative knowledge, supporting methodological transparency, and ensuring scientific accountability. It also highlights how the principles of Open Science are embedded in every methodological and ethical choice proposed throughout the book, transforming Digital Forensics from a procedural craft into an epistemically grounded research field.

In this context, Part IV performs three key functions. First, it offers an integrative synthesis that articulates the relationships among all previous parts and clarifies their shared contribution to the evolution of the field. Second, it provides a critical reflection on the remaining challenges that Digital Forensics must address, including technical, institutional, and philosophical issues. Third, it outlines future perspectives for research, education, and policy, emphasizing the importance of sustained collaboration and the continuous refinement of conceptual and semantic frameworks.

Ultimately, this part invites the reader to view Digital Forensics as a dynamic and evolving scientific ecosystem that unites methodological structure with interpretative flexibility, empirical rigor with ethical responsibility, and technological innovation with epistemological depth. By closing with a comprehensive analysis and forward-looking perspective, Part IV reaffirms the central message of this book: The strength of Digital Forensics lies in its capacity to integrate structure, meaning, and openness in the pursuit of reliable and verifiable knowledge.

Chapter 13
Concluding Remarks: Toward a Scientifically Grounded and Open Digital Forensics

Abstract This final chapter integrates the theoretical, methodological, and semantic foundations developed throughout the book, offering a comprehensive reflection on the evolution of Digital Forensics as a scientific discipline. It revisits the main conceptual trajectories presented in earlier chapters, linking controlled experimentation, conceptual modeling, and ontology engineering under the shared vision of openness, rigor, and reproducibility. Rather than restating individual conclusions, the chapter examines how these contributions collectively establish a coherent epistemological framework for Digital Forensics, capable of bridging empirical investigation with semantic reasoning and ethical responsibility. It discusses the interplay between the ExperDF-CM and ExperDF-Onto models, highlighting their roles in structuring experiments, formalizing knowledge, and promoting interoperability across forensic tools and research environments. The chapter also identifies current gaps and challenges, such as data sensitivity, methodological fragmentation, and the need for community-driven governance of forensic ontologies. Finally, it outlines future perspectives for the field, emphasizing the convergence of Digital Forensics with Artificial Intelligence, Open Science infrastructures, and human-centered ethics. By synthesizing the insights and advances presented in the preceding chapters, this closing reflection positions Digital Forensics as a mature, transparent, and collaborative science dedicated to upholding the integrity and accountability of digital evidence.

13.1 Contextualization

This book was conceived with the ambition of establishing a rigorous, transparent, and epistemologically coherent foundation for Digital Forensics (DF) as both a scientific and a practical field. Emerging from a context where digital evidence plays an increasingly decisive role in judicial processes, cybersecurity operations, and research investigations, DF faces the dual challenge of maintaining operational efficiency while adhering to the principles of scientific inquiry. The book's central objective has been to address this challenge by proposing a structured framework that integrates conceptual modeling, ontology engineering, and open

E. OliveiraJr et al., *Controlled Experimentation of Digital Forensics*,
https://doi.org/10.1007/978-3-032-19951-5_13

science practices. Through seven chapters, it has progressively built theoretical and methodological scaffolding that supports reproducible experimentation, semantic interoperability, and evidence-based reasoning. The underlying hypothesis guiding this work is that the maturation of DF as a discipline depends not only on technological innovation but also on its capacity to systematize knowledge, formalize procedures, and align itself with the broader epistemic norms of science.

The book begins by examining the historical and philosophical roots of experimentation and the emergence of open science as a transformative movement that reshapes the way scientific knowledge is produced, validated, and shared. It then advanced toward developing domain-specific models and ontologies capable of representing the logic and processes of forensic inquiry. In doing so, it articulated a vision of DF that is not merely reactive, responding to incidents and producing isolated analyses, but proactive, cumulative, and verifiable. This concluding chapter synthesizes the contributions of the previous parts, connecting their theoretical premises, methodological innovations, and practical implications. It also explores remaining gaps, tensions, and emerging opportunities, offering directions for future research and institutional development.

13.2 Integrative Synthesis

The conceptual progression of the book unfolds across three major parts, each addressing a distinct yet interdependent layer of the discipline's scientific architecture.

Part I introduced the epistemological and methodological foundations of Digital Forensics experimentation, situating the field within the broader tradition of empirical sciences. It discussed the persistent lack of reproducibility and transparency in DF research and outlined the core principles of controlled experimentation. The emphasis was placed on transforming forensic procedures, traditionally guided by intuition, expertise, or procedural standards, into replicable scientific investigations governed by hypotheses, variables, and evaluation criteria. This part also connected DF with the broader movement of Open Science, arguing that open data, open methodologies, and FAIR (Findable, Accessible, Interoperable, and Reusable) principles are indispensable for establishing cumulative and trustworthy forensic knowledge.

Part II represented the methodological consolidation of this vision by introducing conceptual modeling as a bridge between theoretical reasoning and empirical execution. The ExperDF-CM model proposed therein encapsulates the life cycle of controlled experiments in DF across five interrelated concepts: *Planning*, *Pre-Operation*, *Operation*, *Analysis and Interpretation*, and *Dissemination*. These stages operationalize scientific reasoning into reproducible procedures, ensuring that forensic experiments can be independently verified and accurately interpreted in their context. The model also functions as an educational and organizational tool, helping researchers and practitioners to articulate hypotheses, design protocols, and document findings consistently. By merging principles from software engineering experimentation, forensic methodology, and research ethics, ExperDF-CM creates a foundation upon which more sophisticated forms of empirical DF can be built.

Part III extended this structure into the semantic domain by presenting ontology engineering as a means to formalize and integrate forensic knowledge. Building upon the ExperDF-CM model, the ExperDF-Onto ontology provides a formal representation of entities, relationships, and processes involved in controlled forensic experimentation. It captures not only structural elements (such as artifacts, tools, datasets, and procedures) but also conceptual relations among them, enabling reasoning, validation, and automated query execution through SPARQL- and RDF-based representations. This semantic formalization transforms experimental documentation into machine-readable knowledge, facilitating interoperability between research projects, laboratories, and digital repositories. Together, ExperDF-CM and ExperDF-Onto form a complementary system: One prescribes how to conduct experiments; the other codifies and connects their outcomes in a structured knowledge space.

13.3 Critical Discussion

Despite the theoretical and methodological advances presented throughout the book, significant challenges remain for the full realization of an open and scientifically rigorous Digital Forensics. The first is cultural: DF has traditionally evolved as a practice-oriented discipline, grounded in law enforcement, cybersecurity response, and proprietary technologies. Moving toward an open, evidence-based research paradigm requires shifting from a mindset of procedural compliance to one of methodological reflection and critical thinking. Researchers and practitioners must be trained not only in technical procedures but also in epistemological reasoning, understanding the difference between evidence as data and evidence as scientifically interpretable information.

A second challenge lies in data governance and ethics. Forensic data are often sensitive, legally protected, or contextually bound to ongoing investigations. While Open Science advocates for transparency and data sharing, DF must reconcile these principles with the need to protect privacy, maintain chain-of-custody integrity, and safeguard the interests of individuals involved. Solutions such as synthetic datasets, anonymization techniques, and controlled access repositories represent promising avenues; however, they require institutional frameworks and shared standards that are still underdeveloped.

A third tension concerns the integration of conceptual and semantic modeling with real-world investigative workflows. The creation of ontologies like ExperDF-Onto depends on continuous dialogue between domain experts, data engineers, and legal professionals. Misalignment between terminological precision and operational reality can hinder adoption and reduce semantic consistency. Moreover, maintaining ontologies in dynamic environments, where technologies, threats, and laws evolve rapidly, requires sustainable governance and community-driven maintenance models.

Finally, there remains an epistemological question: ***Can digital forensics truly emulate the ideals of experimental science?*** While controlled experimentation enhances credibility, forensic phenomena often resist strict control or replication due to the uniqueness of digital incidents. This book argues that rather than imposing rigid scientific templates, DF should embrace a pluralistic approach, combining experimental design, case-based reasoning, and probabilistic inference, all under the overarching principles of transparency and reproducibility.

13.4 Implications and Contributions

The contributions of this book extend across theoretical, methodological, and practical dimensions.

Theoretically, it positions Digital Forensics as a legitimate domain of empirical investigation, capable of generating generalizable knowledge rather than isolated case reports. By connecting DF to the traditions of philosophy of science and experimental methodology, the book reframes the notion of digital evidence as a scientific construct, something that is produced, not merely found, through systematic observation and reasoning. It also contributes to ongoing discussions about the ontology of digital entities, causality in computational environments, and the epistemic status of digital traces as evidence.

Methodologically, the ExperDF-CM and ExperDF-Onto frameworks introduce structured instruments for documenting, reasoning, and sharing forensic experiments. These tools can be embedded into data management plans, laboratory workflows, or digital repositories, thereby aligning DF with broader practices of open and reproducible research. They also serve as didactic resources, helping students and early career researchers to internalize principles of scientific documentation and semantic rigor.

Practically, the implications are tangible for laboratories, judicial systems, and policymaking. Standardizing experimental design and documentation in DF can lead to more consistent expert reports, facilitate peer review of forensic methods, and strengthen the credibility of digital evidence in court. The semantic integration of experimental data also opens pathways for large-scale meta-analysis and knowledge discovery, enabling the identification of methodological patterns, error sources, and reliability metrics across studies. This contributes directly to improving the quality and accountability of forensic practice.

Finally, **socially and ethically**, the book underscores the importance of transparency, accountability, and inclusiveness in digital investigations. By promoting openness and methodological rigor, it aligns DF with the broader values of responsible innovation and trustworthy science, ensuring that the pursuit of truth in the digital realm respects fundamental human rights and societal expectations of justice.

13.5 Future Perspectives

The work presented here opens several avenues for future exploration. One immediate direction involves expanding the ExperDF ecosystem toward full interoperability with Open Science infrastructures. Integrating the ExperDF-Onto ontology with provenance ontologies, such as PROV-O, dataset metadata schemas like DataCite, and workflow vocabularies, like RO-Crate, could enable forensic experiments to be published, discovered, and reanalyzed across platforms. Another promising path lies in incorporating artificial intelligence into forensic experimentation. Ontology-driven AI systems could support hypothesis generation, automated consistency checking, and semantic inference, significantly accelerating the validation of forensic procedures.

A second direction concerns community building and governance. For ontologies and conceptual models to remain living artifacts, they must be maintained collaboratively through participatory and open processes. Establishing an international consortium or working group dedicated to the reproducibility of forensic experiments, similar to initiatives in empirical software engineering or bioinformatics, could ensure long-term sustainability and cross-disciplinary alignment.

A third perspective involves pedagogical transformation. Embedding the principles of controlled experimentation, conceptual modeling, and ontology engineering into forensic education would cultivate a new generation of professionals capable of designing scientifically sound investigations. Such integration could occur not only at the graduate level but also in continuing education and professional certification programs, bridging the gap between academia and practice.

Ultimately, the intersection of Digital Forensics and open science prompts reflection on broader societal implications. As digital evidence increasingly influences legal decisions, public policy, and social narratives, the epistemic robustness of forensic claims becomes a matter of democratic accountability. Ensuring that these claims are reproducible, explainable, and open to scrutiny is both a scientific imperative and an ethical responsibility. Future research should therefore engage with interdisciplinary fields such as philosophy of technology, computational ethics, and law, ensuring that DF remains anchored in human-centered and socially responsive principles.

13.6 Closing Message

This book closes with a vision of Digital Forensics as a science of integrity, one that integrates rigor, openness, and ethical consciousness. Its models and ontologies are not end points but stepping stones toward a more transparent, collaborative, and reflexive discipline. By aligning forensic investigation with the ideals of Open Science, it seeks to elevate DF from a reactive craft to a proactive science capable of self-correction, cumulative learning, and societal contribution. The pursuit of truth in the digital age requires not only better tools but also better epistemologies. In embracing structured experimentation, semantic modeling, and open collaboration, Digital Forensics can serve as both a guardian of evidence and a paradigm of scientific integrity. The spirit of this work can thus be summarized in a single conviction: The strength of digital evidence lies not in secrecy or authority, but in transparency, reproducibility, and shared understanding.

The manufacturer's authorised representative in the EU is Springer
Nature Customer Service Centre GmbH, Europaplatz 3, 69115 Heidelberg,
Germany. If you have any concerns regarding our products, please
contact ProductSafety@springernature.com

Printed and bound by CPI Group (UK) Ltd, Croydon, CR0 4YY
07/10/2026
02229351-0010

Acknowledgments

My sincere gratitude goes out to all those who contributed to the completion of this volume. Special thanks are due to Janet Kim and Dhivya Savariraj of Springer Nature for their attentive support throughout the publication process. I am grateful to Professor Dr. Ilse Derluyn, Dr. Floor Verhaeghe, Dr. Filiz Comez Polat, and all co-authors for their valuable contributions during the chapter review process. My thanks also go to Anne Bultinck for her meticulous and articulate assistance with the layout of this work.

I wish to thank the Belgian Science Policy Office (Belspo), Ghent University Special Research Fund (BOF), the Federal Agency for the Reception of Asylum Applicants (Fedasil), and the European Drugs Agency (EUDA), which have funded research projects throughout the past decade that feed into this volume, and the Research Foundation—Flanders (FWO) [12AFB24N-7028], which funds my current postdoctoral fellowship appointment.

Finally, I wish to acknowledge my colleagues at the Institute for Social Drug Research, in particular Professor Dr. Tom Decorte, Dr. Marthe Ongenaert, Angel Maginet, Herman Wolf and Tamie Wuytjens, for their ongoing support and collaboration.

I would also like to express my heartfelt gratitude to those cherished souls, both in professional and personal life, who embrace beauty, wisdom, strength, and vulnerability alike, with openness and a growth mindset—offering understanding, support, and respect. Thank you.

I am deeply grateful to the women who form my village—steadfast in support and solidarity. Thank you for standing together and sharing strength.

May 2026 Charlotte De Kock

analyses, intervention strategies and health system responsiveness in this field, this volume represents only a starting point for sustained engagement.

We hope this book informs and inspires researchers, practitioners, policymakers, and advocates working to improve health outcomes for refugees and displaced populations in Europe. To carry this commitment further, the book concludes with research and policy recommendations designed to guide ongoing work within the European Migration and Substance Use (EUMISU) research network, established in conjunction with this publication.

Ghent, Belgium Charlotte De Kock
May 2026

Preface

In a time of unprecedented global displacement, complex humanitarian crises, and ongoing human rights violations, *Substance Use Among Refugees in Europe* addresses a critically underexplored intersection between substance use and displacement in Europe. It is the result of a collaboration among more than thirty scholars across Europe.

I hope it stands as a meaningful contribution to the field—timely, comprehensive, and committed to fostering deeper understanding and collective action. After a decade of research on the migration–substance use nexus in Europe, I am deeply grateful to publish this work alongside so many dedicated co-authors.

As editor, I have sought to frame substance use within an ecosocial perspective inspired by Nancy Krieger's *Epidemiology and the People's Health*, underscoring how political, structural, social, and psychological determinants intertwine and manifest throughout displacement. Guided by a health equity and rights-based approach, contributors aim not only to avoid harm but to generate reciprocal benefit for the populations involved. This inevitably means that while attention to pre displacement factors is important, a focus on post displacement factors such as reception conditions and integration into society are key factors in reducing mental health and substance use-related problems among refugees and other displaced populations in Europe.

While research on the prevalence and more importantly aetiology of substance use remains one of the foundations that can inform logical models in intervention development, much more of it is still needed. Yet, prevalence studies alone are insufficient. The study of prevalence and aetiology must indeed be complemented by research on the effectiveness of prevention, harm reduction, treatment, and recovery approaches as well as the impact of context such as migration and integration policies—using multiple methods that include first-person perspectives and lived experiences. This combination, I believe, offers a fuller understanding of substance use as both a public health and social equity concern, demanding nuanced, inclusive, and context-sensitive responses.

Readers will find analyses of mental health vulnerabilities influencing substance use, barriers to service access, policy and research gaps, and pathways forward across diverse European contexts. As the first European collection to map situational from evidence in non-displaced settings and populations, and refugees may have specific needs not addressed by host populations or excluded from host population efforts. Population-specific understandings of substance use contexts and cultures are required to implement and monitor effectiveness of interventions. Documentation of underlying protectors and drivers such as hope and despair, strength of social supports, economic constraints and opportunities in illicit drug markets can assist in better understanding and improved program design.

Indeed, substance use disorders among refugees are doubly neglected. Few health and welfare systems are sufficiently resourced to meet population needs of host populations without the additional complexities of refugee population needs. Yet to date our policy and practitioner responses have been limited, and the evidence on which to base our responses is weak.

Substance Use Among Refugees in Europe is the first to comprehensively explore substance use among refugees in Europe and public health approaches. It is an important contribution to understanding substance use, substance use disorders, opportunities and challenges to implementing effective policy and practice. This book brings together evidence and thinking from diverse settings that have relevance for policy makers and practitioners. Most importantly it provides a basis from which to develop an emerging research agenda, within Europe and internationally. This edited volume book provides important insights that will inspire new collective research and intervention efforts. Readers should find it a catalyst to inquiry, reflection, and action.

October 2025

Nadine Ezard
National Centre for Clinical Research
on Emerging Drugs
University of New South Wales
Sydney, Australia

Foreword

Increasing global crises are forcing population movement at a scale never seen before in human history. Around 50 million people are currently seeking refuge in countries of which they are not citizens; a third of those are in Europe. These refugees, asylum seekers and stateless people must navigate loss of home and community, while securing safety, establishing livelihoods, and accessing basic rights in unfamiliar—and often unwelcoming—environments.

Within the dynamics of negotiating the displacement experiences, one issue remains persistently neglected: the place of alcohol and other substance use. While increasing attention is paid to health needs of displaced populations, substance use and substance use disorders remain largely overlooked.

This edited volume, *Substance Use Among Refugees in Europe*, signals an important development in scholarly inquiry. It brings together academic and practitioner exploration of substance use among a range of populations, and looks at a range of interventions to reduce harm and treat disorder.

Relationships between displacement, refugee status, substance use patterns, benefits and harms, and substance use disorders are complex, context specific and not well-described. Previous substance use disorder can be continued or exacerbated, and impact all other areas of health and wellbeing. New onset disorders can arise in the refugee setting. Trauma, particularly repeated trauma and trauma in early life, can underlie use disorders.

In some settings the formal recognition of refugee status and accompanying legal and social protections is associated with lower rates of substance use disorder than host populations. In other settings such as among undocumented migrants and statelessness or protracted displacement with limited rights to movement, the inverse might be observed. Harms related to use are typically exacerbated in contexts of poverty and social exclusion, and where access to services and supports are constrained.

Data for decision making (substance use patterns, affected ages and genders and minority sub-populations, harms associated with substance use, prevalence and incidence of substance use disorder) may be absent and challenging to collect in the context of dynamic situations of displacement. Interventions may be adapted

This book is dedicated to all those who have lost their lives to human rights violations—in war, in the waters of the Mediterranean, and in other rough seas. It honours, in particular, the children who were denied the chance to grow up and help build a more just world.

With solemn hope, I also dedicate this work to all humanity. It is our shared, enduring responsibility to pursue a more just and equitable world with clarity, strength, and determination—honouring those who have perished by securing a better future for all.

To my cherished daughter, the spark of my life—L.L.

Editor
Charlotte De Kock
Institute for Social Drug Research (ISD)
Department of Criminal Law, Social Law
and Criminology
Faculty of Law and Criminology
Ghent University,
Ghent, Belgium

ISBN 978-3-032-32398-9 ISBN 978-3-032-32399-6 (eBook)
https://doi.org/10.1007/978-3-032-32399-6

This work was supported by Research Foundation Flanders (FWO), Belgium, grant number 12AFB24N-7028.

This Springer imprint is published by the registered company Springer Nature Switzerland AG
The registered company address is: Gewerbestrasse 11, 6330 Cham, Switzerland

Charlotte De Kock
Editor

Substance Use Among Refugees in Europe

Emerging Research Directions From Social Epidemiology to Structural Prevention

Springer

Substance Use Among Refugees in Europe

Contents

Editor and Contributors

About the Editor

Charlotte De Kock, PhD is Visiting Professor in Criminology and senior researcher at the Faculty of Law and Criminology, Institute for Social Drug Research (ISD), Ghent University (Belgium). She teaches qualitative methods and critical criminology, and pioneered Belgium's first course on diversity and migration in criminology (Ghent University). Her research focuses on equitable and evidence-based substance use prevention, early intervention, harm reduction and recovery capital in migration contexts, as well as research ethics and critical criminology. Her work has been funded by the Belgian Science Policy Office, Research Foundation Flanders (FWO), the Federal Agency for the Reception of Asylum Applicants (Fedasil), Ghent University (Belgium) and the European Union Drugs Agency (EUDA). She is a deputy member of the Ghent University Board of Governors, the faculty diversity coordinator and the faculty representative in the Centre for the Social Study of Migration and Refugees (CESSMIR). Knowledge translation is a key thread throughout her work.

Contributors

Frederick L. Altice, MD, MA, is Professor of Medicine and of Epidemiology at the Yale School of Medicine (USA), where he also directs the Centre for Clinical & Community Research and the HIV in Prisons Program. His research investigates the interface between infectious diseases and substance use disorders—specifically HIV, TB, and hepatitis in populations with substance use disorders, including incarcerated individuals and key populations globally. He has led implementation-science and intervention studies across multiple countries (Ukraine, Malaysia, Peru, Kyrgyzstan, Armenia) to scale up evidence-based strategies such as medication-assisted therapies, integrated care and mobile health approaches.

Till Bärnighausen, MD, ScD, MSc, MSc, is the Alexander von Humboldt University Professor and Director of the Heidelberg Institute of Global Health at the Faculty of Medicine, Heidelberg University, Germany, and serves as Adjunct Professor of Global Health at the Harvard T.H. Chan School of Public Health (USA). His research focuses on establishing the causal impacts of large-scale global-health interventions (such as HIV treatment, HIV prevention, and childhood vaccination) on health, economic, and social outcomes, and on innovating health-system delivery and methods for applied population-based health research.

Miroslav Barták, PhD (Public and Social Policy), is a lecturer and researcher at the Department of Addiction, First Faculty of Medicine, Charles University and General Teaching Hospital in Prague, Czech Republic, and social worker. His research focuses on alcohol epidemiology, social problems, and, since 2007 also on migration and health. He leads several research projects, lectures to foreign doctors preparing to work in healthcare in the Czech Republic, and is currently working with colleagues on the EU PEACHD project, which focuses on brief lifestyle interventions for cancer prevention in people who have come to the Czech Republic from Ukraine since 2022.

Iwona Bielska, PhD, is an epidemiologist and health services researcher with experience in academic and government settings. She is an Assistant Professor at the Institute of Public Health at Jagiellonian University (Poland), and an Assistant Professor (Part-Time) in the Department of Health Research Methods, Evidence and Impact at McMaster University (Canada). Her research focuses on health care access and utilization patterns among vulnerable population groups. Dr. Bielska is leading the Polish-Ukrainian arm of the Lancet Commission on Health, Conflict and Forced Displacement's qualitative study and a project for WHO Poland on access to mental health and psychological support services among Ukrainian refugees.

Daniel J. Bromberg, PhD, is a postdoctoral researcher at Yale University (USA) whose work focuses on substance use disorders, HIV, incarceration and displacement, and global health implementation science. He has led and published studies on expanding access to medications for opioid use disorder in prison and post-release settings, and during conflict settings in Ukraine.

Jannet M. de Jonge, PhD, is a senior researcher at Amsterdam University of Applied Science (The Netherlands), research group Integrated Complex Care. She is also a trainer Motivational Interviewing and member of the Motivational Interviewing Network of Trainers (MINT Inc) and a mental health psychologist. Her research focuses on prevention and treatment of substance use problems, especially on applying motivational interviewing to special groups young people with a mild intellectual disability, comorbid mental health problems and minority groups. She leads several projects concerned with these topics.

Clara De Ruysscher, PhD, is senior researcher at the Recovery and Addiction research cluster of the Department of Special Needs Education at Ghent University (Belgium), as well as at EQUALITY//Research Collective of the University of Applied Sciences and Arts Ghent (Belgium). Her expertise is situated at the crossroads of mental health and addiction, as a large part of her research focuses on recovery in persons with complex mental health needs. By using action-oriented, ethnographic and co-creative research methods, she aims to place the lived experiences of persons in recovery at the heart of the evidence created.

Sergii Dvoriak, MD, PhD, DMSc, is a psychiatrist and addiction-medicine specialist who has worked in HIV/AIDS prevention and substance use treatment across Eastern Europe and Central Asia. He co-founded the Ukrainian Institute on Public Health Policy (UIPHP) and serves as its Head of the Board and Senior Scientist, where he has led the development of national protocols for treating opioid dependence and HIV-positive people who inject drugs in Ukraine. He has worked internationally—as a consultant to United Nations Office on Drugs and Crime (UNODC), and through collaborations with Yale University and other institutions—to advance opioid substitution treatment, harm reduction, and health-system integration in complex legal and policy environments.

Anna Dzielska, PhD, is a public health, health promotion and health education specialist, and Assistant Professor and Head of the Department of Child and Adolescent Health at the Institute of Mother and Child in Warsaw, Poland. Since 2020, co-Principal Investigator of the international Health Behaviour in School-aged Children (HBSC) study in Poland and a member of the WHO Childhood Obesity Surveillance Initiative (COSI). Active in scientific societies, including the EUSPR. Her research focuses on health behaviour change in children and adolescents, intervention design, and promoting youth participation in research and public health initiatives.

Thomas Heidenreich, PhD, is a psychologist and cognitive-behavioural therapist. Since 2006, he is a professor of Psychology for Social Work and Care at Esslingen University (Germany). Among his research interests are approaches for prevention of SU in various populations.

Mirrian Hilbink-Smolders, PhD, is an epidemiologist and health services researcher with experience in both academic and non-academic healthcare settings. She is a senior research staff member of the Integrated Complex Care research group at the Amsterdam University of Applied Sciences (The Netherlands). Her research focuses on assessing and improving mental health care, especially for hard-to-access and vulnerable populations dealing with complex health problems. Among her research interests are strategies to prevent substance use in young status holders. From 2018 to 2023 she was editorial board member of a monthly published scientific journal of the Dutch College of General Practitioners (NHG). Furthermore, she is member of a regional Health Care Complaints Commission in The Netherlands.

Esben Houborg, PhD, is a sociologist and associate professor at the Centre for Alcohol and Drug Research, School of Business and Social Sciences at Aarhus University, Denmark. His main areas of research are drug policy in a historical and contemporary perspective, criminological research particularly concerning law enforcement, sociological research in the areas of drug treatment and harm reduction, and urban studies of drug-related issues

Anna-Karin Ivert, PhD, is an associate professor in criminology at the Department of Criminology, Malmö University (Sweden). Her research concerns studies on how the social environment affects the development of criminality and mental health problems, as well as studies on collaboration in crime prevention.

Marion Laging, PhD, is a social worker with experiences in addiction aid and prevention. Since 2005, she is a professor of Social Work at Esslingen University (Germany) leading research projects with special focus on setting-oriented concepts of SU prevention, participation, and empowerment.

Corine Latour, PhD, has been the research leader of the Integrated Complex Care research group at the Amsterdam University of Applied Sciences (The Netherlands) since 2018. Her research focuses on biopsychosocial issues and consultative liaison psychiatry. She is a co-founder of the INTERMED consortium. She is a member of the scientific advisory board of the professional association for Caregivers & Nurses. Furthermore, she is a member of the Supervisory Board of Lentis GGZ.

Miriam Hedwig Lorenz, PhD, is a social worker (M.A.) with experiences in (international) youth work and care of immigrant families. She studied in Stuttgart and Esslingen, Germany, and is currently working as a research assistant in a participatory project with refugees while doing her PhD.

Mia-Maria Magnusson, PhD, is a police detective and holds a PhD in Criminology. She works part time for the police as a crime analyst and part time at Malmö University (Sweden) as a lecturer and researcher. Her research mainly concerns gang violence and drug markets.

Johannes Michalak, PhD, is a psychologist and cognitive-behavioural therapist. Since 2014, he is a professor of Clinical Psychology and Psychotherapy at Witten/Herdecke University (Germany). His research interests focus on mindfulness-based approaches, embodiment in psychological disorders and clinical approaches for underserved populations.

Benjamin M. Nikitin, BA, is a medical student at the Icahn School of Medicine at Mount Sinai (USA) and is actively engaged in interdisciplinary health research. His research interests include addiction medicine and HIV in several global health settings, including Ukraine, Peru, Malaysia.

Judith Noijen, MA, PhD candidate, is a senior quality and policy advisor at the Jellinek prevention department in The Netherlands, specializing in both substance use and behavioural addictions such as gambling and gaming. Since 2005, she has worked on the development, implementation, standardization and evaluation of preventive interventions. She focusses on building bridges between science and practice, aiming to translate research into effective prevention implementation. Judith represents prevention within the Academic Workplace Addiction related to the Amsterdam Institute for Addiction Research (AIAR) and the Innovation Lab Mental Health, Shift Left at Arkin/Jellinek. Judith is a certified national trainer of the European Prevention Curriculum (EPC) by the European Union Drugs Agency (EUDA).

Martina Novopacká, PhD, is a sociologist and criminologist, and an assistant professor teaching criminology, statistics, and research methods at Charles University and the University of Ostrava (Czech Republic). She also serves as Head of the Analytical Unit at the Ministry of Justice, where she leads research projects on criminal justice and evidence-based policymaking. Her research focuses on prison studies, substance use, and domestic violence.

Katarzyna Okulicz-Kozaryn, PhD, is a psychologist, assistant professor in the Institute of Mother and Child (IMC, Warsaw, Poland). Before joining IMC she was the Head of the Department of Public Education, Analysis and International Cooperation in the State Agency for Solving Alcohol-Related Problems (PARPA) and assistant professor in the Department of Public Health in the Institute of Psychiatry and Neurology (IPiN). She was the funding member and first treasurer of the European Society for Prevention Research (EUSPR). Her research focuses on risk behaviours among children and adolescents and alcohol use among pregnant women.

Klaudia Palczak, MA, graduated in sociology and political science and has over 17 years of experience in the field of substance use on the national and European level. She was head of the Polish National Drug Monitoring Centre. Since 2007 she's been working at the European Monitoring Centre for Drugs and Drug Addiction (EMCDDA), focusing on EU justice and home affairs, and the implementation of the EU migration and security agendas in particular. Most recently, she's been involved in research on migrants' access to drug-related health care.

Konrad Pędziwiatr, PhD, is Deputy Director of the Center for Advanced Studies of Population and Religion (CASPAR), professor in the Department of International Relations at the Cracow University of Economics (Poland) and coordinator of the Multiculturalism and Migration Observatory (MMO). Associate researcher in the Centre for Migration Research (CMR) at the University of Warsaw. Author of numerous publications on migrations, religion and ethnicity in the processes of migration, migration policy and the politicization of Islam in Europe and the Middle East and North Africa.

Benjamin Petruželka, PhD, is a Czech social scientist and addiction researcher whose work focuses on the epidemiology of substance use, drug policy and public health and the intersection of social disadvantage and substance use. His academic background includes doctoral studies in Addictology and master's-level training in Sociology from Charles University. He is currently a Research and Teaching Assistant at the Department of Addictology, First Faculty of Medicine, Charles University in Prague. Beyond academia, he regularly collaborates with government agencies and

NGOs, contributing to needs assessments for addiction services, cannabis regulation analyses and administrative and register data analysis.

Aline Pouille, PhD, is a postdoctoral researcher at Ghent University (Belgium). Her doctoral research explored substance use recovery through the eyes and lived experiences of persons with a migration background. Since then, she has contributed to various national and European research projects exploring the intersectional experiences and support needs of people in socially or structurally disadvantaged situations. Her work centres on topics such as peer support, addiction recovery, and healthcare in forensic settings, with a strong commitment to integrating experiential knowledge into both research and practice. She was involved in the European SEMID-EU project, which examined the service needs of people with a migration background who use drugs across Europe, applying a community-based participatory research approach.

Vladimir Rogalewicz, PhD, graduated in mathematics and statistics from Charles University, Czech Republic. At present he focuses above all on health systems research, tracing real-world patient pathways, quality indicators in healthcare, cost-effectiveness of health technologies, HTA, mapping and prevention of excessive drinking, and other public health issues. In the past, he was also interested in mathematical foundations of quantum theory, genetic resources of cultivated plants, chemical and biomedical engineering.

Mark Schlessinger, PhD, is Professor of Health Policy and Department Chair at the Yale School of Public Health (USA), a Fellow of the Institution for Social & Policy Studies at Yale University, and former Editor of the *Journal of Health Politics, Policy & Law*. His research investigates how public opinion, bounded rationality in medical decision-making, nonprofit health care organization roles, and the availability of provider information, shape health and social policy. He has contributed to major national and state-level health policy initiatives, consulting with federal agencies, numerous state governments, and nonprofit organizations.

Arash Setoodeh, PhD candidate, is a master in both Law and Migration Studies and a PhD fellow at the Center for Alcohol and Drug Research at Aarhus University (Denmark). His research interests focus on SU among irregular migrants and migration/drug policies. Arash has worked on the topic of the integration of marginalized migrants at both Copenhagen and Frederiksberg municipalities, on advocacy and migration policies at Danish Refugee Council, and on drug research at the Center for Drug and Alcohol Research at Aarhus University

Chico Taguba, MSc, RN, is a Professional Doctorate (PD) candidate at the Integrated Complex Care research group at the Amsterdam University of Applied Sciences (The Netherlands) and a practising mental health nurse. His doctoral research focuses on improving access to mental health and addiction prevention services for young adult refugees in the Amsterdam area.

Birgitte Thylstrup, PhD (master in Psychology), is an associate professor at the Centre for Alcohol and Drug Research, School of Business and Social Sciences at

Aarhus University (Denmark). Her main research areas are substance use disorders and mental health among youth and adults. Birgitte Thylstrup has a long record in prevention and treatment research, risk factors, related harms, marginalization, as well as psychopathology/dual diagnosis. She has worked in depth on developing an effective brief intervention for antisocial personality disorder tested in RCT, the Impulsive Lifestyle Program.

Jonathan Uricher, PhD, is a social worker and sociologist (MA) with experiences in addiction aid and SU prevention. He studied in Stuttgart and Heidelberg, Germany, and worked as a research assistant in a participatory project with refugees while doing his PhD. He is a research assistant at the Institute for Transcultural Health Science in Stuttgart.

Wouter Vanderplasschen, PhD, is associate professor and head of the Department of Special Needs Education (Orthopedagogiek) at Ghent University (Belgium). He is a senior researcher in the field of substance use treatment and recovery. For the past 20 years, Wouter Vanderplasschen has studied the accessibility, effectiveness and quality of care in substance use treatment and addiction recovery in general. His core research interests are vulnerable groups, recovery, case management, continuity of care, quality of life and evaluation of treatment. Recently, he was involved in international studies on continuity of care in and after prison ('My first 48 hours out'), recovery pathways of persons who use drugs in Belgium, The Netherlands and the UK (REC-PATH) and recovery capital among substance users with a migration background. Vanderplasschen has authored more than 150 publications in international peer-reviewed journals about addiction, treatment and recovery. He wrote several books and book publications and is a co-editor of the journal *Drugs: Education, Prevention, Policy*.

Michał Wanke, PhD, is a sociologist and an Assistant Professor at the Department of Cultural Studies of the University of Opole, Poland. He studies people who use drugs, especially cannabis in non-Western contexts. He also conducts research on migration, most recently as a postdoctoral fellow at the Cracow University of Economics in a Horizon Europe PREMIUM_EU project. He published in and guest edited international and Polish journals alike. He received funding from Erasmus+, National Science Centre in Poland and the Polish National Centre for Addiction Prevention. Dr. Wanke acts as an advisor to the Opole Province Self Government for Addiction Prevention.

Estera Wieczorek, PhD, is a public health expert and an Assistant Professor at the Department of Health Economics and Social Security at Jagiellonian University (Poland). She lived in six different countries across Europe and Asia, where she gained knowledge of the specificities of various health systems and cultures. Dr. Wieczorek has expertise in long-term care and care transitions of vulnerable patient groups. Her research focuses on the provision and financing of health and long-term care systems and their impact on care transitions and access to care. Beyond her academic work, she has supported refugees as part of a humanitarian response.

Chapter 1
Introducing the Emerging Research Domain of Substance Use among Refugees in Europe

Charlotte De Kock and Klaudia Palczak

1.1 Situating Refugee and Displaced Populations in Europe

At the time of finalising this introduction, ongoing conflicts such as the genocide in Gaza, instability in north-east Syria and Afghanistan, Sudan's escalating civil war, human rights violations in Venezuela and military coups in West Africa mark the global political arena. These are but some of the ongoing humanitarian crises and geopolitical drivers that shape displacement trends and migration flows in Europe. Indeed, these conflicts are directly reflected in the nationalities of those applying for international protection in Europe.

The highest numbers of applications in 2024 were from nationals of Syria, Venezuela and Afghanistan (European Migration Network, 2025), while total first-time asylum applications in the European Union (EU) and Norway decreased by 13% in 2024 compared to 2023. Historically, these fluctuations are influenced mainly by ongoing conflicts, regional political changes and events such as the displacement caused by the Russian invasion of Ukraine, which involved around 4.4 million people under temporary protection in the EU+ area in 2024.

On 1 January 2024, the total share of third-country nationals in the European population (EU and Norway) was 6.4% (29 million). Although the inflow of displaced populations in Europe is steadily decreasing and is relatively low compared to both total populations and to the uptake of refugees in countries neighbouring the countries of origin, migration has re-emerged as a politically salient and polarising topic across Europe. At the same time, much work remains to be done in the domain of health

C. De Kock (✉)
Faculty of Law and Criminology, Institute for Social Drug Research, Ghent University, Ghent, Belgium
e-mail: charlotte.dekock@ugent.be

K. Palczak
European Union Drugs Agency (EUDA), Partnerships and Innovation Unit, Lisbon, Portugal
e-mail: Klaudia.Palczak@euda.europa.eu

C. De Kock (ed.), *Substance Use Among Refugees in Europe*,
https://doi.org/10.1007/978-3-032-32399-6_1

equity for displaced populations in Europe, which is but one of the reasons why we decided that this book on substance use-related phenomena and needs is timely and necessary.

Despite growing research on refugee health and mental health, substance use among displaced populations in Europe remains poorly understood, under-researched and rarely addressed in policy or practice. This book argues that substance use related problems should be examined ecosocially as a product of the structural (macro), social (meso) and psychological (micro) pressures (De Kock, 2022) experienced before, during and after displacement. By situating substance use related problems within these intersecting contexts, the volume frames it as both a public health and social equity issue, calling for inclusive, evidence-informed interventions across European settings.

Throughout this book different terms are used to describe displaced populations, reflecting the disciplinary focus or empirical scope of each chapter. Authors refer to refugees, asylum seekers, undocumented migrants, non-nationals and persons with a migration background who use drugs (PMWUD).

Following the United Nations' definition, refugees are individuals who have been forced to live outside their country of origin due to a well-founded fear of persecution based on race, religion, nationality, membership of a particular social group or political opinion. In this volume the term 'refugee' is used in an analytical rather than legal sense: it encompasses all displaced populations—independent of their formal legal status—including asylum applicants, persons under temporary or subsidiary protection and those without documentation. This inclusive definition aligns with the book's broader aim to examine displacement and substance use through a structural and human rights lens, rather than through legal categorisation.

In what follows we will first describe mental health risks among displaced populations, followed by an insight into risk factors across migration phases, after which mental health and policy gaps for these populations in Europe will be discussed. The introduction concludes with a chapter overview.

1.2 Increased Mental Health Risks

Forcibly displaced populations are at risk of developing mental problems or disorders (Barbui et al., 2022) due to the stressors they are faced with pre-, during and post-migration. It is well established that there is a high prevalence of post-traumatic stress and related disorder (PTSD), depression and anxiety symptoms and disorders among conflict-affected populations (Charlson et al., 2019), refugees and internally displaced persons after forced displacement (Blackmore et al. 2020; Morina et al., 2018).

Giacco et al. (2018) found that, in the first years of resettlement, only PTSD rates are higher in refugees compared to host countries' populations. Five years after resettlement, rates of depressive and anxiety disorders also increased, drawing the attention to the importance of post-migration stressors. In later work, Giacco

(2020) identified critical time points for mental health that can inform the content and timing of prevention: before the travel, during the travel, at initial settlement in the host country, when attempting to integrate into the host country and, finally, when the immigration status is challenged or revoked.

Whereas PTSD is clearly related to increased risk of substance use (and related problems and disorders) among general populations, the nature and direction of this causal relation is less clear among displaced populations. In Sweden, Harris et al. (2019) observed in a nationwide cohort study that although PTSD diagnosis was over five times more common in refugees than in the Swedish-born population, it was more strongly associated with increased rates of substance use disorders in the Swedish-born population.

Cook et al. (2021) established that second-generation immigrants in Sweden are at increased risk of developing alcohol and drug use disorders, particularly if they have lower socioeconomic status (SES). Solfrank and colleagues (2023), in their study among 238 asylum seekers recruited in psychosocial and general medical outpatient clinics in Germany, pointed out that low educational level, lower sense of coherence and mental distress were associated with substance use disorders.

Although research on the prevalence of substance use (and related disorders) among refugees is scant in Europe, studies do indicate that the observed substance use and related disorders are lower shortly after arrival in Europe compared to general populations and that it increases under the influence of post-migration stressors and a new substance use culture, over time (De Kock & EUDA, 2022). Najdini and colleauges' systematic review and meta-analysis (2025) indeed indicates a higher risk of substance use among second compared to first migration migrants, particularly for drug use and among women for alcohol use. This trend has also been evidenced outside Europe and tentatively explained based on the healthy migrant hypothesis, cultural inoculation and deterrence theory (Salas-Wright & Schwartz, 2019). Increased substance use was hypothesised by Salas-Wright and Schwartz (2019) to be caused by the co-occurrence of discrimination, reception conditions and bicultural stress, which they combined in their theory of cultural stress. However, more studies are needed across European member states, focussing on these substance use trajectories and distinguishing between types of substance use (e.g. medication, illicit substances, alcohol) and related problems and disorders.

The evidence on elevated rates of PTS(D), depression and anxiety symptoms and diagnoses among displaced populations has important implications for understanding substance use-related phenomena. Mental health conditions and exposure to trauma not only increase vulnerability to substance use-related problems but also influence its forms and functions—ranging from self-medication and coping strategies to social adaptation in new environments, including new substance use cultures. At the same time, post-migration stressors such as uncertainty about legal status, isolation and discrimination, in combination with economic status, can exacerbate both mental distress and substance use transitions, creating mutually reinforcing trajectories. Understanding these interrelations requires a perspective that integrates mental health and substance use within the broader continuum of pre-, during—and post-migration experiences.

1.3 Determinants Across Migration Phases

Substance use transitions thus depend on a combination of pre-, during—and post-displacement factors at intersecting micro, meso and macro levels. Substance use disorders pre-displacement, for instance, likely predispose an individual to substance use disorders following displacement (Ezard et al., 2020).

Substance use may also have become a part of life to cope with war or to function in such conditions before displacement, in combination with the availability of substances in new drug markets nested in warfare economies, as documented in Ukraine, Syria and Afghanistan (Hall & Degenhardt, 2014; Molina-Fernández et al., 2025; Steenkamp, 2025). Additionally, displaced populations may initiate substance use in transit as a self-medication strategy (Thin et al., 2025) or because of (involuntary) involvement in drug markets (Daniel et al., 2022; Ivert & Magnusson, 2019).

Besides these pre—and during-migration factors, understanding how post-displacement factors potentially impact substance use transitions is key because these are the factors directly influenced by policy and intervention choices in European host countries. Andersen (1995) referred to these as 'mutable factors'—those health determinants that remain amenable to change, in this case, after displacement.

Several factors have been outlined as key drivers, such as parental PTSD among youth (Ludvigsson & Loboda, 2022; Nielsen et al., 2019), the relation between stigma and the avoidance of services, emotional distress, isolation and loneliness (Douglass et al., 2023), the combined effect of trauma and perceived discrimination (Salama et al., 2020), the housing situation (Horyniak et al., 2016; Szczepanikova, 2013) and unemployment (López-Atanes et al., 2025).

Indeed, migration and displacement in themselves are not consistently linked with substance use (disorders), but rather occur under specific combined circumstances (Elkholy et al. 2023). Subsequently, with an eye on understanding and developing appropriate interventions, it is important to not only focus on the prevalence of substance use (disorders), but prioritise understanding the reasons, contexts and triggers that underly substance use trajectories in specific populations. While these determinants reveal the complexity of substance use transitions, their implications can only be fully understood when positioned within the structural and policy environments of European health systems.

1.4 Mental Health Systems and Policy Gaps

1.4.1 General Health

Although it is widely accepted that migrant-inclusive healthcare policies are essential to ensure that all residents—regardless of legal status, nationality or language—can access timely, affordable and culturally appropriate medical care, health policies vary greatly across the European member states. Despite the aspiration to ensure Universal Health Coverage (Papanicolas et al., 2022), there is evidence of persistent inequalities between migrants and non-migrants in access to European (mental) healthcare services. Indeed, the conventional response to refugee health needs is to address acute and basic needs by means of urgent medical care, yet this often excludes mental health care (Bilican et al., 2025) or overcomplicates it administratively, thereby indirectly restricting access.

1.4.2 Mental Health

Language and communication barriers, overuse of emergency services, underuse of primary healthcare services, in-service discrimination and waiting lists are well documented in European mental health care (Lebano et al., 2020; Satinsky et al., 2019). Travel, translators, out-of-pocket payments and knowledge-related barriers in turn contribute to a mismatch between provided and required services (De Kock, 2022; Woodward et al., 2024). A recent study focussing on the barriers for Ukrainian refugees to health care access and continuity of care (Kardas et al., 2025), for instance, identifies waiting times, information barriers and high service costs as the main barriers for these populations. Strikingly, although these barriers to (mental) health care services for refugees and asylum applicants have long been documented in high-income European countries, little has changed over time (Nowak et al., 2022). Indeed, initiatives tend to remain at project levels, and as Savas (2024, p. 1) puts it: for refugees and migrants, it is still a matter of chance whether they will enjoy people-centred health care that adequately responds to their individual needs.

1.4.3 Substance Use Treatment

The structural inequalities and service barriers described earlier in the chapter intersect profoundly with substance use treatment (SUT) needs among displaced populations. Barriers such as limited entitlements to care, long waiting lists, communication difficulties and discrimination are not only obstacles to mental health services, but likewise prevent timely identification and treatment of substance use problems. In many European contexts, SUT remains administratively and institutionally separated from general or mental health care, resulting in fragmented pathways for displaced persons whose needs often cut across these boundaries.

Due to a large variation in monitoring client migration backgrounds in European substance use treatment (De Kock, 2021), there is scant knowledge concerning these populations in European specialised SUT. Nevertheless, because of the overlap between mental health and SUT, the aforementioned systemic barriers in mental health care are likely mirrored and magnified in the SUT domain.

Two European studies found similar results in Belgium and Germany concerning the characteristics of non-nationals in SUT. Significantly higher unemployment as well as unstable housing were documented in Belgium (De Kock et al., 2020) and Germany (López-Atanes et al., 2025) compared to national (or non-migrant) clients, implying different recovery needs for these populations in treatment. Moreover, the Belgian study on non-nationals in SUT observed that females with non-European backgrounds were almost absent in these services. Additional research points out the underutilisation of specialised SUT by migrant populations as well as the insufficient adaptations of SUT for them (Stylianopoulos et al., 2024; van Selm et al., 2023).

Considering these caveats in both research and policymaking, this book presents a first step in understanding substance use-related phenomena, needs and barriers across varying European contexts and among different displaced populations in Europe. Authors also identify ways forward in both policy and interventions. The included chapters describe case studies in the Czech Republic, Denmark, Germany, Sweden and the Netherlands, while three other chapters focus on the situation in Poland, a European country that has been significantly marked by large numbers of Ukrainian displaced populations due to the Russian invasion in 2022.

1.5 Chapter Overview

The chapters included in this volume collectively explore substance use phenomena, needs and intervention responses among displaced populations across different European contexts. Together, they illustrate how pre-, during—and post-migration experiences intersect with social, economic and policy conditions to shape substance use trajectories and related health outcomes.

Petruželka and colleagues (Chap. 2) analyse the relation between alcohol use, depression and sociodemographic factors in a sample of Ukrainian refugees in the Czech Republic. Their results highlight that the combination of depressive symptoms, economic hardship, being male and having a refugee status significantly increases the risk of alcohol use.

Setoodeh, Houborg and Theylstrup (Chap. 3) in turn present a policy analysis concerning substance use-related responses targeting undocumented migrants in Denmark. The authors triangulate data on the restrictive migration policies, legal impact and the day-to-day practice in deportation camps, prisons and open drugs scenes. They conclude by alerting that a human rights perspective on substance use-related responses for these populations is urgently needed.

Uricher and colleagues (Chap. 4) present their development and evaluation of a participatory prevention concept for hazardous substance use among refugees in shared accommodations in Germany. While the evaluation study did not find significant outcomes, the study did identify the housing situation (prolonged stay in shared accommodation) as a significant moderating factor in the intervention effectiveness and on substance use among the studied populations.

Nikitin and colleagues (Chap. 5) comparatively analyse the resilience of HIV prevention and treatment services for people who inject drugs in Germany and Poland—the countries with the highest Ukrainian refugee populations. The analysis comprises national policy documents and in-depth interviews with stakeholders. They conclude that a rapid policy response to scale up HIV-related services that account for at-risk populations with opioid use disorder is critical to meet the currently rising demand to avoid new HIV outbreaks.

Okulicz-Kozaryn and Dzielska (Chap. 6) present the evaluation of the Add Strength mental health support programme for Ukrainian war refugees in Poland. This intervention was aimed at increasing coping skills and reducing substance use, among other goals. Their pre-post analysis among 630 participants points at a reduction in substance use right after conclusion of the intervention in a small subsample. Their results suggest that structured psychological support potentially mitigates reliance on substance use as a coping strategy, thereby facilitating post-trauma adaptation and well-being, but further evaluation research is needed.

Wanke and colleagues (Chap. 7) also focus on Poland in a qualitative study aimed at identifying barriers to prevention, treatment and harm reduction as well as risk factors for substance use. Based on 28 semi-structured interviews conducted with professionals and refugees, the authors conclude that future strategies should prioritise the consideration of the unique needs, experiences and cultural contexts of alcohol users, youth and injecting drug users with Ukrainian backgrounds.

Ivert and Magnusson (Chap. 8) focus on mental health problems among unaccompanied refugee minors treated for substance abuse. They observe the underuse of child and adolescent psychiatric (CAP) clinics among participants in outpatient treatment in Stockholm, Sweden. Drawing on existing knowledge on the association between mental health problems and drug use, they advocate for more collaboration between SUT on the one hand and CAP clinics on the other.

De Jonge and colleagues (Chap. 9) report on two complementary studies in the Netherlands. They first identify barriers to substance use prevention and services based on a qualitative study among refugees and professionals. Second, they describe the cultural adaptation of a brief intervention based on motivational interviewing, with a focus on feasibility, cultural relevance and effectiveness, integrating the identified communication, knowledge, expectation, trust and organisational barriers.

Pouille and colleagues (Chap. 10) report on focus groups conducted within the framework of the SEMID-EU study undertaken in Amsterdam, Athens, Berlin and Paris. These focus groups targeted the identification of support needs of persons with a migration background who use drugs, availability and accessibility of services and recommendations to improve substance use treatment for PMWUD. They conclude that to improve outcomes for PMWUD, investment in accessible health and social care, culturally and linguistically accessible practices, outreach and harm reduction efforts as well as interdisciplinary cooperation are key.

De Kock (Chap. 11) presents a scoping review of substance use-related interventions implemented in European reception settings. Twenty-one interventions are described and their evaluation evidence rated. A large potential for upscaling professional training and prevention (such as Problem Management Plus) in the reception setting is reported. The chapter concludes by recommending the integration of substance use(rs) in inclusive mental health interventions and trials; prioritising prevention and early intervention; strengthening experimental evaluations; promoting knowledge and skills transfer across reception and treatment; use of digital tools as bridges towards services; and investing in structural and inclusive prevention infrastructures.

Taken together, the chapters in this volume offer a comparative and multi-level perspective on substance use among refugees in Europe, demonstrating the field's diversity and framing directions for inclusive policy and practice. This volume represents a time-specific snapshot of an emerging field. It is the first work that brings together knowledge in the emerging field of substance use-related phenomena and interventions among refugees as a result of the joint effort of over 30 scholars with diverse European backgrounds (Czech Republic, Belgium, Denmark, Germany, the Netherlands, Poland, Sweden and Ukraine).

The concluding chapter (Chap. 12) outlines directions for advancing research and policy making concerned with substance use among refugees in Europe, to be further developed within the European Migration and Substance Use research network (EUMISU), established alongside this publication.

Building on the empirical and conceptual groundwork presented in this volume, the proposed agenda spans intervention and implementation studies as well as social epidemiology, aetiology, sociology, criminology, and research ethics. In doing so, this collective effort responds to Greene and colleagues' (2024, p. 1) call to move beyond questioning the feasibility of providing substance use services to displaced populations and to instead promote their integration as essential components of humanitarian and public health responses. This volume and the EUMISU network thus represent a first step towards consolidating existing knowledge and catalysing future research and policy engagement in this rapidly evolving field.

Competing Interests The authors declare that they have no competing interests. The first author is funded by a postdoctoral fellowship from the Research Foundation—Flanders (FWO) [12AFB24N-7028].

References

Andersen, R. M. (1995). Revisiting the behavioral model and access to medical care: Does it matter? *Journal of Health and Social Behavior, 30*(1), 1–10.

Barbui, C., Purgato, M., Acarturk, C., Churchill, R., Cuijpers, P., Koesters, M., Sijbrandij, M., Välimäki, M., Wancata, J., & White, R. G. (2022). Preventing the mental health consequences of war in refugee populations. *Epidemiology and Psychiatric Sciences, 31*, e24. https://doi.org/10.1017/S2045796022000102

Bilican, S., Irfan, M., Cox, A., Salaets, H., Sabbe, M., & Schoenmakers, B. (2025). Access to mental healthcare for refugees, asylum seekers and migrants: An umbrella review of barriers. *BMJ Open, 15*(6), e096267. https://doi.org/10.1136/bmjopen-2024-096267

Björkenstam, E., Helgesson, M., Norredam, M., Sijbrandij, M., de Montgomery, C. J., & Mittendorfer-Rutz, E. (2020). Differences in psychiatric care utilization between refugees, non-refugee migrants and Swedish-born youth. *Psychological Medicine, 52*(7), 1365–1375. https://doi.org/10.1017/S0033291720005482

Blackmore, R., Gray, K. M., Boyle, J. A., Fazel, M., Ranasinha, S., Fitzgerald, G. & Gibson-Helm, M. (2020). Systematic review and meta-analysis: The prevalence of mental illness in child and adolescent refugees and asylum seekers. *Journal of the American Academy of Child & Adolescent Psychiatry, 59*(6), 705–714.

Charlson, F., Van Ommeren, M., Flaxman, A., Cornett, J., Whiteford, H., & Saxena, S. (2019). New WHO prevalence estimates of mental disorders in conflict settings: A systematic review and meta-analysis. *The Lancet, 394*(10194), 240–248.

Cook, W. K., Li, X., Sundquist, K., Kendler, K. S., Sundquist, J., & Karriker-Jaffe, K. J. (2021). Drinking cultures and socioeconomic risk factors for alcohol and drug use disorders among first-and second-generation immigrants: A longitudinal analysis of Swedish population data. *Drug and alcohol dependence, 226*, 108804.

Daniel, M. I., Oluwakemi, O., & Oluwasola, Y. V. (2022). Irregular migration, drug use and drug trafficking in sub-Saharan Africa; Libya and Nigeria. In I. Muenstermann (Ed.), *The changing tide of immigration and emigration during the last three centuries* (pp. 131–148). IntechOpen.

De Kock, C. (2021). Migration and ethnicity related indicators in European drug treatment demand (TDI) registries. *Journal of Ethnicity in Substance Abuse, 20*(3), 444–470. https://doi.org/10.1080/15332640.2019.1633549

De Kock, C. (2022). Equitable substance use treatment for migrants and ethnic minorities in Flanders, Belgium: Service coordinator and expert perspectives. *Substance Abuse: Research and Treatment, 16*, 11782218221097390. https://doi.org/10.1177/11782218221097390

De Kock, C., Blomme, E., & Antoine, J. (2020). Non-national clients in Belgian substance use treatment. *Drugs & Alcohol Today, 20*(2), 157–171. https://doi.org/10.1108/DAT-12-2019-0074

De Kock, C. & EUDA (2022). *Responding to drug-related problems among migrants, refugees and ethnic minorities in Europe*. European Union Drugs Agency. https://www.euda.europa.eu/drugs-library/responding-drug-related-problems-among-migrants-refugees-and-ethnic-minorities-europe_en

Douglass, C. H., Win, T. M., Goutzamanis, S., Lim, M. S., Block, K., Onsando, G., ... & Horyniak, D. (2023). Stigma associated with alcohol and other drug use among people from migrant and ethnic minority groups: Results from a systematic review of qualitative studies. *Journal of Immigrant and Minority Health, 25*(6), 1402–1425.

Elkholy, H., Tay Wee Teck, J., Arunogiri, S., Asaad, M. R., Baessler, F., Bhad, R. & Baldacchino, A. M. (2023). Substance use disorders among forcibly displaced people: A narrative review. *Current addiction reports, 10*(2), 341–352.

European Migration Network. 2025. Asylum and Migration Overview 2024. Available at https://homeaffairs.ec.europa.eu/news/asylum-and-migration-overview-amo-2024-and-statistical-annex-key-developmentsmigration-policy-2025-07-09en

Ezard, N., Manji, H., & Busse, A. (2020). Substance use disorders in conflict-displaced populations. In J. C. M. Mariani & K. M. Flaherty (Eds.), *Textbook of addiction treatment: International perspectives* (pp. 1463–1475). Springer.

Giacco, D. (2020). Identifying the critical time points for mental health of asylum seekers and refugees in high-income countries. *Epidemiology and Psychiatric Sciences, 29*, e61. https://doi.org/10.1017/S2045796020000539

Giacco, D., Laxhman, N., & Priebe, S. (2018). Prevalence of and risk factors for mental disorders in refugees. *Seminars in Cell & Developmental Biology, 77*, 144–152. https://doi.org/10.1016/j.semcdb.2017.08.003

Global Initiative Against Transnational Organized Crime. (2023). Ukraine's criminal ecosystem and the war: Ukrainian organized crime in 2022. In *Ukraine's patronal democracy and the Russian invasion: The Russia-Ukraine war* (Vol. 1, pp. 263–294). Routledge.

Greene, M. C., Busse, A., Ventevogel, P., Kane, J., & Ezard, N. (2024). Moving from feasible to essential: Progress and future directions for promoting the implementation of substance use services for forcibly displaced populations in humanitarian settings. *Addiction, 119*(3), 408–410. https://doi.org/10.1111/add.15869

Hall, W. D., & Degenhardt, L. (2014). Afghanistan has a sizeable problem with opioid use. *The Lancet Global Health, 2*(10), e557–e558. https://doi.org/10.1016/S2214-109X(14)70353-1

Harris, S., Dykxhoorn, J., Hollander, A.-C., Dalman, C., & Kirkbride, J. B. (2019). Substance use disorders in refugee and migrant groups in Sweden: A nationwide cohort study of 1.2 million people. *PLoS Medicine, 16*(11), e1002944. https://doi.org/10.1371/journal.pmed.1002944

Horyniak, D., Melo, J. S., Farrell, R. M., Ojeda, V. D., & Strathdee, S. A. (2016). Epidemiology of substance use among forced migrants: A global systematic review. *PLoS One, 11*(7), e0159134. https://doi.org/10.1371/journal.pone.0159134

Ivert, A.-K., & Magnusson, M.-M. (2019). Drug use and criminality among unaccompanied refugee minors: A review of the literature. *International Journal of Migration, Health and Social Care, 16*(1), 93–107. https://doi.org/10.1108/IJMHSC-12-2018-0074

Kardas, P., Mogilevkina, I., Aksoy, N., Ágh, T., Garuoliene, K., Lomnytska, M., Istomina, N., Urbanaviče, R., Wettermark, B., & Khanyk, N. (2025). Barriers to healthcare access and continuity of care among Ukrainian war refugees in Europe: Findings from the RefuHealthAccess study. *Frontiers in Public Health, 13*, 1516161. https://doi.org/10.3389/fpubh.2025.1516161

Lebano, A., Hamed, S., Bradby, H., Gil-Salmerón, A., Durá-Ferrandis, E., Garcés-Ferrer, J., Azzedine, F., Riza, E., Karnaki, P., & Zota, D. (2020). Migrants' and refugees' health status and healthcare in Europe: A scoping literature review. *BMC Public Health, 20*, 1039. https://doi.org/10.1186/s12889-020-09193-x

López-Atanes, M., Rosenkranz, M., Erkoreka, L., Recio-Barbero, M., Bari, M., Hiller, P., Penka, S., Lindert, J., Martens, M., & Schäfer, I. (2025). Special needs of refugees with substance use disorders from conflict-affected countries: A comparison with German-born individuals. *Social Psychiatry and Psychiatric Epidemiology., 60*(7), 1563–1572. https://doi.org/10.1007/s00127-025-02842-2

Ludvigsson, J. F., & Loboda, A. (2022). Systematic review of health and disease in Ukrainian children highlights poor child health and challenges for those treating refugees. *Acta Paediatrica, 111*(7), 1341–1353. https://doi.org/10.1111/apa.16133

Molina-Fernández, A. J. M., Ayllón-Alonso, E., & Mena-García, B. (2025). *Wars, substances and addictions: Perspectives and solutions from public health to a global problem*. PrePrints.org. https://doi.org/10.20944/preprints202504.2495.v1

Morina, N., Akhtar, A., Barth, J., & Schnyder, U. (2018). Psychiatric disorders in refugees and internally displaced persons after forced displacement: A systematic review. *Frontiers in psychiatry, 9*, 433.

Najdini, M., Mathieu, J., Shadili, G., Frigaux, A., Ménauges, M., Mouton, C., et al. (2025). Substance use prevalence among immigrants by generational status in Europe: A systematic review and meta-analysis. *Alcohol: Clinical and Experimental Research, 49*(7), 1381–1391.

Nielsen, M. B., Carlsson, J., Rimvall, M. K., Petersen, J. H., & Norredam, M. (2019). Risk of childhood psychiatric disorders in children of refugee parents with post-traumatic stress disorder: A nationwide, register-based, cohort study. *The Lancet Public Health, 4*(7), e353–e359. https://doi.org/10.1016/S2468-2667(19)30102-X

Nowak, A. C., Namer, Y., & Hornberg, C. (2022). Health care for refugees in Europe: A scoping review. *International Journal of Environmental Research and Public Health, 19*(3), 1278. https://doi.org/10.3390/ijerph19031278

Papanicolas, I., Rajan, D., Karanikolos, M., Soucat, A., & Marimont, J. F. (Eds.). (2022). Health system performance assessment: A framework for policy analysis. WHO.

Pouille, A., De Kock, C., Vander Laenen, F., & Vanderplasschen, W. (2020). Recovery capital among migrants and ethnic minorities: A qualitative systematic review of first-person perspectives. *Journal of Ethnicity in Substance Abuse*, 1–31. https://doi.org/10.1080/15332640.2020.1710700

Salama, E. S., Castaneda, A. E., Lilja, E., Suvisaari, J., Rask, S., Laatikainen, T., & Niemelä, S. (2020). Pre-migration traumatic experiences, post-migration perceived discrimination and substance use among Russian and Kurdish migrants—A population-based study. *Addiction, 115*(6), 1160–1171. https://doi.org/10.1111/add.14942

Salas-Wright, C. P., & Schwartz, S. J. (2019). The study and prevention of alcohol and other drug misuse among migrants: Toward a transnational theory of cultural stress. *International Journal of Mental Health and Addiction, 17*(2), 346–369. https://doi.org/10.1007/s11469-018-9955-0

Satinsky, E., Fuhr, D. C., Woodward, A., Sondorp, E., & Roberts, B. (2019). Mental health care utilisation and access among refugees and asylum seekers in Europe: A systematic review. *Health Policy, 123*(9), 851–863. https://doi.org/10.1016/j.healthpol.2019.07.009

Savas, S. T., Knipper, M., Duclos, D., Sharma, E., Ugarte-Gurrutxaga, M. I., & Blanchet, K. (2024). Migrant-sensitive healthcare in Europe: Advancing health equity through accessibility, acceptability, quality, and trust. *The Lancet Regional Health–Europe, 41*, 100905. https://doi.org/10.1016/j.lanepe.2023.100905

Solfrank, M., Nikendei, C., Zehetmair, C., Friederich, H. C., & Nagy, E. (2023). The burden of substance use and (mental) distress among asylum seekers: A cross sectional study. *Frontiers in psychiatry, 14*, 1258140.

Steenkamp, C. (2025). Captagon and conflict: Drugs and war on the border between Jordan and Syria. *Mediterranean Politics, 30*(3), 478–502. https://doi.org/10.1080/13629395.2024.992725

Stylianopoulos, P., Hertner, L., Heinz, A., Kluge, U., Schäfer, I., & Penka, S. (2024). Good practice in reaching and treating refugees in addiction care in Germany—A Delphi study. *BMC Public Health, 24*(1), 30. https://doi.org/10.1186/s12889-023-17446-1

Szczepanikova, A. (2013). Between control and assistance: The problem of European accommodation centres for asylum seekers. *International Migration, 51*(4), 130–143. https://doi.org/10.1111/imig.12006

Thin, S. M., Phanudulkitti, C., Zaw, M. T., Saengungsumalee, S., Sorofman, B. A., Theeraroungchaisri, A., & Kittisopee, T. (2025). Determinants of self-medication in immigrants: A systematic review. *Journal of Immigrant and Minority Health, 27*(2), 366–385. https://doi.org/10.1007/s10903-024-01256-8

van Selm, L., White, T. M., Picchio, C. A., Requena-Méndez, A., Busz, M., Bakker, I., Romero, D., Gayo, R. P., Pouille, A., & Vanderplasschen, W. (2023). Drug use and access to drug dependency services for vulnerable migrants who use drugs in the European Union: Consensus statements and recommendations from civil society experts in Europe. *International Journal of Drug Policy, 118*, 104087. https://doi.org/10.1016/j.drugpo.2023.104087

Walg, M., Rosenbusch, S., Bender, S., & Hapfelmeier, G. (2024). Unhealthy substance use among unaccompanied refugees in Germany. *Drugs: Education, Prevention and Policy, 31*(5), 584–594.

Woodward, A., Fuhr, D. C., Barry, A. S., Balabanova, D., Sondorp, E., Dieleman, M. A., Pratley, P., Schoenberger, S. F., McKee, M., & Ilkkursun, Z. (2024). Health system responsiveness to the mental health needs of Syrian refugees: Mixed-methods rapid appraisals in eight host countries in Europe and the Middle East. *Open Research Europe, 3*, 14. https://doi.org/10.12688/openreseurope.14631.1

Chapter 2
Ukrainian Refugees in Czechia: The Relationship between Alcohol Use and Motives, Symptoms of Depression, and Sociodemographic Factors

Benjamin Petruželka, Martina Novopacká, Vladimír Rogalewicz, and Miroslav Barták

2.1 Introduction

Migrants and forcibly displaced populations are heterogeneous and the links between migration, displacement, and substance use are complex (EUDA, 2023; Elkholy et al., 2023). Generally, there is a lower prevalence of substance use among migrants than among the population in the host country (EUDA, 2023). However, it does not mean that some migrants did not use substances before their arrival to the host country and were in need of care (EUDA, 2023). There are a number of risk factors that migrants and forcibly displaced people may experience that could lead to an increase in the prevalence of substance use (EUDA, 2023; Elkholy et al., 2023). These include unemployment and poverty, loss of family and/or social support networks, or the move to a cultural setting where substance use may be more socially tolerated. Other risk factors have also been identified, including adverse socioeconomic living conditions, traumatic experiences, low educational levels, family separation, family

B. Petruželka (✉) · V. Rogalewicz · M. Barták
Department of Addictology, First Faculty of Medicine, Charles University, Prague, Czech Republic
e-mail: benjamin.petruzelka@lf1.cuni.cz

V. Rogalewicz
e-mail: vladimir.rogalewicz@lf1.cuni.cz

M. Barták
e-mail: miroslav.bartak@lf1.cuni.cz

M. Novopacká
Faculty of Social Studies, Department of Social Work, Ostrava, University of Ostrava, Ostrava, Czech Republic
e-mail: martina.novopacka@osu.cz

C. De Kock (ed.), *Substance Use Among Refugees in Europe*,
https://doi.org/10.1007/978-3-032-32399-6_2

and socioeconomic status, work environment, stress, or social exclusion (EUDA, 2023; Elkholy et al., 2023).

With the outbreak of the war in Ukraine (24 February 2022), many inhabitants of Ukraine were displaced and some of them relocated to Czechia, and in this chapter we will focus on them. In Czechia, non-EU nationals predominate among foreigners, with Ukrainians clearly dominating. Slovaks constitute the largest group among foreigners from EU countries (CZSO, 2024). At the end of 2023, there were 573,976 Ukrainians living in Czechia (CZSO, 2024). Most of them came to Czechia due to the war, but Ukrainians made up a significant proportion of foreigners living in Czechia already before the war began (CZSO, 2024). The composition of the Ukrainian population, as well as any research on their alcohol use or mental health in the period before and after the outbreak of the war, are fundamentally incomparable (Barták et al., 2023). War refugees from Ukraine have been granted the same healthcare rights as Czech citizens, which paradoxically has put them in a better position than previous migrants (Dlouhý et al., 2022).

The size of Ukrainians refugee population has been relatively stable over time. A total of 90% of refugees since 2022 have repeatedly applied for an extension of the temporary protection (Červenka, 2024). Most refugees live in the three largest Czech cities with more than a quarter of refugees living in Prague (Červenka, 2024, CZSO, 2024). The population is relatively well educated, with a high proportion of university graduates (46%) (Červenka, 2024). The population is not gender-balanced; Ukrainian women (75%) significantly outnumber men (Červenka, 2024). Theory suggests that women may face a number of stressors (also mentioned above) such as high levels of social isolation, low socio-economic status, insufficient social support, and poor adaptation to the host culture, even if the host culture is relatively similar and there is already a Ukrainian community in the country (Dlouhý et al., 2022).

The socioeconomic situation is considered a risk factor for alcohol consumption among migrants, especially in the acute phase of displacement, and is one of the micro-level factors of vulnerability to substance use disorder among migrants (Elkholy et al., 2023). In terms of socioeconomic status, a 2023 survey showed that two-thirds of Ukrainian refugees in Czechia lived below the income poverty line, and the share of refugees with the lowest income (less than 50% of the median equivalent income) increased (Kavanová et al., 2023). Single parents are among the most vulnerable (Kavanová et al., 2023). The latest survey shows that two-thirds of people over the age of 15 are currently employed, almost 86% of working refugees have full-time jobs, just over a tenth have part-time jobs, and 3% are engaged in casual work (Červenka, 2024). However, uncertainty in the labor market remains a problem. Up to 58% of working Ukrainians have very insecure jobs. New workers are more likely to end up in poor working conditions. A third of them are not entitled to vacation, and a similar proportion can only find out shortly in advance whether they will have work (Kavanová et al., 2023). The share of refugees working in jobs requiring significantly lower qualifications was even higher in 2023 than in 2022. Sixty-one percent of refugees were underemployed, with older people, women, and new entrants to the labor market being the most affected (Kavanová et al., 2023).

The largest study on the mental health of Ukrainian refugees in Czechia was conducted relatively soon after their arrival (Kavanová et al., 2022). The survey revealed a fairly high prevalence of mental illness symptoms, 45% of refugees reported problems corresponding to at least moderate depression or anxiety (Kavanová et al., 2022). The self-evaluation of depression should be taken into consideration because of the high-stress burden assumed among those who have recently fled the war in their country (Mesa-Viera et al., 2022). In 2022, further research was conducted (Mazhak et al., 2024), when 52.7% of respondents rated their emotional and psychological status as fair, 26% as bad, and 7.7% as very bad. The share of respondents who reported using alcohol or other drugs to feel better about their situation was 22% (assessed as a little), 8.2% (moderately) and 3.1% (a lot).

Access to healthcare for Ukrainian refugees is relatively poor. Available evidence shows that 62% of Ukrainian refugees do not have a general practitioner (Kavanová et al., 2022). However, another researcher shows that almost three quarters (72%) of respondents have visited a doctor at least once, with the majority of them seeking medical assistance repeatedly (Červenka, 2024).

In the context of war-related displacement, Ukrainian refugees in Czechia face a combination of stress factors—cultural dislocation, economic hardship, and traumatic loss—which intensifies symptoms of depression and can influence problematic alcohol use. Research on alcohol use has increasingly recognized that sociodemographic factors affect not only consumption patterns, but also the psychological drivers underlying risky drinking (Cooper, 1994; Khantzian, 1997; Kuntsche et al., 2006). However, the literature has not yet systematically examined how these sociodemographic vulnerabilities intersect with motives for alcohol use, symptoms of depression, or alcohol use. The aim of this research was first to describe the alcohol use and its motives, symptoms of depression and sociodemographic characteristics of Ukrainian refugees in Czechia in two waves of the survey. Second, we focused on the relationship between alcohol use and motives, symptoms of depression and sociodemographic factors.

2.2 Methods

2.2.1 Data Collection

Data collection of the first wave took place in the second half of 2022 (Barták et al., 2023) and the second wave was carried out at the end of 2024. The same inclusion criteria were used in both waves, namely age above 18 years, being a Ukrainian refugee who arrived in Czechia after 24 February 2022, and willingness to take part in the survey based on informed consent. Participants were informed about the purpose of the survey, the possibility of withdrawing from the survey at any time, as well as about the option not to answer any questions if they are not comfortable with them. All the participants in both waves gave their informed consent, which was the first part of the research questionnaires.

Data collections were conducted online using Google (first wave) and Survio (second wave) questionnaires in the Ukrainian language. Czech language was used as a source text for translation into Ukrainian by bilingual speakers working with the research team. Convenience sampling was chosen for both rounds of the survey, as this was the only way to contact respondents in the case of this sensitive topic. Hence, no power analysis was performed during the preparatory phase, and the researchers focused on collecting as many responses as possible as the situation and conditions at the time allowed. Therefore, both data collections were carried out directly by the research team with support from members of the Ukrainian community, who helped distribute links to the questionnaire. In the first survey, respondents were recruited through the Institute of Postgraduate Medical Education, where language courses for Ukrainian health professionals were held, and through the authors' social contacts (Barták et al., 2023). For the second survey, the social media (Facebook) distribution of questionnaires was also used (however with very limited results). Both questionnaires included similar questions. All major data collection agencies refused to carry out the collection, citing bad experiences with collecting data from people from Ukraine. The reason given by the agencies is that people from Ukraine are afraid to report their data, even anonymously, due to concerns about maintaining their residence status. We were therefore unable to use the existing panel of Ukrainian respondents in the Czech Republic (the panel established by the Institute of Sociology, Czech Academy of Sciences) for our research. However, our data collection showed that the agencies' concerns may be ungrounded and that respondents can be found for this type of research. This possible limitation in data collection with regard to certain topics may be important information for further research in the field in Czechia.

2.2.2 Measures

We used measures in three areas: alcohol use, symptoms of depression, and sociodemographic status.

Alcohol use in the last 12 months was measured using the alcohol screening instrument AUDIT (Alcohol Use Disorders Identification Test) (Babor et al., 2001). For the descriptive analysis of both waves, we used the following categories of alcohol risk consumption: likelihood of alcohol dependence (score of 20 or more points), hazardous or harmful alcohol consumption (score of 8–19 points), low risk (score of 0–7 points), and in the second wave we used actual exact scores for the in-depth analysis. To evaluate the reasons for alcohol use, we used the Modified Drinking Motives Questionnaire (Gavrilova et al., 2021). In the second wave, specifically, we constructed four categories of drinking motives—Social, Coping, Conformity, and Enhancement—based on Kážmér et al. (2024). These indices were computed by summing the items assigned to each domain in accordance with their validated factor structure. Furthermore, we present only selected items from the Modified Drinking Motives Questionnaire for both waves in the descriptive analysis because there were missing data for some questions in the first wave. Respondents were also asked about changes in alcohol use after their arrival in Czechia.

BDI—Beck Depression Inventory (Jackson-Koku, 2016) was used to provide participants' self-estimation of characteristic attitudes and symptoms of depression. For the descriptive analysis of both survey waves, we used categories (severe depression (score of 29 or more), moderate depression (score of 20–28), mild depression (score of 14–19), minimal depression (score of 0–13), and we used the actual exact scores for the in-depth analysis in the second wave.

The socio-demographic data included gender, age (categorized for the descriptive analysis), and employment status. For the purposes of in-depth analysis of data from the second wave, financial hardship was coded dichotomously, with 1 indicating respondents who reported that it was difficult or very difficult to make ends meet, and 0 indicating respondents who reported that it was easy or very easy.

2.2.3 Statistical Analysis

Descriptive statistics were calculated for both waves of data collection to summarize the sample characteristics. In-depth analyses were performed on the dataset from the second wave using SPSS and Microsoft Excel.

Pearson's zero-order correlations were calculated to explore associations among AUDIT total scores, BDI total scores, and the four drinking motive indices. Differences in alcohol use, symptoms of depression, and motive scores by gender were examined using one-way analysis of variance (ANOVA).

Finally, hierarchical multiple regression analysis was conducted to predict AUDIT total scores. In the first step, demographic covariates (gender, age, financial hardship), symptoms of depression (BDI total), and the four motive indices were entered as predictors. In the second step, interaction terms were included to assess moderation effects: specifically, interactions between symptoms of depression and each drinking motive, as well as between symptoms of depression and gender, and between financial hardship and gender.

2.3 Results

2.3.1 Two Waves of Research among Ukrainian Refugees

Table 2.1 shows characteristics of the samples from both waves. Data in both waves were collected mainly with help of the Ukrainian community members. The data from the first wave were collected closer to the outbreak of the conflict (2022), while the data from the second wave were collected later (2024). In terms of gender, the results are largely comparable. The second wave sample included a higher proportion of respondents from younger age categories, more respondents had a paid job and experienced less financial hardship.

In the second wave, the lower proportion of respondents was in higher risk alcohol consumption groups and depression. However, in the second wave, a higher proportion of respondents reported drinking slightly more. The motive of alcohol use "to forget your worries" (coping motive) and "because I like the feeling" (en-hancement motive) were more prevalent among respondents in the first wave. Conformity ("because your friends pressure you to drink") and social motives ("as a way to celebrate") were more prevalent among respondents in the second wave.

2.4 Patterns of Alcohol Use and Depression in the Second Wave: The Role of Drinking Motives and Intersectional Factors in a Ukrainian Refugee Sample

2.4.1 *Sample Characteristics*

While the data from the first wave were collected at a time when respondents were experiencing extraordinary stress (related to their immigration to Czechia and to consequences of the new outbreak of the conflict in Ukraine), the second wave took place under more stable conditions (if one can say that). This made it possible to collect a significantly larger number of completed questionnaires that could then be analyzed in greater detail. We will return to this issue in Discussion.

The sample consisted predominantly of women (77.8%, $n = 140$; see Table 2.2) which is in line with findings of Spurný & Tabery (2025). The average age of participants was 36.5 years ($SD = 11.1$), with women slightly older than men (37.0 vs. 34.5 years). When asked to evaluate their financial situation, 63.2% of respondents reported no difficulty, while 36.8% experienced financial hardship. The distribution was comparable across gender groups, showing no statistically significant differences.

2.4.2 *Patterns of Alcohol Use, Depression and Gender*

The analysis using the Alcohol Use Disorders Identification Test (AUDIT) revealed significant gender differences in alcohol-use severity. Men reported notably higher mean AUDIT scores ($M = 6.0$, $SD = 6.4$) compared to women ($M = 2.6$, $SD = 2.8$), with a medium effect size ($r = 0.27$, $p < 0.001$). Post-migration drinking behavior also differed by gender: 26.5% of men reported increased alcohol consumption following their displacement, versus 19.5% of women. Social motives were most frequently

Table 2.1 Characteristics of samples from both waves of research

Variables		First wave		Second wave	
		N	%	N	%
Gender	Female	49	74%	140	77%
	Male	17	26%	40	22%
	Other	0	0%	2	1%
Age	18–35	23	35%	72	46.2%
	36–45	25	38%	48	30.8%
	46–55	13	20%	29	18.6%
	55 and older	5	7.6%	7	4.5%
Employment	Paid job in Czechia	30	45%	108	59.3%
Financial hardship	Strongly agree	14	21%	12	6.6%
	Agree	24	36%	103	56.6%
	Disagree	19	29%	46	25.3%
	Strongly disagree	9	14%	4	2.2%
AUDIT	Likelihood of alcohol dependence	3	5%	2	1%
	Hazardous or harmful alcohol consumption	8	12%	17	9%
	Low risk	55	83%	163	90%
Beck depression inventory	Severe depression	1	1%	0	0%
	Moderate depression	9	14%	15	8.2%
	Mild depression	21	32%	40	22%
	Minimal depression	35	53%	127	69.8%
Change in drinking frequency after entering Czechia	Drinking less	28	42%	44	26%
	Roughly the same	33	50%	90	54%
	Drinking more	5	8%	35	20%
Selected motives of drinking (almost never/ never)	To forget my worries	25	38%	104	57%
	Because your friends pressure you to drink	55	83%	84	48%
	Because I like the feeling	21	32%	110	63%
	As a way to celebrate	8	12%	40	22%

Table 2.2 Second wave of research (totals and results of rank-biserial correlation)

	Total (n = 180)		Female (n = 140)		Male (n = 40)		Effect Size
	N	%/M(SD)	N	%/M(SD)	N	%/M(SD)	U/Eta
Age	180	36.5 (11.1)	140	37.0 (11.0)	40	34.5 (11.4)	Ns
Employment status Student Employed Unemployed	11 120 17	7.4 85.7 11.5	8 94 15	6.8 80.3 12.8	3 22 4	10.3 75.8 13.7	Ns
Financial hardship No Yes	115 67	63.2 36.8	87 53	62.1 37.9	26 14	65 35	Ns
ALCOHOL CONSUMPTION							
AUDIT score	180	3.3 (4.2)	140	2.6 (2.8)	40	6.0 (6.4)	0.27***
Change in drinking frequency after entering **Czechia** More Less No change	35 44 90	20.1 26.1 53.3	26 31 76	19.5 23.3 58.0	9 12 13	26.5 35.3 38.2	0.22**
DRINKING MOTIVES							
Coping	180	0.64(0.8)	140	0.66(0.8)	40	0.57(0.8)	Ns
Enhancement	180	0.71 (0.89)	140	0.54(0.7)	40	0.66(0.6)	Ns
Social	180	1.07 (0.93)	140	0.81(0.7)	40	0.85(0.6)	Ns
Conformity	180	0.21 (0.47)	140	0.26(0.5)	40	0.28(0.4)	Ns
DEPRESSION							
BDI categories							
Minimal depression	127	69.8	93	66.4	33	82.5	0.12*
Mild depression	40	22.0	33	23.6	6	15.0	
Moderate depression	15	8.2	14	10.0	1	2.5	
BDI total scale	180	8.0(7.9)	140	8.9(8.1)	40	5.1	0.24***

Note. ns-p-values were not significant at alfa of 5%

endorsed overall (M = 1.07), followed by enhancement (M = 0.71), coping (M = 0.64), and conformity (M = 0.21). While men showed a descriptive trend toward higher scores in enhancement motives (p = 0.070), formal comparisons using the Mann–Whitney U test (biserial correlation test) revealed no statistically significant gender differences across any of the four motive domains. Despite the aforementioned alcohol use, only 1.1% of respondents reported being ever offered professional support for alcohol-related issues.

The mood was within the normal range in 70% of participants (Table 2.2). Mild depression was more prevalent among women (23.6%) than men (15.0%), while moderate depression was reported by 10.0% of women and only 2.5% of men. The average BDI-II scores further confirmed these trends: women had significantly higher depression scores on average ($M = 8.9$, $SD = 8.1$) than men ($M = 5.1$), with a moderate effect size ($r = 0.24$, $p < 0.001$).

2.4.3 Relation between Symptoms of Depression, Alcohol Use and Alcohol Use Motives

Zero-order correlation analyses revealed significant associations between alcohol use motives, alcohol use, and symptoms of depression (Table 2.3). Both coping ($r = 0.445$, $p < 0.01$) and enhancement motives ($r = 0.551$, $p < 0.01$) demonstrated strong positive correlations with AUDIT scores, indicating that individuals who drink to manage negative emotions or enhance positive feelings are more likely to exhibit problematic alcohol use. Social motives showed a moderate association with AUDIT scores ($r = 0.349$, $p < 0.01$), while conformity motives were only weakly correlated ($r = 0.174$, $p < 0.05$).

The relationship between symptoms of depression and alcohol use was modest but statistically significant ($r = 0.196$, $p < 0.01$). BDI-II scores were most strongly correlated with coping motives ($r = 0.445$, $p < 0.01$), followed by social ($r = 0.218$, $p < 0.01$) and enhancement motives ($r = 0.224$, $p < 0.05$). No significant correlation was observed between symptoms of depression and conformity motives.

Table 2.3 Zero-order correlations among AUDIT total, BDI total, and drinking-motive indices ($n = 180$)

Variable	r (AUDIT)	r (BDI-II)
AUDIT Total score	—	0.196**
BDI-II Total score	0.196**	—
Coping motives	0.445**	0.445**
Enhancement motives	0.551**	0.550***
Social motives	0.349**	0.218*
Conformity motives	0.174*	0.174*

Note. Values represent Pearson's zero-order correlations. Significance: $p < 0.05$*, $p < 0.01$**, $p < 0.001$.***; BDI-II = Beck Depression Inventory-II; AUDIT = Alcohol Use Disorders Identification Test

2.4.4 Drinking Motives and Intersectionality as Moderators in the Depression–Problematic Drinking Relationship

In the first step of modeling, we entered demographic data, symptoms of depression, and the four motive scales. This block accounted for just over 40 percent of the variance in AUDIT scores, with coping and pleasant-feeling motives emerging as the strongest risk factors and male gender associated with lower alcohol-use severity. In the second step, we added interactions between depression and each motive, as well as between depression and gender, and between hardship and gender. The inclusion of these product-term interactions significantly improved the model fit. Notably, the link between financial hardship and problematic drinking was accentuated among men, whereas the association between symptoms of depression and alcohol problems was more pronounced among women. No interactions between depression and drinking motives proved significant (Table 2.4).

Note ns-p-values were not significant at alfa of 5%.

Table 2.4 Hierarchical linear regression predicting AUDIT scores (n = 140)

	Model 1				Model 2			
Predictor	B	SE	β	p	B	SE	β	p
Constant	4,1	1,05	-	***	5.05	1.17	-	***
Gender (1 = female)	−2,9	0.6	−0.3	***	−2.7	0.85	−0.3	**
Age	−0.02	0.02	−0.05	Ns	−0.02	0.02	−0.07	Ns
Depression (BDI)	0.07	0.04	−0.13	Ns	0.22	0.11	0.46	*
Hardship	−1.1	0.6	−0.12	Ns	−3.9	1.17	−0.43	***
Social motives	0.63	0.4	0.15	Ns	−0.1	0.51	−0.03	Ns
Coping motives	0.96	0.30	0.23	**	1.6	0.5	0.37	**
Conformity motives	−1.18	0.63	−0.15	Ns	−1.8	1.16	−0.23	Ns
Enhancement motives	1.31	0.37	0.29	***	0.7	0.61	0.16	Ns
Gender × hardship	-	-	-	-	3.6	1.3	0.36	**
Gender × BDI	-	-	-	-	−0.28	0.1	−0.58	**
BDI × social motives	-	-	-	-	0.08	0.05	0.35	Ns
BDI × conformity motives	-	-	-	-	0.02	0.08	0.06	Ns
BDI × coping motives	-	-	-	-	−0.05	0.03	−0.2	Ns
BDI × enhancement motives	-	-	-	-	0.04	0.05	0.13	Ns
R^2	0.416				0.513			
F	13.01				10.54			
p	***				***			

2.5 Discussion

We identified risk factors that increase the risk of alcohol use among Ukrainian refugees. These include motives for drinking alcohol, symptoms of depression, and financial hardship. This is consistent with the literature showing that socioeconomic living conditions and mental health influence substance use among migrants (EUDA, 2023; Elkholy et al., 2023).

The results show significant developments over the two years in which the surveys were conducted. The second wave showed a lower proportion of respondents reporting higher risk alcohol use and, at the same time, higher proportion of respondents reporting that they drink more since arriving in Czechia. We should consider explanations for this shift to less risky but increasing alcohol use compared to the situation before arriving in Czechia and shortly after it.

Respondents' motives shifted towards social related motives of alcohol use. While in the first wave respondents reported more motives related to coping with problems and enhancement, in the second wave respondents reported more social motives and motives related to conformity. The relationship between alcohol use risk and motives is confirmed by the findings of the second wave, which showed that coping and enhancement motives have a stronger influence on AUDIT scores than social motives and conformity-related motives. Other studies focusing on migrants from different backgrounds also mention the importance of coping motives (Cano et al., 2017; Horyniak et al., 2016). This suggests that, at the beginning, the respondents coming to Czechia were more influenced by their difficult situation (immediate exposure to outbreak of the war and related stress, changes in socioeconomic situation, and migration) and used alcohol to cope with it, while later their situation improved. Respondents in the second wave reported less serious symptoms of depression. The second wave included more respondents who reported having a paid job and being more satisfied with their financial situation, indicating adaptation to the labor market in the country. Similar results were shown by the PAQ Research survey (PAQ, 2024); however, it is important to note that integration has not been that successful in other aspects.

With a high degree of caution, changes in alcohol use patterns among migrants can also be a consequence of acculturation into Czech society, which would be consistent with research of Czaderny (2025). The refugees may have adapted to the culture in Czechia, which is characterized by social aspect of alcohol drinking (Petruželka et al., 2025).

These results may also have been influenced by the non-representative sampling procedure and a low number of responses mainly in wave 1, when some refugees may have been afraid of possible misuse of provided information, e.g., in proceedings for the granting of a visa for the purpose of toleration. While topics such as the labor market, housing, knowledge of Czech, and children's education are regularly surveyed among people from Ukraine, questions concerning alcohol consumption are not included in these surveys (see Spurný & Tabery, 2025). However, some sociodemographic characteristics of the sample did not change over time, suggesting that the samples are comparable. The differences may reflect the improvement in the situation of Ukrainians. The second wave sample included more respondents, who reported having paid employment and being more satisfied with their financial situation, indicating adaptation to the country's labor market. Similar results were shown by PAQ Research (PAQ, 2024).

Despite risky alcohol consumption among some respondents, only 1.1% of respondents reported that they had ever been offered professional help or intervention in connection with alcohol problems in Czechia. This is in line with the literature (Dlouhý et al., 2022) and other sources cited in the Introduction, which suggest that migrants may have difficulties accessing healthcare and other services.

The results of the analysis highlight the importance of symptoms of depression and coping and enhancement motives in driving risky alcohol use and underscore the importance of focusing on these motives in interventions targeting Ukrainian refugees. Pinto et al. (2022) found in their research that drinking motives differed among foreign workers, with positive motives (enhancement and social) and coping being more common among business expatriates; however, this research was conducted in different countries and in an environment that was not affected by war, as is the case with Ukrainian refugees in Czechia.

The findings underscore gender differences in both the frequency of alcohol use and the riskiness of consumption. Women reported more symptoms of depression, while men reported more hazardous drinking. After arriving in Czechia, a higher proportion of men than women reported an increase in alcohol consumption. The motives for drinking were largely the same for both sexes, with no statistically significant differences. This suggests that although the drinking severity differed by gender, the underlying motivating factors were essentially comparable for men and women. However, some different aspects influenced men and women. For men, the link between financial hardship and problematic drinking was emphasized, while for women, the association between symptoms of depression and alcohol problems was more pronounced.

The results of hierarchical regression analysis as a whole demonstrate that drinking motives and social factors moderate the depression–alcohol misuse link in distinct ways. Coping and enhancement motives remain strong predictors of AUDIT scores, even after accounting for intersectional interactions, with gender moderating and amplifying the impact of depression and hardship on drinking risk. Moderation analyses conducted by Cano et al. (2017) showed that immigration-related stress influenced the severity of alcohol use in men, but not in women, and that social support mitigated this stress.

There may be several reasons for the negligible proportion of respondents who were offered brief interventions. The first is the generally low amount of brief interventions provided by primary care providers in the Czech Republic for substance use, which is a long-standing issue (see, for example, Kabíček et al., 2010). It is also necessary to take into account that, unlike smoking cessation counseling, alcohol counseling is not covered additionally and separately, so there is no financial incentive for healthcare professionals to provide counseling on alcohol use. Last but not least, people from Ukraine very often face acute problems rather than prevention of non-communicable diseases, including addiction, unless addiction is the reason why they visit their general practitioner. Furthermore, the health care and its availability for this group might be considered low, and thus receiving brief intervention might be less frequent (Kavanová et al., 2022).

The main limitation of this research is the sampling and data collection. The data were collected online which means that people without access to these technolo-gies or not being able to use them were excluded. We also used convenience sampling which might have led to under or over sampling of certain groups, for example, people experiencing homelessness who are at higher risk of addiction-related issues. The convenience sampling is less reliable than representative sampling. Furthermore, the waves were not collected on the same sample which would allow to measure the change more reliably at the individual level, and this presents limitation of our data. We measure two populations which most likely changed over time. However, our aim was to capture this change. Moreover, we were unable to measure how many refugees received the questionnaire and what percentage of them responded, which could of course have led to sampling bias. There are no strictly representative studies conducted in Czechia, nevertheless, some research (see Spurný & Tabery, 2025) are based on panel data. The so-called panel of the Institute of Sociology of Czech Academy of Sciences was created in cooperation with the Ministry of Labor and Social Affairs of the Czech Republic (MPSV). Recruitment for the panel was conducted from among applicants for humanitarian benefits (HuD). All Ukrainian refugees over the age of 18 who arrived in the Czech Republic after the start of the war in Ukraine on February 24, 2022, and who applied for HuD between March and May 2022, were registered with the MPSV. The MPSV contacted HuD applicants with an offer to join the panel. In the next phase, the panel was supplemented in cooperation with the Ministry of the Interior of the Czech Republic (MV). During online registration for the extension of temporary protection in the first quarter of 2023 and 2024, Ukrainian refugees were offered the opportunity to join the panel (see Spurný & Tabery, 2025). The administrators of the panel of Ukrainian households in the Czech Republic (which is the best source of the data) stated that they were unable to collect data on sensitive topics such as alcohol consumption. This points to another limitation of our data, namely that respondents may be suspicious of official authorities, because they are assessed by the Czech state when applying for temporary protection. This mistrust may have affected their willingness to participate in the survey, and thus the final sample. Furthermore, it may also have affected their willingness to answer questions about health and other sensitive topics accurately. We were able to reduce this mistrust through cooperation with representatives of the Ukrainian community. However, it is possible that the willingness of people with mental health and addiction issues to participate might have been lower and willingness to answer questions acutely have been also influenced and led to underestimation of health-related behavior. In previous research among this group (Barták et al., 2023), some respondents expressed the opinion that this questionnaire is more suitable for people with addictions problems. This also points to the potential stigmatization of this issue among refugees.

2.6 Conclusion

The results show that the situation of Ukrainian refugees may have improved in terms of risky alcohol use and symptoms of depression. However, there are respondents who are at a greater risk and need interventions that are not readily available to them. In this regard, we can recommend brief interventions, which could be a good starting point for vulnerable individuals. Furthermore, we recommend working on the general accessibility of health and social services and on social inclusion. The results showed significant differences within the refugee population. The combination of financial hardship, male gender and refugee status increases the risk of alcohol use, and the combination of female gender, refugee status and symptoms of depression has a similar effect. This needs to be taken into account when planning and providing any interventions.

Competing Interests
The authors declare that they have no competing interests.

Funding This study was funded by Office of the Government of the Czech Republic in 2024, grant no. N-00-20 in 2024, Cooperatio program of Charles University, scientific field Health Sciences (HEAS) in 2022, Cooperatio program of Charles University, scientific field Health Sciences (HEAS) in 2025, and the European Union under the REFRESH - Research Excellence For Region Sustainability and High-tech Industries project number CZ.10.03.01/00/22_003/0000048 via the Operational Programme Just Transition.

References

Babor, T., Higgins-Biddle, J., Monteiro, M., & Saunders, J. (2001). *Audit—The alcohol use disorders identification test: Guidelines for use in primary care*. World Health Organization.

Barták, M., Petruželka, B., Ponomarenko, M., Shuranova, L., & Rogalewicz, V. (2023). Characteristics of alcohol use among migrants from Ukraine to The Czech Republic in the context of the war in Ukraine in 2022. *KONTAKT-Journal of Nursing and Social Sciences Related to Health and Illness, 25*(2), 124–130. https://doi.org/10.32725/kont.2023.019

Cano, M. Á., Sánchez, M., Trepka, M. J., Dillon, F. R., Sheehan, D. M., Rojas, P., et al. (2017). Immigration stress and alcohol use severity among recently immigrated Hispanic adults: Examining moderating effects of gender, immigration status, and social support. *Journal of Clinical Psychology, 73*(3), 294–307. https://doi.org/10.1002/jclp.22330

Červenka, J., M. (2024). Ukrajinští uprchlíci v České republice v roce 2024. In Czech. Retrieved February 14, 2025, from https://mv.gov.cz/clanek/vyzkum-vetsina-z-ukrajinskych-uprchliku-v-cesku-jsou-zeny-zhruba-dve-tretiny-uprchliku-pracuji-a-podnikaji.aspx

Cooper, M. L. (1994). Motivations for alcohol use among adolescents: Development and validation of a four-factor model. *Psychological Assessment, 6*(2), 117.

Czaderny, K. (2025). The longitudinal relationship between acculturation and alcohol use among immigrant adolescents in Europe. *International Migration Review. Advance online publication.* https://doi.org/10.1177/01979183251333767

Czech Statistical Office (2024). Počet cizinců, demografické události. In Czech. Retrieved January 14, 2025, from https://csu.gov.cz/pocet-cizincu-demograficke-udalosti?pocet=10&start=0&podskupiny=291&razeni=-datumVydani

Dlouhý, M., Barták, M., Dobiášová, K., Hnilicová, H., Janečková, H., & Petráková, A. (2022). Health and health care for refugees and migrants. Academicoupcom. [online][2023-12-14].
Elkholy, H., Tay Wee Teck, J., Arunogiri, S., Asaad, M. R., Baessler, F., Bhad, R., & Baldacchino, A. M. (2023). Substance use disorders among forcibly displaced people: A narrative review. *Current Addiction Reports, 10*(2), 341–352.
European Union Drugs Agency. (2023). Migrants and drugs: health and social responses. EUDA. Februady 14, 2025, from https://www.euda.europa.eu/publications/mini-guides/migrants-and-drugs-health-and-social-responses_en
Gavrilova, Y., Blevins, C., & Abrantes, A. (2021). Modified drinking motives questionnaire–revised: Psychometric validation in a psychiatric sample of young adults with predominantly polysubstance use. *Addictive Behaviors, 114*, 106753. https://doi.org/10.1016/j.addbeh.2020.106753
Horyniak, D., Higgs, P., Cogger, S., Dietze, P., & Bofu, T. (2016). Heavy alcohol consumption among marginalised African refugee young people in Melbourne, Australia: Motivations for drinking, experiences of alcohol-related problems and strategies for managing drinking. *Ethnicity & Health, 21*(3), 284–299. https://doi.org/10.1080/13557858.2015.1061105
PAQ. (2024). Integrace ukrajinských uprchlíků: 2 roky poté a výhled na 2024+. In Czech. Retrieved December 14, 2024, from: https://www.paqresearch.cz/content/files/2024/02/PAQ_Hlas_Ukrajincu_Dva_roky_pote-2.pdf
Jackson-Koku, G. (2016). Beck depression inventory. *Occupational Medicine, 66*(2), 174–175. https://doi.org/10.1093/occmed/kqv087
Kabíček, P., Csémy, L., Sulek, Š., & Mizerová, L. (2010). Syndrom rizikového chování dospívajících: Krátká intervence ke snížení zneužívání návykových látek v praxi praktického lékaře pro děti a dorost. *Zaostřeno, 8*(3), 1–8.
Kavanová, M., Marková, L., & Prokop, D. (2023). *Hlas Ukrajinců: Integrace uprchlíků na trhu práce a v bydlení*. In Czech. Retrieved December 14, 2023, from: https://www.paqresearch.cz/content/files/2023/07/PAQ_Hlas_Ukrajincu_PraceBydleni_2023.pdf
Kavanová, M., Prokop, D., Škvrňák, M., & Levínský, M. (2022). Téměř polovina uprchlíků trpí symptomydepresí a úzkostí. O dostupné péči jim chybí informace [almost half of the refugees suffer from symptoms of depression and anxiety. They lack information about available care]. In Czech. PAQ research. Retrieved December 14, 2023, from: https://www.paqresearch.cz/post/dusevni-zdravi-hlas-ukrajincu
Kážmér, L., Csémy, L., & Šíba, O. (2024). Validation of factor structures of the drinking motives questionnaire among the Czech young and adult general population. *BMC Psychology, 12*(1), 505. https://doi.org/10.1186/s40359-024-02002-2
Keyes, K. M., Grant, B. F., & Hasin, D. S. (2010). Evidence for a closing gender gap in alcohol use, abuse, and dependence in the United States population. *Drug and Alcohol Dependence, 93*(1–2), 21–29. https://doi.org/10.1016/j.drugalcdep.2007.08.017
Khantzian, E. J. (1997). The self-medication hypothesis of substance use disorders: A reconsideration and recent applications. *Harvard Review of Psychiatry, 4*(5), 231–244. https://doi.org/10.3109/10673229709030550
Kuntsche, E., Knibbe, R., Gmel, G., & Engels, R. (2006). Replication and validation of the drinking motive questionnaire revised (DMQ-R, Cooper, 1994) among adolescents in Switzerland. *European Addiction Research, 12*(3), 161–168. https://doi.org/10.1159/000092118
Mazhak, I., Paludo, A. C., & Sudyn, D. (2024). Self-reported health and coping strategies of Ukrainian female refugees in The Czech Republic. *European Societies, 26*(2), 411–437. https://doi.org/10.1080/14616696.2023.2203230
Mesa-Vieira, C., Haas, A. D., Buitrago-Garcia, D., Roa-Diaz, Z. M., Minder, B., Gamba, M., et al. (2022). Mental health of migrants with pre-migration exposure to armed conflict: A systematic review and meta-analysis. The lancet. *Public Health, 7*(5), e469e481. https://doi.org/10.1016/s2468-2667(22)00061-5

Mulia, N., Ye, Y., & Greenfield, T. K. (2008). Disparities in alcohol-related problems among white, black, and Hispanic Americans. *Alcoholism: Clinical and Experimental Research, 33*(4), 654–662. https://doi.org/10.1111/j.1530-0277.2008.00880.x
Petruželka, B., Barták, M., Rogalewicz, V., & Babor, T. F. (2025). What drove changes in alcohol sales during the COVID-19 pandemic in Czechia? An interrupted time series analyses. *Drug and Alcohol Review, 44*(4), 1207–1221. https://doi.org/10.1111/dar.14035
Pinto, L. H., Nunes, F., & Bastida Dominguez, M. (2022). "Enhancers" and "copers"? Understanding drinking motives and alcohol use among international workers. *Journal of Ethnicity in Substance Abuse, 21*(4), 1361–1388. https://doi.org/10.1080/15332640.2020.1852145
Spurný, M., Tabery, P. (2025) Integrace ukrajinských uprchlíků: trh práce, bydlení, znalost češtiny a vzdělávání dětí—Výzkum Hlas Ukrajinců. [Integration of Ukrainian refugees: labor market, housing, knowledge of Czech, and children's education—Research by Voice of Ukrainians] (in Czech) Praha. Centrum pro výzkum veřejného mínění. Available from: https://cvvm.soc.cas.cz/images/articles/files/5935/vyzkumnazpravahlasukrajincuvlna8vlna9.pdf

Chapter 3
Responding to Needs Related to Drug Use Among Undocumented Migrants in Policy, Law, and Practice in Denmark

Arash Setoodeh, Esben Houborg, and Birgitte Thylstrup

3.1 Introduction

Rising migration flows globally and across Europe have prompted many states to tighten their migration policies. These shifts have spilled over into welfare and health sectors, where eligibility criteria — often designed around citizenship — have been narrowed (Hacker et al., 2015). For migrants, access to healthcare and social benefits is generally conditioned on lawful residence. Yet, in several European welfare states[1] a significant gap persists between formal inclusion and the effective guarantee of equal access to healthcare and social services among migrant groups (Cuadra, 2012; Dauvrin et al., 2012).

In countries where statutory recognition is decisive for entitlement, migrants without legal residence face additional layers of challenges. Across the European countries, restrictions on undocumented migrants'[2] access to health and social

[1] The European welfare state is commonly defined as a model of governance in which the state assumes primary responsibility for securing the well-being of its population through the provision of healthcare, social services, and income support. These services are not offered as privileges, but as social rights tied to membership in the national community (Marshall, 1950).

[2] Various terms in the relevant literature are used to refer to these individuals, such as irregular/irregularized, or illegalized migrants (Damsa & Franko, 2022; Hacker et al., 2015). However, for ease of reference, we use the term "undocumented migrants", referring to those who either have been rejected for legal stay or have lost their legal status.

A. Setoodeh (✉) · E. Houborg · B. Thylstrup
Dpeartment of Psychology and Behavioral Science, Center for Alcohol and Drug Research, Aarhus University, Copenhagen, Denmark
e-mail: as.crf@psy.au.dk

E. Houborg
e-mail: eh.crf@psy.au.dk

B. Thylstrup
e-mail: bt.crf@psy.au.dk

C. De Kock (ed.), *Substance Use Among Refugees in Europe*,
https://doi.org/10.1007/978-3-032-32399-6_3

services are common but differ in various ways, ranging from near-total exclusion to narrowly circumscribed entitlements limited to emergency care and selected preventive health care services (Hacker et al., 2015).

These general patterns take a concrete form in the Danish welfare system which is built on the principle of universality for those recognized as legal residents (in Danish terms 'Borgere'). Eligibility functions via the PIN (Personal Identification Number; in Danish: Det Centrale Personregister_CPR), which gives an individual access to most essential public services and benefits, such as healthcare, social welfare, banking, and labor market (Damsa & Franko, 2022). For migrants legally residing in Denmark for more than three months, it is required to obtain a PIN in order to access such services and benefits (CPR-loven, 2023, Article 16). Absence of such registration significantly limits one's access to care.

Danish migration policies not only regulate migrants' stay in Denmark but also regulate their rights, including entitlement to health services and welfare benefits. Losing legal stay, whether through asylum rejection or revocation/expiry of a residence permit, places migrants under expulsion and/or return obligations (to the arriving country). In effect, this entails the loss of PIN and transfer to Danish deportation centers, where the rights and access to healthcare and welfare are substantially reduced, regulated primarily by the Aliens Act and the Return Act. This positions these migrants in a gray area between national legislations and Denmark's universal human-rights obligations (Gammeltoft-Hansen & Scott Ford, 2022).

In recent decades, Danish immigration legislation has become significantly more restrictive, narrowing the pathways to legal residence and Danish citizenship. The latest major policy shift, known as the "2019 paradigm change", formally reoriented asylum policy from integration to repatriation (Schwörer, 2025). This frames undocumented migrants as temporary presences—either to be regularized or deported—which justifies withholding welfare support (Damsa & Franko, 2022; Lindberg, 2020). Research shows that these policy shifts often reinforce segregation, stigmatization, and marginalization among undocumented migrants, pushing many into homelessness and encounters with the criminal justice system (Pouille et al., 2023, 2024; Rechel et al., 2011; Winters et al., 2018).

These dynamics have contributed to a growing population of undocumented migrants living in deportation centers; established in 2015, Danish deportation centers accommodate migrants without legal stay, who have received a final expulsion order, and do not cooperate with the return process (Bendixen, 2021). These state-run facilities operate under the Danish Prison and Probation Service, where the residents are subject to strict rules and obligations, including mandatory residence and reporting duties, highly limited mobility, and risk of imprisonment for non-compliance. Basic needs such as food and accommodation are provided, but the residents are denied the right to work, study, and obtain any formal income (ibid). Thus, deportation centers function as sites of control where life is heavily regulated while migrants await their deportation.

Multiple structural barriers, socio-economic inequalities, and personal stressors linked to migration and insecure legal status often increase the risk of initiating and/or intensifying drug use among undocumented migrants (Horyniak et al., 2016; Pouille et al., 2024; van Selm et al., 2023), where risk factors such as trauma, social exclusion, and poverty embedded in pre-, peri-, and post-migration experiences shape the prevalence and patterns of drug use (Pouille et al., 2024). While the current immigration policy landscape in Denmark has been widely criticized for producing a fragmented system in which undocumented migrants routinely fall through the cracks (Damsa & Franko, 2022; Hansen et al., 2006; Jensen et al., 2011), addressing drug-related needs among this group remains essential. However, access to care for drug-related problems, such as prevention, drug treatment, and harm-reduction, is categorized as a social welfare entitlement conditioned on lawful residence in Denmark (Jørgensen & Thomsen, 2016). A further challenge is that this policy stands in marked contrast to human rights principles, which are universal and inalienable, applying to all individuals regardless of legal status (Lister et al., 2024). In consequence, as scholars such as Benhabib (2004) and Soysal (1994) argue, this contrast reveals deeper tensions between the Danish nationally formulated welfare entitlements and post-national human-rights claims. This tension raises a central question that we will pursue in this chapter: how is access to healthcare and social services in response to the drug-related problems for undocumented migrants who use drugs (UMWUD) in Denmark, regulated and translated through the interaction of Danish policy and practice?

3.2 Characterizing UMWUD in Denmark

In this context, the literature on sociodemographic characteristics of undocumented migrants in Denmark is limited (Funge et al., 2021; Jensen et al., 2011), although a recent estimate outlined up to approximately 28,900 individuals (Clausen & Skaksen, 2016), of whom drug users comprise a particularly vulnerable subgroup. Similar to findings from recent European studies (Pouille et al., 2024; European Union Drugs Agency (EUDA), 2021; De Kock, 2020), UMWDU in Denmark are predominantly male and young-to-middle-aged adults (Søgaard et al., 2021; European Committee for the Prevention of Torture (CPT, 2024; Clausen & Skaksen, 2016). This pattern is consistent with official Danish statistics, which show a clear male predominance both in the asylum system and the expulsion process (Udlændingestyrelsen (US), 2025).

Like other undocumented migrants, the UMWUD are formally assigned to Danish deportation centers for expulsion and fast return. In practice, however, the expulsion process is rarely swift, as legal and practical complications such as the principle of non-refoulement[3] and the absence of return agreements with certain countries of origin often delay or even prevent deportation (CPT, 2024). In these cases, undocumented migrants may be placed under "tolerated stay", a status that excludes

[3] In the global context, non-refoulement is a core principle of international refugee and human rights law that prohibits states from returning individuals to a country where there is a real risk of being subjected to persecution, torture, inhuman or degrading treatment, or other serious human rights violations (European Migration Network (EMN), n.d).

them from formal rights while permitting their continued presence in Denmark (Gammeltoft-Hansen & Scott Ford, 2022). As a result, rather than functioning as short-term transit sites for return, deportation centers function as prolonged transits, where the indefinite character of stay intensifies the precariousness of UMWUD's lives. As a result, some UMWUD are left to navigate their lives by moving from the deportation centers into urban environments, particularly in Denmark's two largest cities, Copenhagen and Aarhus. Their mobility is often shaped by overlapping factors, including concerns of expulsion, pursuing involvement in the informal economy, greater accessibility and affordability of drugs, as well as the pursuit of care and peer networks (Setoodeh et al., 2024). However, at the same time, this movement is often constrained by available financial and social resources and the absence of residence documents (Holeksa, 2024). As an example, moving to urban environments means leaving basic guarantees (food and accommodation) behind, increasing drug use through marginalization and street-based survival, as well as the risk of being subjected to law enforcement (see also Rhodes, 2009). For some UMWUD, subsequent movement occurs either voluntarily (returning to deportation centers) or involuntarily by law enforcement (arrest, conviction, and transfer to prison), often as a consequence of involvement in the open drug scene[4] or other criminalized activities (Christoffersen, 2017; Kammersgaard et al., 2024).

The movement away from deportation centers to urban or institutional settings not only affects UMWUD's visibility and exposure to risk, but also their encounter with low-threshold services and/or prison-based healthcare services largely designed for legal residents. It is therefore crucial to study how movement across these constrained environments creates both risks and (potentially) resources (Duff, 2010; Holeksa, 2024; Rhodes, 2009) and how the interaction of policy-practice in each environment impacts UMWUD's lived experiences.

3.3 Methodology

To comprehend the complex matrix of entitlements and examine how the Danish welfare structures regulate and restrict access to healthcare and social services for UMWUD, we investigate the intersection of Danish healthcare, welfare, and migration policies. However, often the gap between policy and practice is not transparent but unfolds in legal and administrative gray zones. Thus, to gain a comprehensive understanding, we must examine how these policies interact on a macro level, and how they are interpreted in the environments that the UMWUDs navigate on a meso level (see also De Kock, 2022). Accordingly, we will focus on three Danish legislative frameworks: the Health Act, the Social Services Act, and the Aliens Act. Further, to understand how these statutory frameworks are interpreted in practice, we analyze

[4] Open drug scenes are urban environments where public or semi-public drug use and drug dealing are visible and concentrated, often linked to informal support networks and harm reduction services (Grønnested, & Lalander, 2015).

six expert interviews with two legal scholars, one street legal-aid professional, and three social and healthcare professionals who work with UMWUD. The rationale for this selection of experts is to capture perspectives from the different urban and institutional settings that shape UMWUD's everyday encounters with healthcare and social provisions in deportation centers, open drug scenes, and prisons. Analytically, these interviews thus function as a lens that identifies how ambiguous policies are applied in practice and traces the discretionary mechanisms through which access to welfare services in Denmark is regulated across the three environments.

Extensive participant observations and interviews with undocumented migrants were also conducted as part of a larger focus on the lives of UMWUD in Denmark. However, to maintain the chapter's focus on macro and meso dynamics, this data will be discussed in a separate publication currently in progress.

The study received approval from Aarhus University's Research Ethics Committee and all participants provided written informed consent including the named individuals in this chapter.

3.4 Analysis

We examine the intersection of migration law, healthcare, and social rights across two analytically distinct environments: institutional settings (deportation centers and prisons) and urban settings (open drug scenes in Copenhagen and Aarhus).

3.4.1 Across Environments: Contexts of (in)visibility

Each environment operates as an arena where Danish healthcare and welfare policies intersect with institutional or urban governance, forming localized regimes of inclusion and exclusion. The intersections between these environments often affect access to care and resources and contribute to the production of risks (Rhodes, 2009). In institutional environments such as deportation centers, social exclusion is often compounded by bureaucratic ambiguity and rigid surveillance— in urban settings, precarious housing, policing, and the absence of legal documentation structure access to e.g., harm-reduction and healthcare services. In navigating urban settings, environmental pull factors, such as proximity to low-threshold services, drug availability, and anonymity, frequently interact with personal push factors such as access to services, drug market, or peer networks to shape mobility decisions. As a result, a transitional commute often emerges where UMWUD circulate between institutional and urban settings in response to shifting levels of law-enforced control and opportunities for support. This movement is typically short-term and results in episodic contact with services, discontinuity in care, and fluctuating visibility. For some UMWUD, the relative autonomy and social community at the open drug scenes may serve as an incentive to leave the more restrictive deportation centers, even when minimal formal health services are available. As Nadir Hamza, a street lawyer from Stenbroens Jurister, a legal aid organization supporting homeless individuals in Copenhagen, noted:

> People have literally told me that the circumstances [in the deportation centers] are so bad and so terrible [that] they would rather live on the street as drug users or die than go back to the deportation centers.

Addressing drug-related problems of UMWUD in deportation centers often involves a bureaucratic process with prolonged waiting times; as Helle Andersen, a nurse who has worked for several years at the Red Cross clinic in the Sjælsmark deportation center, 30 km north of Copenhagen, described:

> They [UMWUD] have to come first to us and say they have a problem…we don't give medicine here, but you come to the nurse and ask for a doctor's appointment - it's a normal doctor [General Physician (GP)] who's here [at the deportation center], and he or she will evaluate if you are qualified for help, and then he or she will send the note to the drug treatment center [in the city nearby]. But there's a very long waiting list, so it can take a long time, and it's not many we get through because they can't wait that long.

Such bureaucratic wait-times to access health resources combined with the restrictive conditions in deportation centers shape the everyday life of UMWUD increasingly difficult to endure, as Helle explained:

> They say this is like prison. There's nothing to do. It's very cold, and there's no color. People get more isolated, and it increases [their] drug use.

In both Nadir and Helle's views, the confinement-like atmosphere of deportation centers, marked by surveillance and restricted mobility, is a strong push factor that prompts UMWUD to leave the center despite the risks that they face in the urban environments; while they may not be guaranteed safety, housing, and access to services in the open drug scene, they may find a stronger sense of agency, accessibility, and social connection. A staff member at a national NGO providing healthcare to migrants in Copenhagen noted that for many UMWUD, the primary driver of movement to this environment is managing drug dependence:

> The deportation centers are not supposed to be a nice place to be. Because then they [UMWUD] probably return home… That's the politics. So of course they move. It's easier to get drugs, to make money, to steal [in open drug scene]. What the hell are you going to do out there [in deportation centers]? If you want drugs delivered, you need a lot of money, and it's not super easy.

She also emphasized that moving to the open drug scene is not only about managing dependence, but also involves seeking a sense of social inclusion, network, and belonging:

> They have different situations and needs, but they have also relations and friendships. You're among others. There is a life [going on]. There might be other people like you. I mean, you wouldn't sit alone in a room and stare at the wall, right?

Nadir's observations from the open drug scene in Copenhagen also highlight the pull of community and peer networks:

> ... so there's a sense of community, they all sit together, they all have relatable friends whom they can relate to, and drugs are accessible (...) they have a drug using room where the drug use is monitored for healthcare purposes and they don't feel judged.

However, as Helle noted, leaving the deportation centers to move to the open drug scenes also exposes UMWUD to environments that involve significant risks related to precarious survival strategies:

> If they don't get the help [in open drug scene] they steal things to sell or sell themselves; that's a very high personal cost.

Besides exposing themselves to risk environments in urban settings, leaving deportation centers is also criminalized in Denmark. As Jakob Fastrup, a lawyer with extensive expertise focusing on Danish deportation centers explained:

> It is said that they have the same rights as everybody else, according to human rights. But the reality is that they have these obligations to stay there [in the deportation center] and to report and tell where they are if they are not there. And if they don't fulfill this, the [deportation center] authorities will send the case to the police, and the police will pick them up. And they will be taken to court and then put in prison. You can be put in prison up to four years if you don't stay at the deportation center, or if you don't report, or if you don't tell where you are. Not the first time, but when you have done it a few times – maybe three or four times. Even if the reason for not being there is because you are afraid, or if you are taking care of your children in Denmark, or any other good reason. If you don't report or show up, you will be punished.

Although some UMWUD sooner or later return to the deportation center for basic care, "mostly they vanish again ... and sometimes I hear they ended up in prison," as Helle noted. However, while imprisonment may secure basic needs, access to drug-related healthcare is also limited during incarceration. Lærke Lund Kjærgaard, a former social worker and consultant in the Danish Prison and Probation Service, explained that all new arrivals in Danish prisons undergo a self-report screening focused on mental health and drug use history, with interpreters used for non-Danish speakers. Inside prisons, however, health and social offers are separated:

> If you have been sentenced to deportation, you aren't allowed (as a main rule) to get the social offer involved in drug treatment, but you can still get the opioid agonist therapy (OAT) in prisons and detention centers, so that's a political decision that we are navigating after.

Lærke clarified that social drug treatment refers to non-medical, psychosocial interventions such as individual or group counseling, rehabilitation programs, and reintegration support, typically delivered by external providers within the Danish prison system. However, while UMWUD are excluded from the social aspects of drug treatment, their right to work is recognized, similar to other inmates:

> If you are serving a sentence in a Danish prison, you have the right and obligation to take part in work and you'll will be paid for this - approximately 12–20 DKK depending on whether you also receive a supplement.

Lærke also reflected on the paradox of prisons where recognition as an inmate can confer limited resources and structure, but where significant risks and vulnerabilities also persist:

> There are drugs available. Of course, not in the same way as outside, but if you want it, you can probably get it. Maybe not the drug you prefer, but something. But you also have to pay extra for it. But if they continue the drug use inside [prison], I think it's for the same reasons; to cope with the consequences of incarceration.

The movement of UMWUD between the three settings shows that boundaries between institutional and urban environments are porous and co-produced by policies, entitlements, and service gaps that lead UMWUD to exercise a sense of individual agency within their constrained life circumstances (Lindberg, 2023). Drawing on her fieldwork, the staff member at the national NGO noted that these movements are predictable yet hard to follow and rarely result in improved life conditions:

> They don't get followed by systems, and when we see them again, they've moved, disappeared, or are in worse health than before.

To understand how the Danish migration, health, and welfare policy frameworks affect the settings that the UMWUD move between, it becomes important to study how the implementation of policies across deportation centers, open drug scenes, and prisons shapes the risks and possibilities that UMWUD encounter. Accordingly, the next section will treat the interaction of Danish policy and practice across institutional and urban environments.

3.4.2 Migration Policy: Production of (in)Visibility

The principal determinant of a migrant's status in Denmark is migration policy, which also determines the consequences of losing legal stay. The basis for expulsion and return to the country of origin is stated in the Aliens Act (Udlændingeloven, 2025) and the Return Act (Hjemrejseloven, 2024) (Gammeltoft-Hansen & Scott Ford, 2022). Status, rights, expulsion procedures, and the conditions of residence pending return are all regulated by these national frameworks.

The Aliens Act defines a series of strict obligations for residents who are under an expulsion or return order. Among these, the duty to reside in a designated return center (Article 33) and the duty to report to authorities at regular intervals (Article 34) form the core of the policy. Further, the Aliens Act includes requirements such as the duty to notify authorities of any change in address or whereabouts, which failure to comply can result in serious legal consequences, including administrative fines, pre-trial detention, and criminal imprisonment (Articles 36–38). Consequently, these articles empower the authorities to criminalize non-compliance, regardless of the underlying reasons, whether related to fear, health, drug dependence, or survival needs.

Under the Danish migration law, migrants without legal residence can be detained if milder measures are not sufficient to ensure that they leave the country. For example, this applies in cases where undocumented migrants scheduled for deportation fail to cooperate with the police in organizing their departure or do not comply with established reporting or residence obligations, as described in the Return Act (Articles

15 and 16). Detention may also be used when there are reasons to suspect that a person has committed a criminal offense that could lead to deportation, or a person has entered Denmark in breach of an existing entry ban (Article 14), or with false identity papers. Asylum seekers may also be detained under specific circumstances in the Aliens Act when they are to be transferred to another EU country under the Dublin Regulation (Article 29a) or when they significantly hinder the processing of their case and detention is considered necessary to ensure they attend the procedure (Article 36) (CPT, 2024). The Aliens Act offers only minimal social protection for undocumented migrants, thus restricting their rights. According to Article 42a, such individuals are entitled solely to basic subsistence and accommodation, with the law explicitly stating that support is limited to essential needs, including necessary healthcare. This safety net (Hacker et al., 2015) only covers urgent or acute medical situations and does not extend to comprehensive healthcare or preventive and rehabilitative services. Furthermore, Article 42b authorizes the authorities to demand reimbursement for support and healthcare costs if the individual possesses the means to do so, thereby placing an additional economic burden on vulnerable migrants.

The national NGO worker at the healthcare clinic in Copenhagen observed that the precarity linked to undocumented status, including fear, trauma, and the risk of deportation, is increased among UMWUD and may deter engagement with national NGO services. She described her encounters with migrants who "avoid services, not just because they don't have a PIN, but because they don't trust that the system will help them or even see them." She also noted that migrants seeking help from the national NGO often come in waves, which may reflect a combination of factors, including shifts in migration policy (e.g., Denmark's 2019 paradigm change), stop-and-search policing in drug hotspots, and capacity pressure on low-threshold services during the cold seasons of the year (see also Biswas et al., 2011).

She also emphasized that, as a frontline professional, her mandate is shaped and constrained by the legal framework established by the state:

> We have to follow the law: our mandate, we support migrants. We are under the Danish health authorities. We cannot just do whatever we want. There are rules and it's regulated.

The NGO worker at the clinic explained that the rules and regulations governing support for migrants determine not only who is eligible for protection, but also what forms of support that can be offered. Moreover, access to harm-reduction services or emergency care in urban settings depends on trust, which is quickly eroded by repeated exclusion and the instability of their status:

> When they come to the city, most of them are pushed into informal or illegal ways of surviving because they are excluded from the system.

Helle also observed that many drug-using residents disappear from the deportation center Sjælsmark:

> They go to Copenhagen to get their drugs, and they don't get the help there either. I know a couple of them; they haven't been here [deportation center], and I haven't been able to get them to come back. Just three, four months ago, we had one, but now he's in Vestre Prison - probably because he didn't get any money, so he had to get his drugs by getting involved in drug dealing.

This (in)visibility dynamic produced by migration policy, as Helle noted, extends into the Danish prison system, as Lærke observes that Danish prisons now hold a growing number of foreign nationals, predominantly men.

Given that this regime means that UMWUD in deportation centers are subjected to surveillance and constant risk of sanctions, movement into high-risk environments like the open drugs scenes presents a survival strategy to UMWUD—a dynamic that underlines the paradox in the migration system: while the law tightly regulates undocumented migrants, it simultaneously produces the conditions that make strict compliance nearly impossible for UMWUD. In consequence, this dynamic produces shifting (in)visibility of UMWUD across the environments they navigate.

3.4.3 Health and Welfare at the Margins: Navigating Drug-Related Needs

While Danish migration policy is the principal determinant of legal status and rights—and thus sets the terms of (im)mobility and deportability—access to healthcare and social support is negotiated at the intersection of the Health Act and the Social Services Act. The next sections therefore trace how navigation of needs for UMWUD in Denmark is shaped by policy interpretation under these two acts, alongside the migration regime.

3.4.3.1 Navigating Healthcare

The Health Act states that "easy and equal" access is among the main goals of the Danish healthcare system (Sundhedsloven, 2025, Article 2), and all individuals "who have residence in this country are entitled to services under this Act" (Article 7). These services include free medical treatment through GPs, specialist consultations, and hospital care, and are often categorized as acute treatment, continued treatment, and planned or non-urgent treatment. However, the entitlement to access is based on legal residence and registration in the PIN system (Article 7, sec. 2). On the other hand, the same Act, in Article 80, obliges regional authorities[5] to provide acute treatment for persons who don't have (legal) residence in Denmark. This includes the right to receive acute treatment for undocumented migrants, but on the condition that it is not reasonable, under the circumstances, to send these individuals to their home country for treatment (Article 80, sec. 2). Thus, although UMWUD are in principle entitled only to acute treatment, access to treatment still depends on the interpretation of the circumstances. Furthermore, Article 81 (sec. 2) allows regions to charge patients for such care, making emergency access formally available but often financially

[5] In Denmark, the country's five administrative regions are responsible for operating and managing the hospital system. They also fund a wide range of primary and specialist healthcare services. Approximately 95% of hospital beds are owned by these regions (Birk et al., 2024).

inaccessible for UMWUD. Reasons such as fear of encountering immigration law enforcement, the criminal justice system, or stigmatization may deter UMWUD from seeking treatment. To address this gap, three clinics have operated in major Danish cities since 2011, in collaboration with the Danish Medical Association, the Danish Red Cross, and the Danish Refugee Council. As they receive undocumented migrants on an anonymous basis, they offer limited healthcare access but fall short in addressing needs beyond acute care (Birk et al., 2024).

This legal framework creates interlinked challenges of how access to health services is determined in practice. First, the healthcare legislation leaves undocumented migrants without guaranteed rights beyond acute care. Secondly, access beyond hospital emergencies depends on the interpretation of acute care in clinical practice, resulting in case-by-case decisions rather than enforceable legal guarantees. As the healthcare worker at the national NGO explained:

> The thing is that we offer basic healthcare, but we don't deal with their drug use. For example, if they inject drugs and they get infections, we treat their wounds and their infections or whatever they have. But we don't do treatment for drug use. We can't - we're not allowed under the Danish health authorities.

Thirdly, the limited rights are implemented unevenly, as laws and policies are interpreted in different ways by different institutions and professionals, producing systemic inconsistency. As Nadir observed:

> The law might say they can access acute treatment, but hospitals read that differently. They ask for a PIN. They ask for payment. Sometimes they bill. And the patient just walks away.

Thus, exclusion from relevant health services is embedded in institutional structures and how frontline actors interpret and apply the law. In contrast, practitioners in urban harm-reduction settings such as the open drug scenes often interpret their mandate to respond through an ethic of care, offering informal help despite legal constraints. As the healthcare worker at the national NGO puts it:

> They [UMWUD] don't qualify for services, but we still see them, still try to help them.

This discretionary practice reflects a pragmatic response to the humanitarian needs of a migrant group excluded by the design of the law. In contrast, institutional environments such as deportation centers and prisons tend to apply the law more rigidly. Helle noted:

> There is no room in the system for flexibility. We can only do what the guidelines allow, and the guidelines are very tight.

Taken together, these dynamics— the legal construction of entitlement and the local interpretations of policy—reveal that exclusion is not merely a result of legal absence, but the outcome of a structurally embedded system of discretion and constrained care. According to the legal scholar, Jens Vedsted-Hansen, the conditionality reflects an even deeper legal structure, as Denmark's international human rights obligations such as non-refoulement, do not impose a positive obligation to provide comprehensive healthcare. Furthermore, Nadir explained that the legal language used in Danish healthcare legislation regarding entitlements complicates access. For instance, he highlighted the discretionary wording in Article 81(2), which states that regions have the option to charge or waive fees, but are not legally required to do so.

> That difference between may and must, that's everything! It leaves it to the hospital to decide, and most of them decide to charge.

Nadir believes that although Article 81(2) of the Health Act authorizes hospitals to charge for treatment, it allows for payment exemption in cases where the individual cannot pay. Yet, this rule is not intended to demand a fee from individuals without legal residence. He further supported his legal interpretation by referencing Article 5 of the Act on Legal Protection (Retssikkerhedsloven, 2022) and Article 7 of the Public Administration Act (Forvaltningsloven, 2014). These provisions impose an obligation on public authorities, including hospitals, to process all requests for assistance (formally or informally), and actively consider all possible means of support:

> Article 5 of the Act on Legal Protection basically says the municipal council has to treat applications and questions regarding help within all the possible means that exist … and the wording … means all authorities, so even public hospitals.

Nadir further explained that an "application" should be interpreted broadly, such that a person does not need to submit a formal request; rather, the presence of need itself should trigger institutional consideration of alternatives, including exemption from payment. Additionally, Article 7 of the Public Administration Act stipulates that public authorities must provide sufficient guidance to individuals they interact with, especially when they are navigating bureaucratic systems. Nadir argued that the mere fact of an individual appearing at a hospital without a PIN should be reason enough to initiate an assessment for exemption:

> As soon as the person comes in without a PIN number and without private healthcare, they need to look into this … They can conclude the person is resourceful and bill them, or they can ask a few questions and find out that the person is homeless and lives on the streets collecting bottle deposits - and that should result in an exemption.

This legal argument is reinforced by practice guidelines from the Danish Agency for Patient Complaints (STPK, 2019), which underline the obligation to apply reasonableness assessments even without a formal application. According to Nadir, this interpretation applies not only to acute care but also to continued and planned treatment, making the law more inclusive in theory than it is in practice. Despite this, however, Nadir noted that most hospital staff are either unaware of these obligations or choose not to act on them, leading to systemic exclusion. The practical outcome is that undocumented migrants are routinely charged, even when legal and ethical justifications exist for exemption. Nadir emphasized that even guidelines meant to permit exemptions in cases of vulnerability or homelessness are poorly communicated and inconsistently applied:

> There's no training, no protocol. One doctor might help. Another might not even let you in.

In contrast, the national NGO worker has observed how practitioners in urban environments in central Copenhagen often compensate for legal exclusions by working around them:

> They [undocumented migrants] avoid the system not only because of lack of rights, but because they don't trust that entering it won't cost them more.

She described a culture of silent resistance among some staff, choosing to assist undocumented migrants with informal referrals and non-institutional care options. In institutional environments like deportation centers, these rights are interpreted far more narrowly than in hospitals. Helle confirmed that even when treatment is technically available, barriers in procedure and communication prevent access:

> We try to help, but they don't come. Some disappear into the city. Others end up in prison.

She explained that a temporary PIN can be issued for very specific purposes, such as collecting prescribed medicine, but they are not transferable across services or institutions:

> One case, one PIN. And when it's over, it's over. If they need something else, we start again.

In sum, while emergency care is formally guaranteed in the Danish healthcare law, the scope of this guarantee is ambiguous. This fragmented recognition is mediated not only by legal status but by environment, institutional culture, and the discretion of individual professionals navigating between ethics and law. As Damsa and Franko (2022) argue, this is a condition of "institutional non-recognition" where needs may be acknowledged informally but not met structurally.

3.4.3.2 Navigating Social-Welfare Care

The Social Services Act is the primary legal framework regulating social welfare rights in Denmark, including financial support, housing, and care for vulnerable groups. It aims to prevent social problems and address individuals' needs arising from reduced physical or mental functioning or particular social difficulties (Article 1, Serviceloven, 2025). Article 2 stipulates that municipalities must provide social services "to persons over the age of 18 who are legally residing in the country," thereby, similar to the Health Act, making legal residence a prerequisite for entitlements.

Drug treatment in Denmark is offered by the municipalities and is regulated through the Social Services Act for psychosocial treatment (Articles 101, 101a, and 102), and the Healthcare Act for OAT (Article 142). The logic of entitlement to drug treatment is mirrored in both acts, applying to individuals with legal residence. In effect, the entire architecture of the Social Services Act and the Health Act at the macro level results in the systematic denial or severe restriction of these rights for UMWUD in Denmark. However, Article 101a in the Social Services Act, which states the possibility of an anonymous drug treatment offer, may function as a de facto access point for UMWUD. While not constituting a formal entitlement, practical access depends on how municipalities interpret and implement the provision.

In Danish deportation centers, access to drug-related resources is extremely limited by both law and institutional practice, as there is no on-site OAT available, and the only possibility is to seek referral to an external clinic. As Helle elaborates the procedure in the Red Cross clinic at Sjælsmark deportation center:

> We don't have medicine that can be used as a substitution [treatment]; we don't have morphine, methadone, or opioids. It's only the doctor who can refer [to the external clinic]. He comes once a week here; our clinic is only open three days a week and only from nine to eleven, so there's not enough money to give [UMWUD] that service so that they can come at any time, so it's a problem. If you don't come to your appointment, the time is gone…The system is built like that there's no room in this system for drug users…Because there's not enough money! [That's why] It's not many we get through because they can't wait that long.

Jakob, the lawyer, confirmed that UMWUD in deportation centers have no specific rights concerning their drug use:

> That's the short answer. They have the right to live out there and get food and a bed, but if they are drug addicts, they will probably need some drugs, and to get money to buy that, their only possibility is to continue their criminality. That is what is happening.

Lærke explained that the prison environment operates according to a more structured logic, and although inmates under expulsion sentences are excluded from most social drug treatments in Danish prisons, exceptions can happen:

> To use the exceptions, they need not only to be here for a long time, but there should be concrete reasons for offering treatment. For example, if it is necessary for the health of the person concerned or to enable the person to participate in daily life together with other prisoners and staff. This is up to the evaluation of the social worker and the treatment offer in conversation with the [prison] management.

However, eligibility for these offers often depends on administrative discretion than enforceable right, and frequently requires that the inmate is highly motivated, able to overcome institutional barriers such as navigating rules, language, and fit specific institutional criteria. As Lærke noted, even those who technically qualify must actively request treatment, and uptake is low:

> It's a very small population that we offer this. And that's also because they aren't interested in receiving the treatment. They have to participate voluntarily. Of course, we are concerned about their needs, all of the population's needs, and we try to motivate (them) into social treatment for drug use. But they have to make the request themselves to get the offer.

Still, for some UMWUD, incarceration represents not only a respite from street-level survival and the coerciveness of the deportation centers but a rare context in which their health, agency, and need for treatment are at least partially recognized, even if this recognition remains conditional and incomplete. As Lærke put it, the experience of having basic needs met and being seen by the system stands in stark contrast to the invisibility and exclusion faced elsewhere:

> Food is free or you get money to buy your own food. It's a safe place and there are other people as well. You might even be able to actually get OAT because prisons have a mandate to do it.

In sum, access to drug treatment for UMWUD remains severely restricted, reflecting broader exclusions from the Danish welfare system. Limited treatment options and bureaucratic barriers in deportation centers often push UMWUD toward urban drug scenes, where survival depends on informal or illegal activities and exposure to multiple social and health-related harms. Paradoxically, incarceration—often a consequence of such marginalization—can provide one of the few institutional contexts in which UMWUD gain access to basic healthcare and drug treatment, albeit under conditions of confinement and control.

3.5 Discussion

Our study shows a fragmented and incoherent welfare landscape facing UMWUD. Entitlements and responding to basic needs are determined as much by local practices and personal judgment as by the formal guarantees of Danish law. In the discussion, we critically examine the interpretation and implementation of acute healthcare, the ethical and practical consequences of legal unclarity, and the tension between the conditional logic of Danish law and the universal human rights.

3.5.1 Interpretation of Acute Healthcare in Practice

A key finding from both our empirical and legal analyses is the central, but also ambiguous category of 'acute' or 'emergency' healthcare for undocumented migrants in Denmark. The Danish legislation, as articulated in the Aliens Act, the Health Act, and the Social Services Act, echoed in institutional policies and guidelines, obliges the state to provide emergency treatment to all individuals regardless of status. Yet, as in many other European countries (Chauvin & Garcés-Mascareñas, 2014; Cuadra, 2012; Willen, 2012), the interpretation of emergency is context-dependent, leaving substantial space for frontline discretion. In particular for UMWUD, this threshold is precarious, as many chronic and compounding drug-related needs are consistently categorized as non-acute, resulting in their exclusion from care until a life-threatening moment arises. This finding contributes to comparative studies on undocumented migrants'healthcare access (Horyniak et al., 2016; Pouille et al., 2023, 2024; van Selm et al., 2023; Winters et al., 2018) by showing how the requirement of legal residence reinforces a gatekeeping logic at the meso level in the Danish welfare context. Health professionals are thus placed in the position as moral and legal arbiters of access and entitlement. This ambiguity contributes to broader debates on "governing through uncertainty" (Ticktin, 2011), illustrating how legal ambiguity functions not merely as a policy flaw, but as a structural feature that regulates access through discretionary and moral reasoning.

3.5.2 *Policy Interpretation: Barrier or Safety Net*

The discretionary, case-by-case interpretation of acute healthcare embedded in Danish policy generates both openings for access and risks of exclusion. This ambiguity can occasionally act as a safety net, enabling healthcare professionals to secure treatment for vulnerable individuals who would otherwise be excluded from formal entitlements. Since the law does not precisely define what constitutes acute care, some professionals interpret current policies broadly, applying their discretion to offer care in situations that may not meet a strict threshold of emergency. Yet, these windows of access to care are highly contingent and may differ significantly between settings, leading to inconsistent application of care. As in other European countries (Karl-Trummer et al., 2009), this fragmentation heightens the risk environment for undocumented migrants. Moreover, discretionary decisions, particularly concerning UMWUD, are often shaped by implicit biases or structural stigma attached to status, drug use, or homelessness (Hacker et al., 2015; Pouille et al., 2023). In this context, discretion can both help and harm, depending on the actors involved. This chapter shows how even in a universal welfare regime, discretion becomes a sorting mechanism, reinforcing selective inclusion rather than universal access. The solution, as Nadir and other experts argue, would require a clearer legislative language and a more inclusive definition of healthcare treatment, including acute and non-acute treatments, that closes the loopholes through which exclusion persists, so that access is not dependent on goodwill but enforceable rights (Biswas et al., 2012; Huschke, 2014).

3.5.3 *Human Rights Versus Social Rights: Entitlement and the Policy Dilemma*

The Danish healthcare system vividly embodies a structural contradiction between two competing frameworks of entitlement: the conditionality of social rights and the universality of human rights. This tension lies at the heart of the access dilemma for UMWUD. In the Danish social rights model, access to healthcare and social services is tethered to formal criteria: legal residence, registration with a PIN, and inclusion within state bureaucracies. Rights are not presumed but granted. This logic, institutionalized through the Aliens Act, the Health Act, and the Social Services Act, restricts healthcare access for UMWUD to emergency needs and systematically excludes non-acute drug-related needs such as social drug treatment services. By contrast, the human rights framework, as set out in Article 25(1) of the Universal

Declaration of Human Rights (United Nations (UN), 1948) and developed in Article 12 of the International Covenant on Economic, Social and Cultural Rights (UN, 1966), affirms healthcare as a right grounded in human dignity, independent of legal status. General Comment No. 14 by the UN Committee on Economic, Social and Cultural Rights (CESCR, 2000) interprets this right to include all persons within a state's jurisdiction, explicitly naming undocumented migrants. As noted in Paragraph 34:

> States are under the obligation to respect the right to health by, inter alia, refraining from denying or limiting equal access for all persons, including asylum seekers and illegal immigrants, to preventive, curative and palliative health services.

General Comment No. 20 further strengthens this reading by classifying legal status as an inadmissible basis for discrimination in accessing Covenant rights (CESCR, 2009). Thus, currently there is a significant normative clash between entitlement through legality and entitlement through humanity in Denmark[6]. For UMWUD, this results in delays, denials, and divergent outcomes across institutional and urban environments, where outcomes are not shaped by needs but by legal ambiguity, interpretation of policy, and institutional culture. European legal institutions increasingly contest this exclusionary logic, as in the case of International Federation of Human Rights Leagues (FIDH) v. France, where the European Committee of Social Rights found that denying healthcare to undocumented migrants violated Article 13 of the European Social Charter[7] (right to social and medical assistance) (European Committee of Social Rights (ECSR), 2004). Further, the European Court of Human Rights, in the case of M.S.S. v. Belgium and Greece, established that neglect of essential healthcare and inadequate living conditions for an asylum seeker amounted to inhuman and degrading treatment, thereby violating Article 3 of the European Convention on Human Rights, which prohibits torture (European Court of Human Rights (ECtHR), 2011). While these rulings are not targeting Denmark specifically, they articulate a growing normative consensus across European states that may breach core human rights standards (Litins'ka, 2018).

In this context, Denmark's approach represents a striking case of policy dissonance: while formally committed to human rights treaties, the country continues to

[6] Denmark has signed and ratified several core international human rights treaties, including the International Covenant on Civil and Political Rights (ICCPR, signed 1966; ratified 1972), the International Covenant on Economic, Social and Cultural Rights (ICESCR, signed 1966; ratified 1972), the Convention on the Elimination of All Forms of Racial Discrimination (ICERD, signed 1966; ratified 1971), the Convention Against Torture (CAT, signed 1985; ratified 1987), and the European Convention on Human Rights (ECHR, ratified 1953). These treaties are legally binding under international law and require Denmark to uphold the rights and obligations they establish.

[7] Denmark signed the original 1961 Charter and later signed the Revised Charter in 1996, but as of now, Denmark has not ratified the Revised Charter. Instead, it continues to be bound by provisions of the 1961 version.

mediate access through a legalistic welfare logic that structurally excludes those most vulnerable.

3.6 Conclusion

This chapter has examined the barriers to healthcare and social support access for UMWUD in Denmark, revealing how various policies, legal ambiguity, institutional discretion, and the absence of enforceable rights produce systematic exclusion. It shows that access is uneven, inconsistent, and often dependent on the individual discretion of frontline professionals rather than on legally guaranteed entitlements. Yet beyond structural exclusion, the chapter has also highlighted how UMWUD navigate and move between fragmented urban and institutional environments - deportation centers, open drug scenes, and prisons - in search of survival and care. These movements are not only spatial but also shaped by the risks and opportunities that each environment presents. In the absence of guaranteed social rights, survival hinges on adaptability within a fractured landscape of care. Such movement within marginality represents both a consequence of systemic ambiguity and exclusion and a form of agency.

At the heart of this exclusion lies a structural contradiction between the conditional logic of national social rights and the universality of human rights. To reconcile this tension and begin aligning practice with international and European legal standards, concrete policy interventions are essential:

- Statutory recognition of a healthcare minimum that ensures access to non-acute but essential services (e.g., harm-reduction, social drug treatment, mental health, chronic care) for all migrants regardless of status while in Denmark (Biswas et al., 2011).
- Binding administrative guidelines that reduce discretion and clarify entitlements for healthcare professionals (Norredam et al., 2006).
- Legal firewalls between healthcare services and immigration enforcement to reduce fear-based avoidance of care, particularly crucial for UMWUD, whose identities are often criminalized and marginalized on multiple fronts (Hacker et al., 2015; Huschke, 2014).
- Municipal initiatives grounded in "urban citizenship" that decouple basic services from national legality and respond to health needs as matters of public concern, not legal worthiness. This idea, increasingly discussed in migration and urban studies, offers a pragmatic way to extend social protections in practice without waiting for national legal reform (Bauböck, 2003; Purcell, 2003).

Crucially, these policy options should not be seen as abstract ideals, but as responses to real tactics of navigation already observed in practice. In reality, UMWUD in Denmark are moving across multiple environments to access care and survive within a contradictory policy system.

Importantly, this chapter reveals a broader European dilemma: how to navigate the contradictions of a rights-based welfare state that universalizes dignity in principle but withholds care in practice. Bridging this gap demands political will and normative clarity - a shift from discretion to duty, from eligibility to entitlement, and from border-making to care-providing. Thus, the question remains: can welfare states like Denmark continue to uphold exclusionary social rights frameworks while claiming adherence to universal human rights? Or must they redefine the social rights of undocumented migrants to make human dignity truly unconditional?

3.7 Competing Interests

This study was funded by the BSS Graduate School at Aarhus University. The chapter is part of Author 1's PhD project, supervised by Author 2 (main supervisor) and Author 3 (co-supervisor). The authors have no conflicts of interest to declare that are relevant to the content of this chapter.

References

Bauböck, R. (2003). Reinventing urban citizenship. *Citizenship Studies, 7*(2), 139–160. https://doi.org/10.1080/1362102032000065946

Bendixen, M. C. (2021). A firm hand: Denmark's policy on rejected asylum seekers and return. Refugees Welcome. https://refugeeswelcome.dk/en/information/reports/.

Benhabib, S. (2004). *The rights of others: Aliens, residents and citizens.* Cambridge University Press.

Birk, H. O., Vrangbæk, K., Rudkjøbing, A., Krasnik, A., Eriksen, A., Richardson, E., & Smith, J. S. (2024). Denmark: Health system review. *Health Systems in Transition, 26*(1), i–152.

Biswas, D., Kristiansen, M., Krasnik, A., et al. (2011). Access to healthcare and alternative health-seeking strategies among undocumented migrants in Denmark. *BMC Public Health, 11*, 560. https://doi.org/10.1186/1471-2458-11-560

Biswas, D., Toebes, B., Hjern, A., Ascher, H., & Norredam, M. (2012). Access to health care for undocumented migrants from a human rights perspective: A comparative study of Denmark, Sweden, and the Netherlands. *Health and Human Rights, 14*(2), 49–60. PMID: 23568947.

CESCR, Committee on Economic, Social and Cultural Rights. (2000). *General Comment No. 14: The right to the highest attainable standard of health (Art. 12).* E/C.12/2000/4. https://undocs.org/E/C.12/2000/4.

CESCR, Committee on Economic, Social and Cultural Rights. (2009). *General Comment No. 20: Non-discrimination in economic, social and cultural rights (Art. 2, para. 2).* E/C.12/GC/20. https://undocs.org/E/C.12/GC/20.

Chauvin, S., & Garcés-Mascareñas, B. (2014). Becoming less illegal: Deservingness frames and undocumented migrant incorporation. *Sociology Compass, 8*, 422–432. https://doi.org/10.1111/soc4.12145

Christoffersen, J. (2017). *Udvisning af kriminelle udlændinge* [Expulsion of criminal foreigners]. Institut for Menneskerettigheder. https://menneskeret.dk/sites/menneskeret.dk/files/media/dokumenter/udgivelser/udvisning_af_kriminelle_udlaendinge_2017.pdf.

Clausen, J. K., & Skaksen, J. R. (2016). *De illegale indvandrere i Danmark* (Arbejdspapir nr. 115). Rockwool Fondens Forskningsenhed. https://en.rockwoolfonden.dk/publications/de-illegale-indvandrere-i-danmark/.

CPR-loven (Lov om Det Centrale Personregister) [The PIN Act]. (2023). *LBK nr. 1010 af 23/06/2023*. Indenrigs og Sundhedsministeriet. https://www.retsinformation.dk/eli/lta/2023/1010.

CPT, European Committee for the Prevention of Torture and Inhuman or Degrading Treatment or Punishment. (2024). *Report to the Danish Government on the visit to Denmark carried out from 23 May to 3 June 2024* (CPT/Inf (2024) 38). Council of Europe.

Cuadra, C. B. (2012). Right of access to health care for undocumented migrants in EU: A comparative study of national policies. *The European Journal of Public Health, 22*(2), 267–271. https://doi.org/10.1093/eurpub/ckr049

Damsa, D., & Franko, K. (2022). 'Without papers i can't do anything': The neglected role of citizenship status and 'illegality' in intersectional analysis. *Sociology, 57*(1), 194–210. https://doi.org/10.1177/00380385221096043(Originalworkpublished2023)

Dauvrin, M., Lorant, V., & Sandhu, S. et al. (2012). Health care for irregular migrants: pragmatism across Europe. A qualitative study. *BMC Res Notes, 5*, 99. https://doi.org/10.1186/1756-0500-5-99

De Kock, C. (2020). *Responding to drug-related problems among migrants, refugees and ethnic minorities in Europe*. European Monitoring Centre for Drugs and Drug Addiction (EMCDDA).

De Kock, C. (2022). Equitable substance use treatment for migrants and ethnic minorities in Flanders, Belgium: Service coordinator and expert perspectives. *Substance Abuse: Research and Treatment, 16*, 1–11. https://doi.org/10.1177/11782218221097390

Duff, C. (2010). Enabling places and enabling resources: New directions for harm reduction research and practice. *Drug and Alcohol Review, 29*(3), 337–344.

ECSR, European Committee of Social Rights. (2004). *FIDH v. France, complaint no. 14/2003, decision on the merits*. https://hudoc.esc.coe.int/eng/?i=cc-14-2003-dmerits-en.

ECtHR, European Court of Human Rights. (2011). *M.S.S. v. Belgium and Greece, Application No. 30696/09*. https://hudoc.echr.coe.int/eng?i=001-103050.

EMN, European Migration Network. (n.d.). *Non-refoulement*. European Commission. https://home-affairs.ec.europa.eu/networks/european-migration-network-emn/emn-asylum-and-migration-glossary/glossary/non-refoulement_en.

EUDA, European Monitoring Centre for Drugs and Drug Addiction. (2021). *Migrants and drugs: health and social responses*. European Union Drugs Agency. https://www.euda.europa.eu/publications/mini-guides/migrants-and-drugs-health-and-social-responses_en

Forvaltningsloven [Public Administration Act], LBK nr 433 af 22/04/2014. (2014). *Retsinformation.dk*. https://www.retsinformation.dk/eli/lta/2014/433.

Funge, J. K., Boye, M. C., Parellada, C. B., & Norredam, M. (2021). Demographic characteristics, medical needs and utilisation of antenatal care among pregnant undocumented migrants living in Denmark between 2011 and 2017. *Scandinavian Journal of Public Health, 50*(5), 575–583. https://doi.org/10.1177/14034948211011400

Gammeltoft-Hansen, T., & Ford, S. S. (2022). Danish immigration law. In P. A. Nielsen & J. Olsen (Eds.), *Public law: Insights into Danish constitutional and administrative law* (pp. 167–208). Hans Reitzels Forlag.

Grønnested, T. E., & Lalander, P. (2015). The bench: An open drug scene and its people. *Nordic Studies on Alcohol and Drugs, 32*(2), 165–182. https://doi.org/10.1515/nsad-2015-001.

Hacker, K., Anies, M., Folb, B. L., & Zallman, L. (2015). Barriers to health care for undocumented immigrants: A literature review. *Risk Management and Healthcare Policy, 8*, 175–183. https://doi.org/10.2147/RMHP.S70173

Hansen, A. R., Krasnik, A., & Høg, E. (2006). Adgang til sundhedsydelser for udokumenterede indvandrere: Rettigheder og praksis [Access to healthcare services for undocumented immigrants: Rights and practice]. *Ugeskrift for Læger, 168*(36), 3011–3013.

Hjemrejseloven [The Danish Return Act], LBK nr 1014 af 27/08/2024 (2024). https://www.retsinformation.dk/eli/lta/2024/1014.

Holeksa, J. (2024). "I knew it was different there": A qualitative study of the motivations and risks of drug policy migrants going to Denmark from Sweden. *Drugs: Education, Prevention and Policy, 32*(1), 72–82. https://doi.org/10.1080/09687637.2024.2307477.

Horyniak, D., Melo, J. S., Farrell, R. M., Ojeda, V. D., & Strathdee, S. A. (2016). Epidemiology of substance use among forced migrants: A global systematic review. *PLoS ONE, 11*(7), Article e0159134. https://doi.org/10.1371/journal.pone.0159134

Huschke, S. (2014). Performing deservingness. Humanitarian health care provision for migrants in Germany. *Social Science & Medicine, 120*, 352–359. https://doi.org/10.1016/j.socscimed.2014.04.046

Jensen, N. K., Norredam, M., & Draebel, T. (2011). Providing medical care for undocumented migrants in Denmark: What are the challenges for health professionals? *BMC Health Services Research, 11*(154). https://doi.org/10.1186/1472-6963-11-154.

Jørgensen, M. B., & Thomsen, T. L. (2016). Deservingness in the Danish context: Welfare chauvinism in times of crisis. *Critical Social Policy, 36*(3), 330–351.https://doi.org/10.1177/0261018315622012.

Kammersgaard, T., Kappel, N., Johansen, K. S., Kronbæk, M., Fahnøe, K. R., & Houborg, E. (2024). 'It has gotten a lot better, but it is still bad': Experiences with the police among marginalized PWUDs in a context of depenalization. *International Journal of Drug Policy, 127*, Article 104393. https://doi.org/10.1016/j.drugpo.2024.104393.

Karl-Trummer, U., Metzler, B., & Novak-Zezula, S. (2009). Health care for undocumented migrants in the EU: Concepts and cases (Background Paper No. 6). International Organization for Migration (IOM).

Lindberg, A. (2020). The production of precarity in Denmark's asylum regime. *Zeitschrift Für Sozialreform, 66*(4), 413–439.https://doi.org/10.1515/zsr-2020-0018.

Lindberg, A. (2023). Bordering Denmark: Deportation, differentiation, and racial formation. In *Border Criminologies from the Periphery: Cross-national Conversations on Bordered Penality* (pp. 266–282). Routledge. https://doi.org/10.4324/9781003333166-17.

Lister, R., Patrick, R., & Brown, K. (2024). *Understanding theories and concepts in social policy* (2nd ed.). Policy Press. https://policy.bristoluniversitypress.co.uk/asset/13528/blad-lister-understanding-theories-and-concepts-2e.pd.

Litins'ka, Y. (2018). Assessing capacity to decide on medical treatment: On human rights and the use of medical knowledge in the laws of England, Russia and Sweden (Doctoral dissertation). Uppsala University.

Marshall, T. H. (1950). *Citizenship and social class*. Cambridge University Press.

Norredam, M., Mygind, A., & Krasnik, A. (2006). Access to health care for asylum seekers in the European Union—a comparative study of country policies. *European Journal of Public Health, 16*(3), 285–289. https://doi.org/10.1093/eurpub/cki191

Pouille, A., De Ruysscher, C., van Selm, L., et al. (2024). Challenges and support needs among persons with a migration background who use drugs in four European metropolitan cities. *Harm Reduction Journal, 21*, 208. https://doi.org/10.1186/s12954-024-01110-x

Pouille, A., De Ruysscher, C., Vander Laenen, F., & Vanderplasschen, W. (2023). "Watch out for the boogieman": Stigma and substance use recovery among migrants and ethnic minorities. *Journal of Community & Applied Social Psychology, 33*(3), 571–586. https://doi.org/10.1002/casp.2657

Purcell, M. (2003). Citizenship and the right to the global city: Reimagining the capitalist world order. *International Journal of Urban and Regional Research, 27*(3), 564–590. https://doi.org/10.1111/1468-2427.00467

Rechel, B., Mladovsky, P., Devillé, W., Rijks, B., Petrova-Benedict, R., and McKee, M. (Eds.). (2011). *Migration and health in the European Union*. Open University Press/WHO Observatory.

Retssikkerhedsloven [Act on Legal Protection and Administration in Social Matters], LBK nr 265 af 25/02/2022. (2022). *Retsinformation.dk*. https://www.retsinformation.dk/eli/lta/2022/265.

Rhodes, T. (2009). Risk environments and drug harms: A social science for harm reduction approach. *International Journal of Drug Policy, 20*(3), 193–201.https://doi.org/10.1016/j.drugpo.2008.10.003.

Schwörer, J. (Ed.). (2025). *New Danish paradigms on asylum and integration: Effects and challenges*. Friedrich-Ebert-Stiftung, Nordic Countries. https://library.fes.de/pdf-files/international/21766.pdf.

Serviceloven [The Social Services Act], LBK nr. 1129 af 22/09/2025. (2025). *Social- og Boligministeriet*. https://www.retsinformation.dk/eli/lta/2025/1129.

Setoodeh, A., Houborg, E., & Thylstrup, B. (2024). Mod Vesterbro, på sporet af afviste asylansøgere. *STOF – Viden om rusmidler og samfund, 2024*(48), 44–49. Center for Rusmiddelforskning.

Søgaard, T. F., Højlund Bræmer, M., & Mulbjerg Pedersen, M. (2021). *Exploring drug supply, associated violence and exploitation of vulnerable groups in Denmark*. European Monitoring Centre for Drugs and Drug Addiction.

Soysal, Y. N. (1994). *Limits of citizenship: Migrants and postnational membership in Europe*. University of Chicago Press.

STPK, Styrelsen for Patientklager. (2019, April 30). *Region havde ikke inddraget alle relevante hensyn og regler ved afgørelse om betaling i forbindelse med ikke-EU-borgers planlagte fødsel i Danmark* (Sagsnummer 18SPS63). https://www.stpk.dk/afgorelser-og-domme/afgorelser-fra-styrelsen-for-patientklager/18sps63/.

Sundhedsloven [The Health Act], LBK nr. 275 af 12/03/2025. (2025). *Indenrigs- og Sundhedsministeriet*. https://www.retsinformation.dk/eli/lta/2025/275.

Ticktin, M. (2011). *Casualties of care: Immigration and the politics of humanitarianism in France*. University of California Press.

Udlændingeloven [The Aliens Act], LBK nr. 1183 af 25/09/2025. (2025). *Udlændinge- og Integrationsministeriet*. https://www.retsinformation.dk/eli/lta/2025/1183.

UN, United Nations. (1948). *Universal Declaration of Human Rights*. https://www.un.org/en/about-us/universal-declaration-of-human-rights.

UN, United Nations. (1966). *International Covenant on Economic, Social and Cultural Rights*. United Nations, Treaty Series, 993, 3. https://www.ohchr.org/en/instruments-mechanisms/instruments/international-covenant-economic-social-and-cultural-rights.

US, Udlændingestyrelsen [Danish Immigration Service]. (2025). *Tal og fakta på udlændingeområdet 2024*. Udlændinge- og Integrationsministeriet. https://us.dk/media/uk0lnhte/tal-og-fakta-10062025_tilgaengelig.pdf.

van Selm, L., White, T. M., Picchio, C. A., Requena-Méndez, A., Busz, M., Perez Gayo, R., et al. (2023). Drug use and access to drug dependency services for vulnerable migrants who use drugs in the European Union: Consensus statements and recommendations from civil society experts in Europe. *International Journal of Drug Policy, 118*, Article 104087. https://doi.org/10.1016/j.drugpo.2023.104087

Willen, S. S. (2012). How is health-related "deservingness" reckoned? Perspectives from unauthorized im/migrants in Tel Aviv. *Social Science & Medicine, 74*(6), 812–821. https://doi.org/10.1016/j.socscimed.2011.06.033

Winters, M., Rechel, B., de Jong, L., et al. (2018). A systematic review on the use of healthcare services by undocumented migrants in Europe. *BMC Health Services Research, 18*, 30. https://doi.org/10.1186/s12913-018-2838-y

Chapter 4
Development and Evaluation of an Evidence-Based Participatory Multi-Component Prevention Concept for Hazardous Substance Use among Refugees in Shared Accommodations

Jonathan Uricher, Miriam Hedwig Lorenz, Johannes Michalak, Thomas Heidenreich, and Marion Laging

4.1 Introduction and Background

4.1.1 Vulnerability of Refugees to Hazardous Substance Use

According to recent systematic reviews and meta-analyses, refugees have a high prevalence of mental disorders (Blackmore et al., 2020; Patanè et al., 2022). Additionally, refugees in Germany often live under precarious housing conditions, especially in the period following their arrival in the host country when they are accommodated in collective or shared accommodations. Schönfeld et al. (2022) analysed data from the socio-economic panel on the mental health of refugees and showed that refugees in shared accommodations have poorer mental health. They demonstrated a connection between accommodation conditions and the mental health of refugees, describing that satisfaction with security and privacy has important effects.

Refugees living in shared accommodations represent a particularly vulnerable group for hazardous and dependent substance use, due to their poorer mental health, frequent traumatic experiences in their country of origin or during flight, and the

J. Uricher (✉) · M. H. Lorenz · T. Heidenreich · M. Laging
Faculty of Social Work, Education and Nursing Sciences, University of Applied Sciences, Esslingen, Germany
e-mail: jonathan.uricher@dhbw.de

J. Michalak
Department of Psychology and Psychotherapy, Faculty of Health, Witten/Herdecke University, Witten, Germany

C. De Kock (ed.), *Substance Use Among Refugees in Europe*,
https://doi.org/10.1007/978-3-032-32399-6_4

psychosocial stress associated with their housing situation in the host country. (Horyniak et al., 2016; Saleh et al., 2023). However, findings to date diverge substantially regarding the reported prevalence of substance use among refugees. Also, some studies point to the vulnerability of refugees, while others demonstrate low prevalence rates among refugees.

Zurhold and Kuhn (2023) collected empirical data on substance use among refugees in shared accommodations and found a lower lifetime prevalence of alcohol and drug use among refugees compared to general German population. Lower prevalence rates for substance use disorders were also observed by Harris et al. (2019) and discussed in the joint report of the European Monitoring Center for Drugs and Drug Addiction (EMCDDA) and the European Union Agency for Asylum (EUAA) (2023). It is striking that after arrival in the destination country, refugee populations showed lower substance use and higher resilience than the general population of the destination country, but the prevalence rates of refugees approach those of the majority population over time (EMCDDA & EUAA, 2023; Harris et al., 2019). The analysis by Zurhold and Kuhn (2023) also shows that substance use among refugees increases after their arrival in Germany.

Refugees often face various barriers to accessing the support system in relation to addiction prevention and addiction support services (Saleh et al., 2023). Zurhold and Kuhn (2023) showed in their study on substance use among refugees that they are largely unfamiliar with the German addiction support system. Aleer et al. (2024) identified in their systematic review that refugee youth have negative experiences or reservations about institutions or are unaware of prevention services, which consequently prevents them from using addiction prevention measures (Aleer et al., 2024). However, the joint report of the EMCDDA and EUAA (2023) points out that professionals in so-called "reception settings" face challenges related to hazardous and dependent substance use, and therefore specific support services are necessary in these settings.

4.1.2 Project PraeWi*: Overview and Objectives*

The research project *PraeWi* addresses the prevention of hazardous and dependent substance use among refugees in shared accommodations.

Developed at Esslingen University of Applied Sciences in cooperation with the Social Welfare Office Stuttgart and various providers of addiction and refugee aid organizations from Stuttgart, the project was designed to be multidisciplinary and participatory. Within the project, hazardous substance use is defined according to the 11th revision of the International Classification of Diseases (ICD-11) definition as "a pattern of psychoactive substance use that appreciably increases the risk of harmful physical or mental health consequences to the user or to others to an extent that warrants attention and advice from health professionals" (WHO, 2024).

The overarching question guiding the project was: "What risks and needs exist among refugees in shared accommodations in relation to hazardous and dependent substance use, and what is central to the design of effective prevention measures so that refugees in shared accommodations can replace dysfunctional coping patterns in the form of hazardous substance use with health-promoting coping strategies?" (The assumptions underlying this question will be substantiated in the following.)

This comprehensive approach allowed for a nuanced understanding of the complex issues surrounding substance use among refugees, while also developing and testing practical interventions. The project's participatory nature ensured that the perspectives and experiences of refugees themselves were central to the research and development process.

The *PraeWi* project aimed to address several key gaps in the existing research and practice:

- The lack of specific, evidence-based prevention measures for refugees in shared accommodations.
- The need for culturally sensitive and linguistically appropriate interventions.
- The importance of considering the unique psychosocial stressors faced by refugees in the context of substance use prevention.
- The potential for participatory approaches to enhance the effectiveness and acceptability of prevention strategies.

By targeting these areas, that are also discussed by other authors as requiring urgent attention (e.g., Saleh et al., 2023; Zurhold & Kuhn, 2023), *PraeWi* aimed to make substantial contributions to the field of substance use prevention among refugee populations, with potential implications and recommendations for policy and practice in Germany and beyond.

4.2 Theoretical Framework

4.2.1 Multifactorial Understanding of Substance Use among Refugees

Substance use among refugees is a complex phenomenon that requires a multifactorial understanding. The bio-psycho-social model provides a comprehensive framework for conceptualizing the various factors that influence substance use in this population (Liel, 2020; Veltrup, 2020).

From a biological perspective, refugees may be at increased risk due to genetic predispositions or physiological changes resulting from trauma and chronic stress. The high prevalence of mental disorders among refugees, including post-traumatic stress disorder, depression, and anxiety, can alter brain chemistry and increase vulnerability to substance use (Blackmore et al., 2020; Patanè et al., 2022).

Psychologically, substance use often serves as a coping mechanism for refugees dealing with traumatic experiences, loss, and the stressors of resettlement. As Horyniak et al. (2016) note, substances may be used for "self-medication" to manage symptoms of mental disorders or emotional distress. The psychological strain of adapting to a new culture and navigating complex administrative asylum processes can also contribute to substance use as a form of escape or relief (Saleh et al., 2023).

Socially, the conditions in refugee camps and shared accommodations can create an environment conducive to substance use. Lack of privacy, prolonged periods of inactivity, and social isolation may increase the likelihood of substance use (Schönfeld et al., 2022). Additionally, changes in cultural norms around substance use between countries of origin and host countries, such as perception and availability of substances, can impact consumption patterns (EMCDDA & EUAA, 2023).

Importantly, substance use among refugees often begins or escalates after arrival in the host country, highlighting the critical role of post-migration factors (Zurhold & Kuhn, 2023). This underscores the need for prevention efforts that address the specific challenges faced by refugees in their new environments.

A multifactorial approach recognizes that substance use among refugees is not simply an individual health issue, but one deeply intertwined with broader social, political, and structural factors. This comprehensive understanding is essential for developing effective, culturally appropriate prevention and intervention strategies for this vulnerable population.

4.2.2 Participatory Health Research and Setting Approach

The theoretical basis for the participatory development and research of the evidence-based prevention concept is the "Model for Participatory Health Research" (Schaefer et al., 2022). The model contains four central components for participatory research projects: the context of the project, its structure in terms of cooperation and collaboration processes, the participatory design, and resulting effects. It was adapted from the original model for community-based research (Wallerstein et al., 2008) for the German-speaking area and aims to provide a conceptual framework for thinking and reflecting in participatory research projects.

Central to the model's approach is the involvement of the very people whose living conditions and areas are being researched. Closely linked to the setting approach, participatory health research aims not only to gain multi-perspective insights that are central to people in the researched setting but also to initiate change processes that improve their living conditions and counteract health inequalities (Abma et al., 2019; Hartung et al., 2020; Schaefer et al., 2022; Wright, 2013).

Knowledge generation in the context of participatory health research is seen as a co-production of the involved actors, whereby all participants can contribute their experiences and thus actively shape the research process together (Hartung et al., 2020). In relation to the processes within the framework of the research and development project *PraeWi*, the participatory project structures should be mentioned here: at the beginning of the project, a steering committee responsible for the strategic direction of the project, which includes all relevant regional stakeholders from the setting of shared accommodations (e.g., refugee and addiction aid organizations as well as representatives of refugees) was constituted. Furthermore, an advisory board was formed for overarching scientific, practice-oriented, ethical, and political reflection and networking. The advisory board comprises representatives from various scientific disciplines, refugees, practice partners, and the project team.

The setting approach (Rosenbrock, 2015) is another key theoretical foundation of the project. This approach focuses not merely on individual behaviour but on the entire setting with all relevant actors and structures, thereby combining behavioural and structural prevention and thus bringing together the individual and structural levels (Hartung & Rosenbrock, 2022). In current professional debates on addiction prevention, the setting approach is considered a core strategy, as it can specifically address socially or health disadvantaged groups in their setting without individual stigmatization and especially focuses on structural living conditions and environmental factors.

By integrating participatory health research with a setting approach, the project aims to develop prevention strategies that are not only evidence-based but also culturally appropriate and responsive to the specific needs and contexts of refugees in shared accommodations. This approach recognizes refugees as active participants in the research and prevention development process, rather than passive recipients of interventions. The combination of participatory health research and the setting approach in the *PraeWi* project offers several advantages:

- It ensures that the prevention strategies developed are grounded in the real-life experiences and needs of refugees.
- It addresses the broader environmental and structural factors that influence substance use beyond individual factors.
- It promotes empowerment and capacity building among refugee communities.
- It facilitates the development of interventions that are more likely to be accepted and effective within the specific context of shared accommodations.

This theoretical framework guided the entire research process of *PraeWi*, from the initial needs assessment to the development, implementation and evaluation of the prevention concept, ensuring that the project remained responsive to the complex realities of refugee life in shared accommodations.

4.3 Needs, Resources and Development

The *PraeWi* research and development project employed a sequential multi-method approach to develop an evidence-based and participatory multi-component prevention concept for hazardous substance use among refugees in shared accommodations. This procedure allowed for gradually gaining insights and incorporating them into the development of the prevention concept, combining qualitative and quantitative research methods to obtain a comprehensive understanding of the complex topic. This approach comprised several consecutive phases.

4.3.1 Phase 1: Systematic Literature Review and Qualitative Exploration

Figure 4.1 depicts the various phases of the study that were designed according to the Exploratory Sequential Design devised by Creswell (2022). The first phase of the project involved a systematic literature review that analysed the current state of research on preventing hazardous substance use among refugees. This review (Lorenz et al. 2021) identified a significant research gap in this area. It revealed that only few empirical studies on the effectiveness of prevention measures for this specific target group were available. However, the review highlighted the great need for target group-specific prevention approaches due to the vulnerability of refugees to hazardous substance use.

Based on the findings of this systematic review, a qualitative exploration phase followed. Semi-structured interviews were conducted with professionals ($n = 5$) and refugees ($n = 8$) from shared accommodations. These interviews were about 1,5 hours long each and aimed to capture the specific situation in the shared accommodations regarding substance use among refugees and to identify resources and challenges. The interviews were recorded, transcribed and transferred to the MAXQDA coding software. Data were coded deductively and then analysed for thematic content (Kuckartz & Rädiker, 2023). The results of the interviews with the professionals (Lorenz et al., 2023) provided important insights into the lifeworld of refugees and the perspectives of professionals. Various risk factors at individual, interpersonal and structural levels that can influence substance use were identified. Additionally, barriers to accessing prevention and support services became evident, such as language barriers and lack of knowledge about the health system.

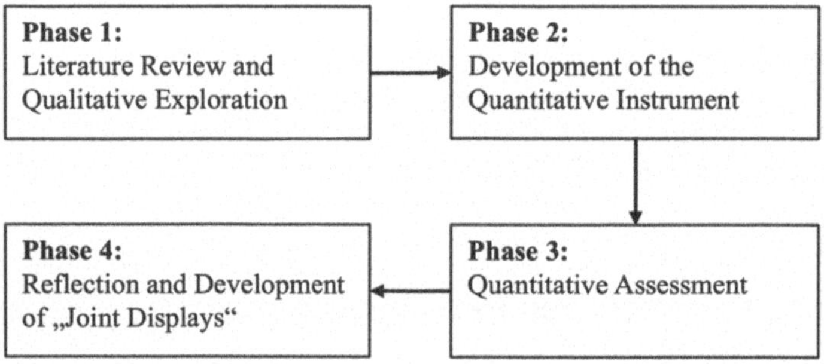

Fig. 4.1 Phases of the exploratory sequential mixed-methods design based on Creswell (2022)

4.3.2 Phases 2–3: Quantitative Needs and Resource Analysis

Based on the results of phase 1, we developed a quantitative instrument that was employed in the field. The third phase of the project encompassed a comprehensive mixed-methods needs and resource analysis. This study (Lorenz et al., 2024b) combined the results of the qualitative interviews with a quantitative cross-sectional study to obtain a comprehensive perspective of the situation. The quantitative part consisted of a cross-sectional study with 185 refugees from 13 different shared accommodations in Stuttgart (Germany). Participants completed questionnaires that were available in various languages and captured various aspects of substance use, mental health and living situation. The data were analysed using bivariate correlations and multivariate logistic regression. The results of the mixed-methods study revealed various risk factors for hazardous substance use:

- Substance use as a coping strategy for flight experiences.
- Presence of suicidal thoughts.
- Length of stay in shared accommodations.

It became evident that with each additional month in shared accommodation, the likelihood of hazardous substance use increased by 2%. These findings underscored the necessity of early prevention measures.

4.3.3 Phase 4: Joining Qualitative and Quantitative Results

The qualitative data from the 13 interviews with professionals and refugees in shared accommodations also provided insights into the complex psychosocial stressors experienced by refugees, such as trauma, uncertainty regarding residence status, and social isolation. At the same time, resources and functional coping strategies were identified that could be incorporated into the prevention concept. In the final phase of the study, joint displays of the qualitative and quantitative results were developed. With this joint display analysis (Guetterman et al., 2015) both qualitative and quantitative data were matched and analysed in a comprehensive manner. A comprehensive joint display of the quantitative correlations and corresponding qualitative quotes is available in Lorenz et al. (2024b).

4.3.4 Participatory and Evidence Based Development of the Multi-Component Prevention Concept

Based on the findings from the previous research phases, the multi-component prevention concept was developed in the fourth phase. This process was highly

Table 4.1 Multi-component prevention concept (Lorenz et al., 2024a)[1]

Component	Measures / *Description*
Health communication through peers	Multilingual information videos Peer counsellor training
Toolkit for professionals	Guide for acute situations E-learning tool for professional training
Bridges in the support system between refugee, addiction and trauma aid	*Cross-sectional component*
Online prevention	Podcast BePrepared app
Target group-specific information and communication strategy	*Cross-sectional component aimed at* e.g. *political and community stakeholders*

participatory and involved various stakeholders who contributed to working groups to the development of the concept:

- Refugees from shared accommodations.
- Professionals from refugee assistance and addiction prevention.
- Representatives of refugee self-organizations.
- Scientists.

The participatory development took place in several steps:

1. Formation of a steering committee and an advisory board as overarching bodies.
2. Establishment of topic-specific working groups (e.g., for creating information videos and a podcast).
3. Regular workshops and discussion groups for joint concept development.
4. Continuous feedback of development steps with target groups.

This participatory approach ensured that the prevention concept considers the needs and perspectives of the target group and is culturally sensitive remaining the theoretical foundations such as the setting approach and the bio-psycho-social model of substance use. At the same time, the scientific findings from the previous research phases were incorporated into the content of the concept development to create an evidence-based foundation. Additionally, insights from trauma research and culturally sensitive addiction prevention were considered. The resulting multi-component prevention concept comprises five main components (see Table 4.1).

These components address different levels of prevention and consider both individual and structural factors. They aim to make health information accessible, qualify professionals, reduce barriers in the support system, and provide low-threshold prevention services.

Emphasis was placed on psychoeducation and the provision of health information (e.g., in the information videos or in the podcast) to empower refugees to make

[1] Adapted from Lorenz et al. (2024a, Table 2). Some modifications were made. https://doi.org/10.1186/s13063-024-08558-z,

informed decisions regarding their substance use. At the same time, the concept aimed to promote alternative coping strategies and strengthen the existing resilience of the target group.

The participatory development made it possible to identify and address potential barriers early on. For example, great emphasis was placed on the linguistic and cultural adaptation of materials to achieve high acceptance in the target group.

Overall, the developed multi-component prevention concept represents an innovative approach that considers the specific needs and life circumstances of refugees in shared accommodations while being based on scientific evidence. The combination of evidence-based research and participatory development provides a promising foundation for implementing and evaluating the concept in practice.

4.4 Implementation and Evaluation

4.4.1 Implementation Strategy

The implementation of the multi-component prevention concept developed in the *PraeWi* project required a comprehensive and carefully planned strategy to address the complex setting of shared accommodations for refugees. This strategy was designed to overcome potential barriers and facilitate the sustainable integration of the prevention concept into the shared accommodation settings.

A key element of the implementation strategy was stakeholder engagement from the early stages of the project. Relevant stakeholders including refugee assistance organizations, addiction prevention services, and refugee self-organizations were involved in the planning and implementation process. This participatory approach ensured that the implementation was responsive to the needs and realities of both refugees and staff working in the accommodations. Regular meetings and workshops were held with stakeholders to gather feedback and make iterative improvements to the implementation approach.

The concept was implemented using a phased roll-out across different shared accommodations within the time frame of the project. This gradual implementation allowed for learning and adaptation based on experiences in the initial sites before scaling up to additional locations. The phased approach also helped manage the workload for staff and avoid overwhelming the system with too many changes at once.

Extensive training was provided for social workers and other professionals in the accommodations to enable effective delivery of the prevention concept. This included workshops on the theoretical background, practical application of the prevention materials, and culturally sensitive approaches to working with refugees. Ongoing support and supervision were offered to staff to address any challenges that arose during implementation.

A core component of the implementation strategy was the involvement of refugees themselves as peer educators. Selected refugees were trained to help disseminate health information and facilitate prevention activities within their communities. This peer-based approach aimed to increase the cultural appropriateness and acceptability of the prevention efforts.

To address language barriers, all prevention materials and activities were provided in multiple languages relevant to the refugee populations in the accommodations. Professional translators were utilized to ensure accuracy and cultural sensitivity in the translations. Visual materials were also developed to support communication with refugees with limited literacy.

Where possible, the prevention concept was integrated into existing health and social services in the accommodations rather than being implemented as a standalone program. This integration approach aimed to enhance sustainability and avoid duplication of efforts. Regular coordination meetings were held with other service providers to align activities.

An implementation team provided continuous support and guidance to staff implementing the concept. This team conducted site visits, offered troubleshooting assistance, and facilitated sharing of best practices across locations. The team also collected ongoing feedback to identify any needed adjustments to the implementation approach.

Recognizing the diverse backgrounds of the refugee population, implementation methods were adapted to be culturally appropriate for different groups. This included consideration of cultural norms around substance use, mental health, and help-seeking behaviours. Gender-sensitive approaches were also incorporated to ensure the prevention activities were accessible and acceptable to both men and women.

To maximize accessibility, prevention activities and materials were designed with low-threshold access in mind. This included offering flexible scheduling of activities, providing childcare during sessions, and ensuring physical accessibility of spaces used. Online and mobile-based components were also developed to allow access to prevention information outside of formal prevention interventions.

Throughout the implementation process, regular monitoring and evaluation activities were conducted to assess fidelity of implementation and identify any emerging challenges or unintended consequences. This allowed for ongoing refinement of the implementation strategy to optimize its effectiveness in the dynamic setting of refugee accommodations.

By employing this multi-faceted and adaptive implementation strategy, the project aimed to overcome the numerous barriers to prevention efforts with refugee populations and ensure the sustained uptake of the multi-component prevention concept across shared accommodation settings. The strategy's emphasis on stakeholder engagement, cultural sensitivity, and flexibility was designed to maximize the relevance and impact of the prevention efforts for this vulnerable population.

4.4.2 Evaluation of the Multi-Component Prevention Concept

The evaluation of the prevention concept was conducted through a cluster-randomized controlled trial, as described in the study protocol by Lorenz et al. (2024a) and reported in the publication by Uricher et al. (In Publication). The study was originally designed as a stepped-wedge trial involving nine shared accommodations, with data collection at various time points. The accommodations were assigned to three clusters, with the prevention concept introduced gradually across clusters.

Due to organizational and structural challenges in three of the nine participating accommodations, the planned stepped-wedge design could not be fully realized. During the study, organizational and structural factors emerged as significant barriers to the implementation of the prevention concept, necessitating adjustments to the study design. The staff was unable to support the implementation as initially planned due to unforeseen challenges. This highlights that the prevailing conditions in shared accommodations pose difficulties not only for residents but also for employees. At the same time, staff members in these settings are essential for facilitating access to preventive interventions, as they are integral to the support structures for refugees. Therefore, future research projects should allocate increased personnel and financial resources to support both implementation and data collection. Consequently, the analysis was conducted using a cluster-randomized pre-post design with linear and logistic multi-level regression analysis models (Hox, 2010). The prevention concept was implemented in four shared accommodations and compared with two control facilities before and after implementation. Key findings from the evaluation study include:

- No significant effect was found for the primary outcome (knowledge about hazardous substance use and its consequences), indicating that the effectiveness of the prevention concept could not be demonstrated.
- Models including structural variables showed a stronger, albeit still non-significant, effect.
- A relationship was found between unclear residence status and increased scores for depression, anxiety, and stress.
- Length of stay in shared accommodations was associated with increased scores for depression, anxiety, and stress.
- High housing satisfaction was associated with lower scores for depression, anxiety, and stress.

The lack of significant results may be attributed to the small sample size and low statistical power. Alternatively, it is possible that the prevention concept was not effective due to refugees' limited capacity to engage with additional topics given their psychosocial stress.

Despite the lack of demonstrated effectiveness, the evaluation provided valuable insights into the importance of contextual factors in shared accommodations regarding the mental health burden of refugees. The study highlighted the complex interplay between structural conditions (e.g., residence status, length of stay) and mental health outcomes.

The evaluation process also revealed methodological challenges in conducting research with refugee populations in shared accommodations. These included difficulties in achieving representative sampling due to the heterogeneity of the target group, language barriers, and the need for culturally sensitive research instruments.

4.5 Discussion

4.5.1 Synthesis of Key Findings

The *PraeWi* project has provided valuable insights into hazardous substance use among refugees in shared accommodation settings, employing various methodological approaches. A key finding is the particular risk situation and structural vulnerability of refugees for hazardous and dependent forms of substance use, aligning with findings from Horyniak et al. (2016). The complex burden of stress experienced by refugees is associated with an increased risk of hazardous substance use (Saleh et al., 2023).

The systematic literature review (Lorenz, 2021) highlighted the interdependencies between mental health burden, structural conditions, and hazardous or dependent substance use. It also revealed the intertwining of the topics of flight, trauma, and addiction, which is hardly adequately addressed in existing care structures. The qualitative study with professionals in shared accommodation settings (Lorenz et al., 2023) paints a picture of the burden on refugees and describes various barriers to assistance services.

Interestingly, this contrasts with the low prevalence rates of hazardous substance use among refugees found in several recent studies (EMCDDA & EUAA, 2023; Harris et al., 2019; Zurhold & Kuhn, 2023). However, all these studies demonstrated that prevalence rates increase with length of stay, and the *PraeWi* project found that the relative probability of hazardous consumption increases by 2% with each additional month. This suggests that even though prevalence rates are relatively low, they remarkably increase during the stay in shared accommodations and therefore the risk factor in the setting should be taken seriously and addressed as early as possible to maintain existing resilience (Walther et al., 2021). Furthermore, we could identify other risk factors for hazardous substance use in the mixed-methods study (Lorenz et al., 2024b) such as substance use due to flight experience (meaning it begins during flight or after arrival in Germany) and suicidal plans. The connection between suicide plans and hazardous substance use illustrates once again the intertwining of mental health and substance use.

4.5.2 Limitations and Methodological Challenges

The *PraeWi* project faced several methodological challenges that need to be considered when interpreting the results. Participatory research with refugees "has special potentials, but also comes with challenges" (Odukoya & von Unger, 2023). While the participatory design allowed for the inclusion of refugees' perspectives and experiences, it also presented challenges in terms of access to the target group and navigating power dynamics.

Access to the target group was complicated by numerous barriers and restrictions due to their structural disadvantage, including linguistic and cultural obstacles or reservations about state organizations (Von Köppen et al., 2020). Power dynamics played a central role and could potentially prevent people from participating (Roura et al., 2021). The initial phase should ensure that the definition of the target group aligns precisely with the intended sampling frame. Early identification and engagement of relevant gatekeepers—such as decision-makers are crucial, as is establishing clear and open channels of communication. Collecting all available information about residents in advance, for example for weighting procedures or language selection, is essential. It is important to communicate transparently with gatekeepers about the necessity of this data and to guarantee robust data protection measures. Existing structures within the field, such as volunteers, facility staff, or social workers, can provide valuable support but may also introduce bias or ethical challenges.

The heterogeneity of the refugee population in terms of origin and flight experiences posed challenges for achieving representative sampling in quantitative research and theoretical saturation in qualitative research (Borde & Blümel, 2020; Fetz, 2018; UNHCR, 2024).

Despite these challenges, the *PraeWi* project's multi-method approach allowed for field exploration and a multi-perspective capture of the burden on refugees in shared accommodations. The systematic sequence of research work, starting with a literature review and progressing through qualitative and quantitative studies, provided a comprehensive understanding of the issue.

4.5.3 Implications and Recommendations for Research, Prevention Practice and Policy

The results of the *PraeWi* project have significant implications for both practice and policy in substance use prevention for refugees. The interdependencies of mental health burden, structural framework conditions, and hazardous or dependent substance use highlight the need for early intervention and prevention measures immediately after refugees' arrival. It is crucial to recognize the functionality of substance use for refugees as a dysfunctional coping behaviour and to address risk factors while offering functional alternatives from a multifactorial perspective. The influence of conditions in shared accommodations on refugees' well-being cannot be overlooked. To determine whether the housing situation in shared accommodation or the length of stay in Germany can be considered risk factors in themselves, future studies should include comparisons with samples of refugees living in alternative types of accommodation. As a policy implication, this suggests the need for alternative forms of accommodation and an acceleration of asylum processes to help refugees more quickly transition to private housing and escape the burden of the shared accommodation setting. Prevention practices should be designed with consideration for the limited capacity refugees may have for engaging with additional topics outside their often energy-sapping asylum process. This has implications for the scope, didactics, and content of prevention concepts.

The *PraeWi* project has opened up several avenues for future research. There is a need for further investigation into how much capacity refugees have for additional topics outside their asylum process and what implications this has for the design of prevention concepts. Future research should focus on developing and evaluating culturally appropriate prevention interventions tailored to the unique needs and experiences of refugees. Longitudinal studies examining changes in substance use patterns and risk factors over time as refugees transition through different stages of resettlement would provide valuable insights. Additionally, implementation science approaches could help identify best practices for integrating prevention programs into existing refugee services and overcoming barriers to access and engagement. There is also a need for research on how to implement culturally sensitive data collection that incorporates concepts from both the global South and the global North while still generating comparable data.

4.6 Conclusion

The *PraeWi* project has made significant contributions to our understanding of hazardous substance use prevention among refugees in shared accommodations. Through its multi-method sequential approach, the project has provided valuable insights into the complex interplay of factors influencing substance use in this vulnerable population.

One of the key findings is the paradoxical relationship between the high-stress situation experienced by refugees and the initially low prevalence rates of hazardous substance use. While refugees face numerous psychosocial stressors and traumatic experiences, studies have shown that their substance use rates are often lower than those of the host population upon arrival. However, the project revealed that the relative probability of hazardous consumption increases by 2% with each additional month spent in shared accommodations. This highlights the critical importance of early prevention efforts to maintain the existing resilience of refugees and address risk factors in their new environment.

The project's comprehensive approach, combining a systematic literature review, qualitative exploration, mixed-methods needs and resource analysis, and a cluster-randomized evaluation study, has provided a nuanced understanding of the challenges faced by refugees in relation to substance use. It has identified key risk factors, including substance use as a coping mechanism for flight experiences, the presence of suicidal thoughts, and the length of stay in shared accommodations.

Moreover, the *PraeWi* project has underscored the importance of addressing structural factors in prevention efforts. The findings suggest that the conditions in shared accommodations, unclear residence status, and prolonged asylum processes significantly impact refugees' mental health and potential substance use. This calls for policy changes to improve housing conditions and accelerate asylum procedures, allowing refugees to transition more quickly to private housing and escape the burden of the shared accommodation setting.

The participatory approach employed in the project has proven valuable in developing culturally appropriate and relevant prevention materials. By involving refugees in various working groups and implementation teams, the project ensured that the perspectives and experiences of the target group were central to the research and development process. This approach has the potential to enhance the effectiveness and acceptability of prevention strategies.

However, the project also faced significant challenges, particularly in the implementation and evaluation phases. The ongoing "crisis mode" in these settings, combined with staff shortages, created a highly stressful environment that affected the project's implementation. These challenges highlight the complexity of conducting research and implementing interventions in the dynamic setting of refugee accommodations. Future studies should consider that both financial and personnel resources are crucial for successful data collection in shared accommodations. Adequate funding and staffing of the professionals in shared accommodations not only facilitate access to these settings but are also essential for reaching the desired sample size. Addressing these resource requirements will enhance the feasibility and reliability of research conducted in this context.

The evaluation study, while not demonstrating significant effects of the prevention concept, provided important insights into the methodological challenges of researching refugee populations. It highlighted the need for larger sample sizes, longer follow-up periods, and more sensitive outcome measures to detect potential effects of prevention interventions in this context.

Looking forward, the *PraeWi* project has opened several avenues for future research and practice. There is a need for further investigation into the capacity of refugees to engage with prevention programs alongside their often energy-sapping asylum processes. Future studies should focus on developing and evaluating culturally appropriate prevention interventions tailored to the unique needs and experiences of refugees, considering the temporal aspects of their resettlement journey.

Implementation science approaches could help identify best practices for integrating prevention programs into existing refugee services and overcoming barriers to access and engagement. Additionally, there is a need for research on how to implement culturally sensitive data collection that incorporates concepts from both the global South and the global North while still generating comparable data.

As global conflicts and climate change continue to drive forced migration, the need for effective substance use prevention strategies for refugees will only grow. The

PraeWi project has laid a foundation for future work in this critical area, emphasizing the need for interdisciplinary collaboration, participatory approaches, and a focus on both individual resilience and structural change. By building on these insights, future efforts can work towards creating more effective, equitable, and compassionate support systems for refugees, ultimately contributing to better health outcomes and successful integration in their new communities.

Acknowledgments We would like to thank all participants of this study. Thank you for giving your necessary and important insights of substance use behaviours among refugees in shared accommodations.

Competing Interests The authors have no conflicts of interest to declare that are relevant to the content of this chapter.

Ethics Approval The underlying studies were performed in line with the principles of the Declaration of Helsinki. Approval was granted by the Alice Salomon University Ethics Committee in Berlin, approval numbers 01–2020/31 and 01–2024/62. Participants in the studies could choose to give informed consent written or online.

References

Abma, T., Banks, S., Cook, T., Dias, S., Madsen, W., Springett, J., & Wright, M. (2019). *Participatory research for health and social Well-being*. Springer Nature. https://doi.org/10.1007/978-3-319-93191-3

Aleer, E., Alam, K., & Rashid, A. (2024). A systematic literature review of substance-use prevention programs amongst refugee youth. *Community Mental Health Journal, 60*, 1151–1170. https://doi.org/10.1007/s10597-024-01267-6

Blackmore, R., Boyle, J. A., Fazel, M., Ranasinha, S., Gray, K. M., Fitzgerald, G., Misso, M., & Gibson-Helm, M. (2020). The prevalence of mental illness in refugees and asylum seekers: A systematic review and metaanalysis. *PLoS Medicine, 17*(9), e1003337. https://doi.org/10.1371/journal.pmed.1003337

Borde, T. & Blümel, S. (2020). Gesundheitsförderung und Migrationshintergrund. In: Bundeszentrale für gesundheitliche Aufklärung (BZgA) (Ed.). *Leitbegriffe der Gesundheitsförderung und Prävention. Glossar zu Konzepten*, Strategien und Methoden. https://doi.org/10.17623/BZGA:Q4i047-2.0

Creswell, J. W. (2022). *A concise introduction to mixed methods research* (2nd ed.). Sage Publications.

EMCDDA, & EUAA. (2023). *Professionals working in reception centres in Europe: An overview of drug-related challenges and support needs. Joint report by the EMCDDA and EUAA.* Publications Office of the EU. https://doi.org/10.2810/82540

Fetz, K. (2018). "Die sind doch alle gleich!"—Warum geflüchtete Menschen oft als homogene Gruppe betrachtet werden und welche Maßnahmen zu einer individuelleren Wahrnehmung beitragen können. *Fachnetz Flucht, 1*. Retrieved March 25, 2025, from http://www.fachnetzflucht.de/die-sind-doch-alle-gleich-warum-gefluechtete-menschen-oft-als-homogene-gruppe-betrachtet-werden-und-welche-massnahmen-zu-einer-individuelleren-wahrnehmung-beitragen-koenne/

Guetterman, T. C., Fetters, M. D., & Creswell, J. W. (2015). Integrating quantitative and qualitative results in health science mixed methods research through joint displays. *Annals of Family Medicine, 13*(6), 554–561. https://doi.org/10.1370/afm.1865

Harris, S., Dykxhoorn, J., Hollander, A. C., Dalman, C., & Kirkbride, J. B. (2019). Substance use disorders in refugee and migrant groups in Sweden: A nationwide cohort study of 1.2 million people. *PLoS Medicine, 16*(11). https://doi.org/10.1371/journal.pmed.1002944

Hartung, S. & Rosenbrock, R. (2022). Settingansatz–Lebensweltansatz. In: Bundeszentrale für gesundheitliche Aufklärung (BZgA) (Ed.). *Leitbegriffe der Gesundheitsförderung und Prävention.* Glossar zu Konzepten, Strategien und Methoden. https://doi.org/10.17623/BZGA:Q4-i106-2.0

Hartung, S., Wihofszky, P., & Wright, T. (2020). Partizipative Forschung—ein Forschungsansatz für Gesundheit und seine Methoden. In S. Hartung, P. Wihofszky, & T. Wright (Eds.), *Partizipative Forschung—ein Forschungsansatz für Gesundheit und seine Methoden.* Springer VS. https://doi.org/10.1007/978-3-658-30361-7

Horyniak, D., Melo, J. S., Farrell, R. M., Ojeda, V. D., & Strathdee, S. A. (2016). Epidemiology of substance use among forced migrants: A global systematic review. *PLoS One, 11*(7). https://doi.org/10.1371/journal.pone.0159134

Hox, J. J. (2010). *Multilevel analysis. Techniques and applications* (2nd ed.). Routledge Taylor & Francis.

Kuckartz, U., & Rädiker, S. (2023). *Qualitative content analysis—Methods, practice and software* (2nd ed.). Sage Publications.

Liel, K. (2020). Theorie und Praxis des bio-psychosozialen Modells: Rolle und Beitrag der Sozialen Arbeit. In: Rummel, C. & Gaßmann, R. (Eds.). Sucht: bio-psychosozial: Die ganzheitliche Sicht auf Suchtfragen–Perspektiven aus Sozialer Arbeit, Psychologie und Medizin (69–79). Kohlhammer.

Lorenz, M. H. (2021). Prävention des riskanten und abhängigen Substanzkonsums bei geflüchteten Menschen: Eine systematische Übersicht. *SUCHT, 67*(5), 255–271.

Lorenz, M. H., Ensle, A., Taggert, J., Uricher, J., Heidenreich, T., & Laging, M. (2023). Professionals' perspectives on substance use among refugees in shared accommodations: A qualitative study. *Health & Social Work, 48*(3), 188–197. https://doi.org/10.1093/hsw/hlad017

Lorenz, M. H., Uricher, J., Michalak, J., Heidenreich, T., & Laging, A. M. (2024b). Hazardous substance use among refugees in shared accommodations: A mixed-methods study. *Zeitschrift für Klinische Psychologie und Psychotherapie, 53*(4), 187–204. https://doi.org/10.1026/1616-3443/a000778

Lorenz, M. H., Uricher, J., Pauzar, M. I., Michalak, J., Laging, M., & Heidenreich, T. (2024a). Evaluation of a multi-component prevention concept for hazardous substance use among refugees in shared accommodations: Study protocol for a cluster randomized controlled trial. *Trials, 25*(1), 770. https://doi.org/10.1186/s13063-024-08558-z

Odukoya, D., & von Unger, H. (2023). Partizipative Forschung. In T. Scharrer, B. Glorius, J. O. Kleist, & M. Berlinghoff (Eds.), *Flucht—und Flüchtlingsforschung. Handbuch für Wissenschaft und Studium* (pp. 153–158). Nomos. https://doi.org/10.5771/9783748921905

Patanè, M., Ghane, S., Karyotaki, E., Cuijpers, P., Schoonmade, L., Tarsitani, L., & Sijbrandij, M. (2022). Prevalence of mental disorders in refugees and asylum seekers: A systematic review and meta-analysis. *Global Mental Health, 9*, 250–263. https://doi.org/10.1017/gmh.2022.29

Rosenbrock, R. (2015). *Prävention in Lebenswelten—der Setting-Ansatz* (pp. 213–219). Deutscher Ärzte Verlag. https://doi.org/10.3238/zfa.2015.0213-0219

Roura, M., Dias, S., LeMaster, J. W., & MacFarlane, A. (2021). *Participatory health research with migrants: Opportunities, challenges, and way forwards.* Health Expectations published by John Wiley and Sons Ltd. https://doi.org/10.1111/hex.13201

Saleh, E. A., Lazaridou, F. B., Klapprott, F., Wazaify, M., Heinz, A., & Kluge, U. (2023). A systematic review of qualitative research on substance use among refugees. *Addiction, 118*(2), 218–253. https://doi.org/10.1111/add.16021

Schaefer, I., Allweis, T., Dresen, A., Amort, F.M., Wright, M. T. & Krieger, T. (2022). PartNet-Methodenpapier: Modell für Partizipative Gesundheitsforschung (PGF-Modell). Deutschsprachige Fassung des "Community-Based Participatory Research Model" und

Hinweise zur Anwendung. “PartNet Perspektiven. Beiträge zur partizipativen Forschung” 02/ 2022—Schriftenreihe des Netzwerks für Partizipative Gesundheitsforschung.

Schönfeld, S., Sauzet, O., & Razum, O. (2022). Gibt es einen Zusammenhang zwischen der Zufriedenheit mit der Unterkunft und der psychischen Gesundheit Geflüchteter in Deutschland?—Eine Querschnittstudie. *Thieme. Gesundheitswesen, 84*, 617–624. https://doi.org/10.1055/a-1802-4530

UNHCR. (2024). *Figures at a glance.* UNHCR Global Trends 2023. Retrieved March 25, 2025, from https://www.unhcr.org/about-unhcr/who-we-are/figures-glance

Uricher, J., Lorenz, M. H., Michalak, J., Heidenreich, T., & Laging, M. (In publication). Evaluation of a Multicomponent Prevention Concept for Hazardous Substance Use Among Refugees in Shared Accommodations: Results from a Cluster-Randomized Controlled Trial and Implications for Living Conditions.

Veltrup, C. (2020). Theorie und Praxis des bio-psychosozialen Modells: Rolle und Beitrag der Psychologie. In C. Rummel & R. Gaßmann (Eds.), *Sucht: bio-psychosozial: Die ganzheitliche Sicht auf Suchtfragen–Perspektiven aus Sozialer Arbeit, Psychologie und Medizin* (pp. 59–68). Kohlhammer.

Von Köppen, M., Schmidt, K., & Tiefenthaler, S. (2020). Mit vulnerablen Gruppen forschen—ein Forschungsprozessmodell als Reflexionshilfe für partizipative Projekte. In S. Hartung, P. Wihofszky, & T. Wright (Eds.), *Partizipative Forschung—ein Forschungsansatz für Gesundheit und seine Methoden.* Springer VS. https://doi.org/10.1007/978-3-658-30361-7

Wallerstein, N., Oetzel, J., Duran, B., Tafoya, G., Belone, L. & Rae, R. (2008). What predicts outcomes in CBPR? In: Minkler, M. & Wallerstein, N. (Eds.). Community-based participatory research for health. From process to outcomes (371–392). 2nd ed. San Francisco, Calif.: Jossey-bass.

Walther, L., Amann, J., Flick, U., Ta, T. M. T., Bajbouj, M., & Hahn, E. (2021). A qualitative study on resilience in adult refugees in Germany. *BMC Public Health, 21*, 828. https://doi.org/10.1186/s12889-021-10817-6

World Health Organization. (2024). *Hazardous substance use.* https://icd.who.int/browse/2024-01/mms/en#1466350777

Wright, M. T. (2013). Was ist Partizipative Gesundheitsforschung? Positionspapier der International collaboration for participatory Health Research. *Präv Gesundheitsf, 8*, 122–131. https://doi.org/10.1007/s11553-013-0395-0

Zurhold, H., & Kuhn, S. (2023). Alkohol und illegale Drogen unter Geflüchteten in Gemeinschaftsunterkünften. *SUCHT, 69*(5), 214–223. https://doi.org/10.1024/0939-5911/a000834

Chapter 5
The Ukrainian Refugee Crisis: Assessing Resilience of HIV Prevention and Treatment Services Targeted for People Who Inject Drugs in Germany and Poland

Benjamin M. Nikitin, Daniel J. Bromberg, Till Bärnighausen, Mark Schlessinger, Sergii Dvoriak, and Frederick L. Altice

5.1 Introduction

The 2022 Russian invasion of Ukraine triggered the worst refugee crisis in Europe since World War II (Balmer, 2022), with over six million Ukrainians being displaced (Ukraine Emergency, n.d.). Displacement during crisis poses a major disruption to individuals' lives, leading to high prevalence of post-traumatic stress disorder, depression, and/or anxiety (Bogic et al., 2015). Mass displacement can also trigger strains on health systems, like those observed during the Syrian crisis, where policymakers and providers implemented emergency measures and invested extensive resources to prevent healthcare disruptions for refugees. Despite these changes to European healthcare systems in response to the Syrian crisis, structural barriers

B. M. Nikitin · D. J. Bromberg · M. Schlessinger · F. L. Altice (✉)
School of Public Health, Yale University, New Haven, CT, USA
e-mail: Frederick.altice@yale.edu

B. M. Nikitin
Icahn School of Medicine at Mount Sinai, New York, NY, USA

F. L. Altice
School of Medicine, Yale University, New Haven, CT, USA

D. J. Bromberg · T. Bärnighausen
Institute for Global Health, Heidelberg University, Heidelberg, Germany

T. Bärnighausen
T.H. Chan School of Public Health, Harvard University, Cambridge, MA, USA

S. Dvoriak
Ukrainian Institute for Public Health, Kyiv, Ukraine

C. De Kock (ed.), *Substance Use Among Refugees in Europe*,
https://doi.org/10.1007/978-3-032-32399-6_5

emerged, including lack of language interpreter services and delays in needed treatment (Aljadeeah et al., 2021). Restrictions in access were most pronounced early in the host European countries, often due to delayed implementation, resulting in harm to individual and public health, with outbreaks of infectious diseases like measles and varicella and inadequately managed non-communicable diseases (NCDs) among refugees (Naja et al., 2019; Pavli & Maltezou, 2017).

The current refugee crisis involving Ukrainians, however, differs in ways that pose distinct and challenging risks. Ukraine has intertwined and volatile HIV and opioid use disorder (OUD) epidemics—the worst in Europe (260,000 people with HIV [PWH] and 350,300 people who inject drugs [PWID]); women account for 20%–25% of PWID and, unlike men, can cross the border freely (Antonenko & Martsynovska, 2022; "Helping Ukrainian Refugees with HIV Treatment and Support in Berlin," 2022; Horyniak et al., 2016). Unlike during the Syrian crisis, PWH and PWID are highly represented among Ukrainian refugees, and constitute stigmatized populations that require innovations in health service delivery to ensure adequate engagement. A rapid and holistic strategy for engaging large numbers of PWH and PWID entering host countries is therefore needed (Nikitin, Bromberg, Madden, et al., 2023).

To ensure continuity of HIV prevention and treatment, the resilience of host country HIV services is essential. To define resilience, we apply the WHO definition: "The ability of a health system exposed to a shock to resist, absorb, accommodate, and recover from the effects of the shock in a timely and efficient manner, including through the preservation and restoration of its essential basic structures and functions through risk management" (*WHO EMRO—Health Systems Resilience*, n.d.). Evidence-based HIV prevention strategies available in Ukraine include pre-exposure prophylaxis (PrEP), which reduces real-world transmission in PWID by 49% (Choopanya et al., 2013), and opioid agonist therapies (OAT) using methadone or buprenorphine, which reduce transmission by 59% (Stone et al., 2021) and for PWH, improves HIV treatment along the entire HIV care continuum, including treatment adherence (Bromberg et al., 2025; Mazhnaya et al., 2018). Not only are such services needed, but they must be timely. For example, even a few days' interruption in OAT can result in agonizing withdrawal symptoms that can lead to recidivist opioid injection, overdose, and death (Carroll, 2019), while discontinuations of antiretroviral therapy (ART) for a week can lead to loss of viral suppression and the potential for HIV transmission (Parczewski et al., 2023). More prolonged delays in ART may accelerate HIV progression and the development of resistant strains of HIV (Parczewski et al., 2023; Taylor et al., 2007).

Much of the European response to the Ukrainian refugee crisis differed substantially from the response during the Syrian crisis and, while some of the initial responses to Ukrainian refugees have been explored in Europe (Biesiada et al., 2023; Davitian et al., 2024; Spiegel, 2022), little is known specifically about how PWH and PWID were treated or whether they could rapidly access life-saving services as demand increased. To assess whether HIV systems have successfully ensured continuity of care for refugees, this study provides an estimate for changes to service demand and a description of health system responses to this disruption in Germany and Poland, the two European Union (EU) countries with the highest populations of Ukrainian refugees (1.2 million and one million, respectively, as of spring 2025) (Ukraine Refugee Situation, 2023).

While the refugee population from Ukraine includes individuals of diverse backgrounds (Ukraine Refugee Situation, 2023), this study places specific emphasis on PWID and PWH, who are both medically vulnerable and highly stigmatized. Intersectional factors such as gender, legal residence status, and language barriers further compound these vulnerabilities. For instance, women who inject drugs may have been more able than men to cross the border, yet they face compounded stigma and may be less likely to seek services due to childcare responsibilities or fear of legal consequences. Similarly, refugees without formal residence status face greater bureaucratic delays in obtaining insurance or accessing treatment. These overlapping identities and statuses can interact to either amplify or constrain individuals' access to care and must be considered in any resilient health systems response. Based on our findings in this study, we identify opportunities for solutions that would improve the resilience of the HIV prevention and treatment systems in Germany and Poland for the Ukrainian refugee crisis and for future migratory crises.

5.2 Methods

5.2.1 Study Design

To evaluate the capacity of German and Polish systems to rapidly provide HIV services amid an unanticipated shock, we applied the World Health Organization (WHO) Health System Performance Assessment (HSPA) framework, which assesses health system capacity for universal care using four interconnected factors: governance, resource generation, financing, and service delivery (Papanicolas, 2022). These factors are embedded in a socioecological context, such as a refugee crisis, including patient-, clinician-, community-, health system-, and structural-level factors. For example, at the patient level, delayed insurance or OAT interruptions create immediate risks, while at the clinician level, specialist-only prescribing limits care. Community non-governmental organizations (NGOs) bridge gaps in linkage, but their reach is constrained by funding, and structural policies like EU directives and drug patents ultimately shape service access.

Given the influx of refugees, we estimated the increased demand for each HIV service, as detailed below. Based on these estimates, the governance of the health system was evaluated through existing national policy documents that dictated HIV service delivery in both countries. Financing for these policies was identified based on publicly available documents. To understand resource generation and service delivery, in-depth interviews were completed with purposively selected stakeholders. Assessed HIV system resources included access to insurance, interpreter services, and community infrastructure for linking patients to services. Service delivery examined patient and provider experiences with providing care to patients for key prevention/treatment strategies: OAT, PrEP, and ART.

5.2.2 Context: Estimating the Shock to the System

To gauge the increased demand for HIV services, we compared current estimated demand for HIV services with demand before the 2022 refugee crisis. For OAT, the estimated number of displaced PWID was known in Poland (EMCDDA Trendspotter Briefing: Responsiveness and Preparedness in Addressing Drug-Related Needs of Displaced Ukrainians in EU Countries Bordering Ukraine, n.d.); the number of PWID in Germany was derived proportionally from refugee population estimates in Poland versus Germany (Ukraine Refugee Situation, 2023). Though a 2016 study from Ukraine estimated the percent of PWID willing to start OAT as 36% (Makarenko et al., 2016), OAT scale-up in Ukraine increased dramatically since then; demand for OAT is now estimated at 72% in individuals who have previously received or are currently receiving OAT based on a 2021 biobehavioral survey (Bromberg et al., 2025). As PWID migrate, stress increases and their social networks are dismantled (West, 2019), creating disruptions in PWID's access to illicit drugs and potentially leading them to legal and safer treatment options. To adjust for unanticipated changes in demand amid displacement, an upper/lower bound was added (±10%) (Horyniak et al., 2016). By multiplying the upper and lower bound by the number of externally displaced PWID in each country, the number of refugees from Ukraine willing to receive OAT was determined. This was then compared against the existing number of OAT patients per country prior to the Russian invasion. These values were applied to Eq. 5.1 to determine the increase in demand (Viral Hepatitis Elimination Barometer among People Who Inject Drugs in Europe, 2023).

$$\%\ \textit{estimated demand increase} = \frac{\textit{estimated number of displaced individuals seeking services}}{\textit{number of people receiving services before invasion}} \tag{5.1}$$

For PrEP, no data were available for the overall population of refugees engaging in high-risk behavior. Because the proportion of male refugees was low, and therefore the likely number of male refugees who have sex with men was also limited (on behalf of the Dynamics Study Team et al., 2019; Ukraine Refugee Situation, 2023; Yayboke et al., 2022), the number of PWID in each country served as a sufficiently reliable (albeit imperfect and conservative) metric. As PrEP scale-up was low in Ukraine before the war (Cairns, 2022), potential demand for PrEP was unknown. To more accurately measure demand, the percentage of PWID in Ukraine who were willing to start OAT (72%; ±10%) was used (Bromberg et al., 2025) and subsequently adjusted to account for the proportion of people on OAT who reported willingness to start PrEP (65%; ±10%) (Ni et al., 2021). Using these estimates, the likely number of PWID wanting PrEP in Poland and Germany was calculated. This was then compared against estimates for the number of people in both countries receiving PrEP prior to the Russian invasion using Eq. 5.1 (Country Factsheets: Germany, 2022; Country Factsheets: Poland, 2022).

For ART, the coverage rate in Ukraine (83%) (Antonenko & Martsynovska, 2022) was adjusted (±10%) to account for anticipated changes in demand and was then used to estimate absolute demand among displaced PWH ("Helping Ukrainian Refugees with HIV Treatment and Support in Berlin," 2022; Ukraine Refugee Situation, 2023); this estimated demand was compared against the number of people in each country receiving ART prior to the refugee crisis using Eq. 5.1. Next, the number of externally displaced PWH from Ukraine was derived from a UNAIDS estimate ("Helping Ukrainian Refugees with HIV Treatment and Support in Berlin," 2022). Based on the proportions of refugees from Ukraine in Poland and Germany (Ukraine Refugee Situation, 2023), the number of externally displaced PWH in each country was calculated. The coverage rate in Ukraine was used to determine the number of displaced PWH in each country who would be seeking ART. This number was compared against the host country population receiving ART (Eq. 1).

5.2.3 Assessing Governance, Financing, Resources, and Service Delivery

All webpages of the German and Polish ministries of health and drug policy were searched to compile existing documents related to HIV services. Only national policies were recorded. Interviews with key informants, however, were used to understand how policies in various regions were enacted. When necessary, policy documents were translated through the DeepL software (version 23.9). As with interview transcripts, policy documents were coded for key themes using NVivo (Release 1.7.1). Coding was completed separately by BMN and DJB and was subsequently cross-referenced. If disagreement emerged, FLA broke the tie. Interviews were transcribed verbatim, translated (when necessary), and back-translated for content in real time (Brislin, 1970); three participants did not consent to being recorded, so extensive notes were used instead. After all transcripts and interview notes were de-identified, they were coded for key themes in NVivo (Release 1.7.1).

From June 2022 to November 2023, semi-structured interviews were completed in both Poland and Germany (N = 30; 45 minutes each) with a purposively selected sample of stakeholders across the socioecological model, including policy officials, providers of HIV services, HIV refugee organization (HRO) employees, displaced PWH from Ukraine, and researchers (Table 5.1).

Participant phenotypes accounted for all steps in the process of HIV policymaking and implementation. For each phenotype, a separate interview guide was developed to direct questions during the interview that evaluated governance, financing, system resources, and service delivery. The interview guides were informed by prior studies of HIV and refugee health (Nikitin, Bromberg, Madden, et al., 2023;

Table 5.1 Participant characteristics

Country	Policy official	Provider of HIV services		HIV refugee organization employee	Displaced HIV patient/clients from Ukraine		Researcher
		Prevention	Treatment		Male	Female	
Germany	2	3	1	3	1	5	2
Poland	4	4	2	1	2	0	0

Nikitin, Bromberg, Pykalo, et al., 2023), reviewed by external experts in HIV and migrant health, and piloted with two informants to refine clarity and sensitivity. Interview guides are available upon request to the corresponding author. Participants were recruited through purposive and snowball sampling, including outreach via ministries, NGOs, academic networks, and peer referrals from refugee organizations. Because most refugees were from Eastern Ukraine and author resources were limited, refugee participants were interviewed in Russian; all other participants were interviewed in English.

5.2.3.1 Ethics

The Yale Institutional Review Board (IRB) deemed the study low risk and therefore exempted it from review. All consent for interviews was obtained verbally using a script as approved by the Yale IRB. Any identifying information was redacted prior to interview transcription.

5.2.4 Results

Using the WHO HSPA Framework, findings are reported across its four pillars.

5.2.4.1 Demand for HIV Services

While the number of displaced PWH and PWID from Ukraine was relatively similar (Table 5.2), the proportionate increase in demand for services was substantially higher in Germany (55% to 289% for OAT, 30% to 218% for PrEP, 25% to 27% for ART) than in Poland (2% to 12% for OAT, 3% to 18% for PrEP, 5% to 6% for ART).

Table 5.2 Estimated number of people with HIV and people who inject drugs in Germany and Poland before and after the war

Country	Number of PWH before the invasion	Estimated number of displaced PWH from Ukraine (incremental percentage)	Estimated number of displaced PWID from Ukraine
Germany	91,000 (Country Factsheets: Germany, 2022; Country Factsheets: Poland, 2022)	5310 (+5.8%)	3035 to 12,139
Poland	19,000 (Country Factsheets: Germany, 2022; Country Factsheets: Poland, 2022)	4650 (+24.5%)	2658 to 10,630

Legend PWH: People with HIV, PWID: People who inject drugs

5.2.4.2 Financing

In both Germany and Poland, HIV prevention and treatment were financed by a combination of NGO programs and, from the national level, each country's respective public health insurance plan. In Germany, stakeholders reported that clinics and NGOs were sufficiently funded to cover the prevention and treatment services that were offered. Funding for HIV treatment (ART) and OAT increased by 16% and 17%, respectively, between 2020 and 2023. Funding for HIV prevention between 2021 and 2023, however, decreased by 12% (Table 5.3).

Individual state funding, a potential source of significant funding for these services, was not assessed.

In Poland, funding for both HIV prevention and treatment increased between 2020 and 2023 by 36% (Table 5.4). The increase in national funding for HIV treatment (36% between 2020–2023, including allocations from the Ukraine Relief Fund) suggests a strategy to expand access, which likely encouraged refugees with HIV to seek care by signaling system readiness to absorb new patients. However, because prevention budgets remained comparatively low, many displaced PWID and PWH still encountered barriers to engagement, underscoring the gap between national-level strategies and on-the-ground resilience.

Table 5.3 Spending for HIV prevention services, opioid agonist therapies, and antiretroviral therapy in Germany from 2020 through 2023, in thousands of USD (1 EUR = 1.12 USD)

Treatment type	2020	2021	2022	2023
HIV prevention*	Unknown	$39,395	$35,028	$34,478
HIV treatment (antiretroviral therapy)*	$50,810	$55,282	$58,141	$59,354
Opioid agonist therapies	$50,797	$55,272	$58,130	$59,336

*HIV treatment included PrEP and PEP. HIV prevention included national funding for HIV/STI education, drugs and substance use education, implementation of the national strategy on drugs and addiction policy, and migration and integration in the German system (2025)

Table 5.4 HIV prevention services, opioid agonist therapies, and antiretroviral therapy in Poland from 2020 through 2023, in thousands of USD (1 PLN = 0.25 USD)

Program type	2020	2021	2022	2023
HIV prevention	$749	$779	$1110	$1019
HIV treatment*	$86,999	$97,500	$99,983	$117,923*

*In 2023, $9.750 million of the $117.923 million disbursed from the Ukraine Relief Fund (FPU) was used for HIV treatment of Ukrainians (National AIDS Center, 2022; 2024)

Despite this substantial increase, absolute funding for HIV prevention services remained low relative to Germany. Funding for HIV treatment, however, was higher than in Germany, likely reflecting the higher prevalence of HIV in Poland.

> In Poland, prevention is very weak… 90% of all the prevention budget goes to testing. (HIV services provider, Poland)

NGOs in Poland that provided OAT were underfunded and lacked long-term support. This was further impacted by the political climate in Poland, with NGOs being targeted by the country's right-leaning leadership.

> My organization is on the list of the "dangerous" organizations in Poland. Because of the very right-wing government… they have tried to cut our supply of money off… so for sure we cannot get support from the national government. (Provider, Poland)

Due to insufficient resource infrastructure as per participant interviews, several NGOs were founded in Germany and Poland to help link refugees from Ukraine to HIV services, including HelpNow. Though operating in EU host countries, HelpNow received funding from the Ukraine-based NGO Alliance for Public Health—one of the major recipients of funding from the Global Fund Against AIDS, Tuberculosis and Malaria (GFATM). Funding that was budgeted for this organization, as well as for many others, was exhausted, and HelpNow started operating on a volunteer basis. Employees from NGOs attributed the lack of funding to a perceived lack of need and a dense bureaucracy.

> Germany doesn't see this as a problem [for linking the patient to care]. "We have medications, what's the problem?" they say. (HRO Employee, Germany)
>
> They [Polish officials] tell us: "We give ART, we do all the necessary testing, what else do you want from us?" (HRO Employee, Poland)

Being unpaid, employees became increasingly exasperated.

> I'm burnt out. I can't do this anymore. There is no end in sight. (HRO Employee, Germany)

Lacking any source of funding, these organizations continued to face an increasing demand, with displaced Ukrainians encountering serious problems with accessing the HIV services system within their host country.

5.2.4.3 Governance and Resource Generation

The various policies that defined resource generation and their perceived impact are outlined in Table 5.5.

Policies for access to health insurance in both Germany and Poland for Ukrainians were relatively similar, requiring approval of residency paperwork, which was often delayed access to health services. Bureaucratic backlogs in Germany slowed the process further. Participants reported that, upon submission of their application, receiving a plastic insurance card could take two weeks to six months and that to their knowledge, they could not access any health services until this approval. There were, however, some exceptions.

> We needed health insurance [for OAT], and we got it in a day or two… That is at an accelerated pace, because everyone else had to wait a month, a month and a half, for all this registration [to be completed] … There is a long queue (Displaced Ukrainian, Germany). (Nikitin, Bromberg, Madden, et al., 2023)

To offset federal delays, some German states provided temporary insurance vouchers for up to 1 month, though this information was not widely accessible to patients or insurance offices. In addition, not all German states provided temporary insurance cards.

> If the patient doesn't know about their rights, they won't get [the temporary insurance card]. (HRO Employee, Germany)

In Poland, insurance access was processed quickly. In cases where delays occurred, several providers agreed to make exceptions if refugees could show proof that they were refugees and that they had crossed the border on or after February 24, 2022 (providers in Germany also made this exception, but only for the early days of the invasion). For patients on OAT, this exception was common, as discontinuation could lead to immediate and severe clinical withdrawal side effects.

> Regardless of whether they have access to insurance, [refugees] get access to OAT… People understand how urgent this treatment is. (HRO Employee, Poland)

No policies in either country required healthcare services to provide translation services, reducing access to healthcare for refugees. Consequently, many refugees opted to make long commutes to clinics with Ukrainian- or Russian-speaking providers, while others opted to receive care in Ukraine either by telemedicine or frequent border crossings.

In Poland, efforts to address language barriers had been attempted through the creation of Ukrainian/Russian-language provider databases and a smartphone app, *LikarPL*, that served as a two-way communication platform between patients and providers, though uptake was limited. In Germany, no such platforms were identified and, in some cases, refugees had to find and pay a private translator (10 euros per hour) for each clinical encounter. When translation services were available, some refugees reported discriminatory practices from interpreters.

Table 5.5 Insurance and linkage to HIV services: policies and perceived implementation

Jurisdiction	Policies and government actions	Perceived implementation of the policy	Policy source
European Union	All Ukrainian citizens who entered European Union countries on or after February 24, 2022, have the legal right to a residence permit and all healthcare services	This directive has been implemented through different laws and actions in Germany and Poland, as described below	Council Implementing Decision (EU), 2022/382 ("COUNCIL IMPLEMENTING DECISION (EU), 2022/382 of 4 March 2022," n.d.)
	Patient privacy is protected. It is illegal to divulge the health status of any patient	Despite this regulation, there have been reports of refugee health status being divulged in both Germany and Poland	General Data Protection Regulation (EU) ("REGULATION (EU) 2016/679 OF THE EUROPEAN PARLIAMENT AND OF THE COUNCIL of 27 April 2016 on the Protection of Natural Persons with Regard to the Processing of Personal Data and on the Free Movement of Such Data, and Repealing Directive 95/46/EC (General Data Protection Regulation)," 2016)
Germany	For Ukrainian citizens: Statutory health insurance is granted after temporary residency is processed	Though insurance is indeed granted, processing times can take from 2 weeks to 6 months. German states have responded by providing temporary insurance vouchers to refugees who need access to care more urgently. However, knowledge of these vouchers among refugees and even refugee counselors is reportedly limited	Residence act (paragraph 24) (social code (SGB) fifth book (V)—statutory health insurance - (article 1 of the law of December 20, 1988, BGBl. I p. 2477), 1988); Social code (book V) (social code (SGB) fifth book (V)—statutory health insurance—(article 1 of the law of December 20, 1988, BGBl. I p. 2477), 1988)
	For non-Ukrainian nationals from Ukraine: Asylum application must be completed. If accepted, protections are granted through the asylum act, which only provides insurance for "acute illness or pain during the first 18 months" of residence	Completion of an asylum application is a lengthy and often unsuccessful process	Asylum Act ("Asylum Act in the Version Promulgated on 2 September 2008 (Federal Law Gazette I, p. 1798), Last Amended by Article 2 of the Act of 11 March 2016 (Federal Law Gazette I, p. 394," 2016)

(continued)

Table 5.5 (continued)

Jurisdiction	Policies and government actions	Perceived implementation of the policy	Policy source
	Ukrainian citizens with registered residency in Germany can leave the country for up to 6 months. After 6 months, however, they lose their right to re-entry	Many Ukrainians have opted to continue receiving healthcare in Ukraine and then to return to Germany	Ukraine residence transition ordinance ("Vierte Verordnung Zur Änderung Der Ukraine-Aufenthalts Übergangsverordnung," 2023)
	Laws requiring interpretation in healthcare were not found	Access to interpretation is limited and dependent on volunteers and imperfect translation apps like Google translate. Interview participants have reported making long commutes to find a provider who speaks their language	N/A
Poland	For Ukrainian citizens: All Ukrainian citizens registered on or after February 24, 2022, are granted a Ukr-PESEL (*Powszechny Elektroniczny system Ewidencji Ludności*; universal electronic system for registration of the population) number, giving them access to public health insurance. This number is valid for 18 months, concurrent with the maximum limit of stay in Poland for Ukrainian nationals. After 18 months, application is necessary via the Office for Foreigners	The UKR-PESEL number is generally issued relatively quickly and efficiently	Act on Assisting Citizens of Ukraine (Article 4) (Fremer, 2022)
	Leaving Poland for greater than 1 month will result in loss of the above legal residency protection	Refugees need to choose between continued access to health insurance and visiting family in other countries	Act on Assisting Citizens of Ukraine (Article 3, 11) (Fremer, 2022)

(continued)

Table 5.5 (continued)

Jurisdiction	Policies and government actions	Perceived implementation of the policy	Policy source
	Non-Ukrainian nationals from Ukraine can be issued a certificate of temporary protection by the Office for Foreigners. Insurance will be provided via the Office for Foreigners and includes coverage for basic and special care/treatment, prescriptions, and dental care	While their applications are submitted and pending approval, individuals still have access to free healthcare, reportedly	Temporary protection for foreigners (temporary protection for foreigners, n.d.)
	Laws requiring interpretation in healthcare were not found	Access to language interpretation is limited and dependent on volunteers and imperfect translation apps. Despite no existing requirements, however, Poland has attempted to ease the interpretation burden by implementing a government-developed platform: LikarPL	N/A

> There were not enough interpreters [at the refugee center] … When she [a volunteer interpreter at the refugee center] heard that I was asking to translate something related to drugs… she was like… "I'm with God, I go to church. I won't translate that, I'm sorry" (Displaced Ukrainian, Germany). (Nikitin, Bromberg, Madden, et al., 2023)

5.2.4.4 Governance and Service Delivery

Opioid Agonist Therapies

Policies that defined OAT service delivery in Germany and Poland, often highly restrictive, are outlined in Table 5.6.

German and Polish guidelines were similar in terms of their stringent qualification requirements to prescribe OAT. Unlike in many other countries, both Germany and Poland mandated providers to have training in addiction medicine. This limited the number of providers in both countries who could prescribe OAT. Neither country changed training/treatment requirements to meet the anticipated increase in demand during the Ukrainian refugee crisis, creating bottlenecks for treatment entry.

Laws in Poland were more restrictive by limiting OAT prescription to limited specialized centers, generally located *only* in urban locations, complicating care for nearly all refugees residing in rural areas. As shown in Fig. 5.1, refugees living in rural areas in both countries may have needed to travel dozens to hundreds of miles to reach the nearest OAT provider, who was likely located in an urban center.

Table 5.6 Opioid agonist therapy policies and perceived implementation issues

Country	Policies and government actions	Perceived implementation of the policy	Policy source
Germany	OAT medication brought from Ukraine must be carried with approved documentation (original prescription and transit documents from the provider). OAT medication can *only* be carried by the patient themself or by their authorized provider. Furthermore, a Schengen certificate for medical treatment is required. Only a limited quantity of medication can be brought in (~30 days, according to interviews)	Many refugees are not made aware of all these rules and required documentations, causing possible delays at the border. No reports of OAT medication seizure were reported, though. Because patients cannot bring in large quantities of take-home OAT medication, they must find an OAT provider in Germany almost immediately upon arrival	The narcotics act ("narcotics act in the version published on march 1, 1994," 2023); Narcotics Foreign Trade Ordinance (Ordinance Concerning the Foreign Trade in Narcotics, 1981)
	Patients in Germany are generally required to take all OAT medication on-site. If the patient demonstrates that (1) they cannot stay on OAT without receiving take-homes, (2) their treatment allows it, and (3) the danger to others is found to be minimal, then they are permitted to be given take-homes by the provider	Most patients arriving from Ukraine, many of whom are already prescribed take-homes, must be re-started as naïve patients and attend the clinic on a daily or multi-weekly basis to receive their medication	Narcotics prescription ordinance (sect. 5, paragraph 9) (ordinance on the prescription, dispensing and proof of the disposition of narcotic drugs (narcotic drugs prescription ordinance), 2009)
	OAT can only be provided by physicians trained in addiction medicine	The number of providers who prescribe is still not high due to training barriers. Many providers also do not acquire this qualification due to perceptions of stigma	Decision of the joint Federal Committee on an amendment to the guideline on methods of contract medical care (MVV-RL): Annex I no. 2 substitution-based treatment of opiate addicts ("announcement a decision of the joint Federal Committee on an amendment to the guideline on methods of contract medical care (MVV-RL): Annex I no. 2 substitution-based treatment of opiate addicts," 2018)

(continued)

Table 5.6 (continued)

Country	Policies and government actions	Perceived implementation of the policy	Policy source
Poland	Access to OAT is free of charge for all individuals with a PESEL (*Powszechny Elektroniczny system Ewidencji Ludności*; universal electronic system for registration of the population) number	There has been confusion over who has access to health insurance, with some physicians at the start of the crisis providing OAT to refugees simply based on the date of entry listed in their passport	*Treatment for Ukraine* (Poland, n.d.)
	OAT medications: "May be provided by a health care center upon license from the provincial governor issued upon positive opinion of the bureau head"	OAT centers are limited and are generally only available in urban areas, making access more difficult for refugees, especially those living in less urban regions	2005 Counteracting Drug Addiction Law (Act of Law of 29 July 2005 on Counteracting Drug Addiction, n.d.)
	OAT centers must have: A pharmacy distributing OAT medication, appropriate rooms, and "proper personnel capacity"	These requirements limit the number of available OAT centers and force many center to turn prospective patients away, putting them on a long waitlist instead	2005 Counteracting Drug Addiction Law (Act of Law of 29 July 2005 on Counteracting Drug Addiction, n.d.)
	With documentation of OAT treatment in Ukraine, patients can start treatment as non-naïve	Many clinics have requested translation of required documents, which is not widely available to refugees free of charge	*Treatment for Ukraine* (Poland, n.d.)
	Prescribing take-home OAT medications is legal	Many providers are reluctant to prescribe take-home medications	*Eurasian harm reduction association* (Poland, 2021)

Legend OAT: opioid agonist therapies

OAT implementation constraints further restricted access. While prescribing take-home OAT was legal in both countries, Germany's requirements were much more stringent, requiring many steps to justify why take-home prescriptions were essential and verify that take-home prescriptions would not pose harm to others. Concerns about violations of this policy among providers created reluctance to prescribe take-home doses even as patients had met the requirements to receive take-home doses in Ukraine. Ukraine had increased access to take-home dosing during the COVID-19

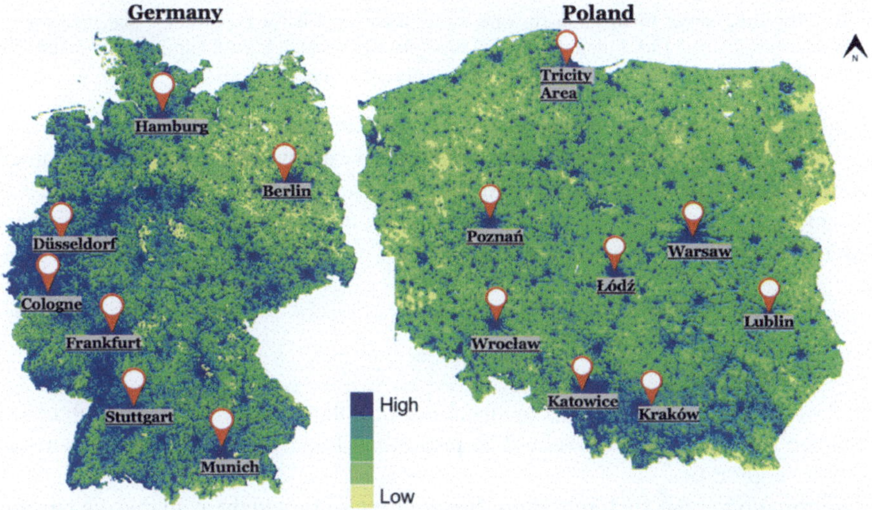

Fig. 5.1 Population density maps of Germany and Poland overlayed with pins of the most populous cities. WorldPop (www.worldpop.org[1]—School of Geography and Environmental Science, University of Southampton; Department of Geography and Geosciences, University of Louisville; Departement de Geographie, Universite de Namur) and Center for International Earth Science Information Network (CIESIN), Columbia University (2018). Global High Resolution Population Denominators Project—Funded by The Bill and Melinda Gates Foundation (OPP1134076)

pandemic (Ivasiy et al., 2024; Meteliuk et al., 2021) and early in the war (Altice et al., 2022), resulting in increased OAT scale-up, improved retention without increasing mortality. This often meant that stable OAT patients from Ukraine, while displaced, had to start treatment anew, with substantial restrictions to take-home dosing until patients were observed daily for variable, but often prolonged, periods of time.

> With a "magic letter" from the Ukrainian doctor, they [OAT patients] can be given take-home medications sooner, but they still have to come in every day at the start. (HRO Employee, Germany)

Patients had to request this letter from their provider in Ukraine before leaving the country, which was not always possible amid the chaos of a full-scale war. One patient who did not know about this type of letter reported that they had to pick up medication daily, for the foreseeable future, from a distant clinic.

> [I must pick up OAT medication] every day… It's very far and very difficult. It's about fifty minutes by bus to Augsburg, and from Augsburg, I take another bus for about an hour to Munich. (Displaced Ukrainian, Germany) (Nikitin, Bromberg, Madden, et al., 2023)

Although less constrained by formal policy restrictions, providers in Poland were still reluctant to prescribe take-homes. Still, they were generally more amenable than in Germany.

---

[1] Source: WorldPop (www.worldpop.org). This work is licensed under the Creative Commons Attribution 4.0 International License (http://creativecommons.org/licenses/by/4.0)

> The first time, I got medication for one week, then I got it for two weeks, and then for two weeks again… I told them that every time my trip takes at least a hundred kilometers. (Displaced Ukrainian, Poland) (Nikitin, Bromberg, Madden, et al., 2023)

In Poland, if paperwork demonstrating that the patient was stable on OAT in Ukraine was provided, the patient could be started on take-home dosing right away, albeit for shorter take-home intervals than in Ukraine. Such documentation, however, was seldom available. Documentation requirements in Poland appeared less stringent than in Germany.

Pre-Exposure Prophylaxis for HIV

PrEP was generally not covered by insurance in Poland (Table 5.7), although newer guidance indicated that PrEP could be prescribed free of charge through insurance in some larger cities.

Information about such programs, however, was not widely available, as government officials stated that the cost of PrEP was 50 euros for consultation and that the medication costs about 3 euros per day. Consequently, several refugees discontinued PrEP after moving to Poland.

> People taking PrEP in Ukraine wanted to continue, but they chose not to because of the price. There were no alternatives for them. (HRO Employee, Poland)

In Germany, by contrast, PrEP had been covered by health insurance since 2019. This allowed refugees greater access. Still, PrEP was only covered by public insurance only when patients saw an infectious disease specialist, who were limited in Germany.

Antiretroviral Therapy for Treating HIV

Table 5.8 provides a summary of ART policies and their perceived implementation. In both countries, only HIV specialists could prescribe ART to patients.

In Poland, specialists had to work in one of the few urban HIV treatment centers; none were available in more rural settings. This created barriers for refugees, many of whom had to commute long distances to reach the nearest HIV center (Fig. 5.1). Disruptions in HIV care consequently led to loss of viral control and possible resistance to ART.

> There have been cases… where [the patients] came back after 2-3 months after stopping treatment when their medications ran out. (Provider, Poland)

> If you're living… in a small city… you could not find any doctor who treats HIV… We have patients who drive 200, 300 kilometers to Frankfurt to get treatment. (Provider, Germany)

In both Germany and Poland, differences in ART regimen were observed. Though the combination of generic tenofovir/lamivudine/dolutegravir (TLD) is a highly tolerated single-pill treatment regimen that has a high barrier to resistance and was

Table 5.7 Pre-exposure prophylaxis policies and perceived implementation

Country	Policies and government actions	Perceived implementation of the policy	Policy source
Germany	At-risk groups (age 16+) have had full insurance coverage for PrEP since 2019	None reported	Agreement on HIV PrEP in accordance with § 20j SGB V (Vereinbarung Über die HIV-Präexpositionsprophylaxe Zur Prävention Einer HIV-Infektion Gemäß § 20j SGB V, 2019)
	To access insurance coverage for PrEP, patients must go to a physician who is an infectious disease specialist or has taken additional training and received certification from the National Association of Statutory Health Insurance Physicians	No patients have reported any barriers, but experts have underlined that this policy may create issues, as the number of physicians that patients can reach is much more limited, and most specialists are in urban centers	Agreement on HIV PrEP in accordance with § 20j SGB V (Vereinbarung Über die HIV-Präexpositionsprophylaxe Zur Prävention Einer HIV-Infektion Gemäß § 20j SGB V, 2019)
Poland	PrEP is generally not covered by public insurance (the National Health Foundation), but there was a small-scale program established in big cities that provides full coverage for PrEP medication	Patients must pay ~50 euros for a consultation plus 30 euros per 90-day supply. Participants reported no knowledge of the free PrEP program	National Programme For Preventing HIV Infections And Combating Aids For 2022–2026 (*SCHEDULE FOR THE IMPLEMENTATION OF THE NATIONAL PROGRAMME FOR PREVENTING HIV INFECTIONS AND COMBATING AIDS FOR 2022–2026*, n.d.)
	PrEP can be prescribed by all physicians	Patients can choose from a much larger range of providers	National Programme For Preventing HIV Infections And Combating Aids For 2022–2026 (*SCHEDULE FOR THE IMPLEMENTATION OF THE NATIONAL PROGRAMME FOR PREVENTING HIV INFECTIONS AND COMBATING AIDS FOR 2022–2026*, n.d.)

Legend PrEP: Pre-exposure prophylaxis for HIV

Table 5.8 Antiretroviral therapy policies and perceived implementation

Jurisdiction	Policies and government actions	Perceived implementation of the policy	Policy source
European Union	A patent by ViiV healthcare protects the sale of dolutegravir in European Union countries	The cost of dolutegravir, a drug that many Ukrainians currently take as part of the one-pill TLD regimen, in European Union countries is relatively high, making it challenging for public insurances to cover the cost	European Patent WO 2010/011812 (European Patent Specification, 2013)
Germany	Medication can be brought in from Ukraine by the patient if they carry documentation of provider prescription	This has created a significant cushion for Ukrainian refugees. Many have completely avoided receiving care in Germany and have instead returned to Ukraine for more medication and/or requested their provider in Ukraine to have it transferred to them	*Treatment for Ukraine* (Germany, n.d.)
	To be covered by health insurance, patients must obtain HIV care from an infectious disease specialist and/or a doctor otherwise certified by the National Association of Statutory Health Insurance Physicians	This significantly limits the number of available providers that refugees can receive care from. Compounding this issue, refugees are further constrained due to language barriers. However, it has been reported that ART can be accessed for free even without insurance, depending on the state	HIV/AIDS quality assurance agreement (agreement of quality assurance measures in accordance with sect. 135 (2) SGB V for the specialized Care of Patients with HIV infection/AIDS disease (HIV/AIDS quality assurance agreement), 2014)
	Single-pill regimens are recommended over multiple	Most providers have elected not to follow this recommendation when treating refugees, for whom they have opted to prescribe the multi-pill equivalent of TLD	German-Austrian guidelines (recommendation 21) (*German-Austrian guidelines on antiretroviral therapy for HIV-1 infection*, n.d.)
	Interruptions in therapy are strongly recommended against	Despite this recommendation, many providers insist that refugees have all insurance paperwork lined up and reportedly do not prescribe ART until this process is completed	German-Austrian guidelines (recommendation 23) (*German-Austrian guidelines on antiretroviral therapy for HIV-1 infection*, n.d.)

(continued)

Table 5.8 (continued)

Jurisdiction	Policies and government actions	Perceived implementation of the policy	Policy source
Poland	Only HIV specialists working in HIV treatment centers can provide care	There are only 15 to 17 treatment centers in the country. This makes it challenging to access treatment centers for some refugees	National Programme for Preventing HIV Infections And Combating AIDS for 2022–2026 (*SCHEDULE FOR THE IMPLEMENTATION OF THE NATIONAL PROGRAMME FOR PREVENTING HIV INFECTIONS AND COMBATING AIDS FOR 2022–2026*, n.d.)
	Patients have the right to full confidentiality of personal data. However, physicians must report HIV diagnoses to the regional sanitary inspector	There have been reports that the HIV status of patients has been exposed by their provider	National Programme for Preventing HIV Infections And Combating AIDS for 2022–2026 (*SCHEDULE FOR THE IMPLEMENTATION OF THE NATIONAL PROGRAMME FOR PREVENTING HIV INFECTIONS AND COMBATING AIDS FOR 2022–2026*, n.d.)
	Patients are required to report their infection status to all sexual partners	None reported	National Programme for Preventing HIV Infections And Combating AIDS for 2022–2026 (*SCHEDULE FOR THE IMPLEMENTATION OF THE NATIONAL PROGRAMME FOR PREVENTING HIV INFECTIONS AND COMBATING AIDS FOR 2022–2026*, n.d.)

(continued)

Table 5.8 (continued)

Jurisdiction	Policies and government actions	Perceived implementation of the policy	Policy source
	ART consultations and prescriptions are fully covered by public insurance	None reported	National Programme for Preventing HIV Infections And Combating AIDS for 2022–2026 (*SCHEDULE FOR THE IMPLEMENTATION OF THE NATIONAL PROGRAMME FOR PREVENTING HIV INFECTIONS AND COMBATING AIDS FOR 2022–2026*, n.d.)
	Ukrainian ART generics were briefly made available but were then overruled in a court due to a lawsuit	The absence of generics now increases the burden for refugees of transitioning to their old treatment regimen in Ukraine	As reported by UNAIDS SitRep (May 9, 2022) (SITREP: UNAIDS' Response to the Crisis in Ukraine, 2022) and as reported by participants; legislation in reference was not identified
	Documentation of refugee status and past treatment records is required for continuation of ART	Due to insufficient communication of these rules, many refugees did not have these documents and have consequently encountered delays in accessing therapy	*Treatment for Ukraine* (Poland, n.d.)

Legend ART: Antiretroviral therapy for HIV

commonly prescribed to patients in Ukraine, this single-pill generic formulation was not available in either Germany or Poland.

In Poland, policymakers initially addressed this issue initially by allowing TLD to be transported into the country, with the World Health Organization (WHO) donating a supply of medications to Poland until the end of 2022, however, because ViiV Healthcare held patent protections for dolutegravir in the EU, the company demanded to ceasedistribution of generic TLD.

> The WHO got a special deal until the end of 2022, and we had TLD available… but one of the pharma companies has written a claim to the WHO that they should not provide Poland with a generic medication that is patented. (Provider, Poland)

Consequently, providers either transferred patients to the Polish standard-of-care regimen or prescribed multiple pills to create a TLD equivalent. This entailed prescribing dolutegravir as a separate medication, which was expensive in EU countries due to dolutegravir's patent-protected status.

Germany used a similar approach with providers prescribing a multi-pill regimen to maintain the TLD regimen, which was contrary to German-Austrian Guidelines, which encouraged single-pill regimens.

> Normally, I ask a patient if they plan to stay for a long time here in Germany or if they plan to go back in a few months. If they plan to go back in a few months, I would stay with the same treatment… If a patient has a plan to live here for a long time, I could even switch treatment using our new modern German treatment. It's the same as TLD but injectable. (Provider, Germany)

5.3 Discussion

Shocks to HIV service delivery systems may result in sustained treatment interruptions, viral rebound, and increased transmission, consequences that compromise both individual and public health (Jewell et al., 2020). As the war in Ukraine continues and its long-term consequences unfold (de Vogel, 2023), linkage to and retention in HIV prevention and treatment services is critical to protecting refugee health and preventing outbreaks in host countries (Global AIDS Monitoring, 2019: Ukraine, 2019; Nikitin et al., 2025).

Findings from this study applying the WHO HSPA framework, which includes governance, resource generation, financing, and service delivery, suggest that in the new context of the Ukrainian refugee crisis, HIV service systems in both Germany and Poland were insufficiently positioned to absorb the shock of providing universal access to HIV services for refugees—both through continuity of existing services or starting patients anew. While stakeholders reported that Germany had sufficient funding, Poland allocated limited funds to prevention, creating a critical gap in access. System resources to ensure continued access to HIV services for refugees were lacking in both countries, with access to insurance being delayed in Germany, language interpreter services being limited in both countries, and patient-to-provider linkage infrastructure being difficult to navigate in both countries. NGOs from Ukraine, in response to the lack of response by the German and Polish governments, reallocated their funding to fill critical gaps of insufficiently adapted system sources. Service delivery barriers, including specialist-only prescribing requirements, resulted in delays and attrition from care. As outlined in the HSPA framework, governance is a critical factor that influences financing, resource generation, and service delivery. Taken together, these results show that national HIV strategies, while formally robust, were not sufficiently flexible to accommodate the unique needs of displaced PWID and PWH. These findings indicte that resilience depends not only on available resources, but on how rapidly policies can adapt to real-world shocks. Based on these findings, we identify policy changes to could build HIV system resilience based on the key strains identified in this study.

5.3.1 *Toward Resilience Through Policy Change*

HIV policies in Germany and Poland provided a foundation but were not implemented sufficiently to ensure timely access, linkage, and retention in care for refugees. Still, many policies were successful in creating a system for enrolling refugees in insurance and providing them (albeit only those with Ukrainian citizenship) with access to the healthcare system, though equity in access varied by gender, language proficiency, and legal status. Impressively, Poland took important steps to create extensive Ukrainian-language resources for linking patients to care. These actions represent the culmination of substantial efforts in both countries to protect the health of thousands of at-risk refugees.

Here, recommendations based on the HSPA framework are offered for some of the most important and politically viable changes that can improve system resilience in Germany and Poland. Nevertheless, it is worth noting that both countries face a challenging balance for shaping health policies aimed at improving HIV services for refugees. With each having received approximately one million refugees (Ukraine Refugee Situation, 2023), Germany and Poland have certainly spent extensive resources on providing assistance to displaced persons and likely face a critical dilemma: the easier the system becomes to navigate and access, the greater the potential uptake of services may become. This could result in strains on Germany's and Poland's resources and is made even more complicated for the population of focus in this study, as PWID and PWH constitute a very stigmatized and high-cost subset of the refugee population (Bromberg et al., 2020; Gesesew et al., 2017). To help relieve this strain, support from international organizations like the EU and UN may be critical. Importantly, the findings underscore that the flexibility and feasibility of HIV service delivery remain limited. In Germany, specialist-only prescribing requirements reduced feasibility by constraining provider capacity, while in Poland, concentration of HIV and OAT centers in urban areas restricted access for refugees in rural regions. These structural features illustrate that without greater flexibility, even well-funded systems may struggle to ensure equitable care in future crises.

5.3.1.1 Resource Generation—Provide Immediate Access Insurance to All Refugees

As the Temporary Protection Directive declares that Ukrainian refugees should have access to healthcare, ensuring that the timing for access to this system is not delayed is critical to ensuring equity. Policies that uphold principles of equity in HIV care are widely supported by the WHO, UNAIDS, and ECDC (*Ensuring High-Quality HIV Care for Displaced People from Ukraine*, n.d.; Guidance on Ethics and Equitable Access to HIV Treatment and Care, 2004). The ECDC emphasizes that access to HIV services should *always* be free (*Ensuring High-Quality HIV Care for Displaced People from Ukraine*, n.d.).

Ensuring immediate and sustained access to health insurance is essential to upholding the Temporary Protection Directive's commitment that Ukrainian refugees receive equitable healthcare. Delays in registration, particularly in Germany, created barriers to care and forced some refugees to travel back to Ukraine to access life-saving services (Furl et al., 2018). According to the UNHCR, 6% of refugees reported returning to Ukraine at least once to seek healthcare (LIVES ON HOLD: INTENTIONS AND PERSPECTIVES OF REFUGEES AND IDPS FROM UKRAINE, 2023), posing unnecessary risks and costs.

Current practices in Germany allow for temporary insurance vouchers in some states, but implementation is inconsistent, poorly communicated, and often limited to 30 days. A national policy that issues temporary insurance cards valid for at least six months upon residency application would substantially reduce delays and avoid harmful treatment interruptions. These cards should be automatically renewable until a final residency determination is made. As many Ukrainians perceived that leaving Ukraine was a short-term solution, having an open-ended policy may have increased the likelihood that many would seek insurance quickly to avoid delays in accessing treatment.

Importantly, continuous access to insurance generates cost savings for the host country. Interruptions in care for HIV and OUD increase the risk of complications requiring emergency services or hospitalizations, which are both more costly than ambulatory care (Gebo et al., 2010). Moreover, untreated HIV among high-risk populations like PWID increases the potential for onward transmission and future outbreaks (Kingori et al., 2016). While limiting insurance access may appear fiscally conservative, failing to immediately insure this population is likely to result in greater long-term health system expenditures.

5.3.1.2 Resource Generation—Mandate Language Interpreter Services in Healthcare Settings

In both Germany and Poland, no policies that coordinated language interpretation within clinics were identified. Patients reported that Google Translate was insufficient, and they were forced to locate interpreters on their own, in many cases having to pay out of pocket for those services and/or experiencing discrimination from the interpreter they received. As PWID and PWH are a high-risk population, miscommunication of their health needs may have dire consequences (Flores, 2005; Handtke et al., 2019). Policies mandating interpreter services in the healthcare setting are needed. This need is especially critical for PWID identifying as women, who may face both gender-based stigma and linguistic exclusion.

This study showed that patients are less likely to pursue care without language interpretation. For patients who pursue care, the quality of care provided may be diminished, as important medical information might be omitted or improperly translated (Flores, 2005; Handtke et al., 2019). This is especially true for patients seeking access to HIV services, as they tend to experience high levels of stigma (Bromberg et al., 2020; Gesesew et al., 2017) and might be less apprehensive if the center offered confidential interpretation (Jacobs et al., 2018). Healthcare-specific translation platforms, including S-MINDS, X-prompt, and iTranslate, as well as virtual tele-interpreters, have been successfully deployed in other parts of the world and have received high rates of patient satisfaction (Ji et al., 2021). These can be particularly useful in Poland and Germany, where the strain on human resources for in-person interpreter services has been high due to the refugee crisis (Lee et al., 2023).

5.3.1.3 Service Delivery: Create Supportive Policies to Encourage Immediate (or Quickly Earned) Take-Home OAT

In both Poland and Germany, take-home dosing was permitted but prescribed conservatively. In Germany, many patients who had previously been on stable, extended take-home dosing were forced to travel daily or many times per week to pick up OAT medication at the clinic. Developing supportive policies like the right to continuity of care that nudge providers to prescribe take-home dosing of OAT for stable patients could have a meaningful impact on access and retention in care for refugees and even the host population.

Greater access to take-home dosing of OAT is safe and improves health outcomes (Bachireddy et al., 2015; Meteliuk et al., 2021). Extending take-home dosing duration and making it available to more patients has been shown to increase retention in therapy (Ivasiy et al., 2022, 2024; Shojaati & Osgood, 2023), improve access for those starting OAT (Russell et al., 2022), and reduce stigma and exposure to illicit substances (Adams et al., 2023), all while leading to very minimal risks (Gomes et al., 2022). Scale-up of OAT through expanded take-homes has been accomplished in Ukraine during the COVID pandemic (Meteliuk et al., 2021). A similar approach in Germany and Poland could prove meaningful for not only refugees but also the host population.

5.3.1.4 Service Delivery—Allow Primary Care Providers to Prescribe Insurance-Covered OAT, PrEP, and ART

In both countries, nearly all prescriptions for OAT, PrEP, and ART came from specialists. In Poland, prescriptions were limited to a handful of centers. In Germany, prescriptions from non-specialists were not covered by public health insurance. As this study found, patients had to make long commutes to receive care, creating risks of treatment dropout. A potential solution would be decentralizing OAT, PrEP, and ART by enabling primary care physicians to prescribe insurance-covered medications under the guidance of specialists. This approach would likely involve in-person visits to a primary care physician who would then link patients to a specialist via telehealth, thereby removing the burden for patients to travel long distances while not displacing specialist authority. In Ukraine, this approach for OAT enabled faster scale-up of OAT programs (Morozova et al., 2020), indicating that linkage to care was likely improved. The decentralization and integration of HIV services has been successfully deployed in Ukraine and other low- and middle-income countries (Cobos Muñoz et al., 2017; Morozova et al., 2017; Pashchenko et al., 2022). Applying this to higher-income settings is likely to achieve similar benefits for linkage to care (Cobos Muñoz et al., 2017; Reidy et al., 2014).

5.3.2 Limitations

This study is not without limitations. Due to the rapidly evolving crisis, the bulk of available data is qualitative and not backed by quantitative metrics, such as the actual number of Ukrainian refugees enrolled in HIV services. This study attempts to compensate for this gap by offering an estimate of changes to HIV service demands; however, these estimates are very broad due to limited available data.

Funding data for both Germany and Poland were also limited. Due to researcher resource limitations, we examined funding only on the national level without examining state or local level funding, which may be a substantial contributor to overall financial strategies for providing HIV services. Stakeholder interviews, however, helped to fill some of the gaps with regard to state and local funding. Nevertheless, future studies should incorporate these data to be more comprehensive.

Moreover, this study does not focus on refugees from Ukraine who are *not* Ukrainian citizens, as this group is affected by a distinct set of rules. An in-depth analysis of HIV service provision for this group is presently lacking but needed.

5.4 Conclusions

The intertwined HIV and OUD epidemics in Ukraine are a major public health crisis. With mass displacement from Ukraine, host countries have experienced an unprecedented shock to their HIV services, requiring immediate adaptations to treating a highly stigmatized subset of the population. In Germany and Poland, national HIV policies and their implementation play an important role in determining if Ukrainian refugees can be linked to care efficiently. This study shows that, although the existing policies and their perceived implementation have generally enabled continuation of HIV services for refugees, significant barriers remain. In the absence of a coordinated policy and implementation strategy to build a more resilient HIV services system, there is a high likelihood that outbreaks of HIV will occur and introduce microepidemics in these countries. While accounting for the already substantial support of refugees by host countries, policy changes that expedite access to insurance; expand take-home OAT; and allow insurance-covered OAT, PrEP, and ART prescriptions by primary care providers will improve system resilience by easing barriers to linkage to care for Ukrainian refugees.

5.4.1 Recommendations

Based on findings from Germany and Poland, we offer the following actionable recommendations to improve resilience of HIV services in the setting of mass displacement.

5.4.1.1 Policy Recommendations

- Streamline access to public health insurance by simplifying registration procedures and expanding automatic eligibility for displaced individuals.
- Revise prescribing regulations to permit non-specialist providers (e.g., general practitioners) to initiate and manage OAT, PrEP, and ART.
- Mandate professional interpreter services or artificial intelligence interpreting solutions to reduce dependence on informal or digital interpreting methods.

5.4.1.2 Practice Recommendations

- Train HIV services providers and clinic staff in culturally responsive, trauma-informed care, including sensitivity to substance use and gender-based stigma.
- Expand mobile outreach services and urban-rural linkages, particularly in areas where OAT and PrEP access is limited.
- Strengthen support for community-based NGOs, including mechanisms to fund Ukrainian-led efforts that are trusted by displaced populations.

5.4.1.3 Research Recommendations

- Conduct further gender-disaggregated and migration status-specific studies on HIV services uptake among refugees.
- Explore longitudinal outcomes for displaced PWH and PWID to assess the impact of early versus delayed service access.
- Evaluate models of task-sharing in HIV service delivery and their scalability in high-burden, low-resource refugee settings.
- Evaluate the feasibility of **Just-in-Time Adaptive Interventions (JITAIs)** and conversational agents (e.g., large-language-model-based tools) to address emotional needs among mobile, hard-to-reach populations.

Competing Interests: The authors declare that they have no competing interests.

Ethics Approval: This study was approved by the Yale University institutional review board.

References

Act of Law of 29 July 2005 On counteracting drug addiction, Republic of Poland.

Adams, A., Blawatt, S., Magel, T., MacDonald, S., Lajeunesse, J., Harrison, S., Byres, D., Schechter, M. T., & Oviedo-Joekes, E. (2023). The impact of relaxing restrictions on take-home doses during the COVID-19 pandemic on program effectiveness and client experiences in opioid agonist treatment: A mixed methods systematic review. *Substance Abuse Treatment, Prevention, and Policy, 18*(1), 56. https://doi.org/10.1186/s13011-023-00564-9

Agreement of Quality Assurance Measures in Accordance with Section 135 (2) SGB V for the Specialized Care of Patients with HIV Infection/AIDS Disease (HIV/AIDS Quality Assurance Agreement), National Association of Statuatory Health Insurance Physicians (2014).

Aljadeeah, S., Wirtz, V. J., & Nagel, E. (2021). Barriers to accessing medicines among Syrian asylum seekers and refugees in a German Federal State. *International Journal of Environmental Research and Public Health, 18*(2), 519. https://doi.org/10.3390/ijerph18020519

Altice, F. L., Bromberg, D. J., Klepikov, A., Barzilay, E. J., Islam, Z., Dvoriak, S., Farnum, S. O., & Madden, L. M. (2022). Collaborative learning and response to opioid misuse and HIV prevention in Ukraine during war. *The Lancet Psychiatry, 9*(11), 852–854. https://doi.org/10.1016/S2215-0366(22)00318-2

Announcement a decision of the joint Federal Committee on an amendment to the guideline on methods of contract medical care (MVV-RL): Annex I No. 2 Substitution-based treatment of opiate addicts. (2018). Federal Law Gazette.

Antonenko, Z., & Martsynovska, V. (2022). *HIV Infection in Ukraine Information Bulletin* (No. 53)..

Asylum Act in the version promulgated on 2 September 2008 (Federal Law Gazette I, p. 1798), last amended by Article 2 of the Act of 11 March 2016 (Federal Law Gazette I, p. 394). (2016). *Federal Law Gazette.*

Bachireddy, C., Weisberg, D. F., & Altice, F. L. (2015). Balancing access and safety in prescribing opioid agonist therapy to prevent HIV transmission. *Addiction, 110*(12), 1869–1871. https://doi.org/10.1111/add.13055

Balmer. (2022, March 9). *Worst refugee crisis since WW2 as Ukrainians flee country*. Reuters.

Biesiada, A., Mastalerz-Migas, A., & Babicki, M. (2023). Response to provide key health services to Ukrainian refugees: The overview and implementation studies. *Social Science & Medicine, 334*, 116221. https://doi.org/10.1016/j.socscimed.2023.116221

Bogic, M., Njoku, A., & Priebe, S. (2015). Long-term mental health of war-refugees: A systematic literature review. *BMC International Health and Human Rights, 15*(1), 29. https://doi.org/10.1186/s12914-015-0064-9

Brislin, R. W. (1970). Back-translation for cross-cultural research. *Journal of Cross-Cultural Psychology, 1*(3), 185–216. https://doi.org/10.1177/135910457000100301

Bromberg, D. J., Mayer, K. H., & Altice, F. L. (2020). Identifying and managing infectious disease syndemics in patients with HIV. *Current Opinion in HIV and AIDS, 15*(4), 232–242. https://doi.org/10.1097/COH.0000000000000631

Bromberg, D. J., Rhoades, D., Madden, L. M., Ivasiy, R., Meteliuk, A., Pykalo, I., Filippovych, M., Nikitin, B. M., Farnum, S. O., Fomenko, T., Dvoriak, S., Altice, F. L., & the ExMAT Consortium. (2025). Transformation of the HIV treatment cascade for people who inject drugs in Ukraine. *AIDS, 39*(3), 306–311. https://doi.org/10.1097/QAD.0000000000004056

Cairns, G. (2022, October 26). *Rapid scale-up of PrEP in Ukraine this year, despite the war*. Nam Aidsmap. https://www.aidsmap.com/news/oct-2022/rapid-scale-prep-ukraine-year-despite-war

Carroll, J. J. (2019). Sovereign rules and rearrangements: Banning methadone in occupied Crimea. *Medical Anthropology, 38*(6), 508–522. https://doi.org/10.1080/01459740.2018.1532422

Choopanya, K., Martin, M., Suntharasamai, P., Sangkum, U., Mock, P. A., Leethochawalit, M., Chiamwongpaet, S., Kitisin, P., Natrujirote, P., Kittimunkong, S., Chuachoowong, R., Gvetadze, R. J., McNicholl, J. M., Paxton, L. A., Curlin, M. E., Hendrix, C. W., & Vanichseni, S. (2013). Antiretroviral prophylaxis for HIV infection in injecting drug users in Bangkok, Thailand (the

Bangkok Tenofovir study): A randomised, double-blind, placebo-controlled phase 3 trial. *The Lancet, 381*(9883), 2083–2090. https://doi.org/10.1016/S0140-6736(13)61127-7

Cobos Muñoz, D., Merino Amador, P., Monzon Llamas, L., Martinez Hernandez, D., & Santos Sancho, J. M. (2017). Decentralization of health systems in low and middle income countries: A systematic review. *International Journal of Public Health, 62*(2), 219–229. https://doi.org/10.1007/s00038-016-0872-2

COUNCIL IMPLEMENTING DECISION (EU) 2022/382 of 4 March 2022. (n.d.). Official Journal of the European Union.

Country Factsheets: Germany. (2022). UNAIDS. https://www.unaids.org/en/regionscountries/countries/germany

Country Factsheets: Poland. (2022). UNAIDS. https://www.unaids.org/en/regionscountries/countries/poland

Davitian, K., Noack, P., Eckstein, K., Hübner, J., & Ahmadi, E. (2024). Barriers of Ukrainian refugees and migrants in accessing German healthcare. *BMC Health Services Research, 24*(1), 1112. https://doi.org/10.1186/s12913-024-11592-x

de Vogel, S. (2023, May 8). *A war with no end in sight*. Davis Center for Russian and Eurasian Studies, Harvard University.

EMCDDA *Trendspotter Briefing: Responsiveness and preparedness in addressing drug-related needs of displaced Ukrainians in EU countries bordering Ukraine*. (n.d.). EMCDDA.

Ensuring high-quality HIV care for displaced people from Ukraine. (n.d.). ECDC; WHO.

European Patent Specification. (2013, December 25). European Patent Office.

Flores, G. (2005). The impact of medical interpreter services on the quality of health care: A systematic review. *Medical Care Research and Review, 62*(3), 255–299. https://doi.org/10.1177/1077558705275416

Fremer, I. (2022, April 27). *Poland: Parliament adopts new law to regulate influx of Ukrainian refugees and provide them with protection and assistance*. Library of Congress.

Furl, R., Watanabe-Galloway, S., Lyden, E., & Swindells, S. (2018). Determinants of facilitated health insurance enrollment for patients with HIV disease, and impact of insurance enrollment on targeted health outcomes. *BMC Infectious Diseases, 18*(1), 132. https://doi.org/10.1186/s12879-018-3035-7

Gebo, K. A., Fleishman, J. A., Conviser, R., Hellinger, J., Hellinger, F. J., Josephs, J. S., Keiser, P., Gaist, P., & Moore, R. D. (2010). Contemporary costs of HIV healthcare in the HAART era. *AIDS, 24*(17), 2705–2715. https://doi.org/10.1097/QAD.0b013e32833f3c14

German-Austrian guidelines on antiretroviral therapy for HIV-1 infection. (n.d.).

Germany. (n.d.). Treatment for Ukraine. Retrieved https://www.treatment4ukraine.com/en/countries/germany/

Gesesew, H. A., Tesfay Gebremedhin, A., Demissie, T. D., Kerie, M. W., Sudhakar, M., & Mwanri, L. (2017). Significant association between perceived HIV related stigma and late presentation for HIV/AIDS care in low and middle-income countries: A systematic review and meta-analysis. *PLoS One, 12*(3), e0173928. https://doi.org/10.1371/journal.pone.0173928

Global AIDS Monitoring 2019: Ukraine. (2019). UNAIDS.

Gomes, T., Campbell, T. J., Kitchen, S. A., Garg, R., Bozinoff, N., Men, S., Tadrous, M., Munro, C., Antoniou, T., Werb, D., & Wyman, J. (2022). Association between increased dispensing of opioid agonist therapy take-home doses and opioid overdose and treatment interruption and discontinuation. *JAMA, 327*(9), 846. https://doi.org/10.1001/jama.2022.1271

Guidance on ethics and equitable access to HIV treatment and care. (2004). Joint United Nations Programme on HIV/AIDS: World Health Organization.

Handtke, O., Schilgen, B., & Mösko, M. (2019). Culturally competent healthcare—A scoping review of strategies implemented in healthcare organizations and a model of culturally competent healthcare provision. *PLoS One, 14*(7), e0219971. https://doi.org/10.1371/journal.pone.0219971

Helping Ukrainian refugees with HIV treatment and support in Berlin. (2022, May 20). *UNAIDS*. https://www.unaids.org/en/keywords/ukraine#:~:text=UNAIDS%20estimates%20that%20260%20000,risk%20of%20progression%20to%20AIDS

Horyniak, D., Melo, J. S., Farrell, R. M., Ojeda, V. D., & Strathdee, S. A. (2016). Epidemiology of substance use among forced migrants: A global systematic review. *PLoS One, 11*(7), e0159134. https://doi.org/10.1371/journal.pone.0159134

Ivasiy, R., Madden, L. M., Farnum, S. O., Shumskaya, N., De Leon, S. J. G., Bromberg, D. J., Kurmanalieva, A., Duishenaliev, A., Tokubaev, R., & Altice, F. L. (2022). Implementation opportunities for scaling up methadone maintenance treatment in Kyrgyzstan: Methadone dosage and retention on treatment over two years. *Drug and Alcohol Dependence Reports, 4*, 100075. https://doi.org/10.1016/j.dadr.2022.100075

Ivasiy, R., Madden, L. M., Meteliuk, A., Machavariani, E., Ahmad, B., Zelenev, A., Desai, M. M., Bromberg, D. J., Polonsky, M., Galvez De Leon, S. J., Farnum, S. O., Islam, Z., & Altice, F. L. (2024). The impact of emergency guidance to the COVID-19 pandemic on treatment entry, retention and mortality among patients on methadone in Ukraine. *Addiction, 119*(9), 1585–1596. https://doi.org/10.1111/add.16565

Jacobs, B., Ryan, A. M., Henrichs, K. S., & Weiss, B. D. (2018). Medical interpreters in outpatient practice. *The Annals of Family Medicine, 16*(1), 70–76. https://doi.org/10.1370/afm.2154

Jewell, B. L., Smith, J. A., & Hallett, T. B. (2020). Understanding the impact of interruptions to HIV services during the COVID-19 pandemic: A modelling study. *EClinicalMedicine, 26*, 100483. https://doi.org/10.1016/j.eclinm.2020.100483

Ji, X., Chow, E., Abdelhamid, K., Naumova, D., Mate, K. K. V., Bergeron, A., & Lebouché, B. (2021). Utility of mobile technology in medical interpretation: A literature review of current practices. *Patient Education and Counseling, 104*(9), 2137–2145. https://doi.org/10.1016/j.pec.2021.02.019

Kingori, C., Esquivel, C. L., Hassan, Q., Elmi, A., Mukasa, B., & Reece, M. (2016). Recommendations for developing contextually relevant HIV/AIDS prevention strategies targeting African-born immigrants and refugees in the United States. *AIDS Patient Care and STDs, 30*(10), 476–483. https://doi.org/10.1089/apc.2016.0171

Lee, A. C. K., Khaw, F.-M., Lindman, A. E. S., & Juszczyk, G. (2023). Ukraine refugee crisis: Evolving needs and challenges. *Public Health, 217*, 41–45. https://doi.org/10.1016/j.puhe.2023.01.016

Lives on Hold: Intentions and Perspectives of Refugees and IDPS From Ukraine (Regional Intentions Report No. 4). (2023). UNHCR.

Makarenko, I., Mazhnaya, A., Polonsky, M., Marcus, R., Bojko, M. J., Filippovych, S., Springer, S., Dvoriak, S., & Altice, F. L. (2016). Determinants of willingness to enroll in opioid agonist treatment among opioid dependent people who inject drugs in Ukraine. *Drug and Alcohol Dependence, 165*, 213–220. https://doi.org/10.1016/j.drugalcdep.2016.06.011

Mazhnaya, A., Marcus, R., Bojko, M. J., Zelenev, A., Makarenko, I., Pykalo, I., Filippovych, S., Dvoriak, S., & Altice, F. L. (2018). Opioid agonist treatment and improved outcomes at each stage of the HIV treatment Cascade in people who inject drugs in Ukraine. *JAIDS Journal of Acquired Immune Deficiency Syndromes, 79*(3), 288–295. https://doi.org/10.1097/QAI.0000000000001827

Meteliuk, A., Galvez De Leon, S. J., Madden, L. M., Pykalo, I., Fomenko, T., Filippovych, M., Farnum, S. O., Dvoryak, S., Islam, Z. M., & Altice, F. L. (2021). Rapid transitional response to the COVID-19 pandemic by opioid agonist treatment programs in Ukraine. *Journal of Substance Abuse Treatment, 121*, 108164. https://doi.org/10.1016/j.jsat.2020.108164

Morozova, O., Crawford, F. W., Cohen, T., Paltiel, A. D., & Altice, F. L. (2020). Cost-effectiveness of expanding the capacity of opioid agonist treatment in Ukraine: Dynamic modeling analysis. *Addiction, 115*(3), 437–450. https://doi.org/10.1111/add.14797

Morozova, O., Dvoriak, S., Pykalo, I., & Altice, F. L. (2017). Primary healthcare-based integrated care with opioid agonist treatment: First experience from Ukraine. *Drug and Alcohol Dependence, 173*, 132–138. https://doi.org/10.1016/j.drugalcdep.2016.12.025

Naja, F., Shatila, H., El Koussa, M., Meho, L., Ghandour, L., & Saleh, S. (2019). Burden of non-communicable diseases among Syrian refugees: A scoping review. *BMC Public Health, 19*(1), 637. https://doi.org/10.1186/s12889-019-6977-9

Narcotics Act in the version published on March 1, 1994. (2023). *Federal Law Gazette*, (204).

National AIDS Center. (2022). *Schedule for the implementation of the National Programme for preventing HIV Infections and Combating AIDS for 2022–2026*. National AIDS Center.

National AIDS Center. (2024). *Report on the Performance of the Tasks Included in the Schedule for the Implementation of the National Program to Prevent HIV Infection and Combat AIDS in 2023*. National AIDS Center.

Ni, Z., Altice, F. L., Wickersham, J. A., Copenhaver, M. M., DiDomizio, E. E., Nelson, L. E., & Shrestha, R. (2021). Willingness to initiate pre-exposure prophylaxis (PrEP) and its use among opioid-dependent individuals in drug treatment. *Drug and Alcohol Dependence, 219*, 108477. https://doi.org/10.1016/j.drugalcdep.2020.108477

Nikitin, B. M., Bromberg, D. J., Ivasiy, R., Madden, L., Machavariani, E., Dvoriak, S., Poole, D. N., Otiashvilli, D., & Altice, F. L. (2025). Disruptions to HIV prevention during armed conflict in Ukraine and other settings. *Current HIV/AIDS Reports, 22*(1), 10. https://doi.org/10.1007/s11904-024-00716-x

Nikitin, B. M., Bromberg, D. J., Madden, L. M., Stöver, H., Teltzrow, R., & Altice, F. L. (2023). Leveraging existing provider networks in Europe to eliminate barriers to accessing opioid agonist maintenance therapies for Ukrainian refugees. *PLOS Global Public Health, 3*(7), e0002168. https://doi.org/10.1371/journal.pgph.0002168

Nikitin, B. M., Bromberg, D. J., Pykalo, I., Ivasiy, R., Islam, Z., & Altice, F. L. (2023). Early disruptions to syringe services programs during the Russian invasion of Ukraine. *Frontiers in Public Health, 11*, 1229057. https://doi.org/10.3389/fpubh.2023.1229057

On behalf of the Dynamics Study Team, Becker, M., Balakireva, O., Pavlova, D., Isac, S., Cheuk, E., Roberts, E., Forget, E., Ma, H., Lazarus, L., Sandstrom, P., Blanchard, J., Mishra, S., Lorway, R., & Pickles, M. (2019). Assessing the influence of conflict on the dynamics of sex work and the HIV and HCV epidemics in Ukraine: Protocol for an observational, ethnographic, and mathematical modeling study. *BMC International Health and Human Rights, 19*(1), 16. https://doi.org/10.1186/s12914-019-0201-y

Ordinance Concerning the Foreign Trade in Narcotics, Federal Republic of Germany (1981).

Ordinance on the Prescription, Dispensing and Proof of the Disposition of Narcotic Drugs (Narcotic Drugs Prescription Ordinance), Federal Republic of Germany (2009).

Papanicolas, I. (with Rajan, D., Karanikolos, M., Soucat, A., & Figueras Marimont, J.). (2022). *Health system performance assessment: A framework for policy analysis* (1st ed). World Health Organization.

Parczewski, M., Jabłonowska, E., Wójcik-Cichy, K., Zhyvytsia, D., Witak-Jędra, M., Leszczyszyn-Pynka, M., Aksak-Wąs, B., Siwak, E., Cielniak, I., Olczak, A., Szymczak, A., Szetela, B., Bociąga-Jasik, M., Kalinowska-Nowak, A., Mularska, E., Witor, A., Jakubowski, P., Hlebowicz, M., Rozpłochowski, B., et al. (2023). Clinical perspective on human immunodeficiency virus Care of Ukrainian war Refugees in Poland. *Clinical Infectious Diseases, 76*(10), 1708–1715. https://doi.org/10.1093/cid/ciad116

Pashchenko, O., Bromberg, D. J., Dumchev, K., LaMonaca, K., Pykalo, I., Filippovych, M., Esserman, D., Polonsky, M., Galvez De Leon, S. J., Morozova, O., Dvoriak, S., & Altice, F. L. (2022). Preliminary analysis of self-reported quality health indicators of patients on opioid agonist therapy at specialty and primary care clinics in Ukraine: A randomized control trial. *PLOS Global Public Health, 2*(11), e0000344. https://doi.org/10.1371/journal.pgph.0000344

Pavli, A., & Maltezou, H. (2017). Health problems of newly arrived migrants and refugees in Europe. *Journal of Travel Medicine, 24*(4). https://doi.org/10.1093/jtm/tax016

Poland. (n.d.). Treatment for Ukraine.

Poland. (2021). Eurasian Harm Reduction Association.

REGULATION (EU) 2016/679 OF THE EUROPEAN PARLIAMENT AND OF THE COUNCIL of 27 April 2016 on the protection of natural persons with regard to the processing of personal data and on the free movement of such data, and repealing Directive 95/46/EC (General Data Protection Regulation). (2016). *Official Journal of the European Union.*

Reidy, W. J., Sheriff, M., Wang, C., Hawken, M., Koech, E., Elul, B., Kimanga, D., & Abrams, E. J. (2014). Decentralization of HIV care and treatment Services in Central Province, Kenya. *JAIDS Journal of Acquired Immune Deficiency Syndromes, 67*(1), e34–e40. https://doi.org/10.1097/QAI.0000000000000264

Russell, C., Lange, S., Kouyoumdjian, F., Butler, A., & Ali, F. (2022). Opioid agonist treatment take-home doses ('carries'): Are current guidelines resulting in low treatment coverage among high-risk populations in Canada and the USA? *Harm Reduction Journal, 19*(1), 89. https://doi.org/10.1186/s12954-022-00671-z

Schedule for the Implementation Of The National Programme for Preventing HIV Infections and combating aids for 2022–2026. (n.d.). National AIDS Centre.

Shojaati, N., & Osgood, N. D. (2023). Evaluating the impact of increased dispensing of opioid agonist therapy take-home doses on treatment retention and opioid-related harm among opioid agonist therapy recipients: A simulation study. *Systems, 11*(8), 391. https://doi.org/10.3390/systems11080391

SITREP: UNAIDS' response to the crisis in Ukraine. (2022). UNAIDS.

Social Code (SGB) Fifth Book (V)—Statutory Health Insurance—(Article 1 of the Law of December 20, 1988, BGBl. I p. 2477), Federal Republic of Germany (1988).

Spiegel, P. B. (2022). Responding to the Ukraine refugee health crisis in the EU. *The Lancet, 399*(10341), 2084–2086. https://doi.org/10.1016/S0140-6736(22)00841-8

Stone, J., Degenhardt, L., Grebely, J., Larney, S., Altice, F. L., Smyrnov, P., Rahimi-Movaghar, A., Alavi, M., Young, A. M., Havens, J. R., Miller, W. C., Hickman, M., & Vickerman, P. (2021). Modelling the intervention effect of opioid agonist treatment on multiple mortality outcomes in people who inject drugs: A three-setting analysis. *The Lancet Psychiatry, 8*(4), 301–309. https://doi.org/10.1016/S2215-0366(20)30538-1

Taylor, S., Boffito, M., Khoo, S., Smit, E., & Back, D. (2007). Stopping antiretroviral therapy. *AIDS, 21*(13), 1673–1682. https://doi.org/10.1097/QAD.0b013e3281c61394

Temporary protection for foreigners. (n.d.). Republic of Poland. Retrieved https://www.gov.pl/web/ochrona-en/social-assistance

Ukraine Emergency. (n.d.). USA for UNHCR. Retrieved https://www.unrefugees.org/emergencies/ukraine/

Ukraine Refugee Situation. (2023). *United nations high commissioner for refugees.* https://data.unhcr.org/en/situations/ukraine.

Vereinbarung Über Die HIV-Präexpositionsprophylaxe Zur Prävention Einer HIV-Infektion Gemäß § 20j SGB V, National Association of Statutory Health Insurance Physicians (2019).

Vierte Verordnung zur Änderung der Ukraine-Aufenthalts Übergangsverordnung. (2023). *Federal Law Gazette.*

Viral hepatitis elimination barometer among people who inject drugs in Europe. (2023). [Data factsheet]. European Monitoring Centre for Drugs and Drug Addiction. https://www.emcdda.europa.eu/publications/data-factsheet/viral-hepatitis-elimination-barometer-among-people-who-inject-drugs-in-europe_en

West, B. S. (2019). Social networks of substance-using populations: Key issues and promising new approaches for HIV. *Current HIV/AIDS Reports, 16*(1), 48–56. https://doi.org/10.1007/s11904-019-00425-w

WHO EMRO—Health systems resilience. (n.d.). Retrieved September 23, 2025, from https://www.emro.who.int/uhc-health-systems/health-systems-in-emergency-lab/health-system-resilience.html?utm_source=chatgpt.com

Wissenschaftliches Institut der AOK (WIdO). (2025). PharMaAnalyst: Analyses of pharmaceutical prescription data. *Wissenschaftliches Institut der AOK (WIdO).*. https://arzneimittel.wido.de/PharMaAnalyst/

Yayboke, E., Sroubouulis, A., & Edwards, A. (2022, October 3). *Update on Forced Displacement around Ukraine.*

Chapter 6
Substance Use as a Coping Strategy Among Ukrainian War Refugees in Poland: Changes Following Participation in a Mental Health Support Program

Katarzyna Okulicz-Kozaryn and Anna Dzielska

6.1 Introduction

The Russian aggression against Ukraine on February 24, 2022, caused a large influx of war refugees to Poland. This humanitarian emergency differed from other migration crises in the world in several respects: scale and rate (over 1.5 million refugees arrived in Poland within 1 month), demographics (women and children predominated among the refugees, including many children without care or under the care of "non-parents," such as siblings), and forms of assistance (tens of thousands of trips were made from the border in private cars, hundreds of thousands of refugees were hosted in private apartments, and massive financial and material collections were organized) (Ociepa-Kicińska & Gorzałczyńska-Koczkodaj, 2022). In a March 2022 poll among Poles, 61% of respondents declared that they themselves had taken part in aid actions; additionally, 49% reported that their close relatives had been involved, and 45% that their friends had provided some form of support (Pacewicz, 2022). Importantly, rather than creating a separate system for refugees, the Polish government immediately offered inclusion in the existing education system, labor market, or healthcare system on an equal footing with Polish citizens (Wojdat & Cywiński, 2022).

At the same time, no sociodemographic or more in-depth information on the psychosocial needs of the incoming refugees was collected. During the first weeks and months of the war, public discourse was dominated by narratives and images aimed at strengthening empathy for refugees and focusing on the assistance provided by Polish citizens, organizations, municipalities, government bodies, and business

K. Okulicz-Kozaryn (✉) · A. Dzielska
Department of Children and Adolescents Health, Institute of Mother and Child, Warsaw, Poland
e-mail: katarzyna.okulicz@imid.med.pl

C. De Kock (ed.), *Substance Use Among Refugees in Europe*,
https://doi.org/10.1007/978-3-032-32399-6_6

(Zawadzka-Paluektau, 2022). Everyday observations (e.g., at railway or bus stations or at information and support points) and the literature on other humanitarian crises (e.g., Turrini et al., 2019) or internally displaced persons in Ukraine after 2014 (Cheung et al., 2019; Roberts et al., 2019) made it clear that mental health support was needed. This was later confirmed by research (Chudzicka-Czupała et al., 2023; Długosz, 2022; Kovács et al., 2023; Ovcharenko, 2024; Predoiu et al., 2024).

In response to these needs, psychological support for refugees from Ukraine in Poland was spontaneously organized and offered at 270 service points, mainly in the form of individual counseling (Mapuj pomoc, 2025). Additionally, EU-funded projects implemented in Poland focused on building the capacity of professionals and of local and national organizations to implement psychological interventions (van der Ven et al., 2025). These projects included workshops and longer training programs designed to strengthen the psychological well-being and mental health of adults and minors (Peace of Mind & Strength of Heart, 2022), as well as distributing the iFightDepression (2025) tool for Ukrainian displaced persons. Mental health support was also offered by international organizations, such as the UNICEF Refugee Response Office in Poland (2025).

The focus on basic psychosocial assistance and professional mental health support in crisis situations has meant that issues related to the use of psychoactive substances by refugees have been relegated to the background. This topic did not attract significant attention from therapists, the media or researchers, either in the first years of the war or later. Available data indicated only rare incidents of alcohol- or drug-related police interventions involving Ukrainians (International Organization for Migration, 2024), and since 2023, the popular media have mentioned alcohol problems among Ukrainian mothers only occasionally (Gmiterek-Zabłocka, 2023a, 2023b). Although some individuals who had started drug therapy in Ukraine sought opportunities to continue it in Poland (Krawczyk, 2022), overall interest in such support was very low. This is evidenced by the closure, in September 2022, of a helpline for people from Ukraine seeking help in connection with the use of psychoactive substances, just a few months after its launch (KCPU, 2022). On the other hand, there is some evidence from other countries pointing to an increase in psychoactive substance consumption since the outbreak of the full-scale war, including among Ukrainian parents (Hyland et al., 2023), women (Reznik et al., 2025) and students (Kurapov et al., 2022). Conversely, the reverse trend was reported among refugees in the Czech Republic (Barták et al., 2023).

Substance use may be one of the "cognitive and behavioral strategies that people use to manage internal and/or external demands in a stressful encounter" (Folkman & Lazarus, 1988: p. 468). The coping strategies applied in reaction to a difficult situation determine resilience, which is the outcome of the process of adapting to difficult or challenging life experiences (Höltge & Ungar, 2022). Task-oriented coping is associated with high resilience, while emotion-oriented coping is associated with low resilience (Campbell-Sills et al., 2006), including in war-affected populations (Al-Krenawi & Bell, 2023; Kovalenko, 2024). However, coping through substance use, considered an emotion-oriented or avoidance strategy (APA Dictionary of Psychology, 2018), may provide short-term relief. For example, binge drinking was associated with less fear of war and high resilience among Ukrainians relocated to Russia (Konstantinov et al., 2023). Repeated use of substances, however, may be detrimental to physical and psychosocial well-being (Magee & Connell, 2021; Wagner et al., 1999), and increase the likelihood of substance use in the future (D'Aquino & Callinan, 2023; Settles et al., 2010). This risk is greater if a person lacks alternative coping strategies (Cooper et al., 1992), which may be the result of socialization from early childhood (Wadsworth, 2015).

One in eight Canadian students reported that they used substances to cope with COVID-19-related changes (Romano et al., 2021) and more than 1 in 2 Polish medical students reported drinking for coping motives (Bryl et al., 2020). Among internally displaced Ukrainians, approximately 4% reported using alcohol or drugs to cope; however, this increased to 27% among those who screened positive for alcohol use disorders (Ramachandran et al., 2019). Only a minority of Ukrainian war refugees in Poland were found to have resorted to sedatives (15%) or alcohol (3%) to cope, mainly employing problem-focused or emotion-focused strategies (Długosz, 2023). This finding is supported by other studies, indicating that substance use in order to cope is rarely reported in surveys (Kovalenko, 2024; Mazhak et al., 2023; Rizzi et al., 2023) and not even mentioned in qualitative studies based on interviews with Ukrainian war refugees (Baran et al., 2024; Chabursky & Walper, 2024; Kölbel, 2023; Oviedo et al., 2022). Furthermore, there is also no mention of substance use in the descriptions of the above-mentioned interventions aimed at supporting the mental health of refugees.

In the Add Strengths (AS) program—developed in the Institute of Mother and Child in cooperation with the Ministry of Health and in partnership with the UNICEF Refugee Response Office in Poland—substance use was not a primary focus. The intervention was designed to support the mental health of Ukrainian parents and caregivers who fled with children to Poland during the first six months following the Russian aggression. A detailed description of the program is provided in "Appendix" and other results of evaluation studies were presented in another text (Okulicz-Kozaryn et al., 2026).

The AS program addresses multiple risk and protective factors that can influence participants' resilience, health, and parenting skills. As a broad intervention, it may therefore lead to multiple outcomes (National Research Council & Institute of Medicine, 2009). The evaluation was designed to assess changes observed in participants after the program in the following areas: health and well-being; coping strategies (active coping, planning, positive reframing, acceptance, humor, religion, emotional support, use of informational support, self-distraction, denial, venting, substance use, behavioral disengagement, self-blame); resilience; and parental attitudes. In this chapter, however, we focus on one specific element of the study—coping through the use of psychoactive substances.

The main objectives were to: (1) evaluate changes in the frequency of coping through substance use among AS program participants in the context of other coping strategies and psychological functioning, including well-being, resilience, and post-traumatic growth; (2) analyze the role of substance use as a coping strategy, in relation to other coping strategies, in predicting resilience, well-being, and post-traumatic growth among Ukrainian war refugees; and (3) determine whether the predictive role of substance use as a coping strategy diminishes following participation in the AS intervention.

6.2 Methods

6.2.1 Setting

The AS program was implemented across Poland in facilities provided by local governments, non-governmental organizations, and in hotels or hostels where Ukrainian refugees were accommodated.

6.2.2 Measures

The studied variables and the instruments used to measure them, along with short descriptions, are presented in Table 6.1. Some scales, such as the Connor–Davidson Resilience Scale (CD-RISC; Shkolina et al., 2020) and WHO-5, were already available in Ukrainian and had recently been used to assess Ukrainians' mental health during wartime (e.g., Asanov et al., 2023; Kovalenko, 2024; Sydorenko et al., 2025). Other items were translated specifically for this study, although prior applications of the PTGI among Ukrainian soldiers have been reported (Kondratiuk & Puchalska-Wasyl, 2020), and the Brief COPE is frequently used to assess the psychological well-being of Ukrainian refugees (e.g., Khailenko & Bacon, 2024; Khan & Altalbe, 2023; Mazhak et al., 2023).

In the pretest, participants also answered basic sociodemographic questions, including age, gender, education, and a description of their current life situation. Specifically, they were asked whether they were parents and/or guardians of children in Poland, the gender and age of the children under their care, whether they had arrived in Poland before or after February 24, 2022, and from which region, as well as their housing, professional, and material situation (both in Ukraine immediately before the war and currently in Poland).

6.2.3 Study Procedure

This study employed a pretest–posttest design. During recruitment (for details on the AS program content and delivery, see "Appendix"), conducted independently by each trainer or with the assistance of representatives of local governments or non-governmental organizations, all participants received written information about the

Table 6.1 Outcome variables and their measurement

Variable	Scale	Description
Well-being	WHO-5 (Topp et al., 2015)	A 5-item scale with a 6-point response format (0 = *never* to 5 = *all the time*) assessing well-being (e.g., relaxation, energy, good mood) during the past two weeks. Scores are obtained by summing responses across items. A total score below 13 indicates risk of depression (Psychiatric Research Unit)[a]
Coping	BRIEF-COPE (Carver, 1997)	A 28-item scale covering 14 coping strategies (2 items each): active coping, planning, positive reframing, acceptance, humor, religion, emotional support, informational support, self-distraction, denial, venting, substance use, behavioral disengagement, and self-blame. Each strategy score is the sum of its two items
Resilience	CD-RISK—Connor–Davidson resilience scale (Campbell-Sills & Stein, 2007)	A unidimensional, 10-item scale measuring resilience. Items are rated from 0 (*not true at all*) to 4 (*true nearly all the time*). The final score is the sum of all items
Post-traumatic Growth	PTGI—Post-traumatic Growth Inventory (Tedeschi & Calhoun, 1996)	A 21-item scale describing positive changes following a traumatic event. Items are rated from 0 (*I did not experience this change*) to 5 (*I experienced this change to a very great degree*). Higher scores indicate greater positive change. Components: (1) Personal strength, (2) Improved relationships, (3) Appreciation of life, (4) Spiritual growth, (5) New possibilities. Component scores are calculated by summing the relevant items

[a] the Psychiatric Research Unit, WHO Collaborating Center for Mental Health, Frederiksborg General Hospital, DK-3400 Hillerød, (https://www.psykiatri-regionh.dk/who-5/Documents/WHO5_Polish.pdf)

program and signed consent forms to participate and complete the surveys. They were also asked to sign a consent form regarding photography during classes and to confirm that they had read the personal data protection procedure. Participants completed an anonymous survey before the first session and after the final session. Depending on the delivery format (one session per week or two sessions per week), the time between pretest and posttest ranged from 5–6 weeks to 10–12 weeks. Respondent anonymity was ensured by marking questionnaires only with a code consisting of a two-digit trainer identifier and a two-digit number assigned to each participant. All materials were provided in Ukrainian. Completing the surveys typically required 30–45 min.

Evaluation data were collected from 53 groups comprising 630 participants (two individuals completed only the posttest survey). In total, 628 participants completed the pretest and 535 completed the posttest questionnaire. Matched pretest–posttest datasets were available for 84.4% of respondents (n = 532) who participated in the pretest.

According to the trainers, the participant attrition was primarily due to illness at the time of the final session, return to Ukraine, or a change in place of residence.

6.2.4 Analysis

In the first step, changes in continuous variables between the pre- and post-intervention assessments—specifically the primary coping strategy (use of psychoactive substances) and psychological outcomes—were analyzed using the Wilcoxon signed-rank test. This nonparametric test compares paired observations without assuming normal distribution of the data, making it suitable for detecting systematic differences between pre- and post-intervention measurements. In addition to test statistics and p-values, effect sizes (r) were calculated for the Wilcoxon signed-rank tests to provide a standardized measure of the observed changes (Cohen, 1988). In the next step, to assess the impact of substance use as a coping strategy in the context of other coping strategies on psychological characteristics, a series of linear regression models was constructed separately for the pre- and post-intervention assessments. All 14 coping strategies were entered simultaneously as predictors, allowing assessment of the unique contribution of each strategy to the psychological outcomes. Separate models were estimated for the two time points to evaluate whether the predictive value of coping strategies differed before and after the intervention. Each model included one psychological variable as the dependent variable and all 14 coping strategies as independent variables. All statistical analyses were conducted using IBM SPSS Statistics for Windows, Version 28.0 (IBM Corp., 2021).

6.3 Results

6.3.1 Participants' Characteristics

The vast majority of participants were women (97.9%) and mothers (89%) who had come to Poland with their children. Nine participants (1.4%) were caring for other children in addition to their own. Caregivers without their own children (e.g., grandmothers) accounted for 4.1% of the sample, and men—fathers—made up 2.1%. The program was also attended by two pregnant women ("future mothers") and 19 participants (3%) who neither had children nor were caring for children.

Approximately half of the participants (53.6%) were aged 35–44 years. Younger individuals (≤34 years) constituted 26.9% of the sample, while older participants (≥45 years) made up 19.4%. Most respondents (65.2%) had a university degree, although 6.3% did not answer this question. In Poland, participants most frequently (43.9%) rented an independent apartment or lived in a hotel, hostel, or refugee shelter (22.5%). Additionally, 11.1% rented an apartment with other Ukrainians, 9.5% rented an independent room, 7.7% lived with a Polish family or friends, and 2.9% lived with Ukrainian friends. Participants reported a significant deterioration in their financial situation after arriving in Poland. On a 5-point scale ranging from 1 (*very good*) to 5 (*very bad*), the mean rating decreased by one full point—from 2.3 (good as the dominant response) to 3.3 (average as the dominant response). This decline was largely associated with housing difficulties as well as changes in professional status. Before arriving in Poland, 41.2% of respondents held permanent employment consistent with their education; in Poland, this rate fell to 9.5%. Unemployment also increased markedly: from 4.9% in Ukraine to 26.3% in Poland.

6.3.2 Changes in Coping Strategy and Psychological Functioning

The use of psychoactive substances was the least frequently reported coping strategy both before and after participation in the AS program.

Prior to the program, nearly 37% of respondents reported using substances at least occasionally; following the intervention, this proportion decreased to 28%. Percentages of respondents reporting the use of each coping strategy at least occasionally, before and after the intervention, are presented in Fig. 6.1.

Further analysis of changes in the frequency of coping strategies, using Wilcoxon signed-rank tests, indicated a significant decrease in the use of substances as a coping strategy. Mean scores declined from $M = 0.71$ ($SD = 1.10$) at pretest to $M = 0.54$ ($SD = 0.99$) at posttest, $Z = -3.08$, $p = .002$, $\Delta = -0.13$ ($SD = 1.07$). Significant reductions were also observed for other negative coping strategies, including denial, behavioral disengagement, and self-blame, while the frequency of positive strategies increased following the intervention. Pre–post-intervention changes in the frequency of use of various coping strategies are presented in Table 6.2, and bar charts (Fig. 6.2) show percentages of respondents who reported less frequent use, no change, or more frequent use of each coping strategy.

Notably, more than 45% of participants reported increased use of positive reframing and emotional support, with similarly high gains for informational support, planning, and active coping. Effect sizes (r) for the Wilcoxon signed-rank tests ranged from.12 to.39. According to Cohen's (1988) guidelines, most changes were of small magnitude, although three strategies—active coping, emotional support, and self-blame—reached the medium range (Table 6.2).

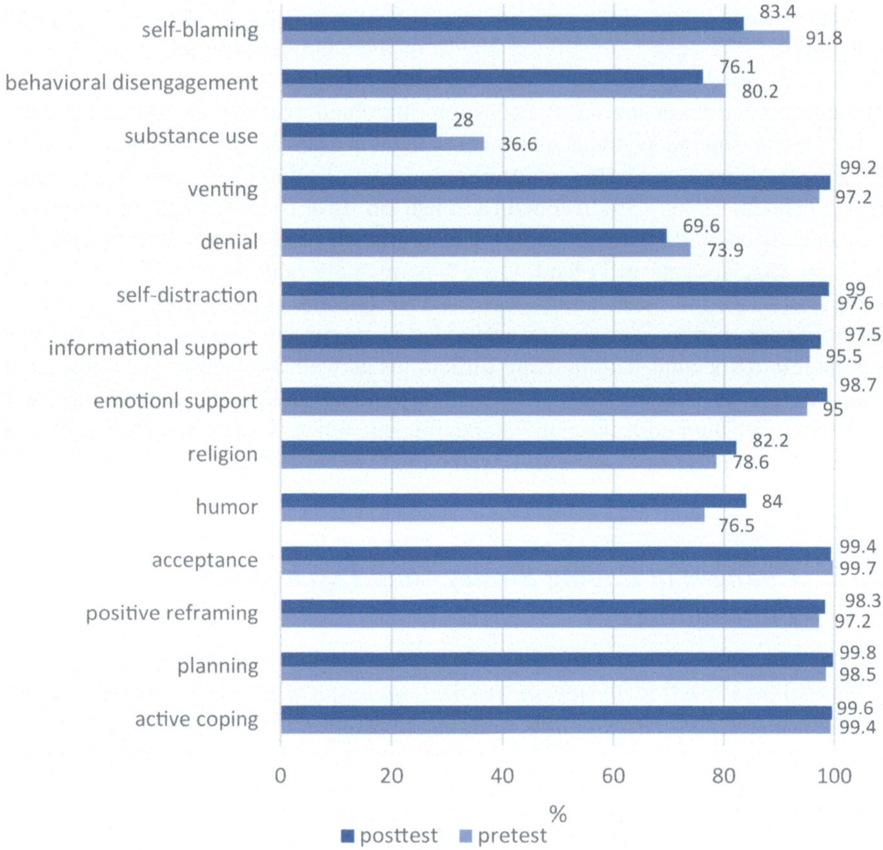

Fig. 6.1 Percentage of respondents reporting the use of each coping strategy at least occasionally, before and after the intervention

Statistically significant changes were observed across all other outcomes (Table 6.3). Psychological well-being, as measured by the WHO-5 index, showed a substantial increase, rising from $M = 10.11$ ($SD = 4.56$) to $M = 15.07$ ($SD = 5.05$), $Z = -16.08$, $p < 0.001$, $\Delta = 5.06$ ($SD = 5.16$). Similarly, participants reported significantly higher levels of resilience post-intervention ($M = 29.06$, $SD = 6.87$) compared to baseline ($M = 25.63$, $SD = 7.56$), $Z = -11.60$, $p < .001$, $\Delta = 3.48$ ($SD = 6.47$). All five domains of post-traumatic growth also improved significantly. Increases were observed in perceived improvement of relationships ($Z = -11.71$, $p < 0.001$, $\Delta = 4.04$, $SD = 6.71$), openness to new possibilities ($Z = -12.06$, $p < .001$, $\Delta = 3.11$, $SD = 5.39$), personal strength ($Z = -11.76$, $p < 0.001$, $\Delta = 2.46$, $SD = 4.33$), spiritual change ($Z = -7.60$, $p < .001$, $\Delta = 0.79$, $SD = 2.27$), and appreciation for life ($Z = -8.60$, $p < .001$, $\Delta = 1.06$, $SD = 2.65$). Taken together, these results suggest that the intervention was associated with a reduction in maladaptive

Table 6.2 Pre–post-intervention changes in the frequency of use of coping strategies

Coping strategy	*N*	*M (SD)* Pretest	*M (SD)* Posttest	Δ*M (SD)*	*Z*	*r*	*p*
Substance use	507	0.71 (1.10)	0.54 (0.99)	−0.13 (1.07)	−3.08	−0.14**	= 0.002
Active coping	516	4.30 (1.24)	4.69 (1.07)	0.39 (1.24)	6.90	0.30***	< 0.001
Planning	517	4.0 (1.36)	4.41 (1.30)	0.42 (1.37)	6.62	0.29**	< 0.001
Positive reframing	517	3.5 (1.43)	3.91 (1.48)	0.42 (1.55)	5.86	0.26**	< 0.001
Acceptance	514	3.96 (1.29)	4.12 (1.29)	0.18 (1.34)	2.82	0.12**	= 0.005
Humor	505	1.70 (1.41)	2.10 (1.45)	0.38 (1.41)	5.84	0.26**	< 0.001
Religion	513	2.26 (1.81)	2.46 (1.82)	0.25 (1.27)	4.33	0.19**	< 0.001
Emotional support	518	3.27 (1.50)	3.84 (1.40)	0.59 (1.46)	8.38	0.37***	< 0.001
Informational support	511	3.17 (1.45)	3.56 (1.40)	0.40 (1.43)	5.77	0.26**	< 0.001
Self-distraction	518	3.75 (1.36)	3.95 (1.31)	0.19 (1.43)	2.66	0.12**	= 0.008
Denial	490	1.81 (1.56)	1.52 (1.37)	−0.24 (1.56)	−3.05	−0.14**	= 0.002
Venting	504	2.97 (1.21)	3.17 (1.21)	0.21 (1.35)	3.49	0.16**	< 0.001
Behavioral disengagement	501	1.79 (1.29)	1.59 (1.24)	−0.19 (1.47)	−3.11	−0.14**	= 0.002
Self-blaming	514	2.94 (1.64)	2.21 (1.50)	−0.71 (1.63)	−8.85	−0.39***	< 0.001

Effect size thresholds: *$0.10 < r \leq 0.30$—small effect; ***$0.30 < r \leq 0.50$—medium effect

coping, improvements in positive coping and multiple dimensions of psychological well-being, resilience, and post-traumatic growth.

Most participants showed improvement across all psychological measures, as illustrated in Fig. 6.3, showing the percentage of respondents who reported that selected psychological outcomes improved, showed no change, or worsened in time.

Specifically, 83.5% reported improvements in well-being, and 69.9% in resilience. Across post-traumatic growth dimensions, between 60.7% and 75.4% of participants experienced positive changes. In contrast, only 19.3% of participants reduced their use of substances as a coping strategy, while 70.4% reported no change and 10.3% indicated an increase. Although the proportion of improvement in substance-related coping was smaller, the high stability likely reflects low baseline scores. These results suggest that while psychological functioning generally improved for most participants, changes in avoidance coping (substance use) were more modest and concentrated among a smaller subgroup.

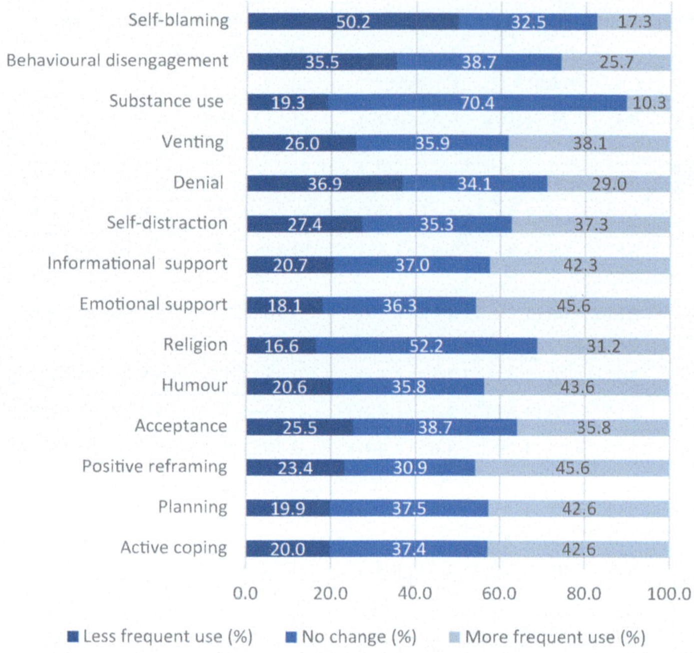

Fig. 6.2 Distribution of change in coping strategies

Table 6.3 Pre–post-intervention changes in psychological outcomes

Variable	*N*	*M (SD)* Pretest	*M (SD)* Posttest	*ΔM (SD)*	*Z*	*p*
Well-being (WHO-5)	496	10.11 (4.56)	15.07 (5.05)	5.06 (5.16)	−16.08	< .001
Resilience (CD-Risk)	495	25.63 (7.56)	29.06 (6.87)	3.48 (6.47)	−11.6	< .001
PTGI—Improved relationships	480	21.95 (6.97)	25.89 (6.08)	4.04 (6.71)	−11.71	< .001
PTGI—New possibilities	494	14.78 (5.74)	17.81 (4.97)	3.11 (5.39)	−12.06	< .001
PTGI—Personal strength	485	12.80 (4.70)	15.29 (3.72)	2.46 (4.33)	−11.76	< .001
PTGI—Spiritual growth	501	4.98 (2.68)	5.78 (2.43)	0.79 (2.27)	−7.6	< .001
PTGI—Appreciation for life	506	11.50 (3.15)	12.42 (2.48)	1.06 (2.65)	−8.6	< .001

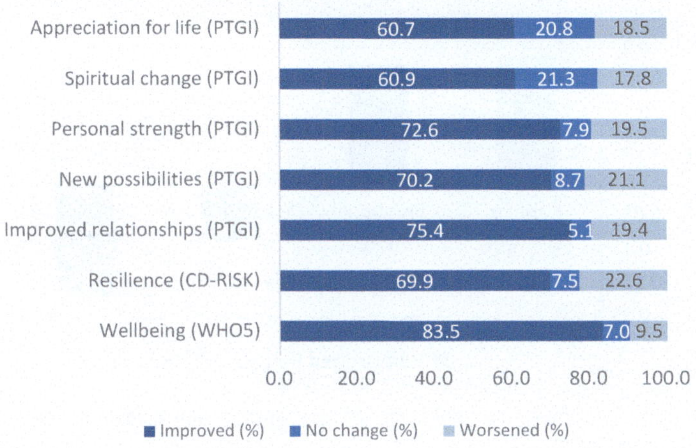

Fig. 6.3 Distribution of change psychological outcomes

6.3.3 Substance Use Coping Strategy Among Predictors of Psychological Outcomes

Multiple linear regression analyses were conducted to examine the predictive value of fourteen coping strategies, including use of psychoactive substances, on psychological outcomes measured before and after the intervention. A significant effect of substance use as a coping strategy emerged only in two pre-intervention models predicting *personal strength* and *appreciation for life*. Figure 6.4 illustrates that substance use is one of the significant coping strategies influencing post-traumatic growth in terms of personal strength. This model was statistically significant, $F(14, 474) = 8.18$, $p < 0.001$, with an adjusted $R^2 = 0.171$, indicating that approximately 17.1% of the variance in personal strength was explained by the coping strategies. Among the predictors, four were statistically significant: positive reframing: $\beta = 0.19$, $p < 0.001$; emotional support: $\beta = 0.18$, $p = 0.001$; substance use: $\beta = -0.09$, $p = 0.046$; behavioral disengagement: $\beta = -0.17$, $p < 0.001$. Notably, substance use strategy emerged as a significant negative predictor, suggesting that individuals who used psychoactive substances to cope reported higher levels of distress.

Figure 6.5 presents standardized beta coefficients for coping strategies significantly associated with appreciation for life after trauma. This model was also statistically significant, $F(14, 487) = 5.24$, $p < .001$, with an adjusted $R^2 = .106$. Six predictors reached statistical significance: positive reframing: $\beta = 0.13$, $p = 0.018$; religious practices: $\beta = 0.12$, $p = 0.009$; emotional support: $\beta = 0.14$, $p = 0.014$; denial: $\beta = 0.10$, $p = 0.03$; substance use: $\beta = -0.09$, $p = 0.048$; behavioral disengagement: $\beta = -0.10$, $p = 0.050$. This model is presented separately because appreciation for life represents a conceptually distinct domain of post-traumatic growth and revealed a unique set of predictors compared to other outcomes. Again, substance use

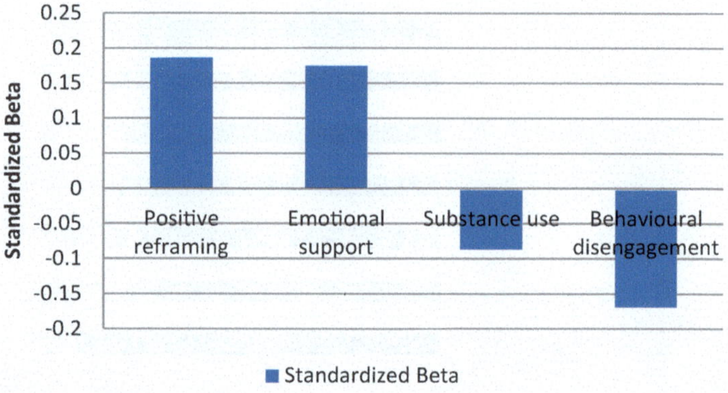

Fig. 6.4 Substance use among the significant coping strategies influencing post-traumatic growth in terms of personal strength

was a significant negative predictor, indicating an association between this strategy and lower levels of appreciation for life.

In all other regression models estimated for the remaining psychological outcomes, the substance use coping strategy did not reach statistical significance. Furthermore, in the post-intervention regression models, the previously observed associations between substance use and these two outcomes were no longer statistically significant. This suggests a potential reduction in the maladaptive impact of substance use following the intervention.

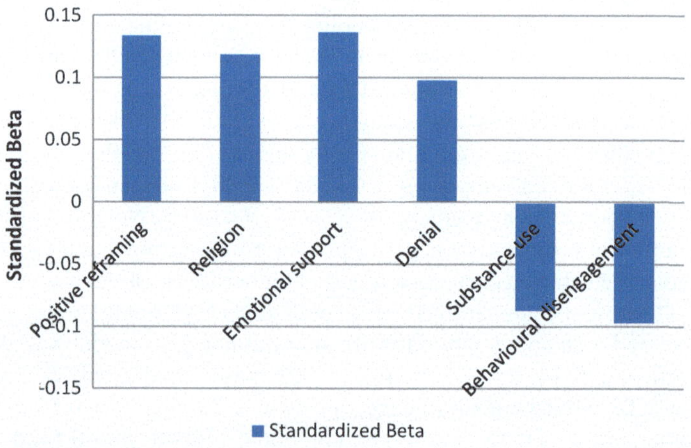

Fig. 6.5 Substance use among the significant coping strategies influencing post-traumatic growth in terms of appreciation for life

6.4 Summary and Discussion

This study demonstrates the positive effects of a psychosocial intervention on the psychological functioning of Ukrainian war refugees. Statistically significant improvements were observed across all measured outcomes, including well-being, resilience, the five domains of post-traumatic growth, increased use of adaptive coping strategies, and decreased use of maladaptive coping strategies, including substance use. These positive effects are comparable to the results of other programs supporting the mental health of Ukrainian refugees (Hillis et al., 2024; Poudel-Tandukar et al., 2024). However, to our knowledge, no previous studies have specifically evaluated the impact of interventions on coping through psychoactive substance use in this population.

In our study, the frequency of substance use as a coping strategy was much lower than that of other coping strategies. Nevertheless, the proportion of respondents reporting its use at least occasionally (37% at pretest and 28% at posttest) was considerably higher than reported in other studies among internally or externally displaced Ukrainians (Długosz, 2023; Kovalenko, 2024; Mazhak et al., 2023; Ramachandran et al., 2019; Rizzi et al., 2023). Indeed, it was even higher than the percentage noted among internally displaced Ukrainians with alcohol use disorders (Ramachandran et al., 2019).

It can be hypothesized that reporting of substance use (both in general and as a coping strategy) is often underestimated due to the tendency to present oneself in a socially desirable manner (Vergés, 2022). The fear of judgment, discrimination, or the creation of records that could reduce chances of securing employment or social support may pose significant barriers to openness in survey responses (ITTC Ukraine, 2022). Service providers have also reported fears among refugees regarding potential legal consequences (e.g., deportation, loss of child custody, difficulties securing employment, or social isolation), a lack of trust in mental health professionals, and reluctance to seek help, which may foster reliance on maladaptive coping mechanisms (Purgato et al., 2024). In this context, the relatively high rates of coping-related substance use reported in our study may indicate the trust that respondents placed in the project team. This trust was largely attributable to the AS trainers, who were not only professionals but also refugees from Ukraine themselves, and thus perceived by participants as "one of us." Their shared experience fostered a strong sense of credibility and rapport with participants.

It is possible that the relatively high rates of coping through substance use observed in this study were also influenced by the fact that only two questions in the otherwise quite extensive questionnaire referred to psychoactive substances. Respondents may therefore have been aware that disclosing problematic behaviors was not the main focus of the study.

Regression analyses did not reveal significant relationships between coping through substance use and participants' resilience or well-being. However, this coping strategy, together with behavioral disengagement, emerged as a significant negative predictor of post-traumatic growth, specifically in the domains of personal strength and appreciation of life. These findings underscore the psychological costs of avoidance coping and highlight the importance of addressing such behaviors in mental health support interventions for displaced populations.

By contrast, the use of emotional support and positive reframing was found to be significant positive predictors of personal strength and appreciation of life after traumatic experiences. These strategies are widely recognized as adaptive responses to stress and trauma (e.g., Aldao et al., 2010; Munroe et al., 2022). More surprising were the positive relationships between post-traumatic appreciation of life and coping through religion and denial. Their beneficial influence may be explained by Bonanno's (2021) argument that the effectiveness of any coping strategy depends heavily on its fit with situational demands, as well as by the possibility that cultural background shapes the perceived adaptiveness of particular strategies (Rizzi et al., 2023).

Importantly, the predictive role of substance use was no longer significant in the post-intervention models, suggesting a reduction in its psychological burden and a potential mechanism of change initiated by the intervention. Although the AS program does not directly address issues related to the use of psychoactive substances, the overall improvement in participants' well-being and mental health resulted in a reduction in the use of this and other avoidance coping strategies. Strengthening participants' ability to adopt positive coping strategies as alternatives to substance use also contributed to the program's success (Cooper et al., 1992).

This study has several limitations, most of which are typical of research conducted in emergency situations. These include the lack of time to await the results of in-depth needs assessments, the allocation of financial resources primarily to interventions intended to reach as many individuals in need as possible rather than to research (Strouse & Moore, 2019), and the instability of the target population, who were frequently on the move in search of new housing (Clark-Kazak, 2021; Gargano et al., 2022). Consequently, it was not possible to randomize participants or recruit a control group. Relocation also contributed to participant dropout, with many individuals replaced by newcomers who joined the program after it had already begun. For the same reasons, long-term effects could not be measured, and within a few months we lost contact with most of the program participants.

Moreover, all posttest assessments were conducted immediately after the end of the intervention program. As such, the pre–post-interval corresponded to the program duration in each group and ranged from 5 to 12 weeks.

The very short planning period and the pressure to launch activities quickly affected the preparation of measurement tools (e.g., proper back-translation was not conducted) and meant that bioethics committee approval was obtained post hoc, reflecting common challenges in the timely review of emergency research protocols (Hunt et al., 2016). Another limitation is the absence of questionnaire items that would allow for a more detailed assessment of behaviors related to psychoactive substance use. However, as noted above, restricting the scope of inquiry may have encouraged greater openness among respondents.

It should also be acknowledged that, to our knowledge, the measurement tools used in this study had not been validated specifically for Ukrainian refugees. Only recently has the validity of the WHO-5 for this population been confirmed (Kurapov et al., 2025). Furthermore, the Brief COPE substance use subscale does not differentiate between types or severity of use, and we did not collect such sensitive data given the refugee context. Finally, the strong gender imbalance (97.9% women) and the use of age categories rather than continuous age further limited the possibility of conducting subgroup analyses.

Despite these limitations, the findings of this study support a number of practical conclusions regarding mental health support, including the reduction of substance use among refugees:

1. Refugees' needs for psychosocial support are enormous; therefore, well-designed interventions can be expected to have significant positive outcomes.
2. Despite the objective difficulties associated with conducting evaluation studies in an emergency context, analyzing the effects of interventions is worthwhile, to better understand their mechanisms and develop the most efficient methods.
3. Besides the program itself, a factor that enhances the effectiveness of an intervention is the credibility and trustworthiness of its providers; in our case, the trainers were professionals in the field of psychology/psychotherapy and refugees themselves, which increased participants' trust.
4. An effective strategy for recruiting parents (who are not always willing to admit that they need psychological support) is to emphasize that by taking care of their own mental health, they can better support their children in coping with stress and difficulties.
5. Substance use is an extremely sensitive issue, especially among people struggling to navigate a new life situation. Interventions aimed directly at reducing substance use may be rejected by refugees. However, generally strengthening coping skills and resilience can also lead to positive changes in substance use.
6. Improving refugees' mental health is only one element of the support they need to adapt to their new environment. However, resilience and social contacts (also established through intervention) likely help them address challenges related to finding employment, healthcare, organizing children's education, etc.

6.5 Conclusions

This study provides preliminary evidence for the effectiveness of a psychosocial intervention in supporting the mental health of Ukrainian war refugees. Statistically significant improvements were observed across all measured outcomes, including well-being, resilience, post-traumatic growth, and coping.

Although coping through substance use was the least frequently reported strategy, a significant post-intervention reduction in its use was nevertheless observed. The significant negative relationship between this coping strategy and post-traumatic growth in the areas of personal strength and appreciation of life underscores the importance of addressing substance use within mental health support interventions.

At the same time, it must be remembered that these are highly sensitive topics that require a foundation of trust and a safe relationship with the target group.

The added value of this study is better understanding of the mechanisms of change that can underlie mental health support interventions, specifically on substance use as a coping strategy.

Acknowledgements This work was supported by the UNICEF Crisis Response Office in Poland (OPK 512-20-01).

Ethics Approval Study approval statement: The study protocol was reviewed and approved by the Ethical Committee of the Institute of Mother and Child (Resolution No. 5/2024 of 23/03/2024). Consent to participate statement: Written informed consent was obtained from all participants.

Competing Interests The authors declare that they have no competing interests.

Appendix The "Add Strength" Mental Health Support Program

Background

Under an agreement with the UNICEF Refugee Response Office in Poland (opened in March 2022), the Ministry of Health designated the Institute of Mother and Child (IMC) to support the mental health of Ukrainian children and their parents and caregivers, helping them recover from the Russian aggression of February 24, 2022. One of IMC's tasks was to develop and implement a mental health support program for parents and caregivers who fled with children to Poland in the first six months after the aggression.

The first step in program planning was an assessment of the needs of the target population. Focus group interviews (FGIs), conducted with four groups of Ukrainian parents ($n = 23$, including one father) who came to Poland with their children after the outbreak of the war, indicated significant deterioration of mental health, marked by flashbacks, feelings of temporariness, detachment from reality, living in limbo, uncertainty, sadness, loneliness, exhaustion, mourning, guilt, and broken or strained relationships with family members. The only positive emotion, although rarely expressed, was hope for the end of the war. Identified coping factors included child-centeredness, spending more time with children, establishing routines, involvement in work, helping others, pursuing hobbies, a sense of being "among one's own," thinking about the future, and self-medication (Ukraińskie matki, 2022).

The key conclusion from the FGIs was that without improvement in their own well-being, parents and caregivers would not be able to support their children in facing adversity and difficulties. Therefore, the concept of resilience (Fleming & Ledogar, 2008; Masten, 2007; Rutter, 1987) was applied as the general theoretical framework for the program. Especially important for the target population were strengthening a sense of hope (Panter-Brick et al., 2015), the ability to use available resources (Panter-Brick & Leckman, 2013), and the appropriateness of parental/guardian responses to children's needs (Kim-Cohen & Turkewitz, 2012).

A second theoretical framework for the program was Cognitive Therapy (Alford & Beck, 1997). Work on recognizing core negative beliefs (considered thinking distortions), reformulating them into more positive ones to build a greater sense of self-efficacy (Morley & Moran, 2011; Osmo et al., 2018), and learning to calm the mind and relax the body using relaxation techniques (Kabat-Zinn, 2016) was incorporated.

The components regarding parent–child relationships and parenting practices were based on the School for Parents and Educators program, which has been implemented in Poland for over 20 years (Sakowska, 2008; Sakowska & Puchała, 2008). This program is grounded in the systemic approach to the family, the psychology of interpersonal communication (De Barbaro, 1999), and Gordon's (1970) Parent Effectiveness Training (PET).

Due to the strong need to be "among one's own" and the excessive time spent on the Internet, clearly expressed in the FGIs, it was decided to deliver the program in the form of on-site workshops.

Content

The intervention program was developed in cooperation with Ukrainian psychologists. It aims to: (1) enhance parents' resilience and mental health and (2) develop parental competencies to support children's mental health and resilience in the face of adversity (Okulicz–Kozaryn et al., 2022). AS consists of 10, 2-h scenarios to be implemented with groups of 10–15 parents/caregivers. The topics and core activities of the meetings are presented in the Table 6.4.

Trainers and Their Training

The recruitment criteria for program trainers/facilitators included a background in psychology or education, fluency in the Ukrainian language, prior experience in conducting workshops, and willingness to participate in a five-day training (two days online and three days on-site, free of charge) and to conduct a full cycle of 10 sessions with at least one group of 10–15 parents. Remuneration was provided for recruiting parents, organizing training venues, conducting sessions, collecting evaluation data, and completing worksheets to monitor activities.

In accordance with the agreement between IMC and UNICEF, training was originally planned for 30 individuals. Following a bilingual (Polish–Ukrainian) announcement on the IMC social media page, shared in Facebook groups focused on Ukrainian refugee support and psychology, 619 applications were received within five days. This made it possible to select 41 candidates— evenly distributed across Poland,

Table 6.4 Add Strengths sessions and content descriptions

No.	Title	Content	Core activities/messages
1	My frontline	Finding strength in the context of experiencing the effects of war and forced migration, learning mechanisms for effective dealing with serious difficulties	Welcome and introduction; Discussion of group norms; Participant's self-introductions (with projection cards); List of expectations for the AS program; Introduction to resilience; "My Frontline" exercise—reflection on one's role as a person and parent in the context of war and refugeeism; "My Battery" exercise—our strengths and resources; Relaxation
2	Strong parent/ caregiver	Strengthening parents' mental health so that they can best support their children	Introduction—joy and self-care during the war, resilient parent as a key resource of children's mental health; "Sensory Awareness" exercise—things/activities that bring us pleasure; "What I Think of Myself"—positive and negative core beliefs; "A Perspective of Hope"—to foster optimism and finding positives
3	Listening	The ability to listen and respond to what we hear in order to support the person speaking to us	Relaxation; "Listening Barriers"—messages that give us a feeling of being or not being listened to; "Listening Button"—importance of the willingness to listen; How to talk with children about the war and other difficult topics
4	Feelings	Recognizing feelings and dealing with them, developing skills needed to accept children's emotions	Relaxation; "Storm of Emotions"—recognizing and naming the feeling; "Anger Circle"—the consequences of suppressing difficult emotions; "Feelings–Thoughts–Body"—to understand their interrelationships; Self-regulation
5	Communication	How to talk so that children will listen and how to listen so that they will talk	Three levels of communication (factual, instrumental, affective); "Facts and Opinions/Opinions and Feeling"—distinguishing facts from opinions and opinions from feelings; Effective communication in the conflict situation (Feeling–Fact–Future formula)

(continued)

Table 6.4 (continued)

No.	Title	Content	Core activities/messages
6	Goals and rules	Setting goals as an element of positive thinking and principles that bring peace and order to an uncertain world	"Changed Situation—Changed Goals"—Importance of getting out from the state of limbo and goals setting; "Our Goals and Goals of Our Children"—internal and external factors that help or hinder their achievement; "Organizing the World"—rules as a factors enhancing a sense of security and how to introduce them; "Daily Routine"—to bring structure and predictability into daily lives
7	Cooperation and consequences	Encouraging the child to cooperate by giving consequences rather than punishing	Relaxation; Discussion about the values that we raise our children for and the traditional methods of enforcing child obedience; Understanding of children's feelings and reactions to the punishment; Parent–Child Collaboration—A New Approach to Discipline; Encouraging Cooperation
8	Conflict solving	5-step method of constructive conflict resolution and how to help children to solve the problems between themselves	Relaxation; Conflict as an opportunity to recognize one's own needs and those of the other person and agree on an acceptable way to meet them; Collaborative approach to problem-solving in conflict situations; Resolving conflicts between children
9	Praises and roles	Strengthening the child's sense of self-esteem and agency by constructive feedback and understanding the impact of the roles we assume on relationships with other people	"Art lesson" exercise to understand the difference between unconstructive praise and positive feedback; Inspiring and motivating children to act and learn; "Six Hats" exercise demonstrating stifling life attitudes and how to step out of roles to enhance self-development and wellbeing
10	Wrap-up	Enhancing awareness of one's own resources in upbringing a child, the sense of agency and self-esteem and knowing where and how to get support and help	Relaxation—"Chocolate Meditation"; "My Persona Resources"—resilience-supporting tools developed during the AS program and how to use these tools to support a child; External Resources—sharing the information on the available support; Reviewing the group's expectations written at the first meeting; Feedback from participants to participants

highly qualified, and themselves war refugees. Training of trainers was conducted in September 2022 by Ukrainian trainers of the School for Parents and Educators program, co-authors of the Add Strength program.

Program Delivery

From October 2022 to January 2023, 41 trainers implemented the AS program with 59 groups of participants ($n = 690$) across Poland. The average number of registered individuals in each group was approximately 12. The average attendance at individual sessions remained at a similar level throughout the program (approximately 10 people per group). The trainers decided when and in what mode (10 sessions × 1 scenario or 5 sessions × 2 scenarios) they would work (the second option was more popular, applied in 45 groups). Their decisions were based mainly on practical reasons: assessment of the needs and capabilities of the participants or the availability of the premises where they worked. Some trainers conducted classes with one group, and others with two or three groups.

The information collected from trainers regarding the process of implementing the program indicated a high level of satisfaction with the sessions and a sense of achieving the program's goals. In their opinion, participants were satisfied with the program and highly involved in all elements of the sessions. Feedback from the participants collected at the end of the program confirmed the observations of the trainers. Participants especially appreciated the efforts of the trainers, the opportunity to establish relationships with other people in the group through the practical applications offered through the sessions, and new, beneficial information and specific algorithms on how to improve their relationships with their children. The main criticism expressed was related to the fact that the program was too short and there was a need for its continuation.

References

Aldao, A., Nolen-Hoeksema, S., & Schweizer, S. (2010). Emotion-regulation strategies across psychopathology: A meta-analytic review. *Clinical Psychology Review, 30*(2), 217–237. https://doi.org/10.1016/j.cpr.2009.11.004

Alford, B. A., & Beck, A. T. (1997). *The integrative power of cognitive therapy*. Guilford Press. Polish edition: Alford, B. A., & Beck, A. T. (2005). *Terapia poznawcza jako terapia integrująca psychoterapię*. Wydawnictwo Uniwersytetu Jagiellońskiego.

Al-Krenawi, A., & Bell, M. M. (2023). Gender differences in Syrian refugees in Jordan: Psychological, self-esteem, family function, marital satisfaction, and life satisfaction. *International Journal of Social Psychiatry, 69*(3), 714–723.

American Psychological Association. (2018, April 19). Avoidance coping. In *APA dictionary of psychology*. https://dictionary.apa.org/avoidance-coping

Asanov, A. M., Asanov, I., & Buenstorf, G. (2023). Mental health and stress level of Ukrainians seeking psychological help online. *Heliyon, 9*, Article e21933. https://doi.org/10.1016/j.heliyon.2023.e21933

Baran, M., Grzymała-Moszczyńska, H., Zjawińska, M., Sugay, L., Pujszo, I., Ovsiienko, Y., Naritsa, V., Niedziałek, J., & Boczkowska, M. (2024). Superhero in a skirt: Psychological resilience of Ukrainian refugee women in Poland. A thematic analysis. *International Journal of Clinical and Health Psychology, 24*(4), Article 100506. https://doi.org/10.1016/j.ijchp.2024.100506

Barták, M., Petruželka, B., Ponomarenko, M., Shuranova, L., & Rogalewicz, V. (2023). Characteristics of alcohol use among migrants from Ukraine to the Czech Republic in the context of the war in Ukraine in 2022. *Kontakt, 25*(2), 124–130. https://doi.org/10.32725/kont.2023.019

Bonanno, G. A. (2021). The resilience paradox. *European Journal of Psychotraumatology, 12*(1), 1942642. https://doi.org/10.1080/20008198.2021.1942642

Bryl, N., Czarnecka-Iwańczuk, M., Romanowska, M., Stanisić, M. G., Michalak, M., & Posadzy-Małaczyńska, A. (2020). Drinking alcohol as a way of coping with stress in students of medical faculties. *Psychiatria Polska, 54*(2), 265–277. https://doi.org/10.12740/PP/99029 (in both English and Polish)

Campbell-Sills, L., Cohan, S. L., & Stein, M. B. (2006). Relationship of resilience to personality, coping, and psychiatric symptoms in young adults. *Behaviour Research and Therapy, 44*(4), 585–599. https://doi.org/10.1016/j.brat.2005.05.001

Campbell-Sills, L., & Stein, M. B. (2007). Psychometric analysis and refinement of the Connor-Davidson resilience scale (CD-RISC): Validation of a 10-item measure of resilience. *Journal of Traumatic Stress, 20*(6), 1019–1028. https://doi.org/10.1002/jts.20271

Carver, C. S. (1997). You want to measure coping but your protocol's too long: Consider the brief COPE. *International Journal of Behavioral Medicine, 4*(1), 92–100.

Chabursky, S., & Walper, S. (2024). Exploring coping strategies among Ukrainian refugee adolescents. *Kindheit und Entwicklung, 33*(4), 236–245. https://doi.org/10.1026/0942-5403/a000462

Cheung, A., Makhashvili, N., Javakhishvili, J., Karachevsky, A., Kharchenko, N., Shpiker, M., & Roberts, B. (2019). Patterns of somatic distress among internally displaced persons in Ukraine: Analysis of a cross-sectional survey. *Social Psychiatry and Psychiatric Epidemiology, 54*(10), 1265–1274. https://doi.org/10.1007/s00127-019-01652-7

Chudzicka-Czupała, A., Hapon, N., Chiang, S. K., et al. (2023). Depression, anxiety and post-traumatic stress during the 2022 Russo-Ukrainian war, a comparison between populations in Poland, Ukraine, and Taiwan. *Scientific Reports, 13*, 3602. https://doi.org/10.1038/s41598-023-28729-3

Clark-Kazak, C. (2021). Ethics in forced migration research: Taking stock and potential ways forward. *Journal on Migration and Human Security, 9*(3), 125–138. https://doi.org/10.1177/23315024211034401

Cohen, J. (1988). *Statistical power analysis for the behavioral sciences* (2nd ed.). Lawrence Erlbaum Associates.

Cooper, M. L., Russell, M., Skinner, J. B., Frone, M. R., & Mudar, P. (1992). Stress and alcohol use: Moderating effects of gender, coping, and alcohol expectancies. *Journal of Abnormal Psychology, 101*(1), 139–152. https://doi.org/10.1037/0021-843x.101.1.139

D'Aquino, S., & Callinan, S. (2023). Drinking to cope as a mediator of the relationship between stress and alcohol outcomes. *Drugs: Education, Prevention and Policy, 31*(5), 516–523. https://doi.org/10.1080/09687637.2023.2236291

De Barbaro, B. (Ed.). (1999). *Wprowadzenie do systemowego rozumienia rodziny* [Introduction to the systemic understanding of the family]. Wydawnictwo Uniwersytetu Jagiellońskiego. (in Polish)

Difference Co. (2022). *Ukraińskie matki: Jak odnalazły się w nowej (polskiej) rzeczywistości?* [Ukrainian mothers: How have they gained their bearings in the new (Polish) reality?] [Unpublished report in Polish].

Długosz, P. (2022). Trauma wojenna ukraińskich uchodźców przebywających w Polsce [War trauma of Ukrainian refugees residing in Poland]. *Studia Polityczne, 50*(4), 15–44. (in Polish).
Długosz, P. (2023). War trauma and strategies for coping with stress among Ukrainian refugees staying in Poland. *Journal of Migration and Health, 8*, Article 100196. https://doi.org/10.1016/j.jmh.2023.100196
Fleming, J., & Ledogar, R. J. (2008). Resilience, an evolving concept: A review of literature relevant to Aboriginal research. *Pimatisiwin, 6*(2), 7–23. PMID: 20963184; PMCID: PMC2956753
Folkman, S., & Lazarus, R. S. (1988). Coping as a mediator of emotion. *Journal of Personality and Social Psychology, 54*(3), 466–475.
Gargano, M. C., Ajduković, D., & Vukčević Marković, M. (2022). Mental health in the transit context: Evidence from 10 countries. *International Journal of Environmental Research and Public Health, 19*(6), 3476. https://doi.org/10.3390/ijerph19063476
Gmiterek-Zabłocka, A. (2023a, February 23). Alkohol i przemoc w rodzinach uchodźczych [Alcohol and violence in refugee families]. *Tokfm*. https://www.tokfm.pl/Tokfm/7,189654,29494933,ukrainskie-dzieci-odbierane-rodzicom-sa-takie-przypadki-bo.html (in Polish)
Gmiterek-Zabłocka, A. (2023b, May 22). Alkohol i przemoc [Alcohol and violence]. *Tokfm*. https://www.tokfm.pl/Tokfm/7,189654,29785124,mamy-problem-z-przemoca-i-alkoholem-w-ukrainskich-rodzinach.html (in Polish)
Gordon, T. (1970). *Parent effectiveness training: The "no-lose" program for raising responsible children*. Peter H. Wyden. Polish edition: Gordon, T. (2002). *Wychowanie bez porażek*. Instytut Wydawniczy Pax.
Hillis, S., Tucker, S., Baldonado, N., Taradaika, E., Bryn, L., Kharchenko, S., Machabelii, T., Taylor, R., Green, P., Goldman, P., Awah, I., Baldonado, J., Gomez, P., Flaxman, S., Ratmann, O., Lachman, J. M., Villaveces, A., Sherr, L., & Cluver, L. (2024). The effectiveness of Hope Groups, a mental health, parenting support, and violence prevention program for families affected by the war in Ukraine: Findings from a pre-post study. *Journal of Migration and Health, 10*, Article 100251. https://doi.org/10.1016/j.jmh.2024.100251
Höltge, J., & Ungar, M. (2022). Quantifying resilience as an outcome: Advancing the residual approach with influence statistics to derive more adequate thresholds of resilience. *Advances in Resilience Science, 3*, 381–390. https://doi.org/10.1007/s42844-022-00078-6
Hunt, M., Tansey, C. M., Anderson, J., Boulanger, R. F., Eckenwiler, L., Pringle, J., & Schwartz, L. (2016). The challenge of timely, responsive and rigorous ethics review of disaster research: Views of research ethics committee members. *PLoS ONE, 11*(6), Article e0157142. https://doi.org/10.1371/journal.pone.0157142
Hyland, P., Vallières, F., Shevlin, M., Karatzias, T., Ben-Ezra, M., McElroy, E., Vang, M. L., Lorberg, B., & Martsenkovskyi, D. (2023). Psychological consequences of war in Ukraine: Assessing changes in mental health among Ukrainian parents. *Psychological Medicine, 53*(15), 7466–7468. https://doi.org/10.1017/S0033291723000818
iFightDepression. (2025). Retrieved May 27, 2025, from https://ifightdepression.com
International Organization for Migration. (2024, January 26). *DTM uchodźcy z Ukrainy i Polska Straż Miejska: Badanie postrzegania, wyzwań i możliwości wzmocnienia relacji*. IOM. https://dtm.iom.int/es/node/34596?close=true
ITTC Ukraine. (2022). *Desk review: Support for people with substance use disorder in Ukraine during the war*. Institute of Psychiatry of the Taras Shevchenko National University of Kyiv.
Kabat-Zinn, J. (2016). *Mindfulness for beginners: Reclaiming the present moment and your life*. Sounds True Inc. [Polish edition: Kabat-Zinn, J. (2021). *Praktyka uważności dla początkujących*. Wydawnictwo Czarna Owca.]
KCPU. (2022, September 30). Krajowe Centrum Przeciwdziałania Uzależnieniom podjęło decyzję o zakończeniu działalności Telefonu Zaufania dla Osób z Ukrainy [The National Centre for Counteracting Addictions decided to close the Helpline for People from Ukraine]. https://kcpu.gov.pl/krajowe-centrum-przeciwdzialania-uzaleznieniom-podjelo-decyzje-o-zakonczeniu-dzialalnosci-telefonu-zaufania-dla-osob-z-ukrainy-z-dniem-30-wrzesnia-2022-r/ (in Polish)

Khailenko, O., & Bacon, A. M. (2024). Resilience, avoidant coping and post-traumatic stress symptoms among female Ukrainian refugees and internally displaced people. *International Journal of Social Psychiatry, 70*(6), 1164–1174. https://doi.org/10.1177/00207640241264662

Khan, A. R., & Altalbe, A. (2023). Potential impacts of the Russo-Ukraine conflict and its psychological consequences among Ukrainian adults: The post-COVID-19 era. *Frontiers in Public Health, 11*, 1280423. https://doi.org/10.3389/fpubh.2023.1280423

Kim-Cohen, J., & Turkewitz, R. (2012). Resilience and measured environment interactions. *Development and Psychopathology, 24*, 1297–1306.

Konstantinov, V., Reznik, A., & Isralowitz, R. (2023). Depression and quality of life among Ukrainian adults relocated to Russia. *Journal of Loss and Trauma, 28*(6), 493–503. https://doi.org/10.1080/15325024.2023.2216986

Kölbel, M. (2023). Ukrainian diaspora: A journey of traumatization, resilience and hope. *Advances in Social Sciences Research Journal, 10*(11), 251–266. https://doi.org/10.14738/assrj.1011.15901

Kondratiuk, V., & Puchalska-Wasyl, M. (2020). Posttraumatic growth, resiliency, and basic hope in soldiers fighting in Eastern Ukraine. *Roczniki Psychologiczne, 22*, 213–231. https://doi.org/10.18290/rpsych.2019.22.3-2

Kovács, J., Csukonyi, C., Kovács, K. E., Liszka, D., & Walawender, P. (2023). Integrative attitudes of Ukrainian war refugees in two neighboring European countries (Poland and Hungary) in connection with posttraumatic stress symptoms and social support. *Frontiers in Public Health, 11*, 1256102. https://doi.org/10.3389/fpubh.2023.1256102

Kovalenko, J. (2024). Surviving the atrocity: A study of resilience and coping behaviour among Ukrainians during the Russo-Ukrainian war. *Journal of Health Psychology, 29*(14), 1688–1703. https://doi.org/10.1177/13591053241274464

Krawczyk, D. (2022, May 27). Uchodźcom z Ukrainy leczącym się z uzależnienia od opiatów pomaga internetowy bot [An online bot helps Ukrainian refugees receiving treatment for opioid addiction]. *Krytyka Polityczna*. https://krytykapolityczna.pl/narkopolityka/polskienarko/uchodzcom-z-ukrainy-leczacym-sie-z-uzaleznienia-od-opiatow-pomaga-internetowy-bot/ (in Polish)

Kurapov, A., Pavlenko, V., Drozdov, A., Bezliudna, V., Reznik, A., & Isralowitz, R. (2022). Toward an understanding of the Russian-Ukrainian war impact on university students and personnel. *Journal of Loss and Trauma, 28*(2), 167–174. https://doi.org/10.1080/15325024.2022.2084838

Kurapov, A., Balashevych, O., Borodko, Y., Vovk, Y., Borozenets, A., & Danyliuk, I. (2025). Psychological wellbeing of Ukrainian civilians: A data report on the impact of traumatic events on mental health. *Frontiers in Psychology, 16*, 1553555. https://doi.org/10.3389/fpsyg.2025.1553555

Magee, K. E., & Connell, A. M. (2021). The role of substance use coping in linking depression and alcohol use from late adolescence through early adulthood. *Experimental and Clinical Psychopharmacology, 29*(6), 659–669. https://doi.org/10.1037/pha0000436

Mapuj pomoc. (2025, May 27). https://mapujpomoc.pl/en/

Masten, A. S. (2007). Resilience in developing systems: Progress and promise as the fourth wave rises. *Development and Psychopathology, 19*(3), 921–930. https://doi.org/10.1017/S0954579407000442

Mazhak, I., Paludo, A. C., & Sudyn, D. (2023). Self-reported health and coping strategies of Ukrainian female refugees in the Czech Republic. *European Societies, 26*(2), 411–437. https://doi.org/10.1080/14616696.2023.2203230

Morley, T. E., & Moran, G. (2011). The origins of cognitive vulnerability in early childhood: Mechanisms linking early attachment to later depression. *Clinical Psychology Review, 31*(7), 1071–1082. https://doi.org/10.1016/j.cpr.2011.06.006

Munroe, M., Al-Refae, M., Chan, H. W., & Ferrari, M. (2022). Using self-compassion to grow in the face of trauma: The role of positive reframing and problem-focused coping strategies. *Psychological Trauma: Theory, Research, Practice, and Policy, 14*(S1), S157–S164. https://doi.org/10.1037/tra0001164

National Research Council, & Institute of Medicine. (2009). *Preventing mental, emotional, and behavioral disorders among young people: Progress and possibilities*. National Academies Press. https://doi.org/10.17226/12480

Ociepa-Kicińska, E., & Gorzałczyńska-Koczkodaj, M. (2022). Forms of aid provided to refugees of the 2022 Russia-Ukraine war: The case of Poland. *International Journal of Environmental Research and Public Health, 19*(12), 7085. https://doi.org/10.3390/ijerph19127085

Okulicz-Kozaryn, K., Sakowska, J., Kondratiuk, V., Zawór, J., Nitkiewicz, H., Węgrzyn-Jonek, E., Zigert, V., Stawecka, E., Nałęcz, H., Andruszczyszyna, T., Sherstyuk, L., & Dzielska, A. (2022). *Dodać Sił. Додати Сил. Podręcznik dla realizatora program* [Programme Textbook]. IMiD. (in Polish and Ukrainian)

Osmo, F., Duran, V., Wenzel, A., Reis de Oliveira, I., Nepomuceno, S., Madeira, M., & Menezes, I. (2018). The Negative Core Beliefs Inventory: Development and psychometric properties. *Journal of Cognitive Psychotherapy, 32*(1), 67–82. https://doi.org/10.1891/0889-8391.32.1.67

Okulicz-Kozaryn, K., Sherstyuk, L., & Dzielska, A. (2026). Evaluation of the emergency response mental health support program for Ukrainian refugee families in Poland. *International Journal of Social Psychiatry*. https://doi.org/10.1177/00207640261438837

Ovcharenko, O. (2024). Zachowanie zdrowia psychicznego uchodźców w warunkach ucieczki przed wojną do Polski z Ukrainy [Maintaining mental health of refugees while fleeing from the war in Ukraine to Poland]. *Przegląd Krytyczny, 6*(1), 31–50. (in Polish).

Oviedo, L., Seryczyńska, B., Torralba, J., Roszak, P., Del Angel, J., Vyshynska, O., Muzychuk, I., & Churpita, S. (2022). Coping and resilience strategies among Ukraine war refugees. *International Journal of Environmental Research and Public Health, 19*(20), 13094. https://doi.org/10.3390/ijerph192013094

Pacewicz, P. (2022, March 12). Aż 91 proc. zaskoczonych, że tak pomagamy uchodźcom. *OKO.press* [As many as 91 percent surprised that we help refugees so much]. https://oko.press/az-91-proc-zaskoczonych-ze-tak-pomagamy-uchodzcom-kobiety-robia-wiecej-a-konfederaci (in Polish)

Panter-Brick, C., Grimon, M. P., Kalin, M., & Eggerman, M. (2015). Trauma memories, mental health, and resilience: A prospective study of Afghan youth. *Journal of Child Psychology and Psychiatry, 56*(7), 814–825. https://doi.org/10.1111/jcpp.12350

Panter-Brick, C., & Leckman, J. F. (2013). Editorial commentary: Resilience in child development—Interconnected pathways to wellbeing. *Journal of Child Psychology and Psychiatry, 54*(3), 333–336. https://doi.org/10.1111/jcpp.12057

Peace of Mind & Strength of Heart. (2022). https://pmsh.iahv-peace.org/pl/strona-glowna/

Poudel-Tandukar, K., Davis, C., Mosijchuk, Y., & Poudel, K. C. (2024). Social and emotional well-being intervention to reduce stress, anxiety, and depression among Ukrainian refugees resettled in Massachusetts. *International Journal of Social Psychiatry, 70*(8), 1461–1469. https://doi.org/10.1177/00207640241270870

Predoiu, R., Piotrowski, A., Makarowski, R., Sygit-Kowalkowska, E., Boe, O., Predoiu, A., & Rawat, S. (2024). Stres, prężność i poczucie własnej skuteczności w okresie wojny rosyjsko-ukraińskiej wśród kobiet z Ukrainy, Polski, Rumunii i ze Słowacji [Stress, resilience, and self-efficacy during the Russo-Ukrainian war among women from Ukraine, Poland, Romania, and Slovakia]. *Psychiatria Polska, 58*(5). (in Polish)

Psychiatric Research Unit, WHO Collaborating Center for Mental Health, Frederiksborg General Hospital. (n.d.). *WHO-5 Well-Being Index*. https://www.psykiatri-regionh.dk/who-5/Documents/WHO5_Polish.pdf

Purgato, M., Bartucz, M., Turrini, G., et al. (2024). Assessing local service providers' needs for scaling up MHPSS interventions for Ukrainian refugees: Insights from Poland, Slovakia, and Romania. *Cambridge Prisms: Global Mental Health, 11*, Article e119. https://doi.org/10.1017/gmh.2024.113

Ramachandran, A., Makhashvili, N., Javakhishvili, J., Karachevskyy, A., Kharchenko, N., Shpiker, M., Ezard, N., Fuhr, D. C., & Roberts, B. (2019). Alcohol use among conflict-affected persons in Ukraine: Risk factors, coping and access to mental health services. *European Journal of Public Health, 29*(6), 1141–1146. https://doi.org/10.1093/eurpub/ckz117

Reznik, A., Pavlenko, V., Kurapov, A., Zavatska, L., Korchakova, N., Pavlova, I., Romem-Porat, S. L., & Isralowitz, R. (2025). War impact on mental health and well-being among Ukrainian and Israeli women: A cross-national comparison. *Global Mental Health, 12*, Article e46. https://doi.org/10.1017/gmh.2025.30

Rizzi, D., Ciuffo, G., Landoni, M., Mangiagalli, M., & Ionio, C. (2023). Psychological and environmental factors influencing resilience among Ukrainian refugees and internally displaced persons: A systematic review of coping strategies and risk and protective factors. *Frontiers in Psychology, 14*, 1266125. https://doi.org/10.3389/fpsyg.2023.1266125

Roberts, B., Makhashvili, N., Javakhishvili, J., Karachevskyy, A., Kharchenko, N., Shpiker, M., & Richardson, E. (2019). Mental health care utilisation among internally displaced persons in Ukraine: Results from a nation-wide survey. *Epidemiology and Psychiatric Sciences, 28*(1), 100–111. https://doi.org/10.1017/S2045796017000385

Romano, I., Patte, K. A., de Groh, M., Jiang, Y., Wade, T. J., Bélanger, R. E., & Leatherdale, S. T. (2021). Substance-related coping behaviours among youth during the early months of the COVID-19 pandemic. *Addictive Behaviors Reports, 14*, Article 100392. https://doi.org/10.1016/j.abrep.2021.100392

Rutter, M. (1987). Psychosocial resilience and protective mechanisms. *American Journal of Orthopsychiatry, 57*(3), 316–331. https://doi.org/10.1111/j.1939-0025.1987.tb03541.x

Sakowska, J. (2008). *Szkoła dla rodziców i wychowawców, część I: Materiały dla prowadzących zajęcia* [School for parents and educators, Part I: Materials for course leaders]. CMPPP. (in Polish)

Sakowska, J., & Puchała, E. (2008). *Szkoła dla rodziców i wychowawców, część II: Materiały dla prowadzących zajęcia* [School for parents and educators, Part II: Materials for course leaders]. CMPPP. (in Polish)

Settles, R. F., Cyders, M., & Smith, G. T. (2010). Longitudinal validation of the acquired preparedness model of drinking risk. *Psychology of Addictive Behaviors, 24*(2), 198–208. https://doi.org/10.1037/a0017631

Shkolina, N. V., Shapoval, I. I., Orlova, I. V., Kedyk, I. A., & Stanislavchuk, M. A. (2020). Adaptatsiia i validizatsiia ukrains'koiu versii shkaly stresostiikosti Konora–Devidsona-10 (CD-RISC-10): aprobatsiia u khvorykh ankylozyruyushchim spondylitom [Adaptation and validation of the Ukrainian version of the Connor–Davidson Resilience Scale-10 (CD-RISC-10): Testing in patients with ankylosing spondylitis]. *Ukrainskyi Revmatolohichnyi Zhurnal, 2*(80). https://doi.org/10.32471/rheumatology.2707-6970.80.15236 (in Ukrainian)

Strouse, D. L., & Moore, K. (2019). Commentary: Contextualizing alternatives to RCTs: Measuring the impact of a non-governmental sponsorship organization's projects to strengthen children's supportive environments. *New Directions for Child and Adolescent Development, 2019*(167), 141–158. https://doi.org/10.1002/cad.20315

Sydorenko, A. Y., Kiel, L., & Spindler, H. (2025). Resilience, psychosomatic health, and support needs of Ukrainian healthcare professionals in wartime: A cross-sectional study. *Journal of Psychosomatic Research, 188*, Article 111995. https://doi.org/10.1016/j.jpsychores.2024.111995

Tedeschi, R. G., & Calhoun, L. G. (1996). The Post-Traumatic Growth Inventory: Measuring the positive legacy of trauma. *Journal of Traumatic Stress, 9*(3), 455–471. https://doi.org/10.1002/jts.2490090305

Topp, C. W., Østergaard, S. D., Søndergaard, S., & Bech, P. (2015). The WHO-5 Well-Being Index: A systematic review of the literature. *Psychotherapy and Psychosomatics, 84*(3), 167–176. https://doi.org/10.1159/000376585

Turrini, G., Purgato, M., Acarturk, C., Anttila, M., Au, T., Ballette, F., Bird, M., Carswell, K., Churchill, R., Cuijpers, P., Hall, J., Hansen, L. J., Kösters, M., Lantta, T., Nosè, M., Ostuzzi, G., Sijbrandij, M., Tedeschi, F., Valimaki, M., … Barbui, C. (2019). Efficacy and acceptability of psychosocial interventions in asylum seekers and refugees: Systematic review and meta-analysis. *Epidemiology and Psychiatric Sciences, 28*(4), 376–388. https://doi.org/10.1017/S2045796019000027

UNICEF. (2025). https://www.unicef.org/eca/pl/polska

van der Ven, E., et al. (2025). *Ukraine's displaced people in the EU: Reach out, implement, scale-up and evaluate interventions promoting mental wellbeing*. Vrije Universiteit Amsterdam. https://research.vu.nl/en/projects/ukraines-displaced-people-in-the-eu-reach-out-implement-scale-up-

Vergés, A. (2022). On the desirability of social desirability measures in substance use research. *Journal of Studies on Alcohol and Drugs, 83*(4), 582–587. https://doi.org/10.15288/jsad.2022.83.582

Wadsworth, M. E. (2015). Development of maladaptive coping: A functional adaptation to chronic, uncontrollable stress. *Child Development Perspectives, 9*(2), 96–100. https://doi.org/10.1111/cdep.12112

Wagner, E. F., Myers, M. G., & McIninch, J. L. (1999). Stress-coping and temptation-coping as predictors of adolescent substance use. *Addictive Behaviors, 24*(6), 769–779. https://doi.org/10.1016/S0306-4603(99)00058-1

Wojdat, M., & Cywiński, P. (2022). *Miejska gościnność: Wielki wzrost, wyzwania i szanse. Raport o uchodźcach z Ukrainy w największych polskich miastach* [Urban hospitality: Rapid growth, challenges, and opportunities. Report on refugees from Ukraine in the largest Polish cities]. Centrum Analiz i Badań, Unia Metropolii Polskich im. Pawła Adamowicza. (in Polish)

Zawadzka-Paluektau, N. (2022). Ukrainian refugees in Polish press. *Discourse & Communication, 17*(6), 761–777. https://doi.org/10.1177/17504813221111636

Chapter 7
Alcohol and Drug Use Among Forcibly Displaced Ukrainians in Poland: At-Risk Groups and Barriers to Accessing Prevention, Treatment, and Harm Reduction Services

Michał Wanke, Iwona Bielska, Estera Wieczorek, and Konrad Pędziwiatr

7.1 Introduction

Historically, Poland has been characterized as a country of emigration with limited experience as a host for forced migrants. Prior to the escalation of Russia's invasion of Ukraine in February 2022, Poland hosted a relatively small refugee population (fewer than 10,000 registered asylum seekers annually), and the national asylum infrastructure lacked the institutional capacity and resources to manage large-scale displacement. Poland was predominantly viewed as a transit country, particularly by asylum seekers who sought protection and long-term resettlement in Western Europe (Górny et al., 2017). The limited material support and integration prospects

M. Wanke (✉)
Department of Cultural Studies, University of Opole, Opole, Poland
e-mail: michal.wanke@uni.opole.pl

I. Bielska
Institute of Public Health, Jagiellonian University Medical College, Kraków, Poland

Department of Health Research Methods, Evidence and Impact, McMaster University, Hamilton, ON, Canada

E. Wieczorek
Department of Health Economics and Social Security, Institute of Public Health, Jagiellonian University Medical College, Kraków, Poland

K. Pędziwiatr
Center for Advanced Studies of Population and Religion (CASPAR), Krakow University of Economics, Kraków, Poland

C. De Kock (ed.), *Substance Use Among Refugees in Europe*,
https://doi.org/10.1007/978-3-032-32399-6_7

in Poland often prompted these migrants to continue their journey westward shortly after lodging initial asylum claims (Sobczak-Szelc et al., 2023).

However, recent developments have fundamentally altered Poland's migration profile. In response to one of the largest forced displacement crises in Europe since the Second World War, Poland emerged as a primary destination for Ukrainian refugees. This led to a pivotal shift in Poland's role from a country of net emigration and transit to one of net immigration and refugee reception-integration. This transformation was not solely driven by geopolitical developments. Domestic policy changes (e.g., the introduction of the "500–800+" child benefit program) and economic growth contributed to Poland's increasing appeal among migrants who considered long-term settlement in Poland (Duszczyk & Matuszczyk, 2022; OECD, 2024; Sobczak-Szelc et al., 2023).

In 2024, there were 990,000 Ukrainian forced migrants (also referred to as refugees) in Poland holding an active temporary protection status (UKR status), which was an increase of approximately 35,000 people over the previous year (Pędziwiatr et al., 2024b). This confirms Poland's continued role as one of the largest host countries for Ukrainian forced migrants in the European Union. For context, Poland's total population is approximately 37.5 million, and foreign-born residents made up just 2.2% of this figure as of 2023—making Ukrainians by far the largest migrant group in the country (OECD, 2024). This population is spatially concentrated in major urban and metropolitan areas in the country (Osica et al., 2024), which is primarily driven by access to services, employment opportunities, and established diaspora networks. The refugee population demonstrates distinct administrative demographic trends: roughly half of all registered individuals are children, while women constitute 61% of the entire population and 77% of all adults (Urząd do Spraw Cudzoziemców [UDSC], 2023).

Refugees from Ukraine are covered by the publicly funded health care system in Poland, including for mental health, at the same level as other Polish residents, on the basis of the March 12, 2022, legal act awarding individuals with temporary protection access to services (Pędziwiatr et al., 2024a). Mental health protection activities are provided by the central government (Ministry of Health), local governments, and institutions. Substance use services are provided by a combination of public and non-governmental organizations. Treatment and recovery services are provided mainly by outpatient and inpatient treatment centers, detoxification wards, day-care centers, drug treatment wards, and rehabilitation facilities (International Society of Substance Use Professionals, 2025). Nevertheless, access to services is hindered due to long wait times, low number of professionals, and an uneven distribution of services, particularly in rural areas. In 2024, patients waited an average of 5.3 months for a psychologist, 1.8 months for a psychiatrist, 1.1 months for treatment of opioid addiction with methadone, and 0.6 months for inpatient alcohol addiction treatment (Fundacja Watch Health Care, 2025).

Since the beginning of the full-scale invasion of Ukraine, many governmental, intergovernmental (INGO), and non-governmental organizations (NGOs) cooperated to provide humanitarian aid, protection, mental health and psychosocial support (MHPSS), and to coordinate and supplement government efforts in Poland (Charycka et al., 2024; Główny Urząd Statystyczny, 2023; IOM, 2024; Save the Children & Klon/Jawor, 2024). The organizations played a crucial role, as many possessed extensive experience in supporting forcibly displaced populations—an area in which the Polish government had limited prior experience (Sibley, 2025). Moreover, NGOs filled funding and service gaps by delivering MHPSS like mental health counseling and trauma support services (Centre for East European and International Studies, 2024; IOM, 2024; Ivashko & Prykhodchenko, n.d.). In 2024, 55% of NGOs whose main goal was to provide aid to refugees offered psychological support to migrants, highlighting the important role of these organizations in delivering mental health services (Charycka et al., 2025).

In Poland, both mental health care and addiction treatment are publicly funded and organized through the National Health Fund (NFZ). The mental health system provides general psychiatric care, while specialized addiction services focus on prevention, treatment, and harm reduction. These services are coordinated by the National Centre for the Prevention of Addictions (KCPU), an agency under the Ministry of Health (KCPU, 2023). Care is delivered through a network of outpatient clinics, inpatient facilities, and therapeutic communities. Despite this formal structure, limited capacity, long wait times, and regional disparities in service availability often lead individuals to seek private care or support from NGOs (Ministry of Health, 2022). In addition, the separation between psychiatric and addiction services can hinder continuity of care for individuals with complex needs.

Although some studies have investigated mental health conditions among Ukrainian refugees in Poland (Kordel et al., 2024; Kovács et al., 2023; Urbański et al., 2024), existing research is largely confined to the early phases of displacement and tends to focus on general psychological distress with limited attention paid to long-term needs or specific issues such as substance use. Moreover, information specific to substance use is sparse. Encounters for psychiatric care and the treatment of substance use disorders accounted for 3% of all publicly funded health care visits among Ukrainian refugees in Krakow, Poland, in 2023, with 59% of them for mental and behavioral disorders due to the use of opioids (Pędziwiatr et al., 2024a). National data shows that the number of refugees receiving substance use treatment in Poland is relatively low with 48 patients receiving outpatient services, 27 receiving treatment for psychoactive substance use other than alcohol, and 137 receiving opioid agonist treatment in 2023 (Krajowe Centrum Przeciwdziałania Uzależnieniom, personal communication, 2025). In a study of displaced female migrants, Venger et al. (2024) found that 25% of the sample reported smoking or using tobacco substitutes, including 9% with systematic use or abuse. Systematic use or abuse of alcohol was reported by 9% of the sample. The use of narcotics, including cannabis and psychostimulants, was less prevalent with 4% reporting episodic, periodic, or systematic use. In a study of coping strategies for negative emotions among Ukrainian refugees, the use of tobacco, alcohol, or other stimulants was the least reported at 3% (Długosz, 2023). In contrast, getting mobilized and focusing on other activities were the most commonly reported coping strategies.

As the available literature demonstrates, little is known about substance use among displaced migrants from Ukraine, as well as the population subgroups that are at highest risk of substance use and abuse. Moreover, the facilitators and barriers to accessing mental health services, specifically related to substance use, are poorly understood. Having information on how forcibly displaced migrants navigate the system and perceive access to it is an essential step toward improving their access to care. Therefore, the aims of this study are to: first, identify the population subgroups at highest risk of substance use and abuse among the Ukrainian forcibly displaced population in Poland, and second, to provide insights on access to substance use prevention and treatment services through a qualitative study.

7.2 Methods

We utilized an exploratory qualitative research design to gain in-depth knowledge about access to MHPSS for Ukrainians forcibly displaced to Poland. The analysis presented in this chapter focuses specifically on substance use prevention and treatment services among this population. We used a purposive sampling method to identify potential participants from across Poland. Participants were selected based on their demonstrated knowledge of the Polish substance use prevention and treatment system, direct involvement in NGO or health care services supporting forcibly displaced Ukrainians, or personal experience with substance use or related service access in Poland as Ukrainian forced migrants. The sample included health professionals and staff working at organizations providing care or services, including in psychiatry, MHPSS, or specialized substance use-related services in front-line and managerial roles, as well as migrants who resided in Poland and had knowledge about forced migrants from Ukraine who sought care in Poland. Thus, this paper is grounded in the perspective of these individuals, who assume different roles among the forcibly resettled Ukrainians, including the perspective of people who have knowledge of those who use substances. A qualitative approach was chosen due to its suitability for exploring complex experiences among hard-to-reach and vulnerable populations, allowing for the collection of rich, contextualized data that would be difficult to obtain through quantitative methods (Ellard-Gray et al., 2015).

All individuals received information about the research team and the study in Polish, English, or Ukrainian, depending on preference. The time and the mode of the interview were agreed on by all the participants. Providing informed consent was mandatory prior to the interview. Semi-structured in-depth interviews were conducted between March and May 2025 by seven interviewers in Polish, Ukrainian, Russian, or English. The interview guide was partially informed by the results of previous studies carried out by the team members. First, the guide explored observations regarding the characteristics of the forcibly displaced Ukrainian population in Poland, specifically in relation to mental health and substance use services. It then examined participants' perspective on motivations for, and methods of, seeking assistance in these areas. Subsequently, it gathered information on the experiences with care and, where applicable, the use of medications. Finally, participants were asked to share their perspectives on adaptations within the health care system. Interviews took place in-person or online. The interviews were video- or audio-recorded and transcribed verbatim. The interviews lasted approximately 60 min. Interviews were analyzed using Atlas.ti and an inductive coding approach. An open coding session, where two authors inductively created codes, was followed by the authors' discussion and thematic analysis that identified six major categories: population groups, substances, challenges related to use, availability of services, transnational differences, and barriers to accessing assistance. The authors developed and defined the codes, and the most prevalent codes within the groups included: for population groups: HIV, user profiles, youth; substances: alcohol, abuse, use before war; challenges related to use: risk factors, homelessness, relationship issues; availability of services: access to MHPSS, access to substance use (SU) services, opioid agonist treatment (OAT), organizing support; transnational differences: difference between Ukraine (UA) and Poland (PL), similarities to PL patients, different medicines; barriers to accessing assistance: language, barriers to access MHPSS, stigma. The Consolidated Criteria for Reporting Qualitative Research (COREQ) checklist served as a guideline for the reporting of the methods and results of this study (Tong et al., 2007).

7.2.1 Ethics Approval

Approval was obtained from the Ethical Committee at the Jagiellonian University in Poland (decision number 118.0043.1.78.2025; 20.02.2025). The procedures used in this study closely followed the Declaration of Helsinki.

7.3 Results

7.3.1 Sample Description

The study included 28 interviews conducted with 37 participants: 27 representatives of organizations and institutions in managerial and front-line positions—INGO (2 participants), NGO (19 participants), healthcare system (6 participants)—and 10 forcibly displaced migrants. Information on their characteristics is presented in Table 7.1.

Ukrainian forced migrants in Poland consist of an array of different population groups. Due to the magnitude and circular nature of Ukrainian migration to Poland prior to 2022 and sometimes an ephemeral migration pattern and changing mobility decisions, the composition of the migrant population is subject to frequent change and lacks clearly defined categories (e.g., between temporary and permanent migrants). Based on our qualitative analysis and coding of interview data, which included

Table 7.1 Participants' characteristics

Health professionals and staff						
Interview count	*Participant count*	*ID*	*Gender*	*Sector of role*	*Type of role*	*Participant code + characteristics*
1	1	P01	F	NGO	Mixed	P01, NGO, front-line and Management role, Female
2	2	P02	M	NGO	Management	P02, NGO, Management role, Male
3	3	P03	F	Healthcare system	Front-line	P03, health care system, Front-line role, Female
4	4	P04	M	INGO	Front-line	P04, INGO, Front-line role, Male
5	5	P05	M	Health care system	Mixed	P05, health care system, Front-line and Management role, Male
6	6	P06	M	Health care system	Front-line	P06, health care system, Front-line role, Male
7	7	P07	F	NGO	Front-line	P07, NGO, Front-line role, Female
8	8	P08	F	INGO	Management	P08, INGO, Management role, Female
9	9	P09	F	NGO	Management	P09, NGO, Management role, Female
10	10	P10	F	Health care system	Mixed	P10, health care system, Front-line and Management role, Female
11	11	P11	M	NGO	Front-line	P11, NGO, Front-line role
12	12	P12	F	NGO	Front-line	P12, NGO, Front-line role, Female
13	13	P13	F	Health care system	Front-line	P13, health care system, Front-line role, Female
14	14	P14	F	Health care system	Front-line	P14, health care system, Front-line role, Female
15	15	P15	F	NGO	Management	P15, NGO, Management role, Female

(continued)

Table 7.1 (continued)

16	16–20	P16	F	NGO	Management, frontline	P16, NGO, Front-line and Management role, Female		
17	21–26	P17	M	NGO	Management, frontline	P17, NGO, Front-line and Management role, Male		
18	27	P18	F	NGO	Front-line	P18, NGO, Front-line, Female		
Forced migrants								
Interview count	*Participant count*	*ID*	*Gender*	*Age*	*Education*	*Arrival date*	*Role*	*Participant code + characteristics*
1	1	REF1	F	44	Higher education	2019	Refugee	R01, Female, 44
2	2	REF2	F	47	Higher education	2014	Refugee	R02, Female, 47
3	3	REF3	F	43	Higher education	2018	Refugee	R03, Female, 43
4	4	REF4	F	43	Higher education	02/2022	Refugee	R04, Female, 43
5	5	REF5	F	46	Higher education	02/2022	Refugee	R05, Female, 46
6	6	REF6	F	39	Higher education	02/2022	Refugee	R06, Female, 39
7	7	REF7	F	45	Higher education	03/2022	Refugee	R07, Female, 45
8	8	REF8	F	37	Higher education	03/2022	Refugee	R08, Female, 37
9	9	REF9	F	62	Vocational	07/2023	Refugee	R09, Female, 62
10	10	REF10	F	42	Higher education	03/2022	Refugee	R10, Female, 42

Source Own elaboration

organizing references to subpopulations into a working group labeled "population groups," three overlapping categories emerged as particularly prominent according to our informants. These were not intended as rigid, mutually exclusive groups, but rather as thematic clusters reflecting the perceptions of experts and forcibly displaced migrants.

First, alcohol use was identified as a widespread and meta-level concern, given its social embeddedness and accessibility, often serving as a coping mechanism. Second, youth were frequently highlighted as a vulnerable subgroup due to ongoing or initiated use of substances such as tobacco, alcohol, and other psychoactive drugs following displacement, though limited knowledge exists about this group's dynamics. Third, a distinct group was recognized comprising individuals dependent on opioids and engaged in opioid agonist treatment, many living with HIV, representing complex health and social needs.

Other subgroups at risk (e.g., people experiencing homelessness or factory workers using stimulants) were also mentioned, but these were less frequently referenced and may be more difficult to identify or reach. While these categories overlap and do not capture the full heterogeneity of the population, they provide a tentative framework grounded in the perspectives of those with direct experience, reflecting patterns observed across multiple interviews.

These subgroups are heterogeneous in that individuals who use illicit substances and those who are undocumented face distinct types of risks related to substance use or abuse, as well as broader social and legal challenges. As a result, they require different types of interventions or, at a minimum, tailored monitoring approaches. As one manager of an NGO providing services to forced migrants put it:

> The diversity is immense. Those individuals who come to seek support for antiretroviral treatment are different from those who use psychoactive substances. After all, those who use substances are very often undocumented migrants. Sometimes they also have problems with the law, who use substances in relation to also experiencing homelessness or housing instability, so these are completely different groups. You really cannot label them in the same manner because there is great diversity among these people. (P15, NGO, Management role, Female)

The chronology and trajectory of the forced migration were noted as being important factors related to substance use. Our participants pointed to an important distinction between individuals who continued substance use from before their displacement and those who initiated or intensified it in the course of the stressful events:

> The stress of war certainly contributed to these people starting to use substances, and they continue to do so here. For some, the living conditions in Poland simply worsened. As a result, they turned to substance use or felt lost in their situation. I don't think that there are any data showing how many of these people had an addiction before coming here and entering the system, and how many became addicted in Poland. (P15, NGO, Management role, Female)

While migration has been identified as a potential trigger for substance use, our data suggest that this behavior may have existed prior to arrival in Poland among some individuals. As the previous participant noted, information on this topic is lacking. These observations point to the importance of screening and monitoring. One of the challenges related to this is the mobility of this population when trying to assess and address substance use.

7.3.2 Alcohol Use

The professionals, as well as the refugees themselves, reported the embeddedness of alcohol in the lifestyles of many forced migrants, pointing to its social acceptance, while also indicating that some individuals turn to it as a stress reliever. Factors that contributed to its use included its accessibility, as well as locations where it was more frequently consumed, including in aggregate accommodation settings. The following excerpt highlights the perceived ubiquity of alcohol use within the daily lives of some displaced persons:

> As for alcohol—unfortunately, everyone drinks. Especially on weekends. On weekdays we work—that's important for all of us: documents, housing, income. On Friday, people drink, recover on Sunday, and are back to work on Monday. (R06, Female, 39)

The risk of alcohol misuse stems from its ubiquity and social acceptability in everyday life. Through its normalization within segments of the displaced population, its use may become problematic, for example, through instrumentalizing it as a coping strategy for forcibly displaced migrants. Some of the study participants described a connection between alcohol consumption and its use for coping with stress, instead of seeking professional support:

> I think that there is still a large group that doesn't come forward. And there are more people who don't come forward than those who do, because when you talk to those who did eventually seek help or treatment, they often say that after work everyone drinks beer, and often these are people who live there, in rented rooms with several other people, and their routine after work is such that they spend their time this way, or they can't cope with their emotions and turn to these substances. (P03, health care system, Front-line role, Female)

Different accounts of alcohol use as an alleged coping mechanism were recorded. Some professionals mentioned this in the context of males in relation to gender roles, broken family ties, and tensions amid those who were not actively involved in supporting the war efforts. Other professionals described alcohol use among female forced migrants, including among those in their 30s and 40s. The disintegration of family connections and the subsequent lack of social support networks that no longer act as protective factors may result in increased drinking, according to some informants. This may be further heightened among women in charge of displaced homes and childcare arrangements on their own. Entangled in poly substance use—for example, mixed with benzodiazepine use—alcohol consumption that is normalized both as a social lubricant and a coping substance presents a great risk to the forced migrant population.

> Alcohol is used in a more subtle manner, high-functioning, drinking alcohol but still managing to take care of everything, so to speak, the home life, kids and so on, but at

> some point, perhaps in a moment of some kind of emotional turmoil, some kind of… I don't know, a breakdown, it sometimes led to suicidal behavior. (P14, health care system, Front-line role, Female)

The shifting boundaries of "sensible" use result in the neutralization of narratives. For example, making comparisons to users of "stronger" substances belittles an increase in alcohol consumption. This is illustrated by the following refugee's reflexive observation:

> People relieve stress in different ways - some drink more alcohol, others use stronger substances. Not me - at most two glasses of wine every couple of months. Lately a bit more often - even with my dad, we sometimes talk over Viber and drink wine. So yes, I started drinking more in the evenings. (R10, Female, 42)

The observations made by service workers and forcibly displaced individuals in our interviews suggest that normalized alcohol use may be an issue especially when it is used in order to relieve stress related to forced migration. As alcohol use is universally accessible and highly normalized in both Ukraine and Poland, it may be considered a risk factor for increased use among the wider forced migrant population.

7.3.3 Substance Use Among Youth

Youth, broadly defined as adolescents, school-aged teenagers, and young adults alike, were identified as another subgroup of focus among forced migrants to Poland in reference to psychoactive substance use. When asked about their observations regarding the subpopulation of substance-using forced migrants, it was suggested that, in some cases, substance use continued after displacement:

> These are often young people… at that age, basically young adults. These are mainly people for whom war was not necessarily the trigger for using these substances, but they are often people who had already used or experimented with psychoactive substances before. (P03, health care system, Front-line role, Female)

However, the interviews suggested that some young people initiated the use of substances (alcohol, cannabis, and mephedrone) despite not having been exposed to psychoactive substances prior to arrival.

Although illicit substance acquisition from the local market was mentioned by health care providers, from the perspective of streetwork and outreach services for youth, substances surfaced incidentally, and alcohol was mentioned as most common amid risk behaviors and recreational use. Cannabis, synthetic cannabis, or other new psychoactive substances were indirectly observed too:

> It seems to me that alcohol is more accessible and more present in their relationships than psychoactive substances. We know this because they talked about it a little and we also had some isolated incidents when they came to [center name] and couldn't function because they were under the influence of something, so we kind of knew that they were using marijuana or something, that could be marijuana, anything chemical, but they're more "soft drugs" than "hard drugs," and actually what they use most are various types of e-cigarettes. Disposable

> ones, snus, anything related to smoking and nicotine rather than alcoholism or psychoactive substances. (P02, NGO, Management role, Male)

However, the widespread use of tobacco and e-cigarettes was noticed. Nonetheless, the informants in our study generally have limited information about prevalence rates among displaced migrants. They suggested that youth are at risk of engaging in substance use due to several factors resulting from the displacement: first, because of the lack of protective factors in the form of "parental supervision"; and second, due to relative isolation or peer rejection in the Polish educational institutions.

Smoking tobacco is mentioned as the most basic form of substance use outside of parental supervision. A participant from an international organization shared an observation of a relationship between smoking and parental disinterest in children's behavior. In the view of our participants, migrant parents are not necessarily ignoring their children on purpose, but rather are structurally less capable of paying enough attention to their offspring. This finding suggests that single parents—predominantly mothers—who participate in the labor market out of economic necessity may experience constrained time and emotional resources.

> And when a mother with these kids has to work from morning till night, where does she get the strength or who is supposed to take care of the children? (P01, NGO, Front-line & Management role, Female)

The service providers that we interviewed also pointed to cases of negative sentiments and peer pressure at schools, allegedly experienced by the Ukrainian forcibly displaced migrant youth. A psychologist working for an NGO highlighted the possibility of conformist attitudes and possible substance use in order to impress peers based on her interactions with Ukrainian youth. She connected this with an observation of a young client who actively attempted to conceal his Ukrainian identity anticipating stigma at school:

> What I hear from these teenage kids is that they sometimes experience bullying, like, "Go back to Ukraine because you're from Ukraine," and stuff like that, and sometimes, to fit in with the group, they try beer or something else, because they want to prove that they're part of the group, and that they're not just some outsiders. (P07, NGO, Front-line role, Female)

Youth are perceived as a subgroup at risk among forced migrants in Poland, including those who had initiated substance use prior to displacement. Additionally, according to observations among our participants, young people are more likely to initiate substance use if they lack parental support or supervision. The social isolation or peer rejection reported by some may also result in taking up risky behavior, including using substances.

7.3.4 People on Opioid Agonist Treatment

Certain groups of individuals may be more likely to be connected to service providers. These include people receiving treatment for opioid use, those enrolled in opioid agonist treatment, or those living with HIV. In some cases, opioid use disorder and HIV infection may co-exist. Services related to HIV care and opioid agonist treatment are usually delivered through established health care systems, NGOs, or international organizations, which often utilize targeted outreach practices. In contrast, individuals who use alcohol or other substances, or youth who are at risk of substance use, may not be as clearly linked to specific services or support networks, making them harder to identify or reach. In our study, we managed to identify specific characteristics of the vulnerable subgroup of people on opioid agonist treatment because there are institutionalized services targeted at it.

In our interviews, references to people living with HIV often overlapped with descriptions of individuals receiving SMT, reflecting a subgroup frequently engaged in both treatments. This aligns with Ukrainian models where HIV care and SMT are integrated, improving antiretroviral therapy (ART) adherence and outcomes (Bachireddy et al., 2013; WHO, 2013).

Professionals in the field point out that a key factor influencing the reception of people who use opioids and those living with HIV in Poland is the significant difference in the size of these populations being larger in Ukraine than in Poland. This disparity has several consequences. It affects the scale of prevention and outreach efforts, the availability of treatment facilities, and the number of trained specialists. It also shapes the broader health care infrastructure. Additionally, some pharmaceuticals commonly used in Ukraine are not registered or available in the European Union, which can further complicate access to care for displaced individuals.

> When it comes to differences between Ukraine and Poland, the main one is in the context of HIV infection: in Ukraine, there are 250,000 people living with HIV, while in Poland at that time there were 25,000 people living with HIV. In Poland, all people who are infected and have Polish public insurance, as this is also important, have access to antiretroviral drugs, because the program itself is for everyone, but you have to go to a doctor in the public health care system, so you need to have insurance in Poland. (…) Secondly, 80% of people in Ukraine have access to generic therapy. In fact, all of them are on the same regimen – those 80%. This regimen does not exist in Poland because these generic companies do not operate in Poland. They do not have a European patent because it is an Indian company. (P15, NGO, Management role, Female)

The generic antiretroviral medications were first conditionally approved and later withdrawn. These changes created dilemmas on how to provide assistance for a highly mobile and vulnerable population, whose settlement status in Poland was not defined:

> The actions of the WHO and UNAIDS led to these drugs being imported in 2022 with the approval of the European Union. But in 2023, these drugs had to be stopped and the original drugs introduced. This is important because these groups migrate, that is, they came to Poland and stayed here for a while, then moved on or returned to Ukraine. This was also a medical dilemma as to what to switch to, whether to change their therapy so that it would be safer for them because everyone was aware that we did not know whether it would be a single visit to us and whether the person would continue this treatment here. (P15, NGO, Management role, Female)

From the perspective of Ukrainian forced migrants living with HIV or using opioids, their relatively small population in Poland also translated into a less extensive support network and availability of services. According to interview participants, people who use opioids and people living with HIV in Ukraine were used to having a dense network of internationally funded specialized facilities providing comprehensive assistance. In contrast to Ukraine, where services were reported to be more accessible and tailored to the needs of people living with HIV or using opioids, in Poland such services are primarily concentrated in major urban areas and delivered through NFZ clinics. While numerous NGOs have provided support to forced migrants since 2022, only a few have specifically focused on this subpopulation. As a result, some individuals had to navigate an unfamiliar and more fragmented system in order to continue their opioid agonist treatment or HIV treatment.

7.3.5 Access to Services and Related Barriers

Our interviewees suggest that connection to services and system navigation among Ukrainian forced migrants who use drugs, are receiving opioid agonist treatment, or are living with HIV may be a challenge upon arrival. In some cases, attachment to care providers may not be well established, resulting in a worsening of symptoms. Several interview participants, particularly those working directly with newly arrived Ukrainian migrants, described situations where individuals already receiving treatment needed to continue or adapt their care after arrival in Poland and this process posed challenges. According to the experiences of one of the participants, there were differences in service navigability between Ukraine and Poland, particularly for those who entered the system:

> In March, I crossed the border and everyone who called me asked where the program was. Because in Ukraine, I have experience with many programs in various organizations supporting people living with HIV, addiction, tuberculosis, or hepatitis. And we have social workers for everything who advise people on what to do, where to go, where to get medication, where to get documents. In Poland, this is not the practice. (P01, NGO, Front-line & Management role, Female)

Patient navigation and connection to services in the public health care system were often facilitated by the NGOs which provided crisis intervention and comprehensive assistance for individuals with mental health or SUD conditions. The sector also acted as a mediator between the forced migrants and the health care system providing orientation and information, and in some cases, services at no or low cost, like for psychotherapy. Some NGOs coordinated assistance between themselves and transferred clients to organizations that were more specialized, for example, in mental health. In the case of supporting people who use drugs, some of the activism and NGO structures were transnationally recreated in Poland.

> The first thing that interests them is the procedure for obtaining treatment, if we are talking about substitution therapy, that is, the procedure for where to go. If they know my phone

> number, they contact me, it doesn't even matter where they are, in which city. I can, for example, immediately provide a list of Polish clinics with addresses and contact details. (P11, NGO, Front-line role, Male)

The transfer of the Ukrainian organizations and activism brought with it the experience and understanding toward best supporting the incoming population of people who use drugs or people living with HIV who were forced to migrate to Poland. These networks included not only staff and volunteers but—importantly—the networks of patients, transferring contacts and trust. Our participants also mentioned transnational activity of religious organizations specializing in crisis intervention services which recreated their activities for people experiencing homelessness or substance dependency in Poland.

Overall, barriers to accessing substance use prevention and treatment services for Ukrainian forced migrants in Poland can be broadly categorized into challenges related to navigating the health care system, structural differences between the Ukrainian and Polish service models, and limitations within existing support networks, including language and cultural barriers.

7.3.6 System Differences and Language Barrier

Challenges stemming from the unfamiliarity with the Polish health care system, as perceived by forcibly displaced Ukrainians themselves, were reported in the interviews. These included differences in administrative procedures, service complexity, and language barriers, affecting access to mental health, psychosocial support, and substance use treatment. These system differences shaped how migrants experienced a range of interventions—from general psychological care to specialized drug treatment.

Forcibly displaced individuals in Poland can access health interventions or treatment through the NFZ-funded public health care system. However, effective use of this system requires not only formal eligibility but also knowledge of its organization, which often differs from the health care system in the country of origin. Some interviewees highlighted that its navigation may be confusing and overwhelming, particularly for those unfamiliar with institutional procedures or administrative expectations. As one participant explained:

> But judging by the issues that people called us about, it seems that they had trouble understanding how the Polish system works. The callers not only needed psychiatric medication, but also insulin and continued oncological treatment. The arrival of patients from Ukraine in the Polish health care system did not follow any clear, established paths that would ensure that this group received adequate assistance for their needs. (P05, health care system, Front-line & Management role, Male)

In certain cases, individuals also face long wait times for appointments, especially in mental health or addiction services. These delays can lead some to seek care in the private sector, which may not be financially feasible for all.

At a more basic level, the language barrier frequently hinders access to NFZ services. Interview participants described situations where displaced individuals were unable to communicate their needs effectively or understand the information provided by staff. One health care worker emphasized how this affects psychiatric care in particular:

> I think what is most important for them - and it's especially critical in psychiatry - is the language barrier. It's difficult for them to communicate, especially during those first months in Poland. They struggle to communicate across many settings, from offices to any kind of health care, and even more so here… in psychiatric care, where the interview is absolutely essential and the diagnosis largely depends on collecting that interview and engaging with the other person. So I think this is the most important challenge. (P03, health care system, Front-line role, Female)

Beyond practical barriers, stigma related to mental health or substance use diagnoses was also reported as a deterrent to seeking care. Some displaced individuals hesitate to approach services due to fear of being judged or misunderstood, both by professionals and their own communities.

These challenges often intersect, creating complex and discouraging situations for people trying to access care. As one participant working within the Polish health care system explained:

> Well, I think it's due to moving to another country where everything works differently. (…) You don't know where to go, which institution to contact, who to talk to, what to do. When it comes to minors, the problem in general with addiction is that people, Poles, bounce from door to door. I don't know, when it comes to accessing psychiatric help for children and young people, it is simply a mission. And it's challenging. And if, on top of that, you're lost in the system, don't understand the reality, have communication difficulties… (P10, health care system, Front-line & Management role, Female)

Access to the public health care system is difficult not only due to the lack of familiarity with it, but also because of the relatively longer wait times for services compared to the ones that the Ukrainians reported having at home. In such cases, those who can afford it switch to the private sector. In the area of mental health support, access to psychiatric care or specialized substance use treatment is possible outside of the public system but relatively expensive. It makes it a highly selective solution for the forcibly displaced population with only a few able to afford it. In fact, some NGOs had time-limited programs that financially supported such visits for forced migrants.

> I know that people try to go to the doctor through the NFZ, but I can't compare here, and they don't say that it's better or worse, but the truth is that in Ukraine you can see a doctor on the same day or I don't know, maybe even during the week. And if that's not possible here, I know that these people often need to pay out of their own pocket to see a private doctor, and most refugees can't afford that, and so we have this possibility to pay for a one-time psychiatric consultation for these people. (P07, NGO, Front-line role, Female)

Paid services are also available from Ukrainian health care professionals through commercial channels, especially in the area of psychotherapy. They include in-person sessions in Poland, or online sessions offered from across the country or from Ukraine.

The Polish health care system plays a crucial role in providing mental health services for forced migrants. However, its complex navigability and accessibility make it not only objectively harder to use—as is the case for Polish patients too—but serve as an additional difficulty for forced migrants who perceive it as being different from their system at home. Although the NGOs were able to provide some services, like psychotherapy, as well as connections with the public system for the newly arrived migrants, the wait times posed challenges.

Not receiving a consultation within a timely manner results in a void that can be filled through the commercial supply, but this imposes financial strain on this vulnerable group. In the case of regulated therapies, such as opioid agonist treatment, the inability to access an immediate supply may result in individuals seeking alternatives on the street market, as was reported by a participant working in an NGO in Poland.

> And Berlin is close by, it's no problem to cross the border, and my clients have told me that while they're waiting here in Poland in line for substitute therapy, they can easily go to Berlin and buy everything [illicit substances] they need there. (P01, NGO, Front-line & Management role, Female)

Regressing to the street supply is a drawback for the substitution treatment and erodes trust, but most importantly, creates serious health risks for the individuals. In terms of the publicly offered services for people who use opioids or for people living with HIV in Poland, our participants reported high effectiveness, citing flexibility and high levels of understanding from the physicians and other health care professionals. Nevertheless, there are differences in the scope and comprehensiveness of the services available to these patients in Poland when compared to Ukraine, particularly around testing, pre-exposure prophylaxis, and treatment regimens. In Poland, their distribution and availability may be affected by a complex system often limited to major urban centers.

For many displaced migrants, interaction with the health care system of a receiving country is further hindered by a language barrier. In the case of patients requiring mental health interventions, such as for patients with psychiatric conditions or substance use disorders, the barrier is significantly greater, requiring deep conversations and the communication of complex information about the persons' emotions and experiences.

> Well, it's also the case that while psychiatric consultations are possible with the help of a translator, therapeutic care is not, so in my opinion, people who require long-term psychotherapy, regardless of the reason, may have a problem in the public system, because there are not many psychotherapists who work under the NFZ and speak Ukrainian or Russian. (P05, health care system, Front-line & Management role, Male)

In the Polish health care system, there is a scarcity of Ukrainian-speaking professionals despite the longstanding presence of these migrants in the country. Community-based support groups in the Ukrainian language for people who use drugs are scarce in Poland.

> [About access] It's difficult. It's difficult with addictions, because often Alcoholics Anonymous and Narcotics Anonymous groups are in Polish, and that's also often a challenge,

> because the group… Well, it's impossible to really operate in two languages, because we discuss such topics in these groups that it's impossible, and often NGOs focus on general psychological care, not on addictions. (P18, NGO, Front-line, Female)

The language barrier intersects all domains of migrant life and can be mitigated with time and language acquisition. However, complex psychiatric diagnoses, interventions, and psychotherapy, as well as system navigation, require good language command or Ukrainian-speaking intermediaries.

In short, participants noted experiencing longer wait times when compared to those in Ukraine, issues with navigating the system, and barriers in communication. Professionals with proficiency of the Ukrainian language were seen as facilitators to receiving care; however, a limited number of them are present in the system.

7.3.7 Anticipated Stigma as a Barrier to Seeking Care

The anticipated stigma surrounding mental health conditions in general, and substance use-related problems, in particular, stands out as the most important culturally constructed barrier to accessing assistance among the displaced people. It is multidimensional and relates to different spheres of forced migrants' activities. The most basic setting is the work environment. As a source of income and relative stability, occupation is seen as fundamental. The prospect of losing a job due to substance dependence, being on treatment for a mental health condition, or living with HIV, makes employed refugees reluctant to disclose such information. According to our study participants, such an anticipation of stigma hinders participation in treatment, as it requires frequent visits for further prescriptions and checkups. Services for patients living with HIV or on opioid agonist treatment are available in the biggest urban centers in Poland, and such visits require making travel arrangements and taking days off work:

> The doctor does not always understand that the patient needs to arrange certain conditions with their employer for not coming to work tomorrow because they have some things to do. Not everyone feels comfortable discussing these topics, (…) people are concerned that they may lose their jobs or housing if others learn that they have an addiction, are living with HIV, or are undergoing treatment for tuberculosis. (P01, NGO, Front-line & Management role, Female)

Based on the interviews with service providers, one of the major factors underpinning the stigma is the fear of formal consequences, including deportation. People who migrate and use opioids are hesitant to disclose any information about their potential dependency, reportedly due to speculation about sharing their medical records with employees which some report occurred in their countries of origin. In the case of infectious diseases, like tuberculosis or infection with hepatitis C virus (HCV), some jurisdictions globally expel such individuals and this reportedly influences the decision of some migrants in Poland to come forward or take tests, despite deportation not being a risk for them.

> We noticed in our harm reduction program that people from Eastern Europe and Central Asia did not want to talk about testing at all and did not want to be tested, even though testing was anonymous and free. Later, they would come to us regularly to exchange equipment, so we talked to them, gave them food, and it only came out during subsequent conversations that in their countries, when people find out that they are addicted, it is recorded in their files, which are then circulated to their employers. Plus, if someone has, I don't know, tuberculosis or HCV, in many countries they are simply deported. So many people are simply afraid of deportation, even though it's not a real possibility in Poland, right? (P15, NGO, Management role, Female)

For many forced migrants, there is a significant barrier to seeking assistance due to a reluctance to be framed as being "mentally ill." This may be rooted in experiences from other countries where surveillance and the criminalization of people who use opioids or who live with HIV has increased the stigma surrounding mental health conditions.

> In Ukraine, it was not common or socially accepted - if someone went to a psychiatrist, there was a stigma, like "you must be mentally ill." I heard that a lot, growing up. Here, in Poland, people are used to the idea from childhood - that it's normal. If there's a problem, they go to a psychologist. And they're not ashamed to say it. They don't have the same kind of mental "frameworks" we were raised with. Younger generations in Ukraine are more relaxed about it, but people born in the 1990s - we were raised in stricter mental patterns. (R08, Female, 37)

The prevailing stigma may also limit opportunities to receive remote assistance. For instance, forced migrants who live in aggregate living arrangements may be reluctant to have phone or video-call consultations with specialists. This hinders the opportunities for these individuals to receive help. Some professionals indicated that in collective shelters, psychological support was provided under different labels, not to stigmatize individuals seeking assistance.

7.4 Discussion

We identified three different subgroups of the Ukrainian forcibly displaced population in Poland, who are vulnerable in relation to substances: individuals who use or abuse alcohol, risk behavior engaging youth and people on opioid agonist therapy. Alcohol use is relatively common, and the risk of its abuse may affect a larger proportion of the population of forced migrants. Youth may be more easily identified through educational institutions, yet many remain out of the Polish system, and their risk behaviors may be unnoticed. In contrast, individuals who are already connected with health care services, such as patients on opioid agonist treatment, are relatively the easiest to follow due to their formal engagement with the system. The former two subgroups are most visible only once abuse occurs, and the individuals report to service providers. Our findings point to challenges in accessing substance use prevention and treatment services, including language barriers, health care system navigation issues, and differences between the systems in Poland and Ukraine. Stigma related to seeking care remains a major issue to be addressed. These structural and cultural issues are in line with those reported in other host countries (Davitian et al., 2024).

The arrival of people who use or are at risk for using psychoactive substances requires appropriate public health responses in terms of prevention, treatment, or harm reduction. This analysis suggests that forced migration may place individuals at risk for psychoactive substance use. Participants indicated that experiencing displacement is related to the disintegration of social support as a protective factor, as well as trauma and loss. In some cases, participants noted that affected groups may seldom seek assistance; rather, it is the health care or prevention systems that reach out to them instead. The gender dynamics of displacement and the single-parent roles that must be fulfilled in conjunction with engagement in the labor market present another issue that should be addressed through gender-sensitive research.

The complex situation of Ukrainian war refugees and the risk factors for substance use and abuse among this population need to be carefully monitored. However, the availability of system-level data to assist with this process is lacking. Monitoring efforts must strike a careful balance with the need for data protection. Alcohol normalization should be studied in the context of similar processes in Poland juxtaposed with its high accessibility. Interwoven in the fabric of daily socializing and dangerously associated with coping, the potential for alcohol abuse should be actively discussed within the forced migrant community. The complex situation of the displaced subgroup of people who use opioids or who are receiving opioid agonist treatment is reportedly well recognized (Karagodina et al., 2023) despite claims of Poland being a post-opioid-crisis state, referring to the country's relatively low rates of opioid overdose and a health care system that has moved beyond the serious prevalence phase (Siuda & Matuszewski, 2025). Their situation seems to be addressed to some extent yet requires even more international coordination, given the differences between Ukraine and countries with less dense support networks like Poland (Nikitin et al., 2023).

Ukrainian forcibly displaced youth and potential risk behaviors remain heavily understudied. In spite of government efforts to have all Ukrainian children enrolled in the Polish educational system, a substantial part (especially older children) remains outside of it, and this presents a significant obstacle to reaching them (Garbicz, 2024). This limited contact with institutional settings—such as schools—not only reduces opportunities for early prevention and monitoring but also makes it difficult to involve this group in traditional forms of research. To overcome these barriers, future studies should apply participatory methodologies, which can help engage youth directly, build trust, and counteract stigma and reluctance to discuss mental health issues (Franczak & Lutz, 2024). Such approaches could also help address peer isolation at schools or early dropout (Van Den Berghe et al., 2024). Studies in other countries show that double-schooling can be challenging, and there are limits of support that can be offered remotely by the Ukrainian schools (Chabursky et al., 2024). Few projects have been successful in activating Ukrainian youth when applying bottom-up strategies (e.g., CARE et al., 2024). Any interventions should address the limited protective factors among this group, which include parental supervision and monitoring, opportunities for involvement in school activities, and social norms that discourage drug use (Hawkins et al., 1992).

The results show that future strategies and programs centered on substance use should take into consideration the unique needs, experiences, and cultural contexts of Ukrainians who were forcibly displaced to Poland to be more effective, equitable, and culturally appropriate. Furthermore, the identification of individuals at highest risk for substance use and abuse can inform tailored interventions, allowing for a more efficient allocation of prevention and treatment services in the country. Our data about stigmatization suggest that any awareness campaigns should be designed with caution, taking into account cultural sensitivity and co-design efforts. Related to this, more research of a participatory character is needed to learn about the circumstances of their stay in Poland.

The findings point to several actionable directions across multiple levels. For service providers, culturally adapted and youth-oriented approaches are essential, especially for reaching individuals outside of formal education systems. Researchers should prioritize participatory and inclusive methods to better engage marginalized groups and generate deeper insights into their needs. At the policy level, efforts should focus on reducing structural barriers, enhancing coordination, and supporting co-designed awareness initiatives that are sensitive to the lived experiences of forcibly displaced populations.

7.4.1 Limitations of the Study

This study employed purposive sampling to engage participants with specific knowledge or involvement in substance use prevention and treatment for forcibly displaced Ukrainians in Poland. The sample was not intended to be representative for these populations, so the results are not generalizable. They are rather a momentary snapshot. The sample included health care professionals, NGO staff, and migrants, but some perspectives, particularly from marginalized or less engaged individuals, may be underrepresented. The qualitative design offers rich contextual data but does not quantify the prevalence of identified barriers. Additionally, the focus on Poland means findings may not be directly transferable to other settings. Participants' knowledge was often specific to their roles or contexts, resulting in some fragmentation of information, which may affect the comprehensiveness of the overall picture.

Despite these limitations, the study provides valuable insights by including multiple perspectives from those directly involved with forcibly displaced Ukrainians and substance use services. Gathering data from both service providers and migrants allowed for the triangulation of findings and a more nuanced understanding, partially addressing the challenge of fragmented knowledge. The qualitative approach was particularly suited to exploring the complex and sensitive experiences of this vulnerable population, yielding information that might be difficult to capture through quantitative methods. While context-specific, the findings offer important guidance for improving services and informing future research in comparable contexts.

To our knowledge, this is the first study to provide insight on access to substance use prevention and treatment services for Ukrainians forcibly displaced to Poland. Furthermore, it identifies three subgroups at risk of substance use or abuse among this population. The participants were identified through purposive sampling, which may limit the scope of the information that was captured. Nonetheless, to arrive at these results, we conducted interviews with over twenty individuals from various governmental, NGO, and INGO organizations across the country, as well as with ten migrants who had first-hand knowledge of the topic. Although our study involved participants with a migration background, it included females, most of whom had a higher level of education, which may limit the findings of our work. However, the expert interviews involved front-line workers and managers, some of whom were Ukrainian refugees themselves, who had knowledge about various population groups that they provide services to.

7.5 Conclusion

While none of the three at-risk groups identified in our interviews (those who use or abuse alcohol, those who engage in risky behaviors, and those receiving opioid agonist treatment) are entirely overlooked by the health care system, the first two appear to be insufficiently recognized within current mental health and prevention efforts. Normalized alcohol consumption and risky behaviors among youth are insufficiently studied despite Ukrainian forced migrants having resided in Poland for three years. Although the third group is reportedly well acknowledged and served by opioid harm-reduction programs despite pronounced systemic differences, it tends to remain socially invisible in what is often described as a post-opioid-crisis society. The findings from this study have important implications for policy and practice given the elevated risk of substance use and abuse among displaced migrant populations.

Acknowledgements The authors want to thank all participants who took part in this study and provided us with their invaluable experiences on the topic. We are grateful to Viktoriia Hurochkina, Viktoriia Yanovska, and Svitlana Luchik-Musiyezdova for assistance in data collection.

Competing Interests The authors have no conflicts of interest to declare that are relevant to the content of this chapter.

References

Bachireddy, C., Soule, M. C., Izenberg, J. M., Dvoryak, S., Dumchev, K., & Altice, F. L. (2013). Integration of health services improves multiple health care outcomes among HIV-infected people who inject drugs in Ukraine. *Drug and Alcohol Dependence, 132*(3), 664–673. https://doi.org/10.1016/j.drugalcdep.2013.09.020

CARE, International Rescue Committee, Save the Children. (2024). *Out of school: Assessment on barriers to school enrolment for Ukrainian refugee adolescents in Poland*

Centre for East European and International Studies. (2024). *Flexible solidarity: Polish and Hungarian responses to forced migration.* ZOiS.
Chabursky, S., Gutt, J., & Guglhör-Rudan, A. (2024). Ukrainian refugee adolescents in Germany—A qualitative study on schooling experiences and the fulfillment of basic psychological needs. *Children and Youth Services Review, 160*, 107582.
Charycka, B., Bednarek, J., & Belina, A. (2025). *Kondycja organizacji pozarządowych działających na rzecz uchodźców w Polsce: Raport z badań 2024.* Stowarzyszenie Klon/Jawor.
Charycka, B., Bednarek, J., & Gumkowska, M. (2024). *Kiedy praca w kryzysie staje się codziennością. Lokalne organizacje społeczne wspierające uchodźców w Polsce.* Stowarzyszenie Klon/Jawor.
Davitian, K., Noack, P., Eckstein, K., Hübner, J., & Ahmadi, E. (2024). Barriers of Ukrainian refugees and migrants in accessing German health care. *BMC Health Services Research, 24*(1), 1112.
Długosz, P. (2023). War trauma and strategies for coping with stress among Ukrainian refugees staying in Poland. *Journal of Migration and Health, 8*, 100196.
Duszczyk, M., & Matuszczyk, K. (2022). Non-salary employment conditions as a factor shaping migration decision-making: An example of workers from Ukraine in Poland. *Migration Letters, 19*(6), Article 6. https://doi.org/10.33182/ml.v19i5.2162
Ellard-Gray, A., Jeffrey, N. K., Choubak, M., & Crann, S. E. (2015). Finding the hidden participant: Solutions for recruiting hidden, hard-to-reach, and vulnerable populations. *International Journal of Qualitative Methods, 14*(5), 1609406915621420. https://doi.org/10.1177/1609406915621420
Franczak, I. B., & Lutz, A. C. (2024). Kids in limbo: War, uncertainty, and the school experiences of Ukrainian refugee students in Poland. *Sociological Forum, 39*(4), 413–426.
Fundacja Watch Health Care. (2025, January). *Barometr WHC 2024: Polacy w kolejkach. Raport dotyczący zmian dostępności do gwarantowanych świadczeń zdrowotnych w Polsce* (No. 01/01/2025). Retrieved May 30, 2025 from https://drive.google.com/file/d/1sIYlpbGXH0aHl25da4ujAxe8tPYatORw/view
Garbicz, K. (2024, October 8). *Mucha: Tylko 20 tys. nowych dzieci z Ukrainy trafiło do szkół. Presja 800 plus nie działa?* https://oko.press/mucha-tylko-20-tys-nowych-dzieci-z-ukrainy-trafilo-do-szkol-presja-800-plus-nie-dziala
Główny Urząd Statystyczny. (2023). *Działalność stowarzyszeń i podobnych organizacji społecznych, fundacji, społecznych podmiotów wyznaniowych oraz samorządu gospodarczego i zawodowego w 2022 r. – wyniki wstępne.*
Górny, A., Grzymała- Moszczyńska, H., Klaus, W., & Łodziński, S. (2017). *"Uchodźcy w Polsce. Sytuacja prawna, skala napływu i integracja w społeczeństwie polskim oraz rekomendacje".* Ekspertyzy Komitetu Badań nad Migracjami PAN. Polska Akademia Nauk, Warsaw.
Hawkins, J. D., Catalano, R. F., & Miller, J. Y. (1992). Risk and protective factors for alcohol and other drug problems in adolescence and early adulthood: Implications for substance abuse prevention. *Psychological Bulletin, 112*(1), 64–105. https://doi.org/10.1037/0033-2909.112.1.64
International Organization for Migration. (2024). *Ukraine and neighbouring countries 2022–2024: Two years of response.*
International Society of Substance Use Professionals. (2025). *Poland.* Retrieved May 30, 2025, from https://www.issup.net/knowledge-share/country-profiles/poland
Ivashko, O., & Prykhodchenko, L. (n.d.). *The role of Polish non-governmental organizations in helping Ukrainian refugees: Social and economic aspects of adaptation.* Lesya Ukrainka Volyn National University. https://evnuir.vnu.edu.ua/bitstream/123456789/26288/1/Ivashko_Prykhodchenko.pdf
Karagodina, O., Kovtun, O., Filippovych, M., & Neduzhko, O. (2023). Qualitative study of barriers and facilitators to HIV detection and treatment among women who inject drugs during the war against Ukraine. *AIDS Research and Therapy, 20*(1), 80.

Kordel, P., Rządeczka, M., Studenna-Skrukwa, M., Kwiatkowska-Moskalewicz, K., Goncharenko, O., & Moskalewicz, M. (2024). Acute Stress Disorder among 2022 Ukrainian war refugees: A cross-sectional study. *Frontiers in Public Health, 12*, 1280236.

Kovács, J., Csukonyi, C., Kovács, K. E., Liszka, D., & Walawender, P. (2023). Integrative attitudes of Ukrainian war refugees in two neighboring European countries (Poland and Hungary) in connection with posttraumatic stress symptoms and social support. *Frontiers in Public Health, 11*, 1256102.

Krajowe Centrum Przeciwdziałania Uzależnieniom. (2023). *System przeciwdziałania uzależnieniom w Polsce*. https://kcpu.gov.pl

Ministry of Health. (2022). *Health needs map: Psychiatric care and addiction treatment 2022–2026*. https://basiw.mz.gov.pl/mapy-informacje/mapa-2022-2026/analizy/opieka-psychiatryczna-i-leczenie-uzaleznien

Nikitin, B. M., Bromberg, D. J., Madden, L. M., Stöver, H., Teltzrow, R., & Altice, F. L. (2023). Leveraging existing provider networks in Europe to eliminate barriers to accessing opioid agonist maintenance therapies for Ukrainian refugees. *PLOS Global Public Health, 3*(7), e0002168.

OECD. (2024). *International Migration Outlook 2024: Poland*. OECD Publishing. https://www.oecd.org/en/publications/international-migration-outlook-2024_50b0353e-en/full-report/poland_f5b1bd47.html

Osica, O., Hamerski, A., & Gawrońska, M. (2024). *Warszawa w kryzysie uchodźczym*. Urząd Miasta Warszawy.

Pędziwiatr, P., Bielska, I., Wanke, M., & Luchik-Musiyezdova, S. (2024a). *Health care provision for economic and forced migrants in Kraków*. CASPAR—OWiM.

Pędziwiatr, K., Stonawski, M., Brzozowski, J., & Szkołut, S. (2024b). *Imigranci ekonomiczni i przymusowi w Krakowie w 2024 roku*. CASPAR—OWiM.

Save the Children & Klon/Jawor Association. (2024). *The condition of non-governmental organisations working with refugees in Poland: Research report*. Save the Children. https://resourcecentre.savethechildren.net/document/the-condition-of-non-governmental-organisations-working-with-refugees-in-poland-research-report-2024/

Sibley, R. (2025). *When Ukrainian refugees in Poland needed help, we were there*. International Medical Corps.

Siuda, P., & Matuszewski, P. (2025). The opioid crisis in Poland? Insights from online forum data. *International Journal of Drug Policy, 142*, 104844.

Sobczak-Szelc, K., Pachocka, M., Pędziwiatr, K., Szałańska, J., & Szulecka, M. (2023). *From reception to integration of asylum seekers and refugees in Poland*. Routledge.

Tong, A., Sainsbury, P., & Craig, J. (2007). Consolidated criteria for reporting qualitative research (COREQ): A 32-item checklist for interviews and focus groups. *International Journal for Quality in Health Care, 19*(6), 349–357.

Urbański, P. K., Schroeder, K., Nadolska, A., & Wilski, M. (2024). Symptoms of depression and anxiety among Ukrainian children displaced to Poland following the outbreak of the Russo-Ukrainian war: Associations with coping strategies and resilience. *Applied Psychology: Health and Well-Being, 16*(3), 851–867.

Urząd do Spraw Cudzoziemców. (2023). Obywatele Ukrainy w Polsce—raport statystyczny. *Biuletyn Informacyjny Urzędu do Spraw Cudzoziemców*. Retrieved May 30, 2026, from https://www.gov.pl/web/udsc/obywatele-ukrainy-w-polsce--raport-statystyczny

Van Den Berghe, L., Pouille, A., Vandevelde, S., & De Pauw, S. S. W. (2024). Looking beyond primary barriers: Support workers' perspectives on school dropout among students with a migration background. *Journal of Ethnic & Cultural Diversity in Social Work, 33*(1), 34–46.

Venger, O., Mysula, Y., Oliynyk, O., Striepetova, O., & Kulivets, O. (2024). Structure and features of psychopathological symptoms in forced migrants and internally displaced persons. *Polish Medical Bibiliography, 77*(2), 225–232.

World Health Organization. (2013). *Consolidated guidelines on the use of antiretroviral drugs for treating and preventing HIV infection: Recommendations for a public health approach*. https://www.ncbi.nlm.nih.gov/books/NBK374288/

Chapter 8
Mental Health Problems Among Unaccompanied Refugee Minors Treated for Substance Abuse

Anna-Karin Ivert and Mia-Maria Magnusson

8.1 Introduction

In 2015, more than 1.2 million people applied for asylum in the European Union (Eurostat, 2025a), and of those almost 90,000 were unaccompanied refugee minors (URM) (Eurostat, 2025b). Sweden, together with Germany, was the country that received the highest number of asylum applications from URMs, with more than 30,000 applying for asylum in Sweden in that year (Eurostat, 2025b). Compared to the total population of asylum seekers in 2015, when people from Syria were in the majority, the majority of URMs had their background in Afghanistan (Swedish Migration Agency, 2025). In Sweden, the vulnerability of URMs received a lot of attention in the following years, both in public debate and by governmental and non-governmental organisations (e.g. Barnombudsmannen, 2017; Länsstyrelsen, 2016, 2022). Two issues that were raised as a source of concern were the mental health of the minors and the occurrence of substance abuse.

Over the ten years that have passed since then, the number of applications for asylum has decreased dramatically as a consequence of more restrictive legislation and increased border controls in both Sweden and the rest of the EU (see e.g. Goverment office of Sweden (2025). In 2024, less than 500 URMs applied for asylum in Sweden, about half of them arriving from Ukraine and applying for protection under the EU´s Temporary Protection Directive (Swedish Migration Agency, 2024). Despite this decline, the health and wellbeing of these children and young adults

A.-K. Ivert (✉)
Department of Criminology, Malmö University, Malmö, Sweden
e-mail: anna-karin.ivert@mau.se

M.-M. Magnusson
Department of Police Work, Malmö University, Malmö, Sweden

Police Department of Stockholm Region, Swedish Police, Stockholm, Sweden

C. De Kock (ed.), *Substance Use Among Refugees in Europe*,
https://doi.org/10.1007/978-3-032-32399-6_8

will continue to present an important concern for societies, both in Sweden and other European countries.

Research on URMs addresses diverse topics such as age assessment (Thevissen et al., 2012), the structure of care and reception (Derluyn & Broekaert, 2008; Kalverboer et al., 2017; Stjerna Doohan et al., 2024; Wimelius et al., 2017), how the children experience their living conditions in the country of destination (Lundberg & Dahlquist, 2012; Malmsten, 2014; Wernesjö, 2014) and how they describe their everyday life and feelings of loneliness and uncertainty about the future (Herz & Lalander, 2017; Lundberg & Dahlquist, 2012; Malmsten, 2014). Much research has focused on the problems encountered by URMs upon arriving in the resettlement country or on difficulties associated with the reception process. However, studies have also discussed the positive relationships, resilience, coping, capacities and strengths found in this group (Eide & Hjern, 2013; Kohli, 2006; Raghallaigh & Gilligan, 2010; Seglem et al., 2014; Solhaug et al., 2025). Studies show that URMs demonstrate capacity and resilience in terms of finding employment and presenting a willingness to work (Çelikaksoy & Wadensjö, 2017), and that positive development is associated with factors such as the use of healthy coping mechanisms, religiosity, involvement in prosocial organisations and a positive outlook (Carlson et al., 2012; Raghallaigh & Gilligan, 2010).

A significant part of the research on URMs has focused on their mental health (see e.g. Ivert & Magnusson, 2020). Over time, a high prevalence of mental health problems among URMs has been found in studies conducted in several European countries, which differ with regard to their immigration policies and the ways in which reception and care are organised and also with regard to the nationalities of the arriving URMs, such as the Netherlands (Bean et al., 2007a, 2007b), Belgium (Derluyn et al., 2009), Austria (Huemer et al., 2011), Norway (Oppedal & Idsoe, 2012), Finland (Sourander, 1998) and Sweden (Ramel et al., 2015; Stjerna Doohan et al., 2024). However, an issue that has been given less attention in the research literature is the issue of how mental health problems are related to substance abuse and criminality among URMs (Ivert & Magnusson, 2020).

In the current chapter, we explore the patterns of substance abuse and mental health problems among URMs who were referred to outpatient clinics for adolescents with substance use problems in the city of Stockholm, Sweden during 2016 and 2017. We describe the patterns of substance abuse and mental health problems found among the URMs, investigate the prevalence of criminality and associations with delinquent peers and experiences of victimisation. Since the importance of access to appropriate care has been stressed in previous research, we also explore to what extent the adolescents had received treatment within the child and adolescent psychiatric (CAP) care. Lessons learned from this period have important implications for society in terms of acknowledging and addressing problems among a group of vulnerable adolescents who, for different reasons, are at increased risk of being exposed to social settings where they risk being abused, becoming involved in drug use and criminality or being recruited into organised crime.

The chapter begins with a brief review of the literature on mental health problems and substance abuse among URMs.

8.1.1 *Mental Health Problems Among URMs*

In the literature, several studies show that many URMs appear to be vulnerable to internalising problems, such as post-traumatic stress disorder, depression and anxiety (Derluyn et al., 2009; Fazel et al., 2012; Prod'hom et al., 2024), but that they report few externalising problems, such as delinquent behaviour (e.g. Bean et al., 2007a, 2007b; Derluyn et al., 2008; Huemer et al., 2011). This is confirmed in a recent review of the literature (Prod'hom et al., 2024). The apparent rarity of externalising problems within this group has been discussed as perhaps being a result of URMs being hesitant to report behaviours that they believe may be considered undesirable (e.g. Derluyn & Broekaert, 2007; Huemer et al., 2011; Prod'hom et al., 2024). The high levels of internalising problems found among URMs are often explained by reference to their experiences of loss of family and friends, trauma prior to and during their flight or a stressful asylum process and the fear of deportation (Derluyn & Broekaert, 2007, 2008; Fazel et al., 2012; Stjerna Doohan et al., 2024). The traumas and mental health problems experienced by many of these children often go untreated (e.g. Stjerna Doohan et al., 2024). Mental health problems being overlooked or not receiving appropriate care also appear to have long-term consequences. Studies that have followed unaccompanied children over time show that their high levels of internalising problems appear to remain years after resettlement (Bean et al., 2007a, 2007b; Jakobsen et al., 2014; Jensen et al., 2014). However, the mental health of unaccompanied minors might also be influenced by their experiences of, for example, racism and discrimination in the country of resettlement (Herz & Lalander, 2021). Experiences of difficulties such as discrimination and economic hardship have been shown to increase depressive symptoms among unaccompanied minors (Keles et al., 2016; Seglem et al., 2014).

8.1.2 *Substance Abuse Among URMs*

Despite the association between mental health problems and substance abuse that has been established in previous research on the general population (Lai et al., 2015; Turner et al., 2018), research focused on substance abuse among URMs remains scarce (Ivert & Magnusson, 2020). Substance abuse is sometimes included as an item in scales aimed at measuring mental health problems (Derluyn et al., 2009; Huemer et al., 2011; Oppedal & Idsoe, 2012; Thommessen et al., 2013) or is occasionally, briefly mentioned in studies investigating the post-migration challenges and conditions of URMs' everyday lives (Auger-Voyer et al., 2014; Herz & Lalander, 2017; Kalverboer et al., 2017). Manhica and colleagues (2017) showed that unaccompanied refugees were at higher risk of hospitalisation due to alcohol-related disorders compared to their accompanied peers, and that unaccompanied male refugees were at higher risk of criminality and hospital care associated with substance abuse than native Swedish males (Manhica et al., 2016). Manhica and colleagues (2017) also found that the longer the male refugees had been resident in Sweden, the higher their risk of substance use. The authors also discuss whether the increased risk for hospitalisation due to alcohol-related disorders among URMs might be explained by a lack of social control from parents or other adult family members, factors which might otherwise function as a buffer against risky behaviours.

In Sweden, the phenomenon of drug use among URMs attracted significant attention in public debate and among Swedish authorities during the years following the refugee crisis in 2015. The police in the metropolitan region of Stockholm, the country's capital, report having witnessed an increase in URMs engaging in crime and spending time in social settings characterised by drug dealing and drug use (Pettersson, 2016). A majority of these children were boys from North Africa, but there was also a smaller group from Afghanistan. The most common drugs used by these children were hashish and benzodiazepines, and some of the Afghan youths also used opiates (Pettersson, 2016). The Swedish National Board of Institutional Care (SiS) reported having witnessed an increase in placements of URMs (Kaunitz & Jakobsson, 2016). More than 60% of these children/adolescents were from North Africa (i.e. Morocco and Algeria). For a majority of the URMs placed in institutional care, substance abuse was named as a reason in the placement application, followed by conflicts or violence at a previous more open institution, and then mental health problems, running away and criminality such as stealing or shoplifting (Kaunitz & Jakobsson, 2016).

The issue of substance abuse among URMs in Sweden is also addressed in reports on children who have gone missing. A report by the County Administrative Boards of Sweden showed that many municipalities identified drug use as a common risk behaviour observed among URMs in connection with their going missing[1] (Länsstyrelsen, 2016, 2022). Further, URMs that go missing may end up on the street, in contexts where they are exposed to abuse, criminality and drugs; these children are also at increased risk of being subjected to human trafficking and exploitation (Barnombudsmannen, 2017; Länsstyrelsen, 2022).

To increase the knowledge on drug use among unaccompanied refugee youth (up to age 21), the Swedish government instructed the Public Health Agency of Sweden, in collaboration with the National Board of Health and Welfare, to investigate drug use among unaccompanied refugee youth in Sweden. Findings from this investigation are inconclusive. However, an analysis of data from outpatient clinics for adolescents with substance use problems shows that patterns of drug use are rather similar between URMs and the other adolescents treated at these clinics (Dahlberg & Anderberg, 2017; Folkhälsomyndigheten, 2017). Although the study does not allow for conclusions about the magnitude of the problem, reports from the social services and from interviews with practitioners working with URMs show that substance abuse does occur, and that the problem is viewed as a cause for concern and as one that needs to be acknowledged (Folkhälsomyndigheten, 2017).

[1] In this case the Swedish Migration Agency considers a child as being missing when there is no knowledge of the child's whereabouts and neither the social services the child's legal guardian or public council have any information (Länsstyrelsen, 2022).

8.1.3 Mental Health Problems and Substance Abuse

The association between mental health problems, internalising as well as externalising problems, and substance use is well established in the research literature on substance abuse among adolescents (Hawkins, 2009; Nawi et al., 2021). Research on adolescents being treated for substance use problems shows that these adolescents report high levels of various mental health symptoms or problems, and that this is particularly true among girls (Anderberg & Dahlberg, 2018) and adolescents with experiences of victimisation (Anderberg & Dahlberg, 2016). In addition, research has also shown that substance abuse during adolescence is associated with mental health problems later in the life course (Degenhardt et al., 2013; Gobbi et al., 2019). The co-occurrence of mental health problems and substance abuse has been identified as an important challenge for both mental health care and substance abuse clinics (Hawkins, 2009). It has been argued that the best way to address this is through a multidisciplinary approach, where both substance use and mental health problems can be addressed simultaneously (Richert et al., 2020), and there is a need for both thorough mental health care screening of adolescents who are referred to substance abuse clinics and integrated treatment programmes that address both problems (Hodgins et al., 2010).

Even if knowledge on substance abuse among URMs is limited, many researchers argue that there is an urgent need to provide sufficient care in relation to the high levels of mental health problems found within the group and also to acknowledge the potential negative consequences of mental health problems going untreated (Derluyn & Broekaert, 2007; Marquardt et al., 2016; Oppedal & Idsoe, 2012; Stjerna Doohan et al., 2024; Thommessen et al., 2013). Appropriate interventions to target mental health problems might prevent the development of more serious social problems, such as delinquency and substance abuse (Huemer et al., 2011). In a study on adaptation among Sudanese URMs in the USA, Luster and colleagues (2010) conclude by noting that 'since substance abuse and mental health problems can be significant barriers to successful adaptation, it is important that service providers find ways to overcome the cultural stigma and offer culturally appropriate support for those experiencing problems' (p. 208).

Substance abuse, or the risk of substance abuse, among URMs is sometimes discussed in terms of self-medication, i.e. that alcohol or drugs are used by the URMs to cope with painful experiences, mental health problems or the challenges of integrating into a new society (e.g. Deveci, 2012; Luster et al., 2010; Manhica et al., 2017). URMs' use of drugs as a means of coping with stressful memories has also been acknowledged by Swedish practitioners working with this group (Pettersson, 2016).

To summarise, knowledge on substance abuse among URMs is limited. However, research has discussed the high levels of mental health problems found in this group in relation to an increased vulnerability for the development of substance abuse problems. In addition, researchers and practitioners underline the importance of acknowledging the occurrence of both mental health problems and substance abuse among

URMs. This is important, not least in relation to adequate care provision, which is crucial for breaking a negative trajectory that might lead to continued substance use and worsen mental health problems, as well as other types of problems such as criminality and victimisation, to prevent negative development. Against this background, the following section will explore different aspects of substance abuse and mental health problems found among URMs who have been referred to outpatient clinics for adolescents with substance use problems in Stockholm, Sweden.

8.2 Data and Methods

The data employed in the present study was collected from the registers of outpatient clinics for adolescents with substance use problems in the city of Stockholm, Sweden, and include all URMs who were referred to these clinics in 2016 and 2017 ($N = 60$), and who participated in an initial screening interview (UngDOK). This data contains no personal information or information that can be linked to a specific individual.

The screening interview was conducted by treatment staff at the clinic and covers the following areas: housing and financial support; occupation; alcohol, drug and tobacco use; treatment history; criminality; childhood; exposure to violence; family and relationships and physical health and mental health. The psychometric properties of the scale measuring alcohol and substance use and the scale measuring mental health problems have previously been tested, with the result that they are generally satisfactory (see e.g. Dahlberg et al., 2017). It is, however, important to remember that this refers to the general population, and validation has not been done in relation to this particular population, i.e. URMs.

Initially, the sample comprised 63 minors, three of whom were excluded following an evaluation of the data, which indicated that these three individuals had most likely been incorrectly categorised as URMs due to a coding error.[2] The final sample consists of 60 URMs.

8.2.1 Measures

The present study includes the screening interview questions covering the adolescents' drug use and their mental health and also questions on criminality, association with delinquent peers, victimisation, problems in the childhood environment and previous and ongoing contacts with CAP care.

[2] In all three cases the adolescents' country of birth was Sweden, and all three reported that they were currently living with their parents and that they had always lived with their parents.

8.2.1.1 Drug Use

The patterns of drug use are described using questions on primary drug (type of drug), frequency of use during the last 30 days, frequency of use during the last three months, age at onset for primary drug use and polydrug use. The questionnaire also includes questions on alcohol use.

8.2.1.2 Mental Health

The interview comprises questions on 11 mental health-related problems, and the extent to which the minors had experienced any of these over the life course and during the last 30 days. The following problems were included: sleep disturbance; depression; anxiety; concentration difficulties; violent behaviour; suicidal thoughts; suicide attempts; hallucinations; medication for psychological disorders; eating disorders and self-harming behaviour. The answers were coded as Yes (=1) or No (=0).

The items measuring mental health problems were also summed to produce an index, measuring overall experiences of mental health problems (alpha = .80; min = 0; max = 12).[3] Prior to constructing the index, missing values were dealt with by replacing them with the mode. This was done in cases in which the distribution of the answers to a given question was 90% versus 10%. For all of the questions included in the index, this resulted in replacing missing values with No = 0. This procedure was only conducted for adolescents who responded to a minimum of 50% of the questions, which meant that index scores were calculated for a total of 48 adolescents.

8.2.1.3 Criminality and Association with Delinquent Peers

To assess criminality, the following questions were used: *have you ever been arrested by the police*? and *have you ever been convicted of a crime*? The answers were coded as Yes (=1) and No (=0). In addition to the minors' own drug use and criminality, we also included measures of association with delinquent peers. These were based on the questions: *do you spend time with peers that use drugs*? and *do you spend time with peers that engage in criminal behaviour?* The answers were coded as Yes (=1) and No (=0).

---

[3] Lifetime experience of mental health problems (alpha = .68; min = 0; max = 8); mental health problems during the last 30 days (alpha = .68; min = 0; max = 6).

8.2.1.4 Victimisation and Experience of Trauma

The questionnaire includes four questions related to victimisation, one generic question (*have you ever been a victim of a crime*?), and three questions associated with exposure to different types of violence: *physical, psychological* or *sexual violence.* Sexual violence was excluded in this study due to low prevalence. The answers were coded as Yes (=1) and No (=0). The latter three were combined to produce a single measure on exposure to violence, where 0 indicates no experience of violence and 1 indicates experience of either physical or psychological violence.

In the screening interview, the minors were also asked about experience of trauma: *have you ever experienced a traumatic event that still affects you psychologically?* The response alternatives were Yes (=1) and No (=0).

8.2.1.5 On-Going and Previous Contacts with CAP Care

To assess the extent to which the minors had received treatment for mental health problems, the screening questions on previous[4] and ongoing contacts with CAP care were used. The answers were coded as Yes (=1) or No (=0).

8.2.2 Statistical Analysis

The analysis begins by describing patterns of drug use and mental health problems, as well as the occurrence of criminality, associations with delinquent peers, victimisation, problems in the childhood environment and contacts with CAP care. Mean values for the summed mental health index were then calculated in order to identify possible differences in mental health in relation to drug use patterns, criminality, associations with delinquent peers, victimisation and contacts with CAP care. The differences were tested by means of a t-test, and Cohen's d was calculated.

8.3 Findings

8.3.1 Descriptives

Table 8.1 presents an overview of the demographic characteristics of the sample. The mean age of the URMs in the sample is 16.5 years (range 14–19). Almost all of the URMs in the sample are male, and a majority has their origins in Afghanistan, followed by Eritrea, Somalia and Morocco. This distribution corresponds to the

[4] This could refer to care received before coming to Sweden.

general distribution of URMs in Sweden during that period (Swedish Migration Agency, 2025). Over the last 30 days, most of the minors had either lived in an institution/home for care and housing or had a family home (i.e. foster care) placement. Almost all of the URMs were enrolled in the educational system, most of them in upper secondary school. Only a few (8%) reported being in neither education, employment nor training. Almost all adolescents (98%) had an ongoing contact with the social services. The interview includes no information on how long the adolescents have resided in Sweden or on their immigration status. In most cases (85%), the minors had been referred to the substance use clinics by the social services or the healthcare sector.

Table 8.1 Descriptive statistics for demographic factors and substance use for total sample ($N = 60$)

	N	% or mean
Demographics		
Mean age		16.5
Gender		
Female	2	3
Male	57	95
Missing	1	2
Country of birth		
Afghanistan	22	37
Eritrea	10	17
Somalia	7	12
Morocco	5	8
Other*	16	26
Living conditions/housing (last 30 days)		
Institution/homes for care and housing	28	47
Family home	23	38
Other	8	13
Occupation		
Compulsory school	17	28
Upper secondary school	23	38
(Language) introduction class	15	25
None	5	8

* Bangladesh, Ethiopia, Iraq, Iran, Yemen, Kurdistan, Saudi Arabia, Sudan, Syria, Thailand and Tunisia

Table 8.2 Patterns of drug use ($N = 60$)

	N	% or mean
Primary drug (N = 57)		
Cannabis	51	85
Alcohol	4	7
Other*	2	3
Frequency of use primary drug (last 30 days) (N = 56)		
No use	41	68
Occasionally/one day a week or less	9	15
2 days a week or more	6	10
Frequency of use primary drug (last 3 months) (N = 55)		
No use	15	25
Occasionally/one day a week or less	28	47
2 days a week or more	12	20
Mean age of onset primary drug ($N = 60$)		15.5
Polydrug use	21	35

* Amphetamines, heroin

8.3.2 *Patterns of Drug Use*

Table 8.2 presents patterns of drug use within the sample. The primary drug for a majority (85%) of the minors was cannabis, though some reported alcohol as their primary drug and a small number reported other drugs. A majority of the minors reported no use of the primary drug during the last 30 days, and almost 50% of the minors reported use of the primary drug on one day per week or less over the last three months. Regular use, two to three days a week or more, was reported by 20% of the minors. Age at onset for primary drug use was on average 15.5 years. About one-third of the sample reported that they used more than one drug; the most common secondary drug was alcohol.

Frequent alcohol use appears to be rather unusual—more than 90% of the URMs reported that they never or almost never (once a month or less) drank alcohol—and alcohol use was therefore excluded from further analysis (data not shown).

8.3.3 *Mental Health Problems*

Table 8.3 presents patterns of mental health problems. Overall, problems such as sleep disturbances, depression and anxiety were common, both during the last 30 days and over the life course. About one-quarter of the minors reported that they had experienced concentration difficulties. Less than 10% reported that they had ever experienced difficulties controlling aggressive or violent behaviour, and very few had experienced this during the past 30 days. Almost one-third of the minors stated that they had experienced serious suicidal thoughts at some point, but only a few had experienced thoughts of this kind during the past 30 days. Suicide attempts, hallucinations (non-drug-related) and eating disorders were uncommon, both during the last 30 days and over the life course. Just over 20% of the minors reported having engaged in self-harming behaviour at some point during their lives, but as with suicidal thoughts, only a few reported having engaged in this behaviour during the last 30 days. About 15% reported that they had been prescribed psychotropic medication at some point.

A categorisation based on the occurrence and severity of reported symptoms among the 48 minors who answered more than 50% of the mental health-related questions showed that 16% reported no problems or only occasional problems/symptoms. Just over 50% reported several common symptoms of stress (sleep disturbance, depression, anxiety and/or concentration difficulties) but no or only occasional serious/severe symptoms/problems (violent behaviour, suicidal thoughts, suicide attempts, hallucinations, eating disorders and/or self-harming behaviour). Almost one-third reported that they had experienced several common stress symptoms and two or more serious/severe symptoms.

8.3.4 Criminality, Victimisation and Psychiatric Care

Table 8.4 presents data on the occurrence of criminality, associations with delinquent peers, victimisation and contacts with CAP care. About 40% of the minors reported that they had experience of being arrested by the police, and 10% reported having a criminal conviction. Only a few (7%) stated that they regularly spent time with friends who engage in criminal activities. One-quarter of the minors reported that they regularly spent time with peers who use drugs.

The items measuring victimisation and exposure to violence indicate that these are rather common experiences among the minors in this study. One-third of the minors reported that they have been victims of a crime, and more than 50% reported that they have been exposed to violence. Experiences of physical violence were most common, followed by psychological violence. Only a few reported experiences of sexual violence. Overall, about 35% of the minors reported that they had experienced two or more forms of violence. About 50% of the minors stated that they have had experiences of traumatic events that still affect them psychologically.

About 30% reported having undergone voluntary psychiatric care at a CAP care clinic in the past, and about 15% reported having ongoing contact with CAP.

The interviews also included questions on whether the minors had at any time been subjected to compulsory custodial care. Only one of the minors had experience of this, i.e. care in accordance with the Care of Young Persons (special Provisions) Act (LVU).

Table 8.3 Descriptive statistics for mental health problems ($N = 60$)

Variable	N	% or mean
Sleep disturbance		
Lifetime	46	77
Last 30 days	38	63
Depression		
Lifetime	40	67
Last 30 days	28	47
Anxiety		
Lifetime	36	60
Last 30 days	26	43
Concentration difficulties		
Lifetime	15	25
Last 30 days	13	22
Violent behaviour		
Lifetime	5	8
Last 30 days	<5	–
Suicidal thoughts		
Lifetime	18	30
Last 30 days	<5	–
Suicide attempts		
Lifetime	5	8
Last 30 days	–	–
Hallucinations		
Lifetime	<5	–
Last 30 days	<5	–
Eating disorders		
Lifetime	<5	–
Last 30 days	<5	–
Self-harming behaviour		
Lifetime	13	22
Last 30 days	<5	–
Medication for psychiatric disorders		
Lifetime	9	15
Last 30 days	5	8
Categorisation based on symptoms*		
No significant symptoms	8	16

(continued)

Table 8.3 (continued)

Variable	N	% or mean
Common stress symptoms, no serious symptoms	25	52
Common stress symptoms and serious symptoms	15	31

* This categorisation only includes minors with data on more than 50 percent of the questions measuring mental health problems ($N = 48$)

Table 8.4 Descriptive statistics for criminality, associations with delinquent peers, victimisation, problems in the childhood environment and contacts with CAP care ($N = 60$)

	N	%
Arrested by the police	24	40
Criminal conviction	6	10
Peers who engage in criminal behaviour*	<5	–
Peers who use drugs	15	25
Victim of crime	20	33
Exposure to violence	32	53
Experience of trauma	32	53
Previous treatment at CAP	18	30
Ongoing treatment at CAP	9	15

* Excluded from further analysis

8.3.5 *Drug Use, Criminality, Victimisation and Utilisation of CAP Care in Relation to Symptoms of Mental Health Problems*

Table 8.5 presents the relationships between the summed index of mental health problems and drug use patterns, criminality, associations with delinquent peers, victimisation and contacts with CAP care. Since the analysis is based on a small sample, and individual observations can therefore have a major impact, the results should be interpreted with caution. The overall differences between subgroups were small. One of the associations that appear to be more pronounced is polydrug use, with minors who reported regular use of more than one substance also reporting more symptoms of mental health problems. Not surprisingly, the findings also show that minors with experience of trauma report higher levels of mental health problems. Finally, minors who had ongoing or previous contacts with CAP care also reported higher levels of mental health problems.

Separate analyses of lifetime experiences of mental health problems and mental health problems during the last 30 days produced similar results to those found for the combined measure.

Table 8.5 Drug use, criminality, victimisation and utilisation of CAP care in relation to symptoms of mental health problems. High values indicate more symptoms. Mean values with standard deviations in brackets

	Mental health problems		
	N	Mean (SD)	*t*-value /Cohen´s d
Primary drug			
Cannabis	39	5.9 (3.3)	-1.087^{ns}/0.50
Other	5	4.2 (3.4)	
Frequency of use			
2–3 days/week or more	7	7.4 (3.2)	-1.400^{ns} /0.59
Less than 2 days/week	35	5.5 (3.3)	
Age at onset			
15 years or younger	13	5.5 (3.4)	0.902^{ns}/0.30
16 years or older	24	6.5 (3.3)	
Polydrug use			
Yes	15	7.4 (2.7)	-1.087^{**}/0.85
No	32	4.8 (3.4)	
Arrested by the police			
Yes	20	5.3 (3.7)	0.231^{ns}/0.06
No	22	5.5 (3.1)	
Criminal conviction			
Yes	5	5.4 (3.1)	0.087^{ns} /0
No	35	5.4 (3.5)	
Peers who use drugs			
Yes	11	6.5 (3.6)	-0.801^{ns} /0.29
No	34	5.5 (3.2)	
Victim of crime			
Yes	19	6.0 (3.5)	-0.779^{ns} /0.26
No	21	5.1 (3.5)	
Exposure to violence			
Yes	27	5.8 (3.5)	-0.539^{ns} /0.2
No	14	5.1 (3.7)	
Experience of trauma			
Yes	27	7.1 (2.8)	−5.428***/1.76
No	15	2.5 (2.4)	
Previous treatment at CAP			
Yes	17	7.8 (2.3)	−3.562**/1.16
No	29	4.5 (3.3)	
Ongoing treatment at CAP			

(continued)

Table 8.5 (continued)

	Mental health problems		
	N	Mean (SD)	*t*-value /Cohen´s d
Yes	7	8.0 (3.5)	−2.069*/0.84
No	40	5.2 (3.2)	

ns = Not significant, *$p < 0.05$, **$p < 0.01$, ***$p < 0.001$

8.4 Discussion

This study aimed to describe patterns of substance abuse and mental health problems among URMs referred to outpatient clinics for adolescents with substance use problems in Stockholm, Sweden. The sample comprised 60 URMs aged 14 to 19 years (mean age 16.5). The majority were male and had their origins in Afghanistan, followed by Eritrea, Somalia and Morocco.

Findings show that many URMs who begin outpatient treatment for substance abuse have significant mental health problems, especially in individuals reporting polydrug use and those reporting experience of trauma. The high levels of what may be considered internalising mental health problems observed in this study are in line with the results of previous research that has investigated the occurrence of mental health problems in other URM populations (Bean et al., 2007a, 2007b; Derluyn et al., 2009; Huemer et al., 2011; Oppedal & Idsoe, 2012; Ramel et al., 2015; Sourander, 1998). The data used in this study only include one measure of what may be considered as an expression of externalising problems, i.e. problems controlling violent behaviour. This is a limitation of this study, and additional measures could have captured more dimensions of externalising behaviour. Less than 10% of the study sample reported having experienced this type of problem. This is also in line with results from previous research, which has shown that URMs report few externalising behaviours or substance-related problems (e.g. Bean et al., 2007a, 2007b, Prod'hom et al., 2024). It has been hypothesised that this might be a result of URMs being hesitant to report behaviours that may be considered undesirable (Derluyn & Broekaert, 2007; Huemer et al., 2011). Another hypothesis presented is that the developmental context shared by URMs enforcing regulatory processes that promote the handling of aggression in order to avoid getting into trouble in a way that might jeopardise the youths' asylum process and future residence status (Oppedal & Idsoe, 2012). The fact that only a few adolescents in the present study reported regular drug use during the past 30 days, as well as during the past three months may indicate a reluctance to disclose socially undesirable behaviours.

The high prevalence of mental health problems in this group implies that substance abuse clinics, as well as other institutions/facilities, need to supplement the provision of treatment for substance abuse with treatment for mental health-related problems. It has been argued that providing adolescents with support for both substance abuse and mental health problems will reduce their need to use drugs to self-medicate (Anderberg & Dahlberg, 2016; Turner et al., 2018). Previous research has also noted that URMs may use drugs to self-medicate or as a means of coping with painful memories (Deveci, 2012; Luster et al., 2010), and it has been stressed that there is a significant need for interventions focused on supporting URMs who suffer from mental health problems, as well as for properly trained care workers and valid diagnostic instruments (Bean et al., 2007a, 2007b; Derluyn & Broekaert, 2007; Marquardt et al., 2016; Oppedal & Idsoe, 2012; Stjerna Doohan et al., 2024; Thommessen et al., 2013). Based on the findings from the present study, only a few (15%) of the URMs have ongoing contacts with CAP clinics, something which must be considered troubling considering the high levels of mental health problems found within this group. However, if mental health problems are identified when the minors begin treatment for substance abuse, this may provide an opportunity to refer them to CAP care and to initiate collaborations that provide support in relation to both substance abuse and mental health.

The URMs included in the present study appear to have become relatively well established in Swedish society—most of them have a stable housing situation and have established contacts with authorities such as the social services. Nevertheless, approximately 40% of the adolescents in the current study report having been arrested by the police.[5] URMs lack social support and social control from parents or other adult family members; factors which might otherwise function as a buffer against risky behaviours (cf. Manhica et al., 2017).

However, URMs who are not part of the system for various reasons may be at even greater risk of exposure to situations in which they may become engaged in criminal activities or addicted to drugs. This has been stressed in relation to URMs who are on the move through Europe, who risk being exploited in various ways and forced to become involved in illegal activities (Beise et al., 2017; Digidiki & Bhabha, 2017). In Sweden, this risk of becoming involved with drugs or other criminal activities and of being exploited in various ways has been recognised by authorities in relation to children who go missing during the reception process (Barnombudsmannen, 2017; Länsstyrelsen, 2016, 2018, 2022). It has, for example, been suggested that URMs are particularly vulnerable in relation to human trafficking but also for being involved in drug dealing and with criminal networks (Länsstyrelsen, 2022). Other vulnerable groups of URMs include those who have never applied for asylum and youths who have turned eighteen or had their age adjusted as a result of age assessments, and who therefore no longer have access to the same resources and support as minors. These individuals might also be particularly vulnerable in relation to mental health problems.

The sample employed in this chapter is small, and single individuals may have an important impact on the distributions of variables within the sample. This means that the findings should be interpreted with caution. Nevertheless, the sample includes all URMs who have been treated at outpatient clinics for minors with substance use problems in the city of Stockholm, Sweden, in 2016 and 2017, and the study therefore reflects the situation of these minors relatively well.

---

[5] In relation to this it is however important to note that in Sweden, the use and consumption of drugs are criminalised.

The lack of a control group may also be seen as a limitation. However, our aim has not been to conduct comparisons with a control group, but rather to describe the patterns of drug use and mental health problems found within this particular group of minors. The report from the Public Health Agency of Sweden referred to above shows that patterns of drug use were rather similar between URMs and other adolescents who receive treatment for substance use problems at outpatient clinics, but that internalising mental health problems and experiences of trauma were more common among URMs (Folkhälsomyndigheten, 2017). At the same time, however, comparisons between URMs and the general population may be difficult due to their different experiences and living conditions.

8.4.1 Conclusion

This chapter has addressed issues related to mental health problems and substance use among URMs in Sweden showing that these adolescents report high levels of mental health problems combined with low levels of contacts with CAP care. Drawing on existing knowledge on the association between mental health problems and substance use, these results need to be taken seriously, and close collaboration is required between substance use clinics and CAP clinics, with more awareness of mental health problems. This would be beneficial in relation to this specific group, but also on a more general level. Successful treatment and access to appropriate care are crucial for positive individual development and successful resettlement for this vulnerable group whose problems risk escalating, and who are at risk of being recruited into organised crime or falling victim to human trafficking.

Ethical Approval The study has been approved by the Regional Ethics Committee in Lund (Dnr. 2017/668).

Competing Interests The authors declare that they have no competing interests.

References

Anderberg, M., & Dahlberg, M. (2016). Experiences of victimization among adolescents with Substance Abuse Disorders in Sweden. *Scandinavian Journal of Child and Adolescent Psychiatry and Psychology*, *4*(3), 123–131. https://doi.org/10.21307/sjcapp-2016-019

Anderberg, M., & Dahlberg, M. (2018). Gender differences among adolescents with substance abuse problems at Maria clinics in Sweden. *NAD Nordic Studies on Alcohol and Drugs, 35*(1), 24–38. https://doi.org/10.1177/1455072517751263

Auger-Voyer, V., Montero-Sieburth, M., & Perez, L. C. (2014). Chasing the European dream: Unaccompanied African youths' educational experience in a Canary Islands' Reception Centre and Beyond. *Education Policy Analysis Archives, 22*(76), 1–19.

Barnombudsmannen. (2017). *Ensamkommande barn som försvinner*. Retrived May 7, 2025, from https://www.barnombudsmannen.se/stallningstaganden/publikationer/ensamkommande-barn-som-forsvinner/

Bean, T. M., Derluyn, I., Eurelings-Bontekoe, E., Broekaert, E., & Spinhoven, P. (2007a). Comparing psychological distress, Traumatic stress reactions, and experiences of unaccompanied refugee minors with experiences of adolescents accompanied by parents. *The Journal of Nervous and Mental Disease, 195*(4), 288–297. https://doi.org/10.1097/01.nmd.0000243751.49499.93

Bean, T., Eurelings-Bontekoe, M. E., & Spinhoven, P. (2007b). Course and predictors of mental health of unaccompanied refugee minors in the Netherlands: One year follow-up. *Social Science and Medicine, 64*(6), 1204–1215. https://doi.org/10.1016/j.socscimed.2006.11.010

Beise, J., Grojec, A. Hansen, C. B. Matthes J., Rosengaertner, S., & You, D. (2017). *A child is a child: Protecting children on the move from violence abuse and exploitation*. Retrived May 7, 2025, from https://data.unicef.org/resources/child-child-protecting-children-move-violence-abuse-exploitation/

BRÅ (The Swedish National Council for Crime Prevention). (2021). *Narkotikamarknader: En studie av smuggling, gatuförsäljning, internethandel och köpare*. (Drug markets: A study of smuggling, street sales, internet trade and buyers). Rapport 2021:10. Retrived May 7, 2025, from https://bra.se/rapporter/arkiv/2021-09-01-narkotikamarknader

Carlson, B. E., Cacciatore, J., & Klimek, B. (2012). A risk and resilience perspective on unaccompanied refugee minors. *Social Work (United States), 57*(3): 259–269. https://doi.org/10.1093/sw/sws003

Çelikaksoy, A., & Wadensjö, E. (2017). Refugee Youth in Sweden who arrived as unaccompanied minors and separated children. *Journal of Refugee Studies, 30*(4), 530–553. https://doi.org/10.1093/jrs/few042

Dahlberg, M., & Anderberg, M. (2017). *Tvärsnittsstudie baserad på uppgifter om ensamkommande barn och unga i databasen IKMDOK*. Linnéuniversitetet.

Dahlberg, M., Anderberg, M., & Wennberg, P. (2017). Psychometric properties of the UngDOK. *Nordic Studies on Alcohol and Drugs, 34*(2), 160–172. https://doi.org/10.1177/1455072516687440

Degenhardt, L., Coffey, C., Romaniuk, H., Swift, W., Carlin, J. B., Hall, W. D., & Patton, G. C. (2013). The persistence of the association between adolescent cannabis use and common mental disorders into young adulthood. *Addiction, 108*(1), 124–133. https://doi.org/10.1111/j.1360-0443.2012.04015.x

Derluyn, I., & Broekaert, E. (2007). Different perspectives on emotional and behavioural problems in unaccompanied refugee children and adolescents. *Ethnicity and Health, 12*(2), 141–162. https://doi.org/10.1080/13557850601002296

Derluyn, I., & Broekaert, E. (2008). Unaccompanied refugee children and adolescents: The glaring contrast between a legal and a psychological perspective. *International Journal of Law and Psychiatry, 31*, 319–330. https://doi.org/10.1016/j.ijlp.2008.06.006

Derluyn, I., Broekaert, E., & Schuyten, G. (2008). Emotional and behavioural problems in migrant adolescents in Belgium. *European Child and Adolescent Psychiatry, 17*, 54–62. https://doi.org/10.1007/s00787-007-0636-x

Derluyn, I., Mels, C., Educ, M., & Broekaert, E. (2009). Mental health problems in separated refugee adolescents. *Journal of Adolescent Health, 44*, 291–297. https://doi.org/10.1016/j.jadohealth.2008.07.016

Deveci, Y. (2012). Trying to understand: Promoting the psychosocial well-being of separated refugee children. *Journal of Social Work Practice, 26*(3), 367–383. https://doi.org/10.1080/02650533.2012.658033

Digidiki, V., & Bhabha, J. (2017). *Emergency within an emergency. The growing epidemic of sexual exploitation and abuse of migrant children in Greece*. Retrived May 24, 2025, from https://fxb.harvard.edu/2017/04/17/new-report-emergency-within-an-emergency-exploitation-of-migrant-children-in-greece/

Eide, K., & Hjern, A. (2013). Unaccompanied refugee children - Vulnerability and agency. *Acta Paediatrica, International Journal of Paediatrics, 102*(7), 666–668. https://doi.org/10.1111/apa.12258

Eurostat. (2025a). *Asylum applicants by type—Annual aggregated data.* Retrived September 25, 2025, https://ec.europa.eu/eurostat/databrowser/view/tps00191/default/table?lang=en&category=t_migr.t_migr_asy

Eurostat. (2025b). *Asylum applicants considered to be unaccompanied minors - annual data.* Retrived May 7, 2025, from https://ec.europa.eu/eurostat/web/products-datasets/-/tps00194

Fazel, M. D., Reed, R. V., Panter-Brick, C., & Stein, A. (2012). Mental health of displaced and refugee children resettled in high-income countries: Risk and protective factors. *The Lancet, 379*, 266–282. https://doi.org/10.1016/S0140

Folkhälsomyndigheten. (2017). *Regeringsuppdrag att kartlägga narkotikavanor bland ensamkommande barn och unga.* Retrived May 25, 2025, from https://www.folkhalsomyndigheten.se/contentassets/05464ec78ae4428d927e2d87c30a1f5f/ensamkommandes-utsatthet-kan-leda-till-okat-narkotikabruk-18034.pdf

Gobbi, G., Atkin, T., Zytynski, T., Wang, S., Askari, S., Boruff, J., Ware, M., Marmorstein, N., Cipriani, A., & Dendukuri, N. (2019). Association of cannabis use in adolescence and risk of depression, anxiety, and suicidality in young adulthood: A systematic review and meta-analysis. *JAMA Psychiatry, 76*, 426–434.

Goverment office of Sweden. (2025). *About the Government's prioritisation: Migration and integration.* Retrieved September 25, 2025, from https://www.government.se/government-policy/the-governments-priorities/migration-and-integration/about-the-governments-prioritisation-migration-and-integration/

Hawkins, E. H. (2009). A tale of two systems: Co-occurring mental health and substance Abuse disorders treatment for adolescents. *Annual Review of Psychology, 60*(1), 197–227. https://doi.org/10.1146/annurev.psych.60.110707.163456

Herz, M., & Lalander, P. (2017). Being alone or becoming lonely? The complexity of portraying 'unaccompanied children' as being alone in Sweden. *Journal of Youth Studies, 20*(8), 1062–1076. https://doi.org/10.1080/13676261.2017.1306037

Herz, M., & Lalander, P. (2021). "I'll Have Security, I'll Go to School, I'll Live My Life"–Unaccompanied Minors on School, Education and Racism. *Violence, Victimisation and Young People: Education and Safe Learning Environments.* Springer, 209–224.

Hodgins, S., Oliver, B. R., Tengström, A., & Larsson, A. (2010). Adolescents who consulted for substance misuse problems: Outcomes 1 year later. *Nordic Journal of Psychiatry, 64*(3), 189–195. https://doi.org/10.3109/08039480903389002

Huemer, J., Karnik, N., Voelkl-Kernstock, S., Granditsch, E., Plattner, B., Friedrich, M., & Steiner, H. (2011). Psychopathology in African unaccompanied refugee minors in Austria. *Child Psychiatry and Human Development, 42*, 307–319. https://doi.org/10.1007/s10578-011-0219-4

Ivert, A.-K., & Magnusson, M.-M. (2020). Drug use and criminality among unaccompanied refugee minors: A review of the literature. *International Ournal of Migration, Health and Social Care, 16*, 93–107. https://doi.org/10.1108/IJMHSC-05-2019-0050

Jakobsen, M., Demott, M. A. M., & Heir, T. (2014). Prevalence of psychiatric disorders among unaccompanied Asylum- seeking adolescents in Norway. *Clinical Practice & Epidemiology in Mental Health, 10*(1), 53–58. https://doi.org/10.2174/1745017901410010053

Jensen, T. K., Bjørgo Skårdalsmo, E. M., & Fjermestad, K. W. (2014). Development of mental health problems -a follow-up study of unaccompanied refugee minors. *Child and Adolescent Psychiatry and Mental Health, 8*(29). https://doi.org/10.1186/1753-2000-8-29

Kalverboer, M., Zijlstra, E., van Os, C., Zevulun, D., ten Brummelaar, M., & Beltman, D. (2017). Unaccompanied minors in the Netherlands and the care facility in which they flourish best. *Child and Family Social Work, 22*(2), 587–596. https://doi.org/10.1111/cfs.12272

Kaunitz, C., & Jakobsson, J. (2016). Ensamkommande barn och ungdomar placerade inom Statens institutionsstyrelse (SiS). *Socialmedicinsk Tidskirft, 93*(1), 43–52.

Keles, S., Friborg, O., Idsoe, T., Sirin, S., & Oppedal, B. (2016). Depression among unaccompanied minor refugees: The relative contribution of general and acculturation-specific daily hassles. *Ethnicity & Health, 21*(3), 300–317. https://doi.org/10.1080/13557858.2015.1065310

Kohli, R. K. S. (2006). The comfort of strangers: Social work practice with unaccompanied asylum-seeking children and young people in the UK. *Child and Family Social Work, 11*(1), 1–10. https://doi.org/10.1111/j.1365-2206.2006.00393.x

Lai, H. M. X., Cleary, M., Sitharthan, T., & Hunt, G. E. (2015). Prevalence of comorbid substance use, anxiety and mood disorders in epidemiological surveys, 1990–2014: A systematic review and meta-analysis. *Drug and Alcohol Dependence, 154*, 1–13.

Lovato, K., Bui, D., & Zaragoza, M. (2025). A systematic literature review: Understanding the mental health and social service needs of unaccompanied immigrant children forcibly separated from their parents during and/or following the "Zero Tolerance" policy in the US. *Children and Youth Services Review*, 108296. https://doi.org/10.1016/j.childyouth.2025.108296

Länsstyrelsen. (2016). *Lost in Migration A Report on Missing Unaccompanied Minors in Sweden.* Retrived May 25, 2025, from https://www.lansstyrelsen.se/stockholm/om-oss/vara-tjanster/publikationer/2016/lost-in-migration---a-report-on-missing-unaccompanied-minors-in-sweden.html

Länsstyrelsen. (2018). *De kan alltid hitta mig " Studie om människohandel och utsatta barngruppers livsvillkor.* Retrived May 25, 2025, from https://www.lansstyrelsen.se/stockholm/om-oss/vara-tjanster/publikationer/2018/de-kan-alltid-hitta-mig---studie-om-manniskohandel-och-utsatta-barngruppers-livsvillkor.html

Länsstyrelsen. (2022). *Ensamkommande barn som avvikit mellan åren 2013 och 2020. Sammanställning av Migrationsverkets statistik över registrerade avvikningar.* Retrived May 25, 2025, from https://integration.lansstyrelsen.se/wp-content/uploads/Ensamkommande-barn-som-avvikit-2013-2020-2.0.pdf

Lundberg, A., & Dahlquist, L. (2012). Unaccompanied children seeking asylum in Sweden: Living conditions from a child-centred perspective. *Refugee Survey Quarterly, 31*(2), 54–75. https://doi.org/10.1093/rsq/hds003

Luster, T., Qin, D., Bates, L., Rana, M., & Lee, J. A. (2010). Successful adaptation among Sudanese unaccompanied minors: Perspectives of youth and foster parents. *Childhood, 17*(2), 197–211. https://doi.org/10.1177/0907568210365664

Malmsten, J. (2014). Unaccompanied children living in transitional houses—voices from Sweden. *International Journal of Migration, Health and Social Care, 10*(1), 18–35. https://doi.org/10.1108/IJMHSC-10-2013-0037

Manhica, H., Gauffin, K., Almquist, Y., Rostila, M., Berg, L., Rodríguez, A., De Cortázar, G., & Hjern, A. (2017). Hospital admissions due to alcohol related disorders among young adult refugees who arrived in Sweden as teenagers -a national cohort study. *BMC Public Health, 17*, 644. https://doi.org/10.1186/s12889-017-4645-5

Manhica, H., Gauffin, K., Almqvist, Y., Rostila, M., & Hjern, A. (2016). Hospital Admission and Criminality Associated with Substance Misuse in Young Refugees—A Swedish National Cohort Study. *PLoS ONE, 11*(11), Article e0166066. https://doi.org/10.1371/journal.pone.0166066

Marquardt, L., Krämer, A., Fischer, F., & Prüfer-Krämer, L. (2016). Health status and disease burden of unaccompanied asylum-seeking adolescents in Bielefeld, Germany: Cross-sectional pilot study. *Tropical Medicine and International Health, 21*(2), 210–218. https://doi.org/10.1111/tmi.12649

Nawi, A. M., Ismail, R., Ibrahim, F., Hassan, M. R., Manaf, M. R. A., Amit, N., Ibrahim, N., & Shafurdin, N. S. (2021). Risk and protective factors of drug abuse among adolescents: A systematic review. *BMC Public Health, 21*, 2088.

Oppedal, B., & Idsoe, T. (2012). Conduct problems and depression among unaccompanied refugees: The association with pre-migration trauma and acculturation. *Anales De Psicología, 28*(3), 683–694. https://doi.org/10.6018/analesps.28.3.155981

Pettersson, M. (2016). Polisens arbete med ensamkommande barn som begår brott. *Socialmedicinsk Tidskrift, 93*(1), 37–42.

Prod'hom, D., Amoussou, J. R., Plessen, K. J., De Grelle, N. C., & Gaultier, S. (2024). Adaptative skills and global functioning of unaccompanied migrant minors in Europe: A Systematised Review. *International Journal of Public Health*, 69, 1606625.

Raghallaigh, M. N., & Gilligan, R. (2010). Active survival in the lives of unaccompanied minors: Coping strategies, resilience, and the relevance of religion. *Child and Family Social Work, 15*(2), 226–237. https://doi.org/10.1111/j.1365-2206.2009.00663.x

Ramel, B., Täljemark, J., Lindgren, A., & Johansson, B. A. (2015). Overrepresentation of unaccompanied refugee minors in inpatient psychiatric care. *SpringerPlus, 4*(131). https://doi.org/10.1186/s40064-015-0902-1

Richert, T., Anderberg, M., & Dahlberg, M. (2020). Mental health problems among young people in substance abuse treatment in Sweden. *Substance Abuse Treatment, Prevention, and Policy, 15*, 43.

Seglem, K. B., Oppedal, B., & Roysamb, E. (2014). Daily hassles and coping dispositions as predictors of psychological adjustment: A comparative study of young unaccompanied refugees and youth in the resettlement country. *International Journal of Behavioral Development, 38*(3), 293–303. https://doi.org/10.1177/0165025414520807

Solhaug, A. K., Oppedal, B., & Røysamb, E. (2025). Life satisfaction, self-efficacy, and depressive symptoms among unaccompanied Asylum-seeking and refugee minors: An exploratory study. *Adversity and Resilience Science*. https://doi.org/10.1007/s42844-025-00169-0

Sourander, A. (1998). Behavior problems and traumatic events of unaccompanied refugee minors. *Child Abuse & Neglect, 22*(7), 719–727. https://doi.org/10.1016/S0145-2134(98)00053-2

Stjerna Doohan, I., Ghazinour, M., Eriksson, M., Padyab, M., & Sundqvist, J. (2024). Challenges for unaccompanied asylum-seeking minors in Swedish compulsory institutional care. *Frontiers in Human Dynamics, 6*, 1411378. https://doi.org/10.3389/fhumd.2024.1411378

Swedish Migration Agency. (2024). *Ensamkommande barn -hur har asylansökningarna utvecklats de senaste 10 åren?* Retrived May 28, 2025 from https://www.migrationsverket.se/om-migrationsverket/migrationsverket-svarar/2024/2024-11-11-ensamkommande-barn---hur-har-asylansokningarna-utvecklats-de-senaste-tio-aren.html

Swedish Migration Agency. (2025). *Statistics/Asylu*m. Retrieved September 25, 2025 from https://www.migrationsverket.se/en/about-the-swedish-migration-agency/statistics/asylum.html. Accessed Access Date 2025.

Swedish National Police. (2017). *Utsatta områden* [Disadvantaged areas]. Swedish National Police.

Thevissen, P. W., Kvaal, S. I., Dierickx, K., & Willems, G. (2012). Ethics in Age estimation of unaccompanied minors. *Journal of Forensic Odonto-Stomatology, 3030*(suppl 1), 85–103.

Thommessen, S., F. Laghi, C., Cerrone, R., Baiocco, B. K. & Todd, B. K. (2013). Internalizing and externalizing symptoms among unaccompanied refugee and Italian adolescents. *Children and Youth Services Review, 35*, 7–10. https://doi.org/10.1016/j.childyouth.2012.10.007

Turner, S., Mota, N., Bolton, J., & Sareen, J. (2018). Self-medication with alcohol or drugs for mood and anxiety disorders: A narrative review of the epidemiological literature. *Depression and Anxiety, 35*, 851–860.

UNHCR. (1994). *Refugee children: Guidelines on protection and care*. Retrived May 24, 2025, from http://www.unhcr.org/3b84c6c67.pdf

Wernesjö, U. (2014). *Listening to Unaccompanied Young Refugees' Voices*. (Doctoral dissertation). Acta Universitatis Upsaliensis.

Wimelius, M. E., Eriksson, M., Isaksson, J., & Ghazinour, M. (2017). Swedish reception of unaccompanied refugee children—Promoting integration? *Journal of International Migration and Integration, 18*, 143–157. https://doi.org/10.1007/s12134-016-0472-2

Chapter 9
Barriers to Substance Use Prevention and Care among Refugees in the Netherlands: Toward a Culturally Sensitive Approach Using Motivational Interviewing

Jannet M. de Jonge, Chico Taguba, Judith Noijen, Corine Latour, and Mirrian Hilbink-Smolders

9.1 Introduction and Background

9.1.1 History of the Refugee Population in the Netherlands

Obtaining an accurate understanding of the number of refugees in the Netherlands requires navigating a complex and evolving landscape. Who you include depends on the definition used. The United Nations Refugee Agency (UNHCR) defines refugees as persons who have fled their countries to escape conflict, violence, or persecution and sought safety in another country (United Nations Convention and Protocol Relating to the Status of Refugees, 1951). According to the UNHCR, there were 237,767 refugees in the Netherlands at the end of 2023: 105,000 (44%) refugees from Ukraine and around 132,000 (56%) refugees from other countries, such as Syria, Eritrea, Afghanistan, Iran, Turkey and Yemen, among others. This is a slight increase compared to 2022 (218,457), when the number more than doubled compared to the previous year (99,586 in 2021), largely due to the arrival of Ukrainian refugees

J. M. de Jonge (✉) · C. Taguba · C. Latour · M. Hilbink-Smolders
Faculty of Health, Sport and Physical Activity, Integrated Complex Care research group, Amsterdam University of Applied Sciences, Amsterdam, The Netherlands
e-mail: j.m.de.jonge@hva.nl

J. Noijen
Jellinek Prevention, Arkin Mental Health Care, Amsterdam, The Netherlands

C. Latour
Inholland University of Applied Sciences, Centre of Expertise Prevention in Health and Social Care, Faculty of Health, Education and Social Work, Amsterdam, The Netherlands

C. De Kock (ed.), *Substance Use Among Refugees in Europe*,
https://doi.org/10.1007/978-3-032-32399-6_9

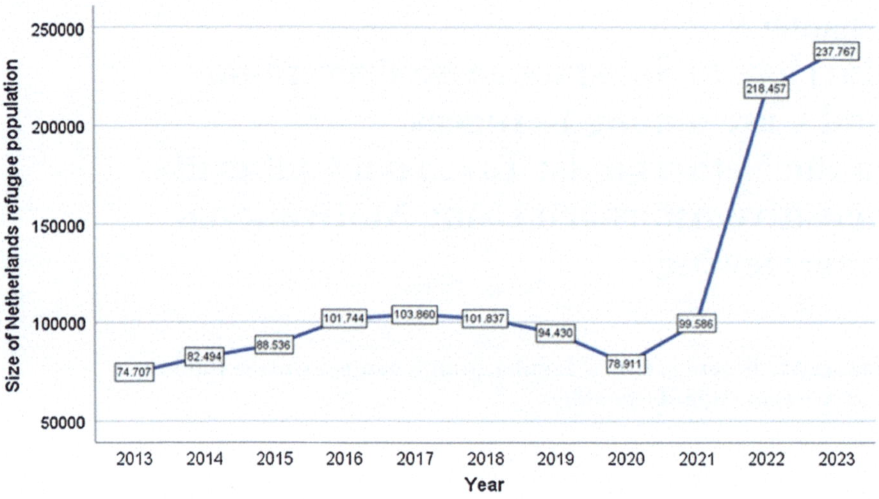

Fig. 9.1 Size of Netherlands refugee population 2013–2023 (based on *Hoeveel vluchtelingen zijn er in Nederland?*, n.d.)

(Hoeveel Vluchtelingen Zijn Er in Nederland? n.d.). Figure 9.1 shows the size of the Netherlands refugee population between 2013 and 2023.

9.1.2 Prevalence of Mental Health and Substance Use-Related Problems among Refugees in the Netherlands

According to healthcare professionals working with refugees, more attention is needed to substance use-related harms within this population. Clinical observations suggest that young adults with a refugee background living in the Netherlands are particularly vulnerable to developing mental health and substance use-related problems. Unfortunately, national data on prevalence remains scarce. Research by the Public Health Service of Amsterdam revealed that young adults with a refugee background living in Amsterdam frequently suffer from emotional distress (60%) and trauma-related symptoms (13%), possibly leading to an elevated susceptibility for substance use. Substance use-related harms and dependence were reported relatively frequent (17%) in this group (Fassaert et al., 2018). Another study among Eritrean and Syrian refugees in the Netherlands revealed high rates of current tobacco smoking (29% and 44%) and hookah smoking (28% and 29%). Almost 5% of the Eritrean refugees and 8% of the Syrian refugees were classified as heavy smokers. Stress relief and reduction of excessive worrying were cited as major reasons for smoking. Alcohol use was reported by 62% of Eritrean and 27% of Syrian refugees, mainly men. Half of the Eritrean alcohol-consuming refugees reported past-month binge drinking. Only a small proportion of the Eritrean and Syrian refugees were current cannabis users (6% and 13%). Neither Eritrean nor Syrian refugees reported opiate use. Non-prescription sleep medication use was rare (6%), while over-the-counter pain medication use was more frequent (18% among Eritrean and 23% among Syrian refugees). However, over-the-counter pain medications were used by 18% of the Eritrean refugees and 23% of the Syrian refugees, respectively. The reasons for using non-prescribed sleep and pain medications are unknown (Speth et al., 2018).

Substance use differs across refugee groups in the Netherlands. Young male refugees appear most at risk of problematic use. Additional risk factors include: long stays in reception centers of the Central Agency for the Reception of Asylum Seekers (COA), mental health problems, social isolation, and boredom (Speth et al., 2018). The high prevalence of substance use problems can be explained in light of pre-migration, migration and post-migration risk factors. If left unaddressed, problematic substance use could lead to well-documented adverse biological, psychological, and social health outcomes. For refugees in particular, it may also hinder the process of civic integration (Razenberg & Asmoredjo, 2019; *World Report on the Health of Refugees and Migrants*, 2022).

9.1.3 Barriers to Prevention and Care

Despite challenges related to mental health and substance use, access to effective prevention and treatment remains limited. Refugees frequently encounter barriers in navigating the Dutch healthcare system, including language and communication difficulties, cultural misunderstandings, unfamiliarity with available services, and stigma related to mental health and substance use. Healthcare professionals likewise report uncertainty about how to address substance use in a culturally sensitive and preventive manner (Van Egten et al., 2023).

9.1.4 Toward Culturally Sensitive Brief Interventions

Several international reports (Kane & Greene, 2018; *World Report on the Health of Refugees and Migrants,* 2022) highlight that substance use problems among refugees and migrants are often under-recognized and undertreated. This underscores the urgent need to integrate substance use prevention and care into broader mental health strategies, particularly through culturally tailored approaches. The lack of refugee-specific interventions in this domain further underscores the importance of adapting existing programs to better reflect the cultural and contextual realities of displaced populations.

While group-based interventions can offer meaningful support, there remains a need for individual, low-threshold options that enable early engagement and help professionals recognize early signs of emotional distress and risk behaviors. Culturally sensitive brief interventions are particularly suitable for refugee populations due to their adaptability to limited time and resources, as well as their applicability across various settings. Both group-based brief interventions, such as Greene et al., 2024 and Bryant et al., 2024, and individual brief interventions (e.g., Shaw et al., 2023) appear feasible and promising. These can be tailored to individual goals and needs, with personalized approaches that take into account specific circumstances, motivational levels, and confidence in behavior change related to substance use. Training professionals to recognize mental health symptoms and risk behaviors, while ensuring access to culturally sensitive care pathways, can support early identification and intervention before problems escalate. Importantly, brief interventions help normalize dialogue around mental health and substance use, thereby reducing stigma and enhancing motivation for further support (Humeniuk et al., 2012).

One valuable approach in this context is motivational interviewing (MI). MI is an evidence-based treatment that has been used effectively in brief interventions and prevention strategies for various substance use disorders (DiClemente et al., 2017; Jiang et al., 2017; Knox et al., 2019). MI is defined as a "particular way of talking with people about change and growth to strengthen their own motivation and commitment" (Miller & Rollnick, 2023). The MI spirit (Fig. 9.2) contains four core elements: collaboration, acceptance, compassion, and empowerment. Collaboration involves joint decision-making, recognizing the client as the expert on themselves; acceptance requires non-judgmental listening and affirmation of the client's experiences; compassion emphasizes alleviating suffering and prioritizing well-being, and empowerment aims to help clients recognize and utilize their strengths and autonomy (Miller & Rollnick, 2023). In practice, MI counselors perform four sequential tasks that guide clients through a stepwise process of behavior change. These steps involve establishing trust (engaging), defining goals (focusing), stimulating motivation through change talk (evoking), and developing practical strategies (planning), with an emphasis on fostering client commitment, confidence, and self-efficacy, as well as supporting their autonomy (Miller & Rollnick, 2023).

MI is particularly suitable for use in culturally diverse contexts, including with refugee communities. However, to be effective in these settings, especially in preventive care, where individuals may not yet perceive their behavior as problematic, MI often requires cultural and contextual adaptation (Lee, 2025; Oh & Lee, 2016). To make MI more culturally sensitive, guidelines suggest that interventions should be grounded in the target group's cultural values, aligned with their norms, and delivered by counselors who are culturally competent, meaning aware of their own biases and knowledgeable about clients' backgrounds (Marín, 1993). However, an overemphasis on cultural competence may inadvertently lead to stereotyping; thus, the concept of cultural humility was introduced, emphasizing ongoing self-reflection, addressing power imbalances, and fostering collaborative relationships that respect clients' cultural identities (Tervalon & Murray-García, 1998). Acting from a stance of cultural humility aligns closely with the MI spirit, promoting a client-centered approach that values what truly matters to the individual.

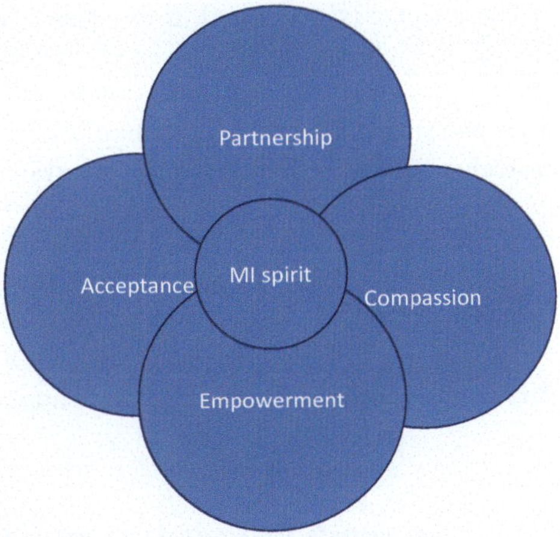

Fig. 9.2. Spirit of motivational interviewing (inspired by Miller & Rollnick, 2023).

9.1.5 *A Brief Intervention in Practice: The Preventive Advisory Conversation*

Guide individuals toward appropriate support (Oudejans et al., 2024). The PAC follows a structured approach informed by the SLP model: symptoms (S), life events (L), and personal characteristics and general functioning (P) (Rijnders & Heene, 2021). This framework emphasizes that individual characteristics significantly influence the emergence and persistence of complaints, helping individuals better understand and address their problems. During PAC sessions, a prevention specialist uses MI to support adults and young people with mental health or addiction concerns, to enhance self-awareness, empower them, and strengthen their confidence in making informed choices. In the Netherlands, PAC (Preventief Adviesgesprek) has been implemented to facilitate early conversations on mental health and substance use.

9.1.6 *Objectives of this Chapter*

This chapter presents two complementary research projects that aim to contribute to a more responsive and culturally appropriate approach to substance use prevention for refugees in the Netherlands:

- First, we present a literature review that explores barriers to prevention and care for mental health and substance use-related problems, from both refugee and professional perspectives.
- Second, we describe the cultural adaptation process of the PAC intervention for young Syrian and Eritrean refugees.

The chapter is structured in two parts: first, an overview of the barriers to care; second, the adaptation process and outcomes of the intervention. Together, these components aim to deepen understanding of the healthcare needs of refugee communities and support the development of more effective, culturally sensitive prevention strategies within the Dutch healthcare system.

9.2 Methods

This section outlines the methodology applied in both research projects.

9.2.1 Research Project 1: Health Challenges of Mental Health and Substance Use among Refugees in the Netherlands

9.2.1.1 Search Strategy

A systematic search was conducted in MEDLINE (via PubMed) and PsycINFO to identify relevant studies. Both databases were searched from inception up to November 15, 2024. The search strategy was developed using the Domain, Determinant, Outcome (DDO) framework. It combined controlled vocabulary (e.g., MeSH and Thesaurus terms) with free-text keywords and applied Boolean operators (AND, OR) to capture key concepts.

Domain terms, included refugees, asylum seekers, displaced persons, status holders, and young adults (18–25 years), operationalized through terms such as refugee, asylum seeker, displaced person, young adult, youth, adolescent, and emerging adult.

Determinant terms addressed substance use, addiction, and mental health problems, using keywords such as drug use, substance misuse, substance use disorder, addiction, substance use prevention/treatment, mental health, mental disorder, psychiatry, and psychological distress.

Outcome terms focused on perspectives and experiences related to healthcare access, operationalized with terms such as health-seeking behavior, attitudes toward health, perspective, experience, lived experience, healthcare utilization, access, barrier, and challenge.

9.2.1.2 Eligibility Criteria

Studies were eligible for inclusion if they focused on young adult refugees aged 18 to 25 years. Studies with a broader age range were also included if this group was represented. Eligible studies addressed mental health and/or substance use, including drug and alcohol consumption, substance misuse, and addiction. Studies had to report relevant outcomes and be published in English or Dutch. No publication date restrictions were applied.

Studies were excluded if they:

Focused exclusively on asylum seekers without official refugee status.
Examined intervention effects.
Consisted solely of questionnaire-based data.

9.2.1.3 Study Selection

The selection process was conducted in two phases. First, titles and abstracts were screened for relevance according to the eligibility criteria. Second, full texts were reviewed to confirm inclusion. Discrepancies in selection were resolved through discussion among the reviewers.

9.2.1.4 Data Analysis

In total, 32 studies met the inclusion criteria. These were subjected to thematic analysis to identify perceived barriers to healthcare access, as reported by refugees and healthcare professionals. The resulting themes are presented in the Results section.

9.2.2 Research Project 2: Mental Health and Substance Use Prevention for Young Refugees

The second part of this study was embedded in the project "Mental Health and Substance Use Prevention for Young Refugees: We Do It Together (MHSUP)" which aimed to bridge the gap between young Syrian and Eritrean refugees and prevention specialists. Funded by FNO Geestkracht, the project ran from late 2021 to June 2024. It was a collaboration between prevention specialists from Jellinek (substance use and addiction expertise), researchers from the Amsterdam University of Applied Sciences, young refugees, and experts from Pharos, the Dutch Centre of Expertise on Health Disparities. This MHSUP project was initiated in response to concerns raised by prevention specialists, who observed that their existing prevention activities were not effectively reaching young refugees. Their request was to make the PAC more culturally sensitive and accessible.

9.2.2.1 Design and Procedure

To enhance the cultural sensitivity of the PAC, we used a design thinking framework focused on understanding user needs and challenges. This approach involves understanding user needs, defining problems, ideating solutions, prototyping, and testing. It emphasizes empathy, creativity, and iterative development to create innovative and effective solutions (Roberts et al., 2016).

1. Problem Definition.

The first phase involved identifying challenges encountered by both prevention specialists and young refugees. Using existing networks within the MHSUP project in the Amsterdam and Utrecht region, Syrian and Eritrean young refugees were recruited for interviews and focus groups, conducted in 2022 and early 2023.

2. Empathy.

In this phase, five prevention specialists were interviewed about their experiences working with individuals from refugee or migration backgrounds. In addition, four experts, professionals with and without a migration background who provide training on culturally sensitive communication, were interviewed to explore common pitfalls and key considerations in prevention practice. Young refugees from Syria and Eritrea ($N = 4$) were also individually interviewed. Five focus groups were conducted: two with Syrian and three with Eritrean participants. All interviews and group discussions were transcribed and analyzed using thematic analysis (Verhoeven, 2020) in MaxQDA. Two researchers independently coded the data. Based on the findings, two personas were developed, fictional but representative profiles of a Syrian and an Eritrean young refugee.

3. Define.

This phase focused on clarifying the specific needs, perceptions, and barriers experienced by young refugees regarding mental health and substance use. Empathy maps of prevention specialists were also created to capture their thoughts, feelings, behaviors, and goals in working with this group. Together, these insights helped identify key issues in communication, trust, and access to care.

4. Ideation.

A culturally sensitive prototype of the PAC was developed using literature on culturally sensitive communication and motivational interviewing, combined with insights from the interviews and focus groups. The development team included a prevention specialist with a migration background, a researcher with a migration background, and an expert in motivational interviewing. The prototype was subsequently tested with prevention specialists and young refugees.

5. Prototype Testing and Training.

Feedback from testing was used to refine the intervention further. A training program on culturally sensitive PAC and motivational interviewing was then designed and delivered to two groups of prevention professionals (N = 20). A young refugee was involved as co-trainer to ensure relevance and accessibility. After the training, participants' experiences and perspectives were evaluated, informing additional refinements to both the training and intervention.

All stages of the project were discussed within the project team. The team members reflected on their experiences during participant recruitment for interviews and focus groups, the conduct of the focus groups, as well as the feedback received on refugee personas and empathy maps from prevention workers. Continuous reflection on these steps facilitated the identification of key lessons learned.

9.3 Results

9.3.1 Research Project 1: Health Challenges of Mental Health and Substance Use among Refugees in the Netherlands

For refugees in the Netherlands who experience mental health or addiction issues, the available healthcare services are not always tailored to their specific needs and circumstances. Various barriers hinder timely access to appropriate care. As shown in Table 9.1, these main barriers can be grouped into five overlapping and interrelated key themes: communication, knowledge, expectations, trust, and the organization of care (Taguba, 2025). They can be understood from both the refugees' and the mental health and addiction care givers' perspectives.

9.3.1.1 Communication

Refugees and mental health and addiction care professionals often face language barriers due to limited proficiency in each other's language. As a result, refugees may struggle to clearly articulate their complaints to professionals, increasing the risk of misdiagnosis or treatment that fails to address underlying issues (Krystallidou et al., 2024). Additionally, refugees may not fully understand the terminology used for mental health and substance use-related issues.

The use of interpreters can be helpful but also has its limitations. They are not always available (Forrest-Bank et al., 2019; Kiliç et al., 2024; Salami et al., 2019), and financial compensation for their service is not always guaranteed (Dressel et al., 2020). Additionally, interpreters do not always have knowledge of mental health and addiction care-specific terminology, which can hinder effective communication

Table 9.1 Health challenges of mental health/substance use issues faced by refugees in the Netherlands

Key themes of barriers	Refugees	Mental health and addiction care professionals
Communication	• Insufficient proficiency of the Dutch language • Do not fully understand the terminology used for mental health and substance use related issues	• Insufficient proficiency of the native language of the refugees • The style of communication does not always align with that of refugees
Knowledge	• Limited health literacy • Lack of knowledge about mental health and substance-use related issues • Lack of knowledge about the accessibility and what mental health and addiction care have to offer	• Lack of knowledge about refugees' lived experience and cultural backgrounds
Expectations	• Unrealistic expectations regarding waiting times • Perception that mental health and substance-use issues will be resolved after only a few sessions • Fear of high out-of-pocket costs • Limited trust in the effectiveness of professional help compared to familiar, community-based support resources • Belief that mental health and substance use-issues will resolve on their own without intervention • Concern that engaging with mental health or addiction care may result in involuntary admission or deportation	• Explicit and implicit bias toward refugees • Discrimination • Over culturalization

(continued)

Table 9.1 (continued)

Key themes of barriers	Refugees	Mental health and addiction care professionals
Trust	• Fear for stigmatization due to violation of their privacy • Lack of familiarity with mental health and addiction care services • Negative experiences with institutions in country of origin • Negative experiences with institutions in the Netherlands	• Inadequate establishment of a relationship of trust due to language related • Mismatch of mutual expectations of health care
Organization of health care	• Geographical distance to care services, in combination with travel expenses • Fragmentation between healthcare and welfare services	• Limited opportunities to enhance integration mental health and addiction care with welfare services due to limited funding • Segmented funding structure between mental health and addiction care, and welfare services • Fragmentation between healthcare and welfare services

(Forrest-Bank et al., 2019). Furthermore, there is a risk that refugees, due to fear of stigmatization, shame, and cultural taboos, may communicate less openly in the presence of an interpreter (Marshall et al., 2016; Poudel-Tandukar et al., 2024; Renner et al., 2020; Salami et al., 2019).

9.3.1.2 Knowledge, Expectations, and Trust

Beyond language barriers, both refugees and mental health and addiction care professionals often experience knowledge gaps. Refugees may have limited health literacy, while professionals may lack understanding of refugees' lived experiences and cultural backgrounds (Forrest-Bank et al., 2019; Posselt et al., 2017; Renner et al., 2020; Salami et al., 2019). These gaps could result in (unspoken) differences in perceptions of mental health and addiction care, leading refugees to hold different expectations of care than professionals can or are willing to provide (Chen et al., 2020; Copolov & Knowles, 2023; Ellis et al., 2010; Fuhr et al., 2019; Posselt et al., 2017; Salami et al., 2019).

Biases among professionals may also influence care. For example, some may assume that certain refugee groups do not struggle with alcohol-related problems due to religious prohibitions, or they may hold discriminatory beliefs that are not explicitly expressed (Posselt et al., 2017).

The level of trust in mental health and addiction care services is crucial in determining whether refugees seek help (Au et al., 2019). Several factors influence this trust. Refugees may experience distrust due to fears that information about their mental health or addiction problems will become known within their community, leading to possible stigmatization. Some fear being labeled as “weak” or “unable to cope with stress” and feel ashamed of their struggles (Fuhr et al., 2019; Salami et al., 2019). Additionally, refugees may worry about the consequences of receiving mental health or addiction care, fearing that it could negatively impact their chances of obtaining residency status (Posselt et al., 2017; Salami et al., 2019). When refugees feel that a professional has little or no knowledge of their specific cultural background and context, it can damage their trust in the care system, as they may feel misunderstood (Ellis et al., 2010, p. 201; McCleary et al., 2016).

Refugees often experience broader challenges such as housing and financial difficulties. Their expectation is often that, when seeking care, they will receive support in all three areas, while care services typically refer them to the welfare sector for such matters. For mental health and addiction care professionals, it is therefore important to also acknowledge and address the broader social needs of refugees and collaborate with organizations within the social domain (Posselt et al., 2015; Posselt et al., 2017).

9.3.1.3 Organization of Care

The last category of barriers pertains to the organization of mental health and addiction care services. Refugees frequently encounter accessibility challenges, such as high travel expenses (Copolov & Knowles, 2023; Kiliç et al., 2024). Additionally, the limitation of service hours often coincides with their work schedules (Copolov & Knowles, 2023; Salami et al., 2019). This issue is particularly significant for refugees, given that many of them are employed part-time and on temporary contracts (Asiel En Intergratie 2024, 2024; Salami et al., 2019). Service providers, wishing to adapt their services to refugee needs, frequently face constraints due to insufficient funding (McCleary et al., 2016; Posselt et al., 2017; Salami et al., 2019).

Furthermore, refugees encounter fragmentation between health care and welfare services (Posselt et al., 2017). Current structures typically require referrals to separate welfare organizations. The absence of an integrated service model, wherein mental health and addiction services are provided alongside welfare assistance within a single access point, may contribute to distrust toward service providers if refugees perceive their broader needs as inadequately addressed (Copolov & Knowles, 2023; Posselt et al., 2017).

This fragmentation is exacerbated by limited collaboration between services characterized by insufficient utilization of each other’s expertise (McCleary et al., 2016; Pavlish et al., 2010). Compounding this issue is a mutual lack of awareness and understanding among service providers regarding the range of available services offered by each sector (Hillhorst & Van Den Wijngaart, 2024; Posselt et al., 2015). Segmented funding structures between healthcare and welfare services perpetuate this fragmented delivery model (Grenzeloos samenwerken?, 2022). Lastly, opportunities to improve integration remain limited due to inadequate financial resources (Hillhorst & Van Den Wijngaart, 2024).

9.3.2 Research Project 2: Mental Health and Substance Use Prevention for Young Refugees

In consultation with the MHSUP project members, five key lessons were distilled from the project experience. These lessons reflect insights gained while adapting the PAC to better suit young refugees from Eritrea and Syria. They are integrated into the training program and align with the four core tasks of MI: engaging, focusing, evoking, and planning.

9.3.2.1 Lesson 1: Engaging with Status Holders

Using MI, the counselor's first task is to engage clients and build a trusting, collaborative relationship. Similarly, our first step in the MHSUP project was to establish trust with Eritrean and Syrian refugees. We learned that trust must be developed on multiple levels, as previous negative experiences with researchers or counselors can lead to suspicion about discussing mental health or addiction issues. To foster collaboration with young Syrian and Eritrean refugees, we needed to engage with trusted community figures. As also noted by Lee (2025), the trust of these community figures in the MHSUP project members was a prerequisite for establishing a trusting relationship with the young refugees. Accepting their pace and valuing their expertise were crucial. Throughout this process, an approach rooted in cultural humility was necessary, emphasizing awareness of our own cultural backgrounds, values, and biases (Tervalon & Murray-García, 1998).

9.3.2.2 Lesson 2: Establishing Shared Goals

In MI, the second task is to determine and focus on shared goals. In the MHSUP project, we aimed to bridge the gap between young Syrian and Eritrean refugees and Jellinek's prevention specialists. However, once conversations began, expectations diverged. Young refugees anticipated receiving information about substances, while project members were primarily interested in understanding the refugees' perspectives on substance use and mental health issues. Establishing a shared understanding of conversation goals was therefore essential. Community figures played a facilitating role by clarifying the expectations to the young refugees and explaining what was expected of them. This collaborative approach to setting the agenda led to more focused and productive conversations.

9.3.2.3 Lesson 3: The Importance of Cultural Values

In MI, the third task is to evoke change talk that reflects a client's desire, ability, reason, or need for change. Counselors empower clients to facilitate their growth. In the MHSUP project, we aimed to actively involve young refugees in transforming the current PAC into a more culturally sensitive intervention. Initially, we assumed this change would be relevant to them; however, we initially overlooked the importance of exploring their perceived benefits of modifying the PAC. We shifted from focusing on a shared goal to actively changing the intervention without fully understanding their perspective. Reflecting on this misstep, we recognized the importance of exploring the values of culturally sensitive counseling with young status holders.

Exploring important values in conversations with young refugees is an expression of culturally sensitive working and cultural humility. In Dutch society, core values include individual autonomy, personal responsibility, and equality among people. Additionally, social connections and enjoying life are often regarded as more important than work performance (Beugelsdijk et al., 2019). While not all values are necessarily shared, some were embraced by Syrian and Eritrean refugees, though the level of importance they assign to these values may vary. Recognizing that culture is what matters to the client helps in understanding their perspectives and fostering motivation that is rooted in their personal values (Lee, 2025). One significant value identified in our MHSUP project was the importance of community. Additionally, when asked about their reasons for collaboration, young refugees valued simply being part of the MHSUP project and appreciated participating together to create positive change.

9.3.2.4 Lesson 4: Ways to Optimize Questioning and Providing Information and Advice

One of the MI skills is asking questions. Dutch communication often relies on direct questions that seek explicit information, but these can be perceived as confrontational. Indirect questions are typically subtler and often embedded within a statement, or another question may be more appropriate in cross-cultural contexts (Bouteh & de Haan, 2019). During our conversations with young refugees, we intentionally used a more indirect approach. For example, instead of directly asking, "What do you think about smoking cannabis?" we reframed it as, "If someone you know smokes cannabis, how do you view that person?". Similarly, we used a more indirect question like, "If someone you know struggles to sleep at night, what do you think could help them?". In the PAC, more indirect questions were integrated when assessing mental health problems or substance use, inspired by questions used in the Cultural Formulation Interview (Aggarwal & Lewis-Fernández, 2020).

Another important MI skill is providing information and advice. In the MHSUP project, there were several instances where we shared information with young refugees, such as practical details about appointment times as well as information related to substance use or mental health issues. Next, we learned that young Syrian and Eritrean refugees highly valued the expertise of counselors and expected sound advice during a PAC. Demonstrating knowledge and competence is beneficial and aligns with the spirit of MI, which recognizes that both counselors and clients are experts in their own right. We found the Teach-Back method particularly useful in this context. This communication technique, widely applied in health care and education, ensures that the client has understood the information correctly. It involves asking the client to restate the information or advice in their own words, which allows the counselor to tailor their communication to the client's needs, improves the effectiveness of educational efforts, and supports better decision-making or behavior change.

Originally developed for communicating with individuals with low health literacy, the Teach-Back method aligns well with culturally sensitive practices (Bouteh & de Haan, 2019; Shersher et al., 2021; Talevski et al., 2020). The core idea is that after providing health-related information or advice, the client is asked to summarize it in their own words (McCaffery et al., 2010). Typical questions include, "Can you tell me in your own words what we just talked about?" or "How would you explain this to someone else?"

In an MI context, the Teach-Back method can be effectively integrated into the ask-tell-ask approach. First, the counselor asks whether the client wants to receive information or if it's okay to share advice. Next, the information is given, followed by the Teach-Back question and a motivational question such as, "What are your thoughts about this information I provided?"

9.3.2.5 Lesson 5: The Role of Community Support

In MI, the final task is to develop a change plan if the client decides to address issues such as substance use. In accordance with MI's spirit of empowerment, the counselor encourages the client's strength and capabilities (Miller & Rollnick, 2023). However, the client's community can significantly influence the change process, either by providing support or creating barriers. In the MHSUP project, we found it essential to discuss the community's role in handling mental health problems and substance use is important. During conversations, both Syrian and Eritrean young refugees mentioned the stigma surrounding substance use within their communities, which can lead to exclusion for those seeking help. On the other hand, family can be very supportive when someone decides to make a change. Community figures also play an important role; gaining their trust can help establish a supportive connection during the help-seeking process. From a perspective of cultural humility, it is important to align the change process with how challenges are typically addressed within the client's community. This recognition not only fosters cultural sensitivity but also increases the likelihood of sustained change.

9.4 Discussion and Recommendations

The barriers perceived by both refugees and professionals, along with the lessons learned from the MHSUP project, overlap in several themes. A central theme is trust in healthcare professionals and organizations. The MHSUP project underscored the essential role of community figures in fostering trust, acting as mediators who encouraged acceptance and engagement. Culturally sensitive communication incorporating MI-techniques such as indirect questioning, exploring personal values, and using the Teach-Back method proved vital for establishing trust and effectively conveying information. Professionals became more aware of both their own and refugees' expectations, which enhanced mutual understanding and engagement.

At the same time, systemic issues such as organizational fragmentation also impacted the MHSUP project's outcomes. Bridging the gap between young Syrian and Eritrean refugees and Jellinek's prevention specialists requires more than culturally sensitive interactions. It calls for structural change within organizations: investing in the development of culturally competent professionals, implementing tailored interventions like PAC, and addressing organizational barriers that limit access and continuity of care. An ongoing research project is focusing precisely on improving pathways between refugees and mental health and addiction services (Taguba, 2024, 2025). Although not all barriers can be fully resolved through direct interaction, the insights gained provide valuable guidance for strengthening cultural sensitivity among mental health and addiction professionals. Further development of PAC and MI training programs is needed to motivate refugees experiencing mental health and substance use challenges toward positive change and growth. Ultimately, well-trained professionals and culturally sensitive prevention strategies are essential to narrowing the gap between refugees and the healthcare system.

Acknowledgments Our thanks go to the following individuals with whom we have worked intensively on this MHSUP project. From Jellinek Prevention: Elske van Putten, Nabil Ben Charif, Shareen Shaban, Youssef El Markous, Driss Kaamouchi; Amsterdam University of Applied Sciences: Eveline Kruse, Sanne Geers; Stichting Ykaello: Mak Yaello and Ali; Here to Support: Adil.

Competing Interests This study was funded by FNO Geestkracht project number 104.232 and Regieorgaan SIA PD 01.010. The authors have no conflicts of interest to declare that are relevant to the content of this chapter.

References

Aggarwal, N. K., & Lewis-Fernández, R. (2020). An introduction to the cultural formulation interview. *Focus, 18*(1), 77–82. https://doi.org/10.1176/appi.focus.18103

Asiel en intergratie 2024. (2024). Centraal Bureau voor de Statistiek. https://longreads.cbs.nl/asielenintegratie-2024/

Au, M., Anandakumar, A. D., Preston, R., Ray, R. A., & Davis, M. (2019). A model explaining refugee experiences of the Australian healthcare system: A systematic review of refugee perceptions. *BMC International Health and Human Rights, 19*(1), 22. https://doi.org/10.1186/s12914-019-0206-6

Beugelsdijk, S., de Hart, J., van Houwelingen, P., & Versantvoort, M. (Eds.). (2019). *Denkend aan Nederland: Publieksmagazine.* SCP. https://www.scienceguide.nl/wp-content/uploads/2019/07/Magazine_SCR-2019_web.pdf

Bouteh, K., & de Haan, A. (2019). Cultuursensitief werken met jeugdigen en gezinnen. *Pharos.*. https://www.pharos.nl/wp-content/uploads/2019/10/Cultuursensitief-werken-met-jeugdigen-en-gezinnen_Pharos_2019-1.pdf

Bryant, R. A., Habashneh, R., Ghatasheh, M., Malik, A., Aqel, I. S., Dawson, K. S., Watts, S., Jordans, M. J. D., Brown, F. L., van Ommeren, M., & Akhtar, A. (2024). Twelve-month follow-up of a controlled trial of a brief behavioural intervention to reduce psychological distress in young adolescent Syrian refugees. *Epidemiology and Psychiatric Sciences, 33*, e80. https://doi.org/10.1017/S2045796024000817

Chen, E., Leos, C., Kowitt, S. D., & Moracco, K. E. (2020). Enhancing community-based participatory research through human-centered design strategies. *Health Promotion Practice, 21*(1), 37–48. https://doi.org/10.1177/1524839919850557

Copolov, C., & Knowles, A. (2023). 'Everything was stuck in my inside and I just wanted to get it out': Psychological distress, coping, and help-seeking for young adult Australian Hazaras from refugee backgrounds. *Transcultural Psychiatry, 60*(1), 114–124. https://doi.org/10.1177/13634615211059684

DiClemente, C. C., Corno, C. M., Graydon, M. M., Wiprovnick, A. E., & Knoblach, D. J. (2017). Motivational interviewing, enhancement, and brief interventions over the last decade: A review of reviews of efficacy and effectiveness. *Psychology of Addictive Behaviors, 31*(8), 862–887. https://doi.org/10.1037/adb0000318

Dressel, A., Falconí, E., Luft, H., Hawkins, M., Noboa, H., Betancourt, Ó., Sedar, A., & Shedlin, M. G. (2020). Attitudes among working professionals toward immigrants and refugees living in Ecuador: Impacts on health and Well-being. *Public Health Nursing, 37*(4), 517–524. https://doi.org/10.1111/phn.12734

Ellis, B. H., Lincoln, A. K., Charney, M. E., Ford-Paz, R., Benson, M., & Strunin, L. (2010). Mental health service utilization of Somali adolescents: Religion, community, and school as gateways to healing. *Transcultural Psychiatry, 47*(5), 789–811. https://doi.org/10.1177/1363461510379933

Fassaert, T., Tuinebreijer, W., Parra, C. L., & De Wit, M. (2018). *Psychosociale screening statushouders.* GGD Amsterdam. https://openresearch.amsterdam/nl/media/inline/2021/11/4/psychosociale_screening_statushouders_ext.pdf?is_http_request=true&auth_replay_token=6pbYJ2K7U2JxDh4iGamo

Forrest-Bank, S. S., Held, M. L., & Jones, A. (2019). Provider perspectives of services addressing the mental health needs of resettled refugee youth. *Child & Adolescent Social Work Journal, 36*(6), 669–684. psyh. https://doi.org/10.1007/s10560-019-00602-1

Fuhr, D. C., Acarturk, C., McGrath, M., Ilkkursun, Z., Sondorp, E., Sijbrandij, M., Ventevogel, P., Cuijpers, P., McKee, M., & Roberts, B. (2019). Treatment gap and mental health service use among Syrian refugees in Sultanbeyli, Istanbul: A cross-sectional survey. *Epidemiology and Psychiatric Sciences, 29*, e70. https://doi.org/10.1017/S2045796019000660

Greene, M. C., Andersen, L. S., Leku, M. R., Au, T., Akellot, J., Upadhaya, N., Odokonyero, R., White, R., Ventevogel, P., Garcia-Moreno, C., & Tol, W. A. (2024). Combining a guided self-help and brief alcohol intervention to improve mental health and reduce substance use among refugee men in Uganda: A cluster-randomized feasibility trial. *Global mental health, 11*, e106. https://doi.org/10.1017/gmh.2024.103

Grenzeloos samenwerken? Adviezen voor het beter mogelijk maken van domeinoverstijgende samenwerking. (2022). Raad voor Volksgezondheid en Samenleving. https://www.raadrvs.nl/documenten/2022/03/04/grenzeloos-samenwerken

Hillhorst, P., & Van Den Wijngaart, M. (2024). *Samenwerken sociaal en medisch domein.* EMMA.

Hoeveel vluchtelingen zijn er in Nederland? (n.d.). Retrieved April 1, 2025, from https://www.unhcr.org/nl/wie-we-zijn/cijfers/

Humeniuk, R., Ali, R., Babor, T., Souza-Formigoni, M. L., de Lacerda, R. B., Ling, W., McRee, B., Newcombe, D., Pal, H., Poznyak, V., Simon, S., & Vendetti, J. (2012). A randomized controlled trial of a brief intervention for illicit drugs linked to the alcohol, smoking and substance involvement screening test (ASSIST) in clients recruited from primary health-care settings in four countries. *Addiction, 107*(5), 957–966. https://doi.org/10.1111/j.1360-0443.2011.03740.x

Jiang, S., Wu, L., & Gao, X. (2017). Beyond face-to-face individual counseling: A systematic review on alternative modes of motivational interviewing in substance abuse treatment and prevention. *Addictive Behaviors, 73*, 216–235. https://doi.org/10.1016/j.addbeh.2017.05.023

Kane, J. C., & Greene, M. C. (2018). *Addressing alcohol and substance use disorders among refugees: A desk review of intervention approaches.* United Nations High Commissioner for Refugee. https://www.unhcr.org/media/addressing-alcohol-and-substance-use-disorders-among-refugees-desk-review-intervention

Kiliç, C., Kaya, E., Karadağ, Ö., & Üner, S. (2024). Barriers to accessing mental health services among Syrian refugees: A mixed-method study. *Turk psikiyatri dergisi = Turkish journal of psychiatry, 35*(2), 87–94. https://doi.org/10.5080/u27044

Knox, J., Hasin, D. S., Larson, F. R. R., & Kranzler, H. R. (2019). Prevention, screening, and treatment for heavy drinking and alcohol use disorder. *The Lancet Psychiatry, 6*(12), 1054–1067. https://doi.org/10.1016/S2215-0366(19)30213-5

Krystallidou, D., Temizöz, Ö., Wang, F., De Looper, M., Di Maria, E., Gattiglia, N., Giani, S., Hieke, G., Morganti, W., Pace, C. S., Schouten, B., & Braun, S. (2024). Communication in refugee and migrant mental healthcare: A systematic rapid review on the needs, barriers and strategies of seekers and providers of mental health services. *Health Policy, 139*, 104949. https://doi.org/10.1016/j.healthpol.2023.104949

Lee, C. S. (2025). Motivational interviewing across cultures: Optimizing practice (pp. xiv, 170). The Guilford Press.

Marín, G. (1993). Defining culturally appropriate community interventions: Hispanics as a case study. *Journal of Community Psychology, 21*(2), 149–161. https://doi.org/10.1002/1520-6629(199304)21:2<149::AID-JCOP2290210207>3.0.CO;2-Y

Marshall, E. A., Butler, K., Roche, T., Cumming, J., & Taknint, J. T. (2016). Refugee youth: A review of mental health counselling issues and practices. Canadian Psychology/Psychologie Canadienne, 57(4), 308–319. Psyh. doi:https://doi.org/10.1037/cap0000068.

McCaffery, K. J., Smith, S. K., & Wolf, M. (2010). The challenge of shared decision making among patients with lower literacy: A framework for research and development. *Medical Decision Making: An International Journal of the Society for Medical Decision Making, 30*(1), 35–44. https://doi.org/10.1177/0272989X09342279

McCleary, J. S., Shannon, P. J., & Cook, T. L. (2016). Connecting refugees to substance use treatment: A qualitative study. *Social Work in Public Health, 31*(1), 1–8. https://doi.org/10.1080/19371918.2015.1087906

Miller, W. R., & Rollnick, S. (2023). *Motivational interviewing: Helping people change and grow* (Fourth ed.). The Guilford Press.

Oh, H., & Lee, C. (2016). Culture and motivational interviewing. *Patient Education and Counseling, 99*(11), 1914–1919. https://doi.org/10.1016/j.pec.2016.06.010

Oudejans, S., van Putten, E., Noijen, J., Spits, M., & el Ouafrassi, M. (2024). *Preventief Adviesgesprek.* Arkin & Mark Bench.

Pavlish, C. L., Noor, S., & Brandt, J. (2010). Somali immigrant women and the American health care system: Discordant beliefs, divergent expectations, and silent worries. *Social Science & Medicine, 71*(2), 353–361. https://doi.org/10.1016/j.socscimed.2010.04.010

Posselt, M., McDonald, K., Procter, N., de Crespigny, C., & Galletly, C. (2017). Improving the provision of services to young people from refugee backgrounds with comorbid mental health and substance use problems: Addressing the barriers. *BMC Public Health, 17*(1), 280. https://doi.org/10.1186/s12889-017-4186-y

Posselt, M., Procter, N., de Crespigny, C., & Galletly, C. (2015). Merging perspectives: Obstacles to recovery for youth from refugee backgrounds with comorbidity. *Australasian Psychiatry: Bulletin of Royal Australian and New Zealand College of Psychiatrists, 23*(3), 293–299. https://doi.org/10.1177/1039856215584512

Poudel-Tandukar, K., Davis, C., Mosijchuk, Y., & Poudel, K. C. (2024). Social and emotional Well-being intervention to reduce stress, anxiety, and depression among Ukrainian refugees resettled in Massachusetts. *The International Journal of Social Psychiatry, 70*(8), 1461–1469. https://doi.org/10.1177/00207640241270870

Razenberg, I., & Asmoredjo, J. (2019). *De rol van gezondheid bij inburgering van statushouders.* Verwey-Jonker Instituut.

Renner, A., Hoffmann, R., Nagl, M., Roehr, S., Jung, F., Grochtdreis, T., König, H.-H., Riedel-Heller, S., & Kersting, A. (2020). Syrian refugees in Germany: Perspectives on mental health and coping strategies. *Journal of Psychosomatic Research, 129*, 109906. https://doi.org/10.1016/j.jpsychores.2019.109906

Rijnders, P., & Heene, E. (2021). *Handboek KOP-model* (1st ed.).

Roberts, J. P., Fisher, T. R., Trowbridge, M. J., & Bent, C. (2016). A design thinking framework for healthcare management and innovation. *Healthcare, 4*(1), 11–14. https://doi.org/10.1016/j.hjdsi.2015.12.002

Salami, B., Salma, J., & Hegadoren, K. (2019). Access and utilization of mental health services for immigrants and refugees: Perspectives of immigrant service providers. *International Journal of Mental Health Nursing, 28*(1), 152–161. psyh. https://doi.org/10.1111/inm.12512

Shaw, S. A., Lee, C., Ahmadi, M., Karim Shor Muluk, H., Mohamed Jibril, Z., Ahmadi, L., Randall, L., Yang, C., & Gilbert, L. (2023). A randomized controlled trial testing the feasibility, acceptability, and preliminary effects of a mental health screening, brief intervention, and referral to treatment among refugees in Malaysia. *The International Journal of Social Psychiatry, 69*(8), 1898–1908. https://doi.org/10.1177/00207640231179323

Shersher, V., Haines, T. P., Sturgiss, L., Weller, C., & Williams, C. (2021). Definitions and use of the teach-back method in healthcare consultations with patients: A systematic review and thematic synthesis. *Patient Education and Counseling, 104*(1), 118–129. https://doi.org/10.1016/j.pec.2020.07.026

Speth, E., Speetjens, P., & Meije. (2018). *Infosheet Vluchtelingen en middelengebruik.* Trimbos-instituut. https://www.trimbos.nl/aanbod/webwinkel/ex016-infosheet-vluchtelingen-en-middelengebruik/

Taguba, C. (2024, 25–10). Towards a better connection [Short communication]. Lisbon Addictions 2024. https://www.lisbonaddictions.eu/presentations/towards-better-connection

Taguba, C. (2025). *Toegankelijkheid van GGZ- en verslavingszorg voor jonge statushouders.* Hogeschool van Amsterdam.

Talevski, J., Shee, A. W., Rasmussen, B., Kemp, G., & Beauchamp, A. (2020). Teach-back: A systematic review of implementation and impacts. *PLoS One, 15*(4), e0231350. https://doi.org/10.1371/journal.pone.0231350

Tervalon, M., & Murray-García, J. (1998). Cultural humility versus cultural competence: A critical distinction in defining physician training outcomes in multicultural education. *Journal of Health Care for the Poor and Underserved, 9*(2), 117–125.

United Nations Convention and Protocol Relating to the Status of Refugees. (1951). https://www.unhcr.org/media/1951-refugee-convention-and-1967-protocol-relating-status-refugees

Van Egten, C., van Bemmel, K., de Gruijter, M. & Hoogenbosch, A. (2023). Opschaling van passende zorg voor vluchtelingen. Verwey-Jonker Instituut https://www.verwey-jonker.nl/wp-content/uploads/2024/03/222380_Opschaling-van-passende-zorg-voor-vluchtelingen.pdf

Verhoeven, N. (2020). *Thematische analyse: Patronen vinden bij kwalitatief onderzoek.* Boom.

Who is an 'asylum-seeker'? (n.d.). Retrieved 1 April 2025, from https://www.unhcr.org/about-unhcr/who-we-protect/asylum-seekers

World Report on the Health of Refugees and Migrants. (2022). *World Health Organisation* (1st ed.).

Chapter 10
Challenges and Needs of Persons with a Migration Background Who Use Drugs: Insights from Multidisciplinary Focus Groups with Professionals in Four European Metropolitan Cities

Aline Pouille, Clara De Ruysscher, and Wouter Vanderplasschen

10.1 Introduction

Even though migration may provide opportunities for safety, education, and work, it also exposes people to instability, social exclusion, and precarious living conditions. These challenges can create vulnerabilities that increase the risk of drug use and dependence, such as poverty, unstable employment, language barriers, discrimination, mental health problems, and trauma experienced before, during, or after migration (De Kock, 2022; Pouille et al., 2020; van Selm et al., 2024).

A considerable proportion of Persons with a Migration background Who Use Drugs (PMWUD) can be considered refugees, either because they meet the legal definition of the 1951 Refugee Convention (UNHCR, 2019) or because they perceive themselves as such after fleeing poverty, violence, or civil unrest in search of safety and a better future (Castañeda et al., 2015). Even when they do not formally qualify for a refugee status, they face similar health and social issues, as well as barriers to treatment and care (WHO Western Pacific Region, 2018). In this chapter, we therefore focus on the broader group of PMWUD, not restricted to the legal definition of refugees.

Reliable data on PMWUD in Europe remain scarce. Contradictory findings on the prevalence of drug use and dependence among migrants highlight the heterogeneity of migrant groups and the importance of considering factors such as socioeconomic position, gender, country of origin, length of residence, and acculturation (European Union Agency for Asylum & European Monitoring Centre for Drugs and Drug

A. Pouille (✉) · C. De Ruysscher · W. Vanderplasschen
Department of Special Needs Education, Ghent University, Ghent, Belgium
e-mail: aline.pouille@ugent.be

C. De Kock (ed.), *Substance Use Among Refugees in Europe*,
https://doi.org/10.1007/978-3-032-32399-6_10

Addiction, 2023; Najdini et al., 2025; van Selm et al., 2023). Overall, although prevalence of drug use appears lower in many groups, migration-related vulnerabilities and structural inequalities create significant risks that demand culturally responsive responses (De Kock, 2022; Pouille et al., 2021).

PMWUD in Europe are frequently deprived of essential healthcare, including specialised and inpatient services, emergency care, and drug treatment (De Kock, 2022; European Union Agency for Asylum & European Monitoring Centre for Drugs and Drug Addiction, 2023; van Selm et al., 2023; van Selm et al., 2024). In addition to insufficient healthcare, individuals with an undocumented or irregular migration status generally have poor or no access to social security facilities such as pensions, sickness benefits, family benefits, and guaranteed minimum resources (Pouille et al., 2024; Rechel et al., 2011). These barriers intersect with other challenges, making PMWUD particularly vulnerable to homelessness, poverty, mental health problems, loss of social networks, and cumulative effects of poor healthcare and chronic stress (European Union Agency for Asylum & European Monitoring Centre for Drugs and Drug Addiction, 2023; European Website on Integration, 2024). At this intersection of migration, homelessness, and drug use, risks of stigmatisation, exclusion, and encounters with the criminal justice system are especially acute (Pouille et al., 2023; Provine, 2011; Rechel et al., 2011). Hence, many PMWUD face precarious situations of destitution and social exclusion (De Kock, 2022).

Despite growing evidence that migration-related stressors, precarious legal and socioeconomic positions, and limited access to health and social services heighten vulnerability to drug use and dependence, little is known about how these aspects influence support needs of PMWUD (De Kock, 2022; Lemmens et al., 2017). Additionally, although professionals directly face the challenges of supporting PMWUD amidst structural barriers, linguistic and cultural difference and service gaps, their perspectives are rarely represented in the literature, resulting in a knowledge gap regarding how European support systems respond to the complex needs of PMWUD (Horyniak et al., 2016; van Selm et al., 2023). Finally, existing research rarely takes into account how the intersection of migration, drug use and destitution impacts the day-to-day realities of PMWUD, their wellbeing and opportunities for recovery and social integration (Pouille et al., 2020). As a result, policy and practice risk overlooking key obstacles and innovative responses to support PMWUD (De Kock, 2022; Lemmens et al., 2017; van Selm et al., 2023).

To enhance knowledge about support needs among destitute PMWUD[1] in Europe, as well as challenges and good practices in addressing these needs, we conducted focus groups with professionals working with PMWUD in four European metropolitan cities hosting a high diversity of destitute PMWUD: Amsterdam, Athens, Berlin and Paris (Lemmens et al., 2017; Pouille et al., 2024). The focus groups answer the following research question: what are the most important support needs of PMWUD according to those working most closely with them, and what challenges

[1] PMWUD in this context refers to the broad and heterogenous group of first-generation migrants who engage in high-risk drug use, meaning that their patterns of use, routes of administration, or the context of use may lead to health or psychosocial problems (Thanki & Vicente, 2013).

and good practices exist in meeting these needs? To offer some background information on these cities, Table 10.1 offers a brief and necessarily simplified overview of these cities along with their regulations on access to healthcare and social security for migrants.

10.2 Methods

In order to explore professionals' perspectives on support needs of destitute PMWUD in Europe, as well as challenges or good practices to meet these needs, we conducted focus groups in Amsterdam, Athens, Berlin and Paris. This focus group study is part of the SEMID-EU project (Services for Vulnerable Migrants Who Use Drugs in the EU)[2] that explored challenges, barriers, and good practices in supporting destitute PMWUD in Europe (see Pouille et al., 2024; van Selm et al., 2023; van Selm et al., 2024). Its aim was to develop recommendations for local services, civil society actors, and EU policymakers.

The study was conducted by a research team of academic and local researchers. The academic researchers were affiliated with European universities and oversaw the research design and coordination. These researchers were also responsible for data analysis and reporting. The local researchers were practitioners working in harm reduction services in each city. They received a two-day training in focus group methodology, were included in the development of the study's protocol, were responsible for recruiting participants and moderating the focus group discussions and were consulted in the data analysis.

10.2.1 Sampling and Recruitment

In each city, local researchers applied purposive sampling to identify professionals with valuable experience or expertise in service provision for destitute PMWUD in their city, including professionals and experts in substance use treatment, harm reduction and social services working with PMWUD. Some focus groups also included persons working with PMWUD from a law enforcement or criminal justice perspective. Efforts were made to ensure diversity in terms of professional background, age, and gender, and to include participants with direct knowledge of, or experience as PMWUD. Table 10.2 offers an overview of the participants per city.

The local researchers sent out an invitation to eligible candidates through e-mail. Depending on the responses and availability of the candidates, they organised one (Amsterdam, Athens and Paris) or two focus groups (Berlin). Each focus group started with an explanation of the research purposes and all participants signed an

[2] More information and resources on the entire SEMID-EU project can be found here: Migrants who use drugs in the EU—Mainline.

Table 10.1 Contextual background of the cities

	Migration and substance use	Access to health care and social security for migrants
Amsterdam (the Netherlands)	In 2022, about 15.8% of the Dutch population was foreign-born. Most common countries of origin among documented migrants are Turkey, the former USSR and Poland (OECD, 2024). In Amsterdam, 59% of the population is noted to have a migration background (i.e., first—or second-generation migrants), mainly from European or Asian descent. 60% of these persons with a migration background are first-generation immigrants (Openresearch.amsterdam, 2024). The Netherlands is known for its liberal drug policy, especially regarding cannabis, and the most commonly used substances are alcohol, cannabis, ecstasy and cocaine (Pomfret et al., 2023)	The legal framework nominally entitles all people to emergency, primary and specialist care, yet financial and bureaucratic hurdles, especially the need for a citizen service number and health insurance, effectively exclude undocumented people and those experiencing homelessness from fuller services and employment-related protections (European Agency for Fundamental Rights, 2016; Médécins du monde, 2017; Pennings, 2020)
Athens (Greece)	Greece has long been known as both a destination and transit country for migrants, with Athens being a key location along many migratory trajectories and one of the main hub cities for migrants in Greece (Martini, 2023). In 2023, 11.3% of the official Greek population was considered foreign-born, with most common countries of birth being Albania, Georgia and Russia (OECD, 2024). The most commonly used substances in Greece are alcohol, marijuana and cocaine (EMCDDA, 2023)	A 2016 law formally opened the public health system to uninsured citizens and vulnerable groups, but service use still requires a social security number, so undocumented migrants and uninsured EU citizens remain largely limited to emergency care (Marini, 2020). Greek nationals and legally resident foreigners may receive benefits, while those without valid residence papers are excluded (Marini, 2020)
Berlin (Germany)	Germany is the main country of destination for humanitarian migrants across the world and EU mobile citizens. In 2023, 18.2% of the German population was foreign-born. The most common countries of birth among foreign-born Germans are Poland, Turkey and Russia (OECD, 2024). Berlin is known as a super-diverse city hosting many residents from different socio-economic classes and migration backgrounds, who suffer from an increasing liberalization of labour, welfare and housing (Hamann & Türkmen, 2020). The most commonly used substances in Germany are alcohol, tabaco, cannabis and cocaine, followed by amphetamine, ecstasy and LSD (EMCDDA, 2023)	Emergency care is guaranteed and some primary or specialist services are formally available to undocumented people for payment, but mandatory health insurance for comprehensive access is typically unattainable without legal status or formal employment. Theoretical reimbursement mechanisms exist but are undermined due to reporting obligations of social service departments to immigration authorities (Médécins du monde, 2017; Schnabel, 2020)

(continued)

Table 10.1 (continued)

	Migration and substance use	Access to health care and social security for migrants
Paris (France)	In 2023, 13.8% of the population was foreign-born, The most common countries of birth of foreign-born French people are Algeria, Morocco and Portugal (OECD, 2024). The urban city of Paris is known as a migration hub. With more than 150 nationalities represented in the city, Paris has the most diverse population in France (OECD, 2018). The most commonly used substances in France are alcohol, tabaco, cannabis, followed by cocaine, ecstasy, LSD and amphetamines (EMCDDA, 2023)	Emergency treatment is supposed to be provided to all, while entitlement to health insurance, similar to social protection, depends on a minimum period of legal residence and a registered address (Isidro & Math, 2020; Médécins du monde, 2017)

Table 10.2 Overview of participants per city

City	Number of participants	Composition of focus group
Amsterdam	8	1 policeman, 1 social worker at a drug consumption room, 1 outreach worker in harm reduction, 1 outreach social worker offering linkage to care for homeless people, 1 person with lived experiences as PMWUD, 1 addiction therapist and counsellor for homeless people, staff member of an interest group for PWUD, 1 care coordinator at a health Centre for people refused by regular healthcare
Athens	7	3 directors of a harm reduction Centre, a therapy Centre for PWUD and national drug policy, 1 sociologist from a specialised therapy Centre for migrants and refugees using drugs with lived experience as PWUD, 1 emeritus professor and infectiologist specialised in working with refugees and migrants with HIV, 1 advocacy officer at an association of people living with HIV
Berlin	FG 1: 8	1 lawyer in criminal and migration low, 4 social workers in harm reduction, health treatment and addiction care, 1 coordinator of homeless care, 1 staff member of the international department of an HIV Centre
	FG 2: 7	5 social workers in harm reduction, drug counselling, harm reduction and psychosocial care, 1 coordinator of intercultural inpatient drug treatment
Paris	9	2 pharmacists, 1 social worker and 1 team manager in harm reduction, 1 person with lived experiences as PMWUD, 1 psychiatrist for young migrants using drugs, 2 project managers of the doctors of the world
Total	39	In the fields of justice (2), harm reduction (15), drug treatment (6), basic need provision (6), healthcare (8), research (2) and other (3)

informed consent form concerning the pseudonymized (re-)use of data from the focus groups and their rights with regard to the study.

10.2.2 Data Collection

The focus group question list and protocol was collaboratively developed by the entire research team and included most important support needs of PMWUD, availability and accessibility of services, and recommendations to improve care for PMWUD. The focus groups were conducted in the national language of each city, except in Amsterdam, where English was used because not all participants spoke Dutch. Each focus group lasted approximately two hours. With permission of the participants, the focus groups were recorded, transcribed verbatim, translated to English and pseudonymised.

10.2.3 Data Analysis

In collaboration with the local researchers, the academic researchers carried out an inductive thematic analysis for each city independently, guided by the six-phase approach of Braun and Clarke (2006). This procedure ensured that coding and theme development were grounded in the data and that the findings reflected the most salient themes within each local context. In a subsequent analytic phase, the city-specific themes were compared, refined, and synthesized into overarching themes that cut across the four cities. This allowed common patterns, divergences, and cross-context dynamics to be identified, while still retaining space to highlight city-specific particularities within each overarching theme. The results of this chapter focus on these overarching results to offer broad insight into good practices, needs and challenges of PMWUD in Europe.

10.2.4 Ethical Considerations

The study was conducted in line with the European Code of Conduct for Research Integrity (All European Academies, 2023). It was approved by the Ethical Commission of the Faculty of Psychology and Educational Sciences at Ghent University (ref. 2022–120).

10.3 Results

Across the focus groups, participants identified the interrelated support needs of PMWUD, along with the challenges and good practices involved in addressing them with regard to: (1) housing, (2) (mental) healthcare, (3) prevention, harm reduction, and substance use treatment, (4) linguistically and culturally accessible services, (5) stigma and criminalisation, and (6) employment, temporality and social integration.

10.3.1 Housing Stability and a Safe Place to Sleep

Across all cities, participants indicated that many PMWUD live on the streets and are in dire need of stable and long-term housing solutions. Stable housing emerged as a fundamental prerequisite for the wellbeing and health of PMWUD as well their opportunities for recovery.

> I think one of the first needs that there is a stable place to sleep... Because if you cannot sleep, you cannot function. (Harm reduction staff member, Paris)

Participants repeatedly stressed that without safe and stable housing, it is nearly impossible for PMWUD to stabilize their health, engage in treatment and care, find employment, and work toward social integration.

Housing insecurity was viewed as both a symptom and a driver of precariousness, feeding into a vicious cycle. Administrative barriers such as registration requirements, identification documents, and proof-of-residence rules were identified as key obstacles to obtaining stable housing. As a result, participants indicated many PMWUD are forced to sleep on the streets. Homelessness was linked to increased drug use and mental and physical health issues, while the absence of a registered address severely limits access to social benefits and health insurance. Participants stressed that this further deepens precariousness and reduces opportunities for recovery and social integration.

The focus groups in Amsterdam, Berlin and Paris touched upon short-term sleeping solutions for PMWUD (e.g., homeless shelters), but participants indicated limited accessibility for PMWUD due to drug use not being permitted in these areas, limited availability (especially in summer), overcrowding and conditions that were considered unsafe and uncomfortable. In Amsterdam and Berlin, temporary housing-first initiatives were described as positive but insufficient, given their limited scale and short duration. In Berlin, a DCR was included in this initiative, with access for PMWUD and opportunities for safe drug consumption. Although these initiatives offer short-term relief for the residents, participants indicated that there was insufficient time to work on underlying issues and offer long-term solutions. This was mentioned to create revolving doors, as individuals are forced back into homelessness after a few months.

> So basically, what you do, you get sick fish out of a sick sea, you try to make them better, and then you throw out back in the sick sea again, hoping they are stronger. (Staff member from an interest group of persons who use drugs, Amsterdam)

Participants in Berlin, Athens and Amsterdam underscored the importance of integrating healthcare and social services into housing initiatives to work towards long-term solutions for the wellbeing, recovery and social integration of PMWUD.

10.3.2 (Mental) Healthcare

Access to healthcare emerged as a central challenge across all cities. Participants underlined that both somatic and mental health needs are common among PMWUD, and that these are interrelated with migration experiences and homelessness.

> We no longer have 'just a homeless person', or 'just a person who consumes alcohol'. No. We have a person who has migrated without health insurance and has psychiatric issues due to trauma while also being homeless. (Social worker drug consumption mobile, Berlin)

The precarious living situation of many PMWUD was mentioned as unhealthy, limiting their opportunity to heal. A lack of health insurance, limited entitlement to public healthcare, and requirements for official residence documents were repeatedly mentioned as key entry obstacles to care. In Athens, participants mentioned that legally, culturally and linguistically accessible care for PMWUD has been getting better due to services specialised in serving PMWUD and measures to support PMWUD in getting health insurance. Yet, bureaucratic and linguistic barriers remain. In Amsterdam, Berlin and Paris, participants discussed that the limited accessibility of (mental) healthcare for PMWUD increases the pressure on low-threshold harm reduction services to help those who can't find help anywhere else, including sometimes even people without drug use or dependence.

Somatic Healthcare. In all contexts, participants described difficulties accessing basic medical care, especially hospital-based services.

> There are very few hospitals that accept migrant addicts and keep them and help them, most hospitals operate in the style of "may this cup be taken from me". (Infectiology specialist in HIV and PMWUD, Athens)

According to participants across the cities, PMWUD without valid health insurance or identification documents were often excluded from treatment or charged fees they could not afford. Participants mentioned that PMWUD were often wrongly denied care, stemming from stigma on drug use, confusion regarding the rights of PMWUD or financial motives. The latter was also linked to structural underfinancing of health services.

In Athens, Berlin and Paris, infectious disease prevention and treatment, such as for HIV and hepatitis C, were noted as areas where late diagnosis and gaps in continuity of care are common for PMWUD.

> Also, budgeting has to be flexible and allow for some breathing room. It has to be able to be replenished, and not allow anyone in charge to make excuses such as 'if the money is no longer there, then we'll ignore the basic right to health, period.' Or, 'We don't care about HIV. Let's just wait until the immunity cells fall below 300,000 and then see what happens.' We see that behaviour every day. (Social worker and coordinator drug consumption mobile, Berlin)

Mental Healthcare. Mental health issues, particularly trauma, psychological distress, depression, and anxiety, were widely reported across the focus groups. Respondents linked these both to pre-migration experiences (e.g., conflict, persecution) and to post-migration conditions (e.g., homelessness, drug use, stigma, criminalisation). However, access to specialised mental healthcare was described as minimal, with long waiting times, language barriers, and limited trauma-informed care and cultural competence among providers.

Across cities rejection due to waiting lists, precarious situations of PMWUD migration (and related legal, language and cultural barriers) and drug use (stigma and exclusion) were mentioned as barriers to mental healthcare. To overcome these barriers and address intersecting problems related to migration, social security, and (mental) health, participants in Berlin proposed on-site specialised mental health support for PMWUD by expanding existing interdisciplinary low-threshold services.

10.3.3 Prevention, Harm Reduction and Substance Use Treatment

Prevention. In Berlin and Amsterdam, participants talked about how PMWUD sometimes get introduced to drugs after their immigration without access to information about (safe) drug use, leading them to start using drugs unaware of their potential consequences. Additionally, participants in Paris emphasised the importance of accessible overdose prevention, noting that misconceptions about dosage can have severe health consequences for PMWUD.

> Many people arrive in the country from the nearby airport. Somebody from their community picks them up, and they stop four blocks down the road, at our premises, and buy heroin and cocaine, which I'm sure isn't in the same dosages as back home, and then they turn blue 3 hours later. (Team manager in an association for persons in precarious situations, Paris)

Therefore, participants in Paris, Berlin and Amsterdam discussed the importance of informing PMWUD about drug policies, (safe) drug use, overdose prevention and treatment options in a linguistically and culturally accessible manner.

Harm Reduction. Participants highlighted that harm reduction efforts, including drug consumption rooms (DCRs), opioid agonist treatment (OAT), and outreach-based harm reduction programmes provide life-saving support and can serve as bridges into broader social care and healthcare.

> "I need an OAT because I've run out of money, I'm in withdrawal," and that's what they need and ask for first. Later, you'll be able to unravel the thread, pull on the wool, and evaluate

specific needs and all that, but that's the need they initially express in 95% of the cases. (Social workers in a harm reduction centre for PMWUD, Paris)

Across all cities, OAT was discussed as an essential stabilising intervention, to increase the health of PMWUD, help them in (re)gaining control over drug use and decrease criminalisation of PMWUD. In Paris' focus group, participants discussed that OAT can be considered essential healthcare, making it accessible to all PMWUD in theory, even when they don't have health insurance or other required documents. In practice, however, lack of time and resources lead to waiting lists for PMWUD. In Berlin, participants discussed that restrictive eligibility criteria and administrative requirements form barriers to OAT for PMWUD. This formed a rationale to develop specific services for PMWUD without health insurance. In the focus groups of Paris and Berlin, outreach, on-site and take-home OAT was mentioned as an effective way to reach destitute PMWUD who experience difficulties in coming to harm reduction centres. In the focus groups of Berlin, DCRs were perceived as safe spaces where individuals can use drugs under supervision, reduce health risks, and connect with care. Yet, current legal restrictions in Germany limit the scope and accessibility of DCRs for PMWUD.

Substance Use Treatment. Even though participants in Paris indicated that sobriety may be a far leap for some PMWUD due to multiple co-occurring underlying issues that need to be resolved first (e.g., homelessness, mental health problems), they also indicated that professionals can support PMWUD to work towards sobriety through residential care or OAT tapering. This was confirmed by participants of the Athens and Berlin focus groups, who advocated for legally and linguistically accessible addiction counselling and residential treatment. In Amsterdam, lengthy enrolment processes, and a lack of health insurance formed barriers towards specialised substance use treatment for PMWUD, while Greek participants indicated strict rules in sobriety-oriented substance use treatment, without the recognition of OAT as a potential recovery pathway, as barriers for many PMWUD.

Integrated, Accessible and Continuous Care. All focus groups addressed the importance of inter-service collaboration in order to offer tailored, continuous and integrated care answering to the complex and interacting needs of destitute PMWUD. Finally, participants across the cities underscored the importance of continuity of care and stable housing to avoid PMWUD to relapse after treatment. In Berlin, a focus group also indicated that collaboration with international services can facilitate continuity of care for PMWUD across countries (e.g., for pre- or post-migration follow-up). Participants across the cities underscored that continuity of care can only be realised when language, legal, social and geographical barriers to care are eliminated.

10.3.4 Linguistically and Culturally Accessible Services

Beyond structural barriers such as housing and legal status, participants across all cities indicated a lack of linguistically and culturally accessible services as barriers for PMWUD toward effective health and social services.

Across all focus groups, language barriers were reported to form major obstacles to social care and healthcare, as well as to necessary information for PMWUD (e.g., about overdose prevention or available services). Increasing the knowledge of the local language among PMWUD was therefore seen as a necessary starting point by participants in Berlin and Athens. However, the focus groups across the cities showed that these barriers can also be overcome by professionals, through the utilisation of translating software and/or the involvement of interpreters or volunteers with a migration background in these services. In Berlin and Athens, participants indicated that enabling PMWUD to communicate in their own language enables feelings of safety and trust.

> The safe space that we provide, that he hears his language from the interpreters, it is the first step in an intimacy. This is very basic. (Psychologist and director in a specialized substance use treatment unit for PMWUD, Athens)

Yet, participants in the focus groups of Athens, Berlin and Paris also underscored the importance of cultural awareness and sensitivity, particularly in navigating differences in moral norms and community practices. Participants from Berlin and Paris referred to community engagement as a possible way to bridge these barriers, though the lack of structural resources to enable this was criticised. Participants in Paris pointed to the inclusion of anthropologists in care teams as a way to bridge cultural barriers.

> Back in the day, with Russian-speaking users generally speaking, and with Punjabis later on, we managed to overcome the language barrier and talk to each other, but that didn't mean we understood each other. So, the involvement of anthropologists in the teams, or of specialists with some knowledge of the communities and the issues at stake, helped the teams to understand why people say yes all the time and then leave and nothing happens. (Pharmacist in a harm reduction centre, Paris)

10.3.5 Stigma and Criminalisation

Participants across all cities described stigma and criminalisation as pervasive forces shaping the lives of PMWUD. They discussed the impact of multiple stigmas on the lives of destitute PMWUD. Stigma related to migration background, drug use, homelessness, residence status and criminal offences were mentioned to compound social exclusion and reinforce mutual mistrust between PMWUD and institutions. According to participants, these stigmas not only shape the interactions of PMWUD with frontline workers but also influence broader public attitudes and political discourses. In Amsterdam and Paris, this public and political reluctance was linked to the shortage of shelter and housing options for destitute PMWUD.

> You feel that it weighs heavily on these users, who know that they're already seen as delinquents because of their drug use, or the fact that they also sell drugs to support themselves, whether it's for food or drink. It's very specific, this deportation, this double delinquency—they don't have accommodation at the moment, at [region], they're homeless. That weighs on them and makes it even harder for them to claim their space because we're already denying them so many. (Coordinator of a drug monitoring centre, Paris)

The criminalisation of drug use, homelessness and irregular migration were mentioned as drivers of precariousness creating barriers for PMWUD toward health and social services. In Berlin, for example, participants noted that even when health or social services were available, PMWUD sometimes stayed away out of fear that personal information could be shared with the authorities, and they would be deported.

> Double stigmatization. Not only are they crack users at [region], but they get woken up. You're not allowed to sleep anywhere. Plus, you're undocumented. It's a double problem. The cops can do whatever they want, they're the ultimate victims of mistreatment. (Coordinator of a drug monitoring centre, Paris)

Across the cities, examples were given of how the precariousness of destitute PMWUD led to contact with law enforcement and the criminal justice system, for example due to drug selling, theft and accumulated fines in combination with a lack of legal support.

Across the four cities, participants addressed the adverse consequences of criminalising PMWUD. In Amsterdam, Athens and Berlin, participants talked about how police custody and prison detainment can lead PMWUD to lose resources for recovery, such as stable health, OAT, employment, social network, housing and access to residence documents (as an empty criminal record may be a requirement), leaving them unsupported upon release. Additionally, participants in Athens, Berlin, and Paris pointed to limited healthcare in detention and prison settings, resulting in communicable diseases going undetected or untreated and leaving PMWUD without access to harm reduction, thereby endangering their health.

> Balanced people, in chronic substitution, who are fine, they have found their families again, they take antiretroviral, they have everything, suddenly they are stopped for old sins, they are stopped by the police, they are locked in, and Golgotha starts all over again. It is Sisyphean this struggle. (Directed of a national focal point for drug policy, Athens)

This is why in all cities, participants discussed the tension between punitive approaches and care provision, with most participants urging a shift from punishment to support.

In Amsterdam and Berlin, participants emphasised the importance of training law enforcement about the rights of PMWUD, how to communicate these rights to them, and the available referral options. In Berlin, collaboration with law enforcement was also discussed as needed to create safe environments for PMWUD around harm reduction centres, making sure that PMWUD are not arrested in front of the centres. Yet, in Amsterdam, Berlin and Paris, participants indicated that collaboration between care and law enforcement remains limited, due to mistrust and negative experiences in the past.

In contrast with the stigmatising and criminalising attitudes PMWUD often face, participants in Paris underscored the importance of openness and non-judgemental attitudes among professionals.

10.3.6 Social Integration, Employment and Temporality

In Athens and Berlin, participants advocated for integration support through education, employment and rehabilitation, enabling PMWUD to overcome language and cultural barriers in the country they reside in. Participants emphasised that employment can provide structure, dignity, (financial) stability and facilitate social integration. In Amsterdam, a person with lived experiences also stressed the importance of 'keeping busy' through work or daily activities, in order to be able 'not to think about drugs'. In Berlin, participants talked about the vicious cycle that comes from not being able to work: people end up homeless, engage in drug use as a survival mechanism on the street, and their opportunities for integration and recovery further declines.

> They want to work, the labour market leads to people having no access, and they end up on the street. They start consuming on the street. This is a chain that absolutely does not break. (Social worker in street work, Berlin)

This was confirmed in Amsterdam, where participants highlighted that long-term employment is often a prerequisite for insurance and other governmental financial and housing resources. Yet, for destitute PMWUD, employment is frequently unattainable due to lack of a work permit or the demands of surviving in precarious conditions. Similarly, participants in Paris emphasised that heavy drug use or homelessness can leave little space or capacity for work, meaning these issues must be addressed before PMWUD can engage in employment.

Across the cities, it became clear that PMWUD often face diverse legal and administrative barriers to entering the labour market. Even when projects exist that offer work opportunities to people without a work permit, e.g., in Amsterdam, they tend to be few in number and often temporary in nature. Therefore, participants in Berlin, Paris and Amsterdam indicate that legal support for receiving work permits as well as more flexible policies regarding work permits or training are needed to enhance opportunities for integration and recovery among PMWUD.

> He was a teacher, but that is not recognized here, and de facto, he is not allowed to work. Then slips into the drug scene, he's homeless, committing petty crimes, getting arrested, and all that while he actually holds a high-quality degree. On the other hand, we have a skills shortage in Germany. It would simply be very clever, also from the point of view of the state, to provide this probationary residence permit with a work permit. (Social worker in a health and social centre with a DCR, Berlin)

The notion of temporality was considered a barrier to social integration, especially in Athens. Participants observed that many PMWUD initially aim to transit through Greece or return home but often end up staying longer than planned. Additionally, when being undocumented, PMWUD can be forced to leave the country at any time. This leaves PMWUD in a constant state of uncertainty, without long-term perspectives. This was confirmed in Amsterdam, where participants stated that many PMWUD, even if they initially planned to stay only temporarily or are forced to leave the country, end up staying, either because they feel ashamed towards their network in their country of origin or because their situation in Amsterdam is still better than the situation they would be in back home. This continuous perception of temporality is mentioned as a driver of drug use as well as a barrier to social integration, care and support. A psychotherapist indicated that this perception cannot function as an excuse not to offer care to PMWUD:

> We need to treat everyone as our tomorrow's neighbour…. and you cannot immobilize a person who is coming as a temporary person who will be here for a little while. (Psychotherapist, Athens)

Additionally, participants in the Athens' focus group identified a "legal gap" for PMWUD facing criminal charges, since they are barred from leaving Greece, but—as was confirmed in Amsterdam—are simultaneously denied basic human rights and the right to work.

> Creative people that did have rights to work and if you give them the opportunity, they will eventually maybe go back to work. But if you [referring to police officer] find 'em enough, they will revoke that [right to work] and you can, you can't fix it. It's like way, way more difficult to them. And if they're not going away and they're going to stay here, yeah. Then you're just piling it up to the debt they have already. The bigger the debt, the further, they will get away building something that allows them to have a normal life again. (Therapist for persons who use drugs and experience homelessness, Amsterdam)

10.4 Discussion

This study shed light on professionals' perspectives on the support needs of destitute PMWUD, including but not restricted to those considered 'refugees' in legal terms. The focus groups in Amsterdam, Athens, Berlin, and Paris provided a comprehensive understanding of the perceived support needs of PMWUD in Europe as well as the barriers and good practices related to meeting these needs. Despite the specific socio-legal configurations of each city, several common themes and systemic issues emerged, offering both critical insights and potential pathways towards more equitable and effective support.

10.4.1 Support Needs of PMWUD in Europe

This study highlighted that PMWUD across Amsterdam, Athens, Berlin, and Paris face overlapping and interconnected needs that are fundamental to wellbeing, recovery, and social integration (Neureiter & Waldmann, 2025; Pouille et al., 2024).

First, housing and a stable place to sleep were confirmed as a precondition for accessing services, improving mental health and social integration, and reducing exposure to violence and exploitation (European Website on Integration, 2024; Pouille et al., 2021). Second, this study confirmed the importance of accessible healthcare that answers to the complex health needs of PMWUD related to drug use, homelessness, and a lack of preventive and continuous care (De Kock, 2022; Neureiter & Waldmann, 2025; van Selm et al., 2024). Additionally, trauma-informed mental healthcare, though not always considered a priority amidst competing needs, has been identified as essential for the wellbeing and recovery of PMWUD (De Kock, 2022; Lebano et al., 2020; Pouille et al., 2024). Third, this study underscored the importance of providing accessible harm reduction, prevention and treatment to PMWUD, in order to increase the health, wellbeing and social situation of PMWUD (Pouille et al., 2024; van Selm et al., 2024). Finally, participants also emphasised the importance of employment, daily structure, and social integration in fostering belonging, self-efficacy, and long-term stability (Pouille et al., 2021). However, these opportunities are often inaccessible due to legal restrictions, social exclusion, or unstable living situations (Neureiter & Waldmann, 2025).

10.4.2 Challenges in Meeting these Support Needs: Legal, Linguistic, Cultural and Social Barriers

This study confirmed multiple and intersecting barriers that undermine access to essential services for PMWUD. First, legal and administrative exclusions, such as the absence of residence status, health insurance, or municipal registration, frequently determine access to housing, healthcare, employment and social protection (Kumar et al., 2024; Lebano et al., 2020; Neureiter & Waldmann, 2025). These systems are often not designed for highly mobile or destitute populations, meaning that even those with legal residence may experience exclusion (Kumar et al., 2024). Linguistic and cultural barriers further impede navigation of services, communication with professionals, and trust-building, especially when translation and culturally competent mediation are unavailable (De Kock, 2022; Lebano et al., 2020; Savas et al., 2024). Finally, stigma and criminalisation were consistently described as shaping both policy responses and day-to-day interactions with institutions, limiting access to support services and reinforcing marginalisation (Neureiter & Waldmann, 2025; Rechel et al., 2011; van Selm et al., 2023). These barriers, in combination with often under-funded health and social services, imply that PMWUD often are excluded from services that address their support needs, even if they—in theory- should have access to them (Kumar et al., 2024; Savas et al., 2024).

Hence, even PMWUD with residence papers frequently encounter multiple barriers to essential support services. Legal complexity, language difficulties, cultural differences, social marginalisation, and stigma associated with drug use intersect to create compounded disadvantages, limiting access to (mental) healthcare, housing, and social services. This intersectionality illustrates that entitlement is shaped not only by formal legal status but also by social, cultural, and structural factors, highlighting the urgent need for integrated, low-threshold, rights-based interventions that respond to both legal and lived realities of PMWUD (Neureiter & Waldmann, 2025; Pouille et al., 2021; Savas et al., 2024). The results of this study confirm multiple exclusionary processes that decrease access for PMWUD to healthcare, social support and recovery. This exclusion reflects processes of 'welfare state bordering', whereby national, regional, and local government practices impose boundaries on access to social rights based on residence status, migration motive, and citizenship (Bendixsen & Näre, 2024).

10.4.3 Promising Practices to Support PMWUD

Despite systemic constraints, participants identified practices that help overcome barriers to care and inclusion. Harm reduction services could sometimes overcome legal constraints because some of their services can be considered essential healthcare, which should be accessible to everyone (Lemmens et al., 2017; Savas et al., 2024). Additionally, participants described creative strategies to reduce legal and administrative barriers for PMWUD, such as providing a temporary residence address or avoiding documentation requirements to access basic care and support. Low-threshold and outreach services that invest in reducing legal, geographical, and cultural barriers through flexible eligibility criteria, outreach and community engagement were described as essential points of contact and important bridges to broader healthcare and social support for PMWUD (Pouille et al., 2024; Regis et al., 2020). Long-term housing opportunities for (undocumented) PMWUD from a housing-first principle were mentioned as offering PMWUD the necessary stability to work towards other (mental) health and social needs (De Kock, 2022; Tumminelli, 2024). To decrease linguistic and cultural barriers, the use of interpreters and community engagement has offered promising solutions for services (Stylianopoulos et al., 2024).

Integrated and collaborative approaches, including cooperation across health, housing, legal, and social services, migrant communities, law enforcement and citizens were seen as crucial to create enabling environments that meet the complex needs of PMWUD (Council of the European Union: General Secretariat of the Council, 2021; Savas et al., 2024).

These practices demonstrate that targeted, person-centred and integrated approaches can mitigate structural exclusion when backed by institutional flexibility and political will. Yet, Savas et al. (2024) note, even highly motivated and well-trained professionals cannot deliver empathetic, person-centred care when working under time pressure, resource constraints, and without backing from their team and institution.

10.4.4 Recommendations for Policy, Practice and Research

Policy. Restricting PMWUD with irregular status to essential healthcare not only leaves substantial space for interpretation, but also fails to answer to the complex needs of PMWUD (Savas et al., 2024). Evidence shows that providing preventive and comprehensive healthcare to people without secure residence status not only upholds human rights but also reduces long-term public expenditure (European Union Agency for Fundamental Rights, 2015). In order to increase the wellbeing of PMWUD, as well as opportunities for recovery and social integration, policies should ensure access for PMWUD to prevention, treatment, harm reduction, and social support (Kumar et al., 2024; Lemmens et al., 2017; Stylianopoulos et al., 2024). This also requires removing administrative and legal barriers that restrict access to housing, healthcare and social services (Kumar et al., 2024). Finally, sufficient funding is needed for services to adequately reach and support destitute PMWUD (Savas et al., 2024).

Practice. Services working with PMWUD should adopt an integrated approach tackling the intersecting challenges PMWUD face, and focus on reducing barriers by offering low-threshold, outreach-based, trauma-informed and culturally responsive care (Kumar et al., 2024). Harm reduction and tailored services are not only vital in addressing immediate physical needs, but also in offering emotional, social, and practical support often lacking in the lives of PMWUD. By maintaining a consistent and non-judgmental presence amid unstable living and health conditions, these services contribute to both physical security and social inclusion. They provide a sense of community, safety, and belonging, fostering hope and enabling positive change across multiple life domains (Brenman, 2021).

Research. This research addressed the broad and heterogeneous group of PMWUD. While this approach allowed us to identify shared challenges, it may have overlooked important details regarding specific substances or particular communities. Future research could focus on the needs and challenges of subgroups, such as gender minorities or communities defined by migration background or type of drug use. Research should also analyse legal and administrative barriers more in-depth and explore feasible policy alternatives from both legal and sociological perspectives. Finally, longitudinal research on existing promising practices would help assess their long-term impact and inform sustainable responses.

10.4.5 Limitations

This chapter has several limitations that should be taken into account when interpreting the findings.

First, this chapter represents the results of five focus groups in four metropolitan cities. These group settings may have inhibited participants from openly discussing highly sensitive or stigmatised issues. Additionally, due to the sampling method (purposive sampling by local researchers) selection bias may have been in place. The varying number and composition of focus groups across cities may have influenced the richness and balance of the data, as well as the prominence of certain themes in the cities. Hence, these results should be interpreted as the views of those participating in the focus groups and not necessarily the general perception of frontline workers on the needs of PMWUD in these cities or across Europe. Second, all focus groups were translated into English, with one focus group conducted in English although this was not the native language of several participants. These translations may have led to certain nuances getting lost. Finally, while the analysis necessarily condenses and reorganises city-level findings into broader themes, some contextual detail is inevitably lost. Moreover, thematic analysis is interpretive in nature; categorisation of themes and subthemes inevitably reflects researcher judgement.

Despite these limitations, the study offers valuable, transferable insights into the support needs of PMWUD, challenges to meeting these needs, and promising practices that can inform more inclusive responses to PMWUD across European contexts.

Acknowledgements This study was funded by the European Union's Justice Programme, Drugs Policy Initiatives (Grant agreement number 101045837). It was carried out by a team of academic, local and community researchers from Amsterdam, Athens, Berlin and Paris, referred to as the SEMID-EU consortium: Joanna Moura, Ingrid Bakker, Roberto Perez, Sultan Baghdadi, Emil, Arturo, Marios Atzemis, Ralf Köhlein, Astrid Leicht, MJ, SK, MC, Mathieu Lovera, Victor Detrez, Elisabeth Avril, Datuna and Ismaël. Special thanks to this exceptional team of researchers for their contribution, commitment and collaboration. We also want to thank all participants of the focus groups for their valuable contributions.

Competing Interests Local researchers were practitioners at harm reduction centres which may have coloured the recruitment and, subsequently, the results. There are no other competing interests to declare.

References

All European Academies. (2023). The European code of conduct for research integrity. https://allea.org/wp-content/uploads/2023/06/European-Code-of-Conduct-Revised-Edition-2023.pdf

Bendixsen, S., & and Näre, L. (2024). Welfare state bordering as a form of mobility and migration control. *Journal of Ethnic and Migration Studies, 50*(11), 2689–2706. https://doi.org/10.1080/1369183X.2023.2298540.

Braun, V., & Clarke, V. (2006). Using thematic analysis in psychology. *Qualitative Research in Psychology, 3*(2), 77–101. https://doi.org/10.1191/1478088706qp063oa

Brenman, N. F. (2021). Placing precarity: Access and belonging in the shifting landscape of UK mental health care. *Culture, Medicine and Psychiatry, 45*(1), 22–41. https://doi.org/10.1007/s11013-020-09683-5

Castañeda, H., Holmes, S. M., Madrigal, D. S., Young, M.-E. D., Beyeler, N., & Quesada, J. (2015). Immigration as a social determinant of health. *Annual Review of Public Health, 36*(2015), 375–392. https://doi.org/10.1146/annurev-publhealth-032013-182419

Council of the European Union, General Secretariat of the Council. (2021). EU drugs strategy 2021–2025. Publications Office of the European Union. https://doi.org/10.2860/736505

De Kock, C. (2022). Responding to drug-related problems among migrants, refugees and ethnic minorities in Europe (background paper commissioned by the EMCDDA for health and social responses to drug problems: A European guide. https://www.emcdda.europa.eu/drugs-library/responding-drug-related-problems-among-migrants-refugees-and-ethnic-minorities-europe_en

EMCDDA. (2023). Statistical bulletin 2023-prevalence of drug use. https://www.euda.europa.eu/data/stats2023_en

European Union Agency for Asylum, & European Monitoring Centre for Drugs and Drug Addiction. (2023). Professionals working in reception centres in Europe: An overview of drug-related challenges and support needs. https://euaa.europa.eu/publications/professionals-working-reception-centres-europe-overview-drug-related-challenges-and-support-needs

European Union Agency for Fundamental Rights. (2015). Cost of exclusion from healthcare—The case of migrants in an irregular situation. Publications Office of the European Union. https://doi.org/10.2811/23637

European Commission's Directorate-General for Migration and Home Affairs (2024). Migrants' access to medium—and long-term housing in the EU: Barriers, governance and good practices. https://home-affairs.ec.europa.eu/whats-new/publications/migrants-access-medium-and-long-term-housing-eu-barriers-governance-and-good-practices_en

European Agency for Fundamental Rights (2016). Healthcare entitlements of migrants in an irregular situation in the EU-28. https://fra.europa.eu/en/publication/2016/healthcare-entitlements-migrants-irregular-situation-eu-28

Hamann, U., & Türkmen, C. (2020). Communities of struggle: The making of a protest movement around housing, migration and racism beyond identity politics in Berlin. *Territory, Politics, Governance, 8*(4), 515–531. https://doi.org/10.1080/21622671.2020.1719191

Horyniak, D., Melo, J. S., Farrell, R. M., Ojeda, V. D., & Strathdee, S. A. (2016). Epidemiology of substance use among forced migrants: A global systematic review. *PLoS One, 11*(7), e0159134. https://doi.org/10.1371/journal.pone.0159134

Isidro, L., & Math, A. (2020). Migrants' access to social protection in France. In J.-M. Lafleur & D. Vintila (Eds.), *Migration and social protection in Europe and beyond (volume 1): Comparing access to welfare entitlements* (pp. 165–178). Springer International Publishing. https://doi.org/10.1007/978-3-030-51241-5_11

Kumar, B. N., Bhopal, A., Blanchet, K., Wickramage, K., & Onarheim, K. H. (2024). Priority setting and migration health policies for European countries. *The Lancet Regional Health-Europe, 41*, 100804. https://doi.org/10.1016/j.lanepe.2023.100804

Lebano, A., Hamed, S., Bradby, H., Gil-Salmerón, A., Durá-Ferrandis, E., Garcés-Ferrer, J., Azzedine, F., Riza, E., Karnaki, P., Zota, D., & Linos, A. (2020). Migrants' and refugees' health status and healthcare in Europe: A scoping literature review. *BMC Public Health, 20*(1). https://doi.org/10.1186/s12889-020-08749-8

Lemmens, P., Dupont, H., & Roosen, I. (2017). *Migrants, asylum seekers and refugees: An overview of the literature relating to drug use and access to services. Background paper commissioned by the EMCDDA for Health and social responses to drug problems: a European guide.* https://www.emcdda.europa.eu/document-library/migrants-asylum-seekers-and-refugees-overviewliterature-relating-drug-use-and-access-services_en

Marini, F. (2020). Migrants' access to social protection in Greece. In J.-M. Lafleur & D. Vintila (Eds.), *Migration and social protection in Europe and beyond (volume 1): Comparing access to welfare entitlements* (pp. 195–209). Springer International Publishing. https://doi.org/10.1007/978-3-030-51241-5_13

Martini, C. (2023). Victoria Square, Athens: Migratory movements and social stratifications in the Centre of the Greek capital. *Identities*, 1–17. https://doi.org/10.1080/1070289X.2024.2406659

Médécins du monde. (2017). Legal report on access to healthcare in 16 European countries. https://www.doctorsoftheworld.org.uk/wp-content/uploads/import-from-old-site/files/2017_final-legal-report-on-access-to-healthcare-in-16-european-countries.pdf

Najdini, M., Mathieu, J., Shadili, G., Frigaux, A., Ménauges, M., Mouton, C., Gressier, F., & Essadek, A. (2025). Substance use prevalence among immigrants by generational status in Europe: A systematic review and meta-analysis. *Alcohol, Clinical and Experimental Research, 49*(7), 1381–1391. https://doi.org/10.1111/acer.70091

Neureiter, M., & Waldmann, G. (2025). Migration and health inequalities in Europe: Examining the impact of discriminatory climates on migrants' unmet healthcare needs. *Journal of International Migration and Integration*. https://doi.org/10.1007/s12134-025-01292-8

OECD. (2018). Working Together for Local Integration of Migrants and Refugees in Paris. OECD Publishing. https://www.oecd.org/en/publications/working-together-for-local-integration-of-migrants-and-refugees-in-paris_9789264305861-en.html

OECD. (2024). International migration outlook 2024. OECD Publishing. https://www.oecd.org/en/publications/international-migration-outlook-2024_50b0353e-en.html

Openresearch.amsterdam. (2024). Population in figures. https://openresearch.amsterdam/en/page/117156/population-in-figures?utm_source

Pennings, F. (2020). Migrants' access to social protection in The Netherlands. In J.-M. Lafleur & D. Vintila (Eds.), *Migration and social protection in Europe and beyond (volume 1): Comparing access to welfare entitlements* (pp. 313–325). Springer International Publishing. https://doi.org/10.1007/978-3-030-51241-5_21

Pomfret, A., Rigoni, R., Busz, M., & Schiffer, K. (2023). *City Report Amsterdam. Shaping the future of drug regulation from the 'bottom-up'. Civil Society Monitoring of Harm Reduction in Europe.* https://correlation-net.org/wp-content/uploads/2024/04/2023_CEHRN-Monitoring_City-Report-Amsterdam_Eng.pdf

Pouille, A., Bellaert, L., Vander Laenen, F., & Vanderplasschen, W. (2021). Recovery capital among migrants and ethnic minorities in recovery from problem substance use: An analysis of lived experiences. *International Journal of Environmental Research and Public Health, 18*(24), 13025. https://doi.org/10.3390/ijerph182413025

Pouille, A., De Kock, C., Vander Laenen, F., & Vanderplasschen, W. (2020). Recovery capital among migrants and ethnic minorities: A qualitative systematic review of first-person perspectives. *Journal of Ethnicity in Substance Abuse*, 1–31. https://doi.org/10.1080/15332640.2020.1836698

Pouille, A., De Ruysscher, C., Van Selm, L., Van Amsterdam, J., Van Den Brink, W., Busz, M., Perez Gayo, R., Atzemis, M., Vanderplasschen, W., The, S. E. M. I. D.-E. U., & consortium. (2024). Challenges and support needs among persons with a migration background who use drugs in four European metropolitan cities. *Harm Reduction Journal, 21*(1). https://doi.org/10.1186/s12954-024-01110-x

Pouille, A., De Ruysscher, C., Vander Laenen, F., & Vanderplasschen, W. (2023). "Watch out for the boogieman": Stigma and substance use recovery among migrants and ethnic minorities. *Journal of Community & Applied Social Psychology, 33*(3), 571–586. https://doi.org/10.1002/casp.2657

Provine, D. M. (2011). Race and inequality in the war on drugs. *Annual Review of Law and Social Science, 7*(1), 41–60. https://doi.org/10.1146/annurev-lawsocsci-102510-105445

Rechel, B., Mladovsky, P., Devillé, W., Barbara Rijks, W., Petrova-Benedict, R., & McKee, M. (Eds.). (2011). Migration and health in the European Union. Open University Press. http://www.euro.who.int/en/about-us/partners/observatory/publications/studies/migration-and-health-in-the-european-union-2011

Regis, C., Gaeta, J. M., Mackin, S., Baggett, T. P., Quinlan, J., & Taveras, E. M. (2020). Community Care in Reach: Mobilizing harm reduction and addiction treatment Services for Vulnerable Populations [community case study]. *Frontiers in Public Health, 8*. https://doi.org/10.3389/fpubh.2020.00501

Savas, S. T., Knipper, M., Duclos, D., Sharma, E., Ugarte-Gurrutxaga, M. I., & Blanchet, K. (2024). Migrant-sensitive healthcare in Europe: Advancing health equity through accessibility, acceptability, quality, and trust. *The Lancet Regional Health–Europe, 41*. https://doi.org/10.1016/j.lanepe.2023.100805

Schnabel, R. (2020). Migrants' access to social protection in Germany. In J.-M. Lafleur & D. Vintila (Eds.), *Migration and social protection in Europe and beyond (volume 1): Comparing access to welfare entitlements* (pp. 179–193). Springer International Publishing. https://doi.org/10.1007/978-3-030-51241-5_12

Stylianopoulos, P., Hertner, L., Heinz, A., Kluge, U., Schäfer, I., & Penka, S. (2024). Good practice in reaching and treating refugees in addiction care in Germany–a Delphi study. *BMC Public Health, 24*(1). https://doi.org/10.1186/s12889-023-17446-1

Thanki, D., & Vicente, J. (2013). PDU (Problem drug use) revision summary. European Monitoring Centre for Drugs and Drug Addiction. https://www.emcdda.europa.eu/drugs-library/pdu-problem-drug-use-revision-summary_et

Tumminelli, G. (2024). Housing first: A system for combatting marginality. In F. Lo Piccolo, A. Mangiaracina, G. Paternostro, & V. Todaro (Eds.), *In and out: Rights of migrants in the European space* (pp. 67–77). Springer Nature Switzerland. https://doi.org/10.1007/978-3-031-51131-8_5

UNHCR. (2019). Handbook on procedures and criteria for determining refugee status and guidelines on international protection under the 1951 Convention and the 1967 Protocol relating to the status of refugees. https://www.unhcr.org/media/handbook-procedures-and-criteria-determining-refugee-status-under-1951-convention-and-1967

van Selm, L., White, T. M., Picchio, C. A., Requena-Méndez, A., Busz, M., Bakker, I., Romero, D., Gayo, R. P., Pouille, A., & Vanderplasschen, W. (2023). Drug use and access to drug dependency services for vulnerable migrants who use drugs in the European Union: Consensus statements and recommendations from civil society experts in Europe. *International Journal on Drug Policy, 118*, 104087. https://diposit.ub.edu/dspace/bitstream/2445/217209/1/870287.pdf

van Selm, L., White, T. M., Picchio, C. A., Requena-Méndez, A., Busz, M., Perez Gayo, R., Pouille, A., Gelabert, P. M., & Lazarus, J. V. (2024). A call to create integrated services to better address the needs of migrants who use drugs in Europe. *Harm Reduction Journal, 21*(1), 9. https://doi.org/10.1186/s12954-023-00923-6

WHO Western Pacific Region. (2018). Health of refugees and migrants: Regional situation analysis, practices, experiences, lessons learned and ways forward. https://cdn.who.int/media/docs/default-source/documents/publications/health-of-refugees-and-migrants-wpro-2018165be999-c496-4779-9b7d-853111f371f9.pdf

Chapter 11
Substance Use-Related Interventions in the European Reception Setting: Let's Prioritise Prevention, Early Intervention and Access to Treatment

Charlotte De Kock

11.1 Introduction

Substance use among (conflict-)displaced populations is attributed to both individual factors—that arise pre, during and after migration—as well as conditions external to the individual, such as reception conditions and the housing situation (Ezard et al., 2020; Horyniak et al., 2016; Chap. 1 in this volume). Indeed, the influences of trauma, loss and displacement or transit-related experiences, in concert with resettlement and acculturation, each play a role in the development of substance use patterns in these populations (Elkholy et al., 2023).

Although epidemiological research points out that substance use is not higher in displaced compared to general populations in Europe (De Kock & EUDA, 2022), substance use-related incidents are a growing concern in the reception setting, following a joint report of the European Drugs and Asylum Agencies conducted among 98 reception professionals in 21 European member states (EUDA & EUAA, 2023). Moreover, substance use becomes more prevalent among second, compared to first generation migrants (Najdini et al., 2025). Nevertheless, little is known concerning the effectiveness of substance use interventions in European reception settings on the one hand (Greene et al., 2021; Lotzin et al., 2021), and strategies for adapting and implementing evidence-based interventions for these populations, on the other.

A recent review on substance use prevention programmes among refugee youth worldwide, for instance, identified only one intervention in Europe (Aleer et al., 2024). Moreover, the above-mentioned joint report by the European Drugs and

C. De Kock (✉)
Faculty of Law and Criminology, Institute for Social Drug Research, Ghent University, Ghent, Belgium
e-mail: Charlotte.DeKock@UGent.be

C. De Kock (ed.), *Substance Use Among Refugees in Europe*,
https://doi.org/10.1007/978-3-032-32399-6_11

Asylum Agency (EUAA & EUDA, 2023) pointed out that professionals in the reception setting want and need more training concerning substance use-related interventions. The majority of respondents (72%) did not receive any training on the topic of substance use and only one in four felt confident about their skills and competences to deal with substance use-related issues, especially prevention and incident management. Over half of the respondents indicated that the reception facility where they work provides substance use-related responses and interventions.

While there is growing academic scholarship on good practices in substance use treatment (Stylianopoulos et al., 2024), as well as growing attention for preventive interventions to strengthen the psychological health and resilience of refugees (Pluck et al., 2022), the evidence base for specific substance use interventions in this setting in Europe remains limited (Aleer et al., 2024; Greene et al., 2018, 2019).

This chapter therefore intends to offer a first comprehensive scoping review that identifies substance use-related interventions in this setting in Europe, outlining key characteristics and analysing their evidence base. We opted for a scoping (instead of a systematic) review because of the dearth of knowledge in the domain of substance use-related interventions in Europe, the rapidly evolving nature of the domain and the fact that previous reviews pointed out the absence of evidence-based interventions in this domain and setting in Europe (Aleer et al., 2024; Greene et al., 2018; Pluck et al., 2022). This qualitative scoping review thus aims to identify the nature and extent of (research) evidence, including ongoing research (Grant & Booth, 2009).

11.2 Method

Searches were first conducted in Web of Science and Scopus using the following search string within the timeframe of 1 January 2014 to 15 April 2025: (drug OR substance) AND (reception OR refugee OR asylum) AND (intervention OR treatment OR prevention OR training).

The inclusion criteria were defined as follows, within the PICO framework:

- Population/Patient/Problem (P): Intervention targets the European reception setting (EU member states, Switzerland and Ukraine) and/or professionals working with, or applicants/refugees/undocumented migrants themselves.
- Intervention (I): Intervention targets prevention, early/brief intervention, screening, treatment, harm reduction, professional training.
- Comparison (C): Considering that this is a scoping review, no comparison group was required.
- Outcome (O): Intervention targets substance use-related outcomes.

Considering the above-mentioned caveats in the current evidence in this domain, an extensive array of purposive sampling methods was used within the same timeframe:

- Bibliography searches in previously identified reports (De Kock, 2022; EUDA, 2013a; Greene et al., 2018; Kane & Greene, 2018; Priebe et al., 2016; Stöver et al., 2018).
- Screening the 2014 Reitox national drug reports[1] (De Kock, 2020)[2] and the 2019 EUDA national monitoring data.[3]
- Follow-up on the relevant responses of an online survey (September 2021) conducted by the EUDA & EUAA (2023).
- Website searches: United Nations High Commissioner for Refugees (UNHCR), Mental Health and Psychosocial Support Network, World Health Organisation, United Nations International Children's Emergency Fund (UNICEF), Médecins Sans Frontières, International Rescue Committee, International Committee of the Red Cross, IOM and Google.
- Follow-up on international meeting reports attended by the author:
  - *Responding to drug-related challenges for Refugees, Migrants and IDPS* (21–23/09/2021, Pompidou Group, Palermo, Italy);
  - *Responding to substance use-related problems in reception settings in EU+ countries* (12/10/2023, EUAA & EUDA, online);
  - *Challenges and lessons in reaching out to undocumented migrants with diverse mental health issues and substance abuse problems* (03/10/2024, Migration Policy Institute, online).

A total of 1076 records were identified after duplicate removal (see Figure 11.1: PRISMA Flowchart). After title screening 80 studies were retained for abstract screening. A total of 36 studies were excluded because they were not conducted in Europe, not published in English, not conducted in the reception setting, excluded substance users as the targeted population, insufficient information on the intervention was available or because the population was not refugees nor professionals in the reception setting. The scoping review includes 43 studies and identifies 21 interventions. In the results section, interventions (and not studies) are the unit of analysis.

The intervention identification phase consisted of gathering administrative data (conveners, implementers, contact information, website) and information on 13

[1] The full method is described in the MATREMI (Mapping and Enhancing Substance Use Treatment for Migrants and Ethnic Minorities) report: www.Belspo.be DR/84. In this study both the 2014 and 2017 Reitox national drug reports submitted by the EU-27 member states to the EUDA were screened using the following queries: ethn*, minorit*, migra*, nationali*, foreign, roma, reception, refugee. The publicly available versions of the 2017 reports contained little to no information on inspiring practices aimed at MEM, and not all of the 2015 and 2016 reports were available online. The focus was subsequently on the 2014 reports for in-depth analysis. Full paragraphs, including the search terms, were listed and read per country. Lastly, inspiring practices related to SUT for MEM were listed.

[2] MATREMI: www.Belspo.be DR/84.

[3] A search was conducted in the Reitox 2019 workbooks received by EUDA using the search terms: migra*, refuge*.

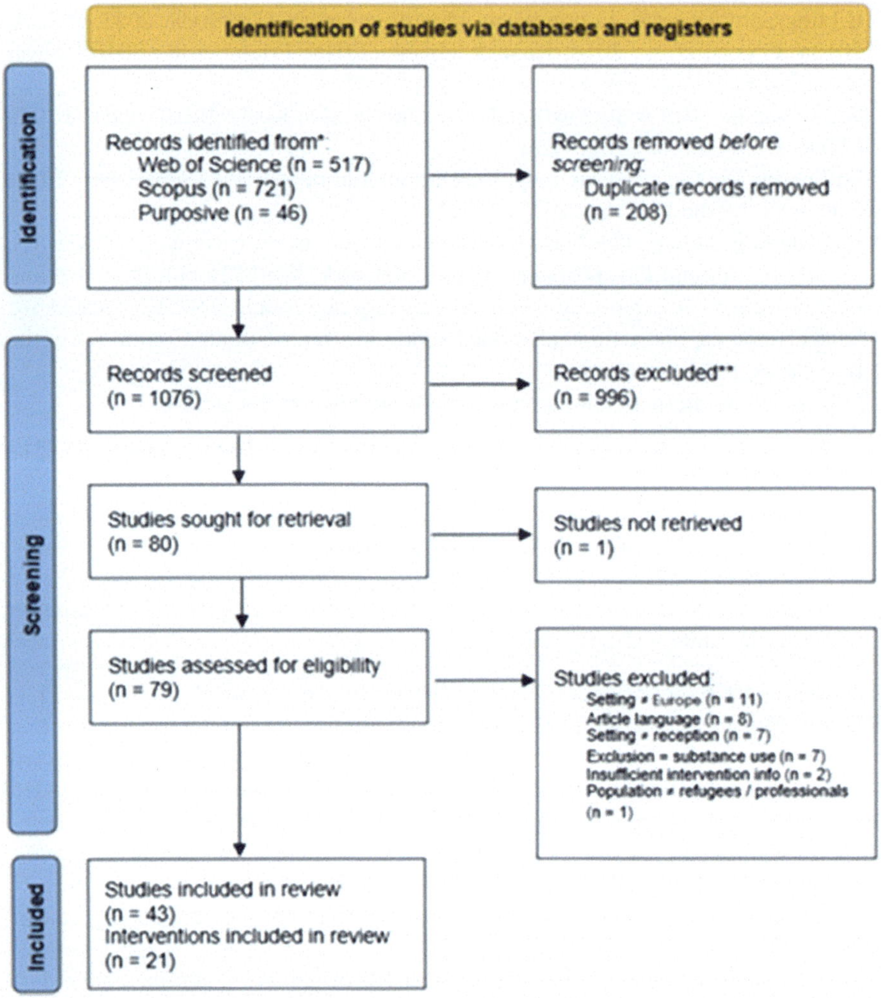

Figure 11.1 PRISMA Flowchart

topics (listed below) related to intervention content, quality and evaluation in an intervention information sheet. This information was gathered by the author and validated by at least one intervention convener in collaboration with EUDA. The intervention information sheets are included in an intervention compendium, publicly available via the EUDA website (suplemented with more recent EUDA monitoring data).

1. Short description.
2. Behavioural, environmental and other change techniques.
3. Main intervention type.
4. Outcomes targeted.
5. Factors targeted.

6. Intervention components/modules.
7. Main target group.
8. Setting.
9. Evaluation study outcomes.
10. Resources: manual/guidelines.
11. Resources: evaluation study.
12. Intervention challenges.
13. Intervention Requirements

The intervention information cited in this chapter stems from the full intervention sheets filled out by intervention conveners or filled out by the author and validated by conveners.

In what follows, we discuss the 21 identified interventions under two categories: the intervention spectrum category (assessment, prevention, and early intervention) targeting displaced populations in the European reception setting, on the one hand, and interventions targeting professionals working with these populations in this setting, on the other hand.

11.3 Results: Interventions in the Reception Setting

11.3.1 Intervention Overview

A total of 21 interventions were identified (Table 11.1). Twelve interventions focus on refugee populations by means of substance use severity assessment ($n = 2$), prevention ($n = 7$) and early intervention ($n = 3$). Nine interventions focus on professionals working with refugee populations by targeting their competences ($n = 7$) and organisational support ($n = 2$).

Of the 21 identified interventions most were developed and implemented in Germany ($n = 6$) and the Netherlands ($n = 4$). Five interventions were initially developed under the impulse of the World Health Organisation (WHO) and implemented across Europe, while specifically focussing on middle-and low-income settings as compared to high-income settings. Three interventions were implemented in Belgium, two in Greece and one in Finland.

Following the Xchange Prevention registry evidence evaluation standards,[4] all interventions were rated as 'additional studies recommended' (Table 11.2: Identified substance use interventions and rating), mainly because of insufficient consistent outcomes in Europe, which makes it difficult to assess if the interventions are effective or not, even if outcomes seem to be in favour of the intervention. For

[4] Xchange ratings include, respectively: beneficial, likely to be beneficial, possibly beneficial, additional studies recommended, unlikely to be beneficial and possibly harmful. Interventions are rated based on rigorous evidence evaluation. More information about the protocol, rating and proceedings can be found on the EUDA Xchange website.

Table 11.1 Identified substance use-related interventions, member states and European studies

Intervention name	Member State (developed)	European (outcome) studies
CUSU-Sy—Assessment	Germany	NA
ASSIST: Screening and brief intervention	*NA (WHO)*	Lee et al. (2023), Greene et al. (2024a), Khan et al. (2011)
BePrepared digital health intervention	Germany	Fischer et al. (2021)
Preventive advisory conversation about psychological issues or substance use	The Netherlands	NA
Step-by-step (SbS)	*NA (WHO)*	Burchert et al. (2019), Cuijpers et al. (2022), Röhr et al. (2021)
Manual for an alcohol and drug policy in the reception setting	Belgium	NA
Professional training—mhGAP	*NA (WHO)*	Purgato et al. (2019)
Mental health and Substance use Animation & Game for refugees	The Netherlands	NA (see chap. 9 in this volume)
MindSpring—Psychoeducation and psychosocial support	Denmark, The Netherlands, Germany	Husby et al. (2020)
Self-help plus (SH+)	*NA (WHO)*	Purgato et al. (2019, 2021), Turrini et al. (2022), Weinreich et al. (2025), WHO (2023), Karyotaki et al. (2023), Acarturk et al. (2024)
Problem management plus (PM+)	*NA (WHO)*	de Graaff et al. (2024), Sever et al. (2024), Knefel et al. (2020), Spaaij et al. (2022), Sijbrandij et al. (2017), Purgato et al. (2019, 2021), Turrini et al. (2025)
Reaching out for minors in Greece	Greece	NA
Origin-arrival-future	Germany	NA
PraeWi prevention and E-learning in the reception setting	Germany	Lorenz et al. (2021, 2023, 2024a, 2024b) (see Chap. 4 in this volume), Uricher (2025)
Professional training—E-learning TAVATA supportive conversational techniques	Finland	NA
Professional training—Perspective 3D	Germany	NA
Professional training—DrugInt basic drug training	Belgium	NA
Professional training—E-learning alto	Belgium	NA

(continued)

Table 11.1 (continued)

Intervention name	Member State (developed)	European (outcome) studies
Professional training—CONSENS mudra	Germany	NA
Professional training—Kethea mosaic	Greece	NA
Professional training—E-learning refugees with psychological complaints and substance use	The Netherlands	NA

Problem Management Plus (PM+), for instance, some effects for relevant outcomes are in favour of the intervention, as found in at least one evaluation study (de Graaff et al., 2024) of acceptable quality in Europe. Intervention rating follows the Xchange prevention rating criteria (protocol 2.0) but has not been endorsed by the Xchange Prevention rating board, at the time of writing. Moreover, the majority of interventions have not been evaluated based on a robust evaluation design (Table 11.1).

11.3.2 Assessment, Prevention and Early Intervention

We identified ten interventions that directly or indirectly target substance use prevention. Additionally, two interventions (ASSIST, CUSU-Sy) primarily target substance use severity assessment. These scopes often overlap in the intervention spectrum (Mrazek & Haggerty, 1994): whereas some interventions focus mainly on preventing use before it occurs, some also include intervening to prevent current use from becoming problematic or harmful. Assessment of substance use severity in turn goes hand in hand with early intervention (e.g., ASSIST-BI). Moreover, some interventions mainly target factors that have been evidenced to influence substance use, such as stress management and coping mechanisms, but not primarily substance use.

As for the quality of evaluation of the interventions, four interventions have undergone rigorous evaluation within the framework of experimental designs in, but mainly outside Europe (Self-Help Plus, ASSIST(-BI), Problem Management Plus and its derivate Step-by-Step). For three interventions, feasibility studies are available and evaluation studies with experimental designs are underway (PraeWi, BePrepared, CUSU-Sy). Descriptive evaluations are available for the remaining five interventions (Preventive advisory talk, Mindspring, Mental Health and Substance Use Animation and Game, Origin-Arrival-Future, Reaching out for minors).

In what follows, we will briefly discuss the nature, theoretical background and evaluation of the interventions based on a categorisation of the available evidence: interventions with outcome studies in Europe, interventions for which outcome or

Table 11.2 Identified substance use interventions and rating

Intervention name	Rating
CUSU-Sy—Assessment	Intervention(s) build(s) on evidenced logical model(s). Evaluation studies are underway. Additional studies recommended
ASSIST: Screening and brief intervention	Intervention(s) build(s) on evidenced logical model(s), descriptive (process) evaluation is available. Outcome studies outside Europe and a validation study in Europe are available. Additional studies recommended
BePrepared digital health intervention	Intervention(s) build(s) on evidenced logical model(s), feasibility study is available. Additional studies recommended
Preventive advisory conversation about psychological issues or substance use	Intervention(s) build(s) on evidenced logical model(s), descriptive (process) evaluation is available. Additional studies recommended
Step-by-step (SbS)	Intervention(s) build(s) on evidenced logical model(s), one RCT in Europe with mixed results is available, others are underway. Additional studies recommended
Manual for an alcohol and drug policy in the reception setting	Intervention(s) build(s) on evidenced logical model(s) but no evaluation studies are available. Additional studies recommended
Professional training—mhGAP	Outcome studies outside Europe are available. Additional studies recommended
Mental health and Substance use Animation & Game for refugees	Descriptive analysis of survey data is available. Additional studies recommended
MindSpring—Psychoeducation and psychosocial support	Intervention(s) build(s) on evidenced logical model(s), descriptive (process) evaluation is available. Additional studies recommended
Self-help plus (SH+)	Two RCT with mixed results are available in Europe. Additional studies recommended
Problem management plus (PM+)	Several outcomes studies outside Europe are available and an acceptable quality RCT with mixed outcomes was conducted in The Netherlands. Additional studies recommended
Reaching out for minors in Greece	Intervention(s) build(s) on evidenced logical model(s) but no evaluation studies are available. Additional studies recommended
Origin-arrival-future	Intervention(s) build(s) on evidenced logical model(s) but no evaluation studies are available. Additional studies recommended
PraeWi prevention and E-learning in the reception setting	Intervention(s) build(s) on evidenced logical model(s). Evaluation studies are underway. Additional studies recommended

(continued)

Table 11.2 (continued)

Intervention name	Rating
Professional training—E-learning TAVATA supportive conversational techniques	Intervention(s) build(s) on evidenced logical model(s) but no evaluation studies are available. Additional studies recommended
Professional training—Perspective 3D	Intervention(s) build(s) on evidenced logical model(s) but no evaluation studies are available. Additional studies recommended
Professional training—DrugInt basic drug training	Intervention(s) build(s) on evidenced logical model(s), descriptive (process) evaluation is available. Additional studies recommended
Professional training—E-learning alto	Intervention(s) build(s) on evidenced logical model(s), descriptive (process) evaluation is available. Additional studies recommended
Professional training—CONSENS mudra	Intervention(s) build(s) on evidenced logical model(s) but no evaluation studies are available. Additional studies recommended
Professional training—Kethea mosaic	Intervention(s) build(s) on evidenced logical model(s), descriptive (process) evaluation is available. Additional studies recommended
Professional training—E-learning refugees with psychological complaints and substance use	Intervention(s) build(s) on evidenced logical model(s), descriptive (process) evaluation is available. Additional studies recommended

process studies are underway and interventions for which only descriptive outcome studies are available.

11.3.2.1 Interventions with Outcome Studies in Europe

Self-Help Plus (SH+)

To counter the challenges related to the limited mental health system capacity in mainly low-income regions, the WHO developed scalable psychological interventions. These interventions target the reduction of psychological distress and improved functioning in people living in communities affected by adversity. The interventions are intended to be delivered through individual, group face-to-face or smartphone formats by non-professionals without specialised mental health training (Sijbrandij et al., 2017). Three interventions were included in this review: Self-Help Plus (SH+), Problem Management Plus (PM+) and Step-by-Step (SbS).

Although these interventions were mainly implemented in low-income settings outside Europe, they are more recently being implemented in Europe. The EU4Health-funded U-RISE and WELL-U projects (Weinreich et al., 2025), for instance, aim to improve the mental health and psychological well-being of displaced people from Ukraine in Europe by implementing these and other interventions (without evaluation). The Horizon2020-funded STRENGTHS[5] (de Graaff et al., 2022; Sijbrandij et al., 2017) and RE-DEFINE[6] (Purgato et al., 2019) consortia are in turn aimed at evaluating these and other interventions in Europe.

SH+ is a guided self-help group intervention that addresses mental health needs in conflict-and disaster-affected low-resource settings. It is designed to provide psychological support to large populations in humanitarian settings, including individuals without formal mental health diagnoses. The intervention design is based on acceptance and commitment therapy (ACT) (French et al., 2017), focussing on mindfulness and psychological flexibility, helping individuals manage distress from adversities.

SH+ combines a five-session pre-recorded audio course with an illustrated self-help book designed for low-literacy populations and can be delivered to groups of up to 30 people. Additionally, the SH+ training for lay facilitators involves a 40-hour workshop over five days, focussing on using SH+ materials (audio recordings and illustrated guides) and practising facilitation skills through role-play.

The intervention has been evaluated in randomised controlled trials (RCT), conducted under the RE-DEFINE project (Purgato et al., 2019) which set up a multinational study investigating the intervention's effectiveness in preventing mental disorders in displaced populations in Italy, Germany, Austria, Finland, Turkey and two sites in the United Kingdom. Although the European RCT demonstrated no positive effect on the targeted outcomes in the primary analysis (Purgato et al., 2021), secondary analyses did report differential outcomes among subgroups and across settings. An individual participant data (IPD) meta-analysis of three of these trials with refugees and asylum seekers (1795 participants) (Karyotaki et al., 2023), showed significantly larger effects on depressive symptoms, self-identified problems and well-being among participants who were not employed and those with lower well-being.

In a subsample, Turrini et al. (2022) equally failed to find a statistically significant long-term preventive effect of SH+ at 12-month follow-up. But in this study, secondary analysis demonstrated that SH+ may have positive long-term prevention effects (psychological distress, depressive symptoms, well-being), provided a sufficient dose of SH+ is received, indicating the importance of implementation context and dosage. Several limitations in the available evaluation studies warrant consideration such as the bias introduced by aggregating data from five countries as well as low sample sizes and attrition. None of the European evaluation studies included outcome indicators or outcomes of substance use at the time of writing.

Problem Management Plus (PM+)

Problem Management Plus (PM+) is an intervention based on cognitive behavioural therapy (CBT) that focusses on stress management, problem solving techniques,

---

[5] Syrian REfuGees MeNTal HealTH Care Systems, Horizon2020, Grant Agreement No. 733337.

[6] Refugee Emergency: DEFining and Implementing Novel Evidence-based psychosocial interventions, Horizon 2020, Grant Agreement No. 779255.

behavioural activation and strengthening social support. The intervention consists of five weekly sessions lasting 90 minutes (Carswell et al., 2018). PM+ is a manualised intervention that can be flexibly and individually adapted to the participant's needs and self-identified practical problems (e.g., unemployment, interpersonal conflicts). Sessions are delivered by trained non-specialist 'helpers' who have a similar cultural background as the participants (Spaaij et al., 2022).

This intervention has been evaluated in different low-resource settings including countries such as Egypt, Ethiopia, Kenya, Malawi, Nepal, Syria, Uganda, Ukraine and Thailand. In Europe PM+ has been evaluated in the context of the STRENGTHS project and disseminated in the context of the U-RISE project. The intervention has been adapted, implemented and evaluated in Austria (Knefel et al., 2020), Switzerland (Spaaij et al., 2022) and in the Netherlands (de Graaff et al., 2022, 2024), mainly targeting Syrian and Afghan forcibly displaced populations. It has also been implemented in Slovakia, Poland and Romania for Ukrainian displaced populations. Further, it has been scaled up in the asylum system in Switzerland where it is routinely accessible (Spaaij et al., 2022).

de Graaf et al. (2022, 2024) studied the effectiveness of Problem Management Plus at 3-month (2023) and 1-year follow-up (2024) for Syrian refugees in a high-income setting (the Netherlands). PM+ reduces psychological distress and anxiety symptoms up to 1 year ($d = 0.28$–0.31), consistent with its behavioural strategies targeting stress management, problem-solving, and behavioural activation. Outcomes for behavioural activation (BA) and social support components however do not align well with the theoretical rationale in these studies. At 12-months, the depression outcome is non-significant. Additional support such as booster sessions or additional (trauma focused) modules were suggested to prolong and consolidate benefits gained through PM+ on other mental health and psychosocial outcomes. The intervention showed particular effectiveness when delivered through hybrid (in-person and online) formats.

PM+ was modified with an Emotional Processing (EP) module for Syrian, Eritrean and Afghan youth (16–25 years) in the Netherlands (Sever et al., 2024). A feasibility study ($n = 90$) found the adapted version culturally acceptable and safe, addressing barriers to mental health access through peer-delivered sessions.

Studies in Austria (Knefel et al., 2020) and Switzerland (Spaaij et al., 2022) confirmed the feasibility and acceptability of PM+ (adapted version in Austria) for refugees in these settings, with significant reductions in common mental health symptoms observed in participants. The Swiss study (Spaaij et al., 2022) demonstrates acceptability and safety when delivered by trained non-specialists. Lastly, an RCT is ongoing in Austria (Knefel et al., 2020) but excludes participants presenting with substance dependence. As substance use is not considered the main focus of PM+, substance use (disorders), and related outcomes have not yet been evaluated in European evaluation studies at the time of writing.

Step-by-Step (SbS)

Step-by-Step (SbS) was conceptualised as an online self-help version of the WHO's PM+ (see supra) within the STRENGTHS consortium (Burchert et al., 2019; Sijbrandij et al., 2017). It is an online and offline computer-and smartphone-based e-mental health programme for Syrian refugees implemented in Lebanon (Cuijpers et al., 2022; Heim et al., 2021), Egypt, Sweden and Germany (Röhr et al., 2021; Woodward et al., 2023) by the STRENGTHS consortium. SbS is rooted in digital cognitive behavioural therapy (CBT) as evidenced by Wright et al. (2019) in the context of primary care in the USA.

SbS consists of three 20-minute segments with visual and audio content, unlocked every four days. The intervention uses illustrated stories with a main character and health professional to teach therapeutic techniques through interactive exercises. Non-specialist helpers with psychology or health backgrounds receive training in emotional support, suicide risk detection and distress management to guide users. They are supervised by a clinical psychologist. SbS thus consists of its content (narratives and exercises), guidance (e-helper support) and delivery (web or app). It can be self-guided or supported by minimal, on-demand or no guidance and is accessible via the website, an app, audio or book.

Eight RCTs were conducted in Jordan, Lebanon, the Netherlands, Turkey, Switzerland, Germany, Sweden and Egypt in the framework of the STRENGTHS project. Although results have been promising, showing improvement in outcomes such as depression, functioning, anxiety, post-traumatic stress, subjective well-being and self-identified personal problems among displaced Syrians in Lebanon (Cuijpers et al., 2022), results of evaluation studies in Europe have so far been inconclusive (see the following).

An SbS app (Sanadak) was qualitatively evaluated through a pilot version in 2019 (Burchert et al., 2019) among 128 Syrian refugees in Germany, Sweden and Egypt, assessing ICT access, usage and barriers through interviews and focus groups. App prototypes were evaluated for usability, user experience and dissemination. Findings highlighted internet access issues and technical literacy as common challenges. While participants identified health benefits because of the app, acceptability, credibility and technical requirements were key implementation barriers (Burchert et al., 2019).

An RCT in Berlin, Germany (Röhr et al., 2021) concluded that Sanadak was not more effective in reducing mild to moderate post-traumatic stress in Syrian refugees than the control condition (psychoeducational reading material) at four months post intervention, nor was it likely to be more cost-effective. While no effectiveness was found as a standalone treatment for reducing post-traumatic stress, it showed potential as a bridging aid within a stepped and collaborative care approach due to good usability and reduction in self-stigma (Röhr et al., 2021). As is the case for PM+ and SH+, substance use is not considered the main focus of SbS and substance use (disorders) and related outcomes have not yet been evaluated in European evaluation studies at the time of writing.

The Alcohol, Smoking and Substance Involvement Screening Test (ASSIST) and ASSIST-Linked Brief Intervention (ASSIST-BI)

The Alcohol, Smoking and Substance Involvement Screening Test (ASSIST) was developed for the WHO by an international group of researchers and clinicians as a technical tool to assist with early identification of substance use-related health risks and substance use disorders in primary health care, general medical care and other settings (Humeniuk et al., 2010).

ASSIST is a screening tool that builds on earlier WHO tools like the Alcohol Use Disorders Identification Test (AUDIT), developed in 1982. ASSIST version 3.1 (considered to be the standard) is a culturally adaptable, 8-item questionnaire administered in 5 to 10 minutes by a health worker to assess the use of a broad range of substances. It assigns a risk score for each substance—categorised as low, moderate or high risk—which guides the appropriate intervention, from no treatment to brief advice or referral to specialised care. Doty et al. (2018) included the ASSIST 3.0 alcohol items in an assessment for mental health and alcohol use problems among conflict-affected adults in Ukraine. The study reported good internal consistency and test-retest reliability for the included outcomes.

Lee et al. (2023) evaluated the ASSIST-11 across 42 countries and found that it is valid and reliable with strong internal consistency and cross-cultural applicability.

The ASSIST-linked Brief Intervention (ASSIST-BI), in turn, is designed to address hazardous and harmful substance use identified through the ASSIST screening tool. It is based on motivational interviewing principles (Rollnick & Miller, 1995) and aims to encourage behavioural change. Greene and colleagues (2024a) found among male refugees in Uganda that the combination of SH+ and ASSIST-BI is feasible, and that if proven effective, it could form a useful first-line intervention approach for male refugees with psychological distress and low-to moderate-level substance use risk. Nevertheless, ASSIST 3.1 and BI have mainly been studied outside Europe in primary health care settings: the interventions have not yet been validated nor evaluated among displaced populations in European reception settings.

11.3.2.2 Interventions for Which Outcome Studies Are Underway in Europe

CUSU-Sy

CUSU-Sy is a culture-sensitive assessment targeted at screening substance use and related behaviours among Syrian refugees (Behr & Lindert, 2024). It was developed together with Syrian refugees with funds from the German Federal Ministry of Education and Research. The instrument assesses substance use and related behaviours and needs, and thereby facilitates referral and health-related monitoring. CUSU-Sy includes 15 items in seven domains of substance use: lifetime use of relevant types of substances, frequency, intensity, self-perception of, and situations posing social and emotional risk factors for substance use-related behaviours, ability to perform, craving, tolerance and intentions to reduce or quit substance use. An evaluation study is underway in Germany.

PraeWi

PraeWi is a multi-component prevention concept which includes a podcast, an app, culturally sensitive information videos in different languages (Arabic, Turkish, Farsi, Ukrainian, Russian, French, German and English), peer education for refugees as well as an e-learning tool and guidelines for the workforce of shared accommodations in Germany.

The intervention is based on a mixed-methods study on the psychosocial situation and substance use among refugees in shared accommodations (Lorenz et al., 2023, 2024a). Insights from these results informed the development of PraeWi.

The intervention was evaluated conducting a multicentre and cluster-randomised controlled trial (Lorenz et al., 2024b) across nine shared accommodations utilising a stepped-wedge design in the pre-registration, with increasing knowledge about substances and substance use as the primary outcome. The analysis was modified to a pre-post study design due to accommodation level dropouts. Although the evaluation study was unable to find a statistically significant effect on the knowledge outcome, secondary analysis did demonstrate that living situation and duration of the residence procedure moderated mental health and well-being. These results are expanded on by Uricher and colleagues in Chap. 4 in this volume.

BePrepared

BePrepared is a brief smartphone intervention for the indicated prevention of substance use disorders (Fischer et al., 2021). It was developed in Germany by the MentalHealth4Refugees consortium funded by the Federal Ministry of Education and Research. The intervention content is based on CBT and Motivational Interviewing. It consists of four intervention modules, which become accessible on a weekly basis over four weeks: diary, change, thinking and doing, and lastly relaxation. The app contains culture-sensitive components and is aimed at young refugees with hazardous use of alcohol and/or cannabis.

The study protocol for a single-armed feasibility trial among 150 young refugees with problematic use of alcohol and/or cannabis was published by Fischer et al. (2021). While the study established usability and acceptance, forming the basis for future efficacy research, substance use-related outcomes post-intervention were not yet published at the time of writing.

11.3.2.3 Interventions with Descriptive or no Evaluation Studies Available in Europe

Preventive Advisory Conversation NL

The Preventive Advisory Conversation (PAC) is a one-time consultation with a prevention specialist for adults and young people who have questions or concerns about psychological issues including substance use-related problems. After identifying the concerns or problems, the PAC provides information about mental health and explores possible solutions or support options. The PAC concludes with tailored advice. By the end of the PAC the client should have increased awareness of their own situation and feel more empowered in their personal choices and options. A culturally sensitive version was developed and is currently implemented for young refugees with residence status in the Netherlands (aged 18–24) (see Chap. 9).

The intervention is based on the I-Change model which combines components of Ajzen's (1991) theory of planned behaviour (attitudes, social norms, perceived behavioural control), Bandura's social cognitive theory (Bandura, 2001) (self-efficacy), Prochaska's transtheoretical model (Prochaska & Velicer, 1997) (stages of change), the health belief model (risk perception, perceived severity/susceptibility) and goal-setting theories (De Vries, 2017; Kasten et al., 2019).

Although detailed process evaluation reports high user satisfaction, and referral to other services after over half of the consultations, the underlying mechanisms of this intervention have thus far not yet been evaluated. This intervention is discussed in Chap. 9 in this volume.

MindSpring

MindSpring (MS) is a community group intervention for refugees with the purpose of strengthening the participants' ability to cope with psychosocial problems, thereby preventing premigration trauma and post-migratory stressors from evolving into psychiatric disorders (Husby et al., 2020). Trained people with refugee backgrounds provide the workshops in their own language with or supervised by a professional coach from a mental health or social service.

The group courses target psychoeducation (awareness concerning trauma, mourning, stress, acculturation, substance use), psychosocial support (coping and referral if needed) and empowerment (focussing on strengths and confidence).

MindSpring exists in many different variants which target adults, children and parents. Websites of the intervention implementers (e.g., Centre General Wellbeing Belgium, Danish Refugee Council, ARQ National Trauma Centre the Netherlands) reveal large implementation differences (e.g., age category 16–30 in Denmark versus 8–13 and 14–18 in Belgium, number of sessions, peer trainers in the Netherlands versus professional trainers in Belgium).

An observational study was conducted in Denmark (Husby et al. 2020) including 92 Arabic-speaking refugees. Participants completed a baseline demographic questionnaire, an outcome questionnaire and the WHO-5 well-being questionnaire in a pre-post design. Paired t-tests showed significant pre-post differences. Nevertheless, outcomes were only measured in the beginning and right after the end of the session series, which is why long-term effects remain unknown. Evaluation studies with experimental designs are underway but not yet available in Europe at the time of writing.

Mental Health and Substance Use Animation and Game

This intervention is implemented in the Netherlands by Jellinek and consists of two components: an animated video and a game aimed at raising awareness and initiating discussions about mental health and substance use among refugees. The intervention is grounded in health education and behavioural change theories, including the health belief model and elements of social cognitive theory. It targets (Arabic-and Tigrinya-speaking) applicants of international protection (AIP) in Dutch reception centres and is designed to improve knowledge, reduce stigma and increase motivation to seek help. The interventions can be executed individually, in pairs or in groups.

The animation provides culturally adapted psychoeducation, while the game stimulates interaction and discussion, but also offers knowledge when played individually. The convener reported in the intervention sheet that descriptive evaluation data from participants and professionals showed the intervention was well received and considered relevant, accessible and culturally appropriate. Positive effects were reported on awareness and attitudes, though structural barriers to care remained. Evaluation studies with an experimental design are not available at the time of writing.

Origin-Arrival-Future

This intervention is implemented by Sucht Hamburg in Germany and focusses on de-tabooing the topic of addiction[7] within various communities. For this purpose, trained key individuals from the respective communities are involved. These volunteers share knowledge in their native language. They facilitate information events within communities, set up information booths in various locations and organise joint activities. The main topics are: What is addiction? How does the addiction support system work in Hamburg? Where can people find help for those affected and their families/friends? Intervention components include but are not limited to an alcohol goggles course, a quiz, videos and disseminating information material.

[7] The word 'addiction' and other wording related to substance use problems, e.g., 'substance abuse', are only used as direct citations from the interventions conveners or authors, as these terms may carry connotations discouraged in modern public health and criminology research in favour of more neutral phrasing such as 'substance use and related problems', 'problematic substance use' or reference to DSM-V categorisations, while ensuring fidelity to original voices.

The convener reported in the intervention sheet that training and information sessions are descriptively evaluated to assess outcomes and success of the project. Six to twelve people take part in an information session. The groups are diverse in terms of age and migration background. Commonly spoken languages include Turkish, Farsi and Arabic and the majority of participants are women. Evaluation studies with an experimental design are not available at the time of writing.

Kethea Mosaic Outreach for Minors

Kethea Mosaic is based in Athens, Greece and provides information, counselling, psychological support and (relapse) prevention services to migrants and refugees with addictions. Kethea Mosaic collaborates with and intervenes in the reception settings and a transcultural high school which hosts unaccompanied minors, where they organise group sessions targeting minors.

Besides this intervention, Kethea Mosaic targets minors and adults in different substance use phases and implements prevention activities (awareness-raising groups for minors— unaccompanied or not). Kethea Mosaic provides counselling services for minors and adults, early intervention for minors at high-risk and supports family members, for instance by means of virtual meetings. Although more in-depth information of targeted interventions was unavailable and evaluation with an experimental design has not yet been conducted, Kethea Mosaic is unique for its high reach among the targeted populations.

11.3.3 Professional Competence Training and Organisational Support

Eight of the identified interventions focus on strengthening professional competences of staff working in or with the reception setting. We located two competence trainings in Germany (Consens Mudra, 3D Perspective), two in Belgium (DrugInt, e-learning Alto) and one each in Greece (Kethea Mosaic), Finland (TAVATA, conversational skills) and the Netherlands (Jellinek). Additionally, the Mental Health Gap Action Programme (mhGAP) (2008) provides a Humanitarian Intervention Guide (mhGAP-HIG) (2015, 2019) that provides evidence-based guidance and tools for assessment and integrated management of priority disorders including substance use-related disorders (Keynejad et al., 2018).

The mhGAP Humanitarian Intervention Guide (2015, 2019 with an expected update in 2026) provides first-line management recommendations for humanitarian emergencies where specialist care is limited. Because the guide mainly targets non-specialist health care providers in low-and middle-income countries and consists of guidelines rather than interventions, we only included behavioural interventions targeting displaced populations in the reception setting in the prevention and early intervention section (see Sect. 11.3.2). Up-to-date interventions and guidelines can be found in the online mhGAP Evidence Resource Centre.

While the interventions discussed in the previous sections may also offer professional competence components, they are not included here because it is not their main focus (e.g., PraeWi and MindSpring; see Sect. 11.3.2).

The identified trainings target both staff in reception settings as well as professionals who work with refugees and AIP outside the reception setting. The identified trainings are mainly face-to-face trainings whereas three also have a dominant e-learning module (Alto e-learning in Belgium; Jellinek in the Netherlands; TAVATA in Finland). The description, targeted factors and outcomes sections of the information sheets demonstrate that all competence trainings have a strong knowledge component.

This shared knowledge component mainly consists of understanding and recognising substance use (related problems). As demonstrated in the below overview, additional knowledge components vary across the trainings. Some trainings focus on treatment service knowledge, others on legal and medical perspectives on substance use, environmental, pre-and post-migration risk factors and behavioural dependencies.

Overview

- **Consens Mudra (Germany):** Knowledge on addiction and support systems, legal foundations and consequences, countries of origin, comorbidity and practical tips on working with non-German speakers.
- **DrugInt (Belgium):** 22 knowledge items including substances and effects, risk and protective factors, intervention spectrum, recovery-oriented principles, partners in and barriers to treatment, professional secrecy, assessment instruments (ASSIST) and the model of behavioural change as a basis of motivational interviewing.
- **E-learning Alto (Belgium):** Learning basic concepts, destigmatisation, building a bond, interventions, working in a team, medical consultation and psychiatric comorbidities.
- **Jellenik e-learning (the Netherlands):** Sub-learning objectives are the purpose and importance of early signalling; what signals of psychological complaints are; what signals of substance use and risky gambling/gaming are; and referring to treatment.
- **Kethea Mosaic (Greece):** The aim of the training is to raise knowledge of professionals working with the population of migrants, refugees and AIP related to drug use, drug-related problems, how to pay attention to addiction and how to face it from specific professional perspectives.
- **Perspective 3D (Denmark):** Knowledge about addiction and its development, especially in relation to the living situation of refugees, of the effects of addictive substances and legal aspects, including (asylum) legal consequences and recognising problematic or addictive substance use.

Besides the knowledge components, trainings also focus—albeit to a lesser extent—on interaction targeting skills and behaviours, be it to varying degrees, ranging from half an hour at the end of the training (DrugInt) to additional multi-day

(Alto) or at-request modules (Perspective 3D, Alto). The methods for achieving this vary significantly across the interventions, as demonstrated below.

- On-site training and peer-review (Alto e-learning in Belgium).
- Conducting a SWOT analysis (DrugInt in Belgium).
- Peer recruitment, exercises on diversity (Consens Mudra in Germany).
- Training about discussion (Jellinek, the Netherlands) and conversational skills (TAVATA in Finland).
- Coaching on addiction prevention topics (Perspective 3D in Germany).

Considering that competences consist of a combination of knowledge, skills, abilities and other characteristics (Arribas-Aguila et al., 2024) such as behaviours, it stands out that the knowledge components are most strongly developed, whereas skills and behavioural components appear more open-ended. Only the TAVATA training (Finland) has a clear skills-related goal by focussing on "supportive conversational skills of professionals working in reception centres to strengthen the mental health of asylum seekers" in the short description in the intervention sheet. Indeed, motivational interviewing as a brief early intervention—the TAVATA goal—is recommended by the WHO as a priority intervention in humanitarian settings in its "Brief psychosocial interventions for people using cannabis or stimulants" (WHO, 2023).

In addition to professional competence training we identified one intervention mainly oriented towards the organisational level of the reception setting: a manual for developing an alcohol and drug policy in the reception setting in Belgium. This guide helps staff in developing a drug policy framework in the reception setting. Such a drug policy consists of 'house rules' concerning substance use as well as installing coherent responses and offering professional guidance.

The conveners of the identified professional trainings are often also available for case-by-case (telephone) consultation by professionals. Additionally, some facilitate active referral to substance use treatment (Kethea Mosaic in Greece; Jellinek in the Netherlands; Alto e-learning in Belgium; Perspective 3D in Germany). Indeed, half of the conveners are substance use-related services that translate parts of their expertise to the reception setting. Additionally, several conveners of professional training also offer tailor-made support to reception centres at their demand. Perspective 3D (Germany), for instance, offers support in "developing prevention structures, and facilitating active referral to the support system" (short description in the intervention sheet).

Concerning the quality of interventions, all identified interventions have an evidenced theoretical background and for some, process or descriptive evaluations are available (DrugInt in Belgium; Alto e-learning in Belgium; Jellinek in the Netherlands; Kethea Mosaic in Greece). Nevertheless, we did not identify any outcome evaluation studies using an experimental design, besides those studies of the mhGAP behavioural interventions discussed previously in the prevention and early intervention section (Sect. 11.3.2).

11.3.4 A Note on the Excluded Interventions

Many practices, interventions, services and materials were not included in this review because of our focus on interventions targeting the European reception setting or (subgroups of) professionals working with applicants/refugees/undocumented migrants themselves. Besides these setting and population criteria we solely focussed on interventions targeting prevention, early/brief intervention, screening, treatment, harm reduction and professional training targeting substance use-related outcomes. Three categories of interventions stand out as relevant adjacent domains in the excluded materials, and directly result in three recommendations for the field:

1. Mental health interventions often exclude substance use(rs) while they are very relevant in preventing substance use-related problems and precursors.
2. Specialised substance use treatment services can inform adaptations in and referral from the reception setting.
3. Visual information materials are useful tools but should be framed in an evidence-based logical model for behavioural or other change.

We will briefly discuss these domains and their relevance for this review.

11.3.4.1 Mental Health Interventions

We excluded several evidence-based mental health interventions because they excluded participants with substance use (characteristics) or were not implemented in the reception setting. Notably, the MentalHealth4Refugees project bolsters seven German nationwide research and implementation projects on innovative mental health care for refugees, funded by the German Federal Ministry of Education and Research. Implementation and evaluation of the included interventions—BePrepared (Fischer et al., 2021; Schäfer et al., 2023), PM+ (de Graaff et al., 2024) and Cusu-Sy (Marth et al., 2021)—were funded in this framework (see supra). Most MentalHealth4Refugees interventions were however not included because of the above-mentioned criteria.

The BETTER CARE consortium (MentalHealth4Refugees) created a stepped intervention targeting unaccompanied minors (Hornfeck et al., 2023; Rosner et al., 2020). Culturally sensitive trauma-focused psychotherapy was integrated into routine clinical care. Additionally, a prevention programme for unaccompanied young refugees with the first symptoms of post-traumatic stress was developed and offered via youth welfare institutions. These interventions are studied in an experimental design and cost effectiveness study. Although the intervention potentially mediated substance use (related problems), this is not considered an intervention target (personal communication 15/04/2025) and remains unevaluated.

The RETREAT consortium (MentalHealth4Refugees) developed culturally adapted cognitive behavioural therapy (CA-CBT) for Farsi or Dari-speaking males with a mental health diagnosis in Germany (Kananian et al., 2022). Study participants with addiction were excluded.

The IMPROVE consortium (Zagha et al., 2024) implemented a 10-week intervention including four GP-delivered, modular CA-CBT sessions focussing on coping with depression, anxiety and stress. It consisted of eight 60-minute online modules from a positive parenting programme (Triple P Online, TPOL) and 10 accompanying protocol-based phone calls with a psychologist. The intervention addresses mental health problems in refugee parents (with children under six years) and aims to prevent their potential impact on the children. The intervention is currently being evaluated using an experimental design. The study does not specifically address substance use (disorders) (personal communication 09/06/2025) but does include its risk factors indirectly, rendering it very relevant to this review.

RefugeesWellSchool is a European-funded Horizon2020 project carried out by seven partners in six European countries (Norway, Finland, Sweden, Denmark, Belgium and the United Kingdom). The consortium implements and evaluates school interventions including a Peer Integration and Enhancement Resource (PIER) and In-Service Teacher Training (INSETT). A three-arm cluster RCT with parallel assignment in 16 Finnish schools (Peltonen et al., 2022) demonstrated that the latter two interventions were not effective in achieving the main goals of decreasing mental health problems and increasing psychosocial resources. Students' age, gender and exposure to socioeconomic daily stressors did however mediate these outcomes. The outcomes emphasise the need to differentiate interventions based on developmental phases and contextual factors.

11.3.4.2 Specialised Substance Use Interventions and Treatment Services

We did not include interventions or services that take place entirely or per definition outside the reception setting. These services and interventions are of course important in terms of referral from the reception setting and relevant for displaced populations who use substances.

ALMAMAR (Reinhardt et al., 2023) was developed within the I-REACH consortium (MentalHealth4Refugees) for Arabic and Farsi-speaking refugees in Germany residing in Rhineland Region inpatient psychiatric settings. ALMAMAR (Arabic for 'path') is an information and psychoeducation tool and an aid for communication between therapists and patients which can prove promising in inpatient substance use treatment. Future research could look into comparing implementation and outcomes of other (preventive) apps (e.g., BePrepared, Sanadak) to inpatient apps.

STARC-SUD (Lotzin et al., 2021) is a cultural-sensitive affect-regulation training that targets male refugees with psychological distress and hazardous substance use or substance use disorders. The intervention is currently being evaluated by Schäfer et al. (2022) in an RCT conducted in six metropolitan regions in Germany. The primary outcome being evaluated is severity of psychological distress.

Lastly, during the exclusion process we also identified many services that target substance use treatment and harm reduction among displaced populations, such as Mount Carmel Hospital (Malta), ADV Nokta (Germany), Kethea Mosaic (Greece),

NHO Chios team (Greece), ONG Lama (Belgium), Reto (Cyprus), Emergency Service Berlin (Germany), IRHH rehabilitation (The Netherlands), and CNAPA (Luxembourg). This list is undoubtedly not exhaustive. It could however be useful to disseminate these services, e.g., via MentalHealth4All.eu or other digital platforms and to establish service learning networks.

11.3.4.3 Visual Information Materials

We identified over 20 sources of translated leaflets and videos aimed mainly at psychoeducation. These materials were not included in the review because they are not per definition interventions. Although these materials can be useful in terms of psychoeducation or briefly informing someone of the characteristics of specific substances or substance related legislation, they should be used carefully and integrated into a theory-based intervention. The full list of these materials can be found via the EUDA website and intervention compendium.

Limiting an intervention to information transfer by handing over a leaflet or referring to a video without follow-up is unlikely to have any effect and can even be harmful (Calam et al., 2022). Impulsive or curious youth may for instance get triggered based on the provided information or recipients may feel misunderstood if they already have basic insights concerning available services and their application-related sources of stress. There are at least two notable stand-alone exceptions that can add value in low-resource settings but need further evaluation: videos on mental health using visual storylines that target mental health-related outcomes (e.g., developed by the EUAA) on the one hand and the WHO leaflet on parenting skills (as embedded in the broader Strengthening Families intervention) on the other.

Lastly, the provision of information to make services more accessible is key. The MentalHealth4All.eu website, funded by the European Asylum, Migration and Integration Fund, is a multilingual, freely accessible digital platform designed to support both health care professionals and migrants/refugees. The platform features practical tools, educational videos and a comprehensive open-access database with information about mental health, translated into multiple languages.

11.4 Discussion

During the past decade there has been a surge in the scientific interest concerning the mental health of and interventions for displaced populations. Financial support by international and European programmes such as Horizon2020, EU4Health, the WHO, the United Nations Refugee Agency as well as national funds such as those of the German Federal Ministry of Education and Research and the Belgian Federal Agency for the Reception of Asylum Seekers gave a clear and necessary impetus to the implementation and evaluation of mental health interventions for displaced populations in Europe. Nevertheless, substance use is often only considered in the margins of, or even excluded from, many such projects. These financial programmes allowed for the evaluation and implementation of interventions in the European reception setting identified in this review, most notably: PM+, Self Help+, SbS and ASSIST(-BI) at the international level.

Nevertheless, much remains to be done in this domain, especially in Europe where evaluation studies of substance-use-related interventions for these populations remain scarce. As posited by Greene et al. (2024b, p. 408), it is key to move beyond asking "whether it is feasible to provide substance use services to displaced populations and begin to promote their adoption as essential components of humanitarian response". The question remains *how* to do this in Europe. We subsequently end this chapter by discussing the review results, centred around six key recommendations.

1. Inclusive mental health interventions do not exclude substance use(rs).
2. Prevention and early intervention are a priority in the reception setting.
3. Experimental evaluations can raise promising ideas to trusted and scalable solutions.
4. The reception and treatment workforce would benefit from intervention knowledge and skills transfer.
5. Digital advances can bridge towards but not replace interventions.
6. Structural prevention and inclusive prevention infrastructures are key.

11.4.1 Inclusive Mental Health Interventions Do Not Exclude Substance Use(Res)

Substance use and its related problems are undeniably related to mental health. As a consequence, interventions aimed at enhancing mental health should equally consider substance use as an outcome and include participants who use substances with or without a DSM-defined diagnosis. In turn, interventions should where possible be adapted or aligned with the needs of these populations. This review shows that the exclusion of substance use-related individual characteristics and the practical divide between substance use and mental health services is deep-rooted in intervention practice, reproduced in evaluation studies and consequently likely reproduces inequity in terms of intervention availability to displaced populations who use substances.

Many of the initially identified studies excluded substance use-related characteristics in participants such as 'severe substance abuse' (Rosner et al., 2020), 'addiction' (Kananian et al., 2022), 'psychotropic medication use' (Röhr et al., 2021), 'usage of neuroleptic drugs, irregular anticholinergic or irregular antiepileptic drug intake' (Zagha et al., 2024) and 'substance dependence' (Knefel et al., 2020). Although there are valid reasons for these exclusions (e.g., homogeneity, intervention goals, etc.), this widespread exclusion hinders the generalisability of findings, albeit limiting intervention applicability to real-world, comorbid populations. Moreover, excluding these participants based on specified characteristics from the already rare ongoing trials among displaced populations risks recreating the image of the 'deserving client' among already severely deprived and at-risk populations.

Additionally, this exclusion may de facto limit the opportunities for targeting substance use in its earlier stages, especially among those at risk—such as youth—by depriving them of interventions that target the underlying mental health issues that likely precede or moderate substance use and related problems. Only one of the identified European mental health intervention evaluation studies specifically included substance use disorders in its trial among inpatient mental health care clients (Lotzin et al., 2021; Schäfer et al., 2022), but was excluded in the review because it did not take place in the reception setting.

Both to advance the field and to do justice to the equitable right to health access among displaced populations who use substances, greater integration and intentional inclusion of substance use(rs) is key in mental health interventions and research. Taking a non-exclusionary stance in study protocols (e.g., Burchert et al., 2019) is a start but does not suffice for in-depth analysis if, for instance, sample power analyses do not include these participant characteristics.

Substance use is more often than not comorbid with other mental health issues, but their interrelation remains understudied (see, e.g., Harris et al., 2019). Therefore both aetiological and substance use intervention research would greatly benefit from the inclusion of substance use-related outcomes and indicators of moderation and mediation in the study of mental health interventions such as CA-CBT for traumatised refugees and asylum seekers (Menon et al., 2024), Hope Groups (Tucker et al., 2024), group therapy for refugees with affective disorders (Wiechers et al., 2023), trauma-focused interventions for children in migration contexts (Becker et al., 2024; Dobler et al., 2025) and especially psychosocial interventions for post-traumatic stress (disorders) for displaced populations (Kip et al., 2020; Nosè et al., 2017; Turrini et al., 2025).

11.4.2 Prevention and Early Intervention Are a Priority in the Reception Setting

Investing in developmentally adapted prevention among at-risk children and their families is key, as demonstrated in earlier work by the European Union Drugs Agency (EUDA, 2013a, 2013b; EUDA & De Kock, 2022; Lemmens et al., 2017). This is especially important in the reception setting. Indeed, family skills programmes such as the United Nations Office on Drugs and Crime's (UNODC) Strong Families and the Triple P adaptation by the IMPROVE consortium (Zagha et al., 2024) are potentially key methods for substance use prevention in both humanitarian (El-Khani et al., 2022) and reception settings.

There is growing evidence that the quality of parenting can for instance be a predictor of the effects on children's mental health of military conflict, making it an important component of the reception of war-affected and other displaced children (Bürgin et al., 2022 in Calam et al., 2022). Also in substance use prevention research, parenting interventions have been evidenced to impact child substance use (Heinrichs et al., 2014). Although scalable preventive interventions for displaced populations are increasingly being evaluated outside Europe (most prominently Strong Families as discussed by El-Khani et al. (2021b), Haar et al. (2020)), these studies remain limited in Europe. Moreover, more intervention studies are needed targeting unaccompanied minors in Europe.

Prevention and early intervention often overlap. In the domain of early intervention we identified ASSIST and ASSIST-BI as scalable evidence-based interventions for respectively the assessment of and early intervention in substance use. Both ASSIST-BI and the Finish TAVATA training for professionals have motivational interviewing and theory of behavioural change as their theoretical basis. The latter are broadly evidenced and referred to in the WHO and UNODC's international standards for the treatment of drug use disorders.

As suggested by Calam et al. (2022), prevention effectiveness might benefit from answering five practical questions before choosing evidence-based interventions in this setting. Dealing with these questions minimises the risk of intervening too soon, (developmentally) inappropriate or without consideration of preconditions, which can lead to negative outcomes. The answers should be anticipated in the intervention design and service support, as well as in structural prevention measures and in prevention infrastructures (see Sect. 11.4).

1. Are the children and their caregivers safe now?
2. Are they in stable living conditions, or are they likely to be moving on soon?
3. How well is the setting where they are currently living resourced to provide support, and who is available to facilitate programmes?
4. How long has it been since the most recent distressing experience?
5. Are there any pre-existing challenges present in the family before the calamity?

11.4.3 *Experimental Evaluations Can Raise Promising Ideas to Trusted and Scalable Solutions*

Based on the identified evaluation studies, all interventions were rated 'additional studies recommended'. Although European professionals in reception settings have little to build on, the unevaluated interventions identified in this review do build on sound theoretical bases. The preventive advisory talk and the mental health and substance use animation game, both implemented in the Netherlands, for instance, build on CBT and the I-Change model, evidence-based health education and behaviour change theories respectively.

Nevertheless, sustained attention is needed to rigorously define programme theory and its logical translation into intervention components. Moreover, manualising interventions, monitoring and evaluation remain key to keep abreast of both effectiveness and programme fidelity, in line with programme theory. As seen in the implementation of MindSpring across several European countries and age groups, adaptations can sometimes blur the definition of core components, reinforcing the need for greater clarity. MindSpring was only evaluated in Denmark (Husby et al., 2020), which raises not only questions of its effectiveness in other populations but also poses risks for professionals because they might be in need of more guidance to implement and adapt the intervention.

Concerning the informative preventive talk implemented in the Netherlands, in turn, it should be noted that although its theoretical foundation links to Prochaska's stages of change, it remains unclear what can be achieved during one scripted conversation. Moreover, although referral is not the goal, it appears to be the main outcome in the descriptive evaluation. Overall, many of the identified interventions dominantly emphasise knowledge components whereas prevention science is clear about the fact that knowledge change alone is insufficient to change behaviour.

Although few evaluation studies have taken place in Europe, the European reception context can learn from scalable interventions tested outside Europe, such as Self-Help+ and the ASSIST alcohol intervention in Uganda (Greene et al., 2024a; Augustinavicius, 2023), PM+ in Turkey (Acarturk et al., 2024), brief interventions in Kenya (Widmann et al., 2017), a transdiagnostic intervention in the prevention of substance use in Uganda (van der Boor et al., 2024), the Common Elements Treatment Approach (CETA) in DRC Congo (Kane et al., 2023) and Zambia (Murray et al., 2020) and UNODC's Strong Families in Lebanon (El-Khani et al., 2021a).

As Calam and colleagues (2022) note, the wealthiest country can become a low-resource setting, especially in times of austerity and pressure on positive integration policies. This means that the above-mentioned interventions that were implemented in low- and middle-income or resource settings will become increasingly relevant for the European context. Mainstreaming the integration of feasible and scalable evidence-based interventions in European reception settings will be key to curb mental health and substance use-related problems during the years to come.

11.4.4 Both the Reception and Treatment Work Force Would Benefit from Intervention Knowledge and Skills Transfer

The majority of professional trainings identified in this review were evaluated in descriptive (formative and process evaluation) designs only. We did not find high-quality experimental evaluation studies of these interventions. Whereas many of these trainings had similar goals, their content and formats varied greatly. Moreover, the trainings tend to be knowledge rather than skills oriented. Subsequently, it is crucial to convey to reception workers, both in their own professional substance use-related training and in the preventive interventions made available to them, the evidence-based prevention principles such as adverted in the European Prevention Curriculum.

Effective prevention focuses on developing practical skills—such as coping, problem solving, and parenting—rather than merely conveying information through passive formats like posters or videos. Interventions should also be developmentally appropriate (Coone et al., 2020) in addition to being adapted to critical moments of mental health transitions (e.g., reception, integration, procedural outcomes) and thus implemented at the right time (Giacco, 2020). The European reception work force would thus greatly benefit from greater access to up-to-date prevention knowledge as well as knowledge transfer between training conveners, mainstreaming and evaluating existing materials.

Beyond workforce training, strengthening supranational networks can enhance knowledge and skills transfer between treatment service experts who operate in specialised care settings. Moreover, the visibility of these initiatives and services is important for the reception setting to be able to refer individuals to such initiatives.

11.4.5 Digital Advances Can Bridge Towards But Not Replace Interventions

Digital advances are currently being taken up in intervention designs and implementation. Two interventions were included in this review: Fisscher and colleagues implemented an early intervention tool (BePrepared) and conducted a feasibility trial (Fischer et al., 2021) and the SbS app (Sanadak) was developed by Burchert et al. (2019). Moreover, professional trainings were linked to an online component in the Netherlands and Belgium, making it more accessible to professionals.

Digital advances can indeed help bridge the treatment gap and facilitate training professionals. Smartphone-delivered mental health care interventions can help those who do not have access to any live interventions (Larsen & Guler, 2024). However, these interventions remain largely unevaluated; implementation is often hampered by technical problems and requirements while drop-out rates in published studies are high (El-Haj-Mohamad et al., 2023).

Besides the use as standalone interventions, digital tools may be used to strengthen live communication, such as with inpatient Arabic and Farsi-speaking patients with substance use (Reinhardt, 2021) and to form a bridge towards inpatient care. Indeed, adding live interaction, co-designing with stakeholders and including the target population involvement might lead to greater acceptance (Bridge et al., 2025; Radu et al., 2023; Woodward et al., 2023) and lower drop-out. Indeed, as many of the included studies had high drop-out rates, future evaluation studies would benefit from anticipating this in their sample power calculations and in all other relevant domains of the study design.

11.4.6 Structural Prevention and Inclusive Prevention Infrastructures Are Key

When theorising substance use interventions in reception environments it is essential to keep in mind that these settings are, ideally, the first safe haven and provisional home for displaced populations. Within this context, the core public health principle requires that interventions prioritise the least invasive, most effective and lowest-cost measures for residents. Applied to substance use prevention, this principle shifts attention upstream, away from individual-level behavioural interventions alone and towards two essential and complementary strategies: structural prevention and inclusive prevention infrastructures.

Structural prevention addresses upstream determinants of health by targeting the broader political, social and economic structures that shape substance use risks (Ingleby, 2019). Rather than focussing directly on individual behaviours, structural prevention emphasises policies and systemic conditions that reduce vulnerability in the first place. In the migration and reception context, this translates into stable housing, access to health care and education, meaningful opportunities for participation and rights-based integration policies. These measures create the conditions for well-being that indirectly but powerfully help prevent substance-related harm:

- Migration and integration policies ensuring basic rights such as housing, health care and education.
- Institutional frameworks such as the WHO mhGAP Humanitarian Intervention Guide, which supports national systems in building scalable mental health and substance use support infrastructures.
- Environmental measures that mitigate risk factors, such as but not limited to reducing frequent relocations between centres, which is shown to disrupt trust, continuity of care and children's mental health.

Without tackling these structural drivers, even evidence-based interventions may fail to achieve their intended outcomes, as living conditions themselves function as upstream risk factors.

While structural prevention emphasises systemic determinants at the policy and societal levels, inclusive prevention infrastructures encompass the institutional, organisational and community-level arrangements that make prevention work possible (Crowley et al., 2024) within reception settings. In other words, they are the enabling frameworks that allow evidence-based interventions to be accessible, trusted and effective. An inclusive prevention infrastructure involves:

- Equipping reception centres and their staff with the capacity to respond appropriately to substance use situations at both the individual and community level.
- Ensuring that prevention and early intervention mechanisms are integrated into wider reception policies and practices, rather than being isolated or ad hoc.
- Establishing frameworks that prioritise prevention and early response over treatment or remediation alone (Crowley et al., 2024).

- Building a safe reception environment where inclusivity—in terms of culture, language and rights—is not incidental but integral.

Thus, inclusive prevention infrastructures function as the operational backbone of prevention. They ensure that reception settings are not merely protective containers but active environments where upstream determinants are addressed, community trust is cultivated and interventions can be implemented effectively.

11.5 Conclusion and Ways Forward

This review highlights the persistent knowledge gap regarding (the effectiveness of) substance use-related intervention for displaced populations in European reception settings. While the identified interventions may be promising, they require additional evaluation studies. Interventions that have been studied extensively outside, or with mixed results in Europe (Strengthening Families, Self Help Plus, Problem Management Plus as well as MindSpring and others) might prove beneficial if their programme theories more clearly relate to substance use outcomes in future long-term evaluation studies.

Despite increased scientific and financial investment in mental health interventions for refugees and applicants of international protection, substance use remains marginally addressed or outright excluded from many studies and intervention designs. The evidence suggests that integrating substance use considerations into mental health interventions, prioritising inclusive approaches and ensuring that interventions are accessible to those who use substances—regardless of diagnosis—are critical steps towards equitable mental health care and research outcomes that are generalisable to real-life comorbid populations.

Investing in prevention and early intervention within reception settings emerges as a key priority. While a range of promising practices and interventions have been identified, only a minority have undergone substance use related evaluation. The review underscores the need for ongoing investment in both the development and evaluation of preventive interventions—such as family and other skills training and affect regulation and motivational interviewing—and in scaling up training for both professionals and refugee peers. Furthermore, digital innovations present new opportunities for expanding intervention and service access, yet these tools require careful evaluation and adaptation to overcome technical and engagement barriers, while they cannot fully replace live interventions.

Importantly, robust prevention infrastructure and structural prevention, both at the state and reception setting levels, are essential for long-term impact. This includes not only behavioural interventions but also broader institutional and policy changes that address structural inequities faced by displaced populations and upstream determinants of health, such as stable housing and access to health care.

This review calls for investing in a true intervention continuum that bridges prevention, early intervention, treatment and harm reduction, while acknowledging the structural and political challenges that persist. Learning from interventions outside Europe and ensuring that future mental health research includes substance use outcomes as well as implementation fidelity will be vital for advancing this field in Europe.

Competing Interests The development of this chapter draws substantively on the European Union Drugs Agency (EUDA)'s institutional resources, including its research infrastructure and funding support (contract CT.21.EU4MD.0034.1.0 and CT.24.SDI.0117.1.0), and is informed by knowledge generated through the Agency's mandate to monitor, assess, and strengthen evidence-based responses in the European context. Previously, the author served as project coordinator of the DrugInt intervention, funded by the Belgian Federal Agency for the Reception of Asylum Applicants (2023–2024), and principal researcher for MATREMI (Belgian Science Policy Office, DR/84, 2018–2020). The author is currently a member of the EUDA XChange Prevention Rating Board, however, rating in this chapter has not been endorsed by the board. The author is currently funded by a postdoctoral fellowship from the Research Foundation—Flanders (FWO) [12AFB24N-7028]. The views, interpretations, and conclusions are those of the author and not those of Belspo, EUDA, or any other EU institution.

References

Acarturk, C., Kurt, G., İlkkurşun, Z., de Graaff, A. M., Bryant, R., Cuijpers, P., Fuhr, D., McDaid, D., Park, A.-L., & Sijbrandij, M. (2024). Effectiveness of group problem management plus in distressed Syrian refugees in Türkiye: A randomized controlled trial. *Epidemiology and Psychiatric Sciences, 33*, e43.

Ajzen, I. (1991). The theory of planned behavior. *Organizational Behavior and Human Decision Processes, 50*(2), 179–211.

Aleer, E., Alam, K., & Rashid, A. (2024). A systematic literature review of substance-use prevention programs amongst refugee youth. *Community Mental Health Journal*, 1–20.

Arribas-Aguila, D., Castaño, G., & Martínez-Arias, R. (2024). A systematic review of evidence-based general competency models: Development of a general competencies taxonomy. *Journal of Work and Organizational Psychology, 40*(2), 61–76.

Bandura, A. (2001). Social cognitive theory: An agentic perspective. *Annual Review of Psychology, 52*(1), 1–26.

Becker, T. D., Castañeda Ramirez, S., Bruges Boude, A., Leong, A., Ivanov, I., & Rice, T. R. (2024). Interventions for prevention and treatment of substance use in youth with traumatic childhood experiences: A systematic review and synthesis of the literature. *European Child & Adolescent Psychiatry, 33*(10), 3419–3438.

Behr, K., & Lindert, J. (2024). Participative development of a culture-sensitive instrument to measure substance use in Syrian refugees. *European Journal of Public Health, 34*(Suppl_3), ckae144.525.

Bridge, L. A., Elsey, J., Pratley, P., & Woodward, A. (2025). Digital mental health tools: A narrative review on overcoming barriers in the age of displacement and disparities. *Maturitas, 198*, 108380.

Burchert, S., Alkneme, M. S., Bird, M., Carswell, K., Cuijpers, P., Hansen, P., Heim, E., Shehadeh, M. H., Sijbrandij, M., van't Hof, E., & Knaevelsrud, C. (2019). User-centered app adaptation of a low-intensity e-mental health intervention for Syrian refugees. *Frontiers in Psychiatry, 9*. https://doi.org/10.3389/fpsyt.2018.00663

Calam, R., El-Khani, A., & Maalouf, W. (2022). Editorial perspective: How can we help the children of Ukraine and others affected by military conflict? *Child and Adolescent Mental Health, 27*(3), 294–296. https://doi.org/10.1111/camh.12581

Carswell, K., Harper-Shehadeh, M., Watts, S., van't Hof, E., Abi Ramia, J., Heim, E., Wenger, A., & van Ommeren, M. (2018). Step-by-step: A new WHO digital mental health intervention for depression. *Mhealth, 4*, 34.

Coone, A., Jongbloet, J., & van de Kreeft, P. (2020). *Europees preventiehandboek. Een leidraad voor wetenschappelijk onderbouwde preventie in de praktijk, vertaling van European Prevention Curriculum (EUDA).* Politeia.

Crowley, D. M., Welsh, J., Meyer Chilenski, S., Gayles, J., Long, E., Jones, D., & Scott, T. (2024). Integrated prevention infrastructure: A framework for addressing social determinants of health in substance use policy making. *Focus, 22*(4), 483–491.

Cuijpers, P., Heim, E., Abi Ramia, J., Burchert, S., Carswell, K., Cornelisz, I., Knaevelsrud, C., Noun, P., van Klaveren, C., & van't Hof, E. (2022). Effects of a WHO-guided digital health intervention for depression in Syrian refugees in Lebanon: A randomized controlled trial. *PLoS Medicine, 19*(6), e1004025.

de Graaff, A. M., Cuijpers, P., Acarturk, C., Akhtar, A., Alkneme, M. S., Aoun, M., Awwad, M., Bawaneh, A. Y., Brown, F. L., Bryant, R., Burchert, S., Carswell, K., Drogendijk, A., Engels, M., Fuhr, D. C., & Hansen, P. (2022). Scalable psychological interventions for Syrian refugees in Europe and the Middle East: STRENGTHS study protocol for a prospective individual participant data meta-analysis. *BMJ Open, 12*(4), e058101. https://doi.org/10.1136/bmjopen-2021-058101

de Graaff, A. M., Cuijpers, P., Elsawy, M., Hunaidy, S., Kieft, B., Gorgis, N., Twisk, J. W., Zakarian, Y., Bouman, T. K., & Lommen, M. J. (2024). The effectiveness of problem management plus at 1-year follow-up for Syrian refugees in a high-income setting. *Epidemiology and Psychiatric Sciences, 33*, e50.

De Kock, C. (2020). European inspiring practices for substance use treatment among migrants and ethnic minorities. In C. De Kock, C. Mascia, F. Laudens, L. Toyinbo, S. Leclerq, D. Jacobs, & T. Decorte (Eds.), *Mapping and enhancing substance use treatment for migrants and ethnic minorities (MEM)* (pp. 87–120). Belspo. https://www.belspo.be/belspo/Fedra/proj.asp?l=de&COD=DR%2F84

De Kock, C., & EUDA. (2022). *Responding to drug-related problems among migrants, refugees and ethnic minorities in Europe*. European Union Drugs Agency. https://www.euda.europa.eu/drugs-library/responding-drug-related-problems-among-migrants-refugees-and-ethnic-minorities-europe_en

De Vries, H. (2017). An integrated approach for understanding health behavior; the I-change model as an example. *Psychology and Behavioral Science International Journal, 2*(2), 555–585.

Dobler, V., Derluyn, I., Draper, A., Marcellino, E., & Pfeiffer, E. (2025). Trauma-focused interventions for children and adolescents in migration contexts. In *Evidence-based treatments for trauma-related disorders in children and adolescents* (pp. 531–553). Springer.

Doty, S. B., Haroz, E. E., Singh, N. S., Bogdanov, S., Bass, J. K., Murray, L. K., Callaway, K. L., & Bolton, P. A. (2018). Adaptation and testing of an assessment for mental health and alcohol use problems among conflict-affected adults in Ukraine. *Conflict and Health, 12*(1), 34.

El-Haj-Mohamad, R., Nohr, L., Niemeyer, H., Böttche, M., & Knaevelsrud, C. (2023). Smartphone-delivered mental health care interventions for refugees: A systematic review of the literature. *Global Mental Health, 10*, e6.

El-Khani, A., Calam, R., Haar, K., & Maalouf, W. (2022). Bridging the gap between the pressing need for family skills programmes in humanitarian settings and implementation. *International Journal of Environmental Research and Public Health, 19*(4), 2181.

El-Khani, A., Cartwright, K., Maalouf, W., Haar, K., Zehra, N., Çokamay-Yılmaz, G., & Calam, R. (2021a). Enhancing teaching recovery techniques (TRT) with parenting skills: RCT of TRT+ parenting with trauma-affected Syrian refugees in Lebanon utilising remote training with implications for insecure contexts and COVID-19. *International Journal of Environmental Research and Public Health, 18*(16), 8652.

El-Khani, A., Haar, K., Stojanovic, M., & Maalouf, W. (2021b). Assessing the feasibility of providing a family skills intervention, "strong families", for refugee families residing in reception centers in Serbia. *International Journal of Environmental Research and Public Health, 18*(9), 4530.

Elkholy, H., Tay Wee Teck, J., Arunogiri, S., Asaad, M. R., Baessler, F., Bhad, R., Borghi, E. N., Busse, A., Ekhtiari, H., & Dave, S. (2023). Substance use disorders among forcibly displaced people: A narrative review. *Current Addiction Reports, 10*(2), 341–352.

EUDA. (2013a). *Drug prevention interventions targeting minority ethnic populations: Issues raised by 33 case studies (P. o. o. t. E. Union, Ed.).* European Monitoring Centre for Drugs and Drug Addiction (EUDA). http://www.EUDA.europa.eu/system/files/publications/736/TDXA13001ENN_412241.pdf

EUDA. (2013b). *Search: Addiction prevention for refugees and asylum seekers.* EUDA. http://www.EUDA.europa.eu/html.cfm/index52035EN.html?project_id=3576&tab=overview

EUDA, & De Kock, C. (2022). *Responding to drug-related problems among migrants, refugees and ethnic minorities in Europe.* Background paper commissioned by EUDA.

EUAA & EUDA. (2023). *Professionals working in reception centres in Europe: An overview of drug-related challenges and support needs.* EUAA & EUDA. https://www.euda.europa.eu/publications/technical-reports/professionals-working-reception-centres-europe_en

Ezard, N., Manji, H., & Busse, A. (2020). Substance use disorders in conflict-displaced populations. In *Textbook of addiction treatment: International perspectives* (pp. 1463–1475). Springer.

Fischer, L. C., Kölligan, V., Wieland, N., & Klein, M. (2021). Development and evaluation of a digital health intervention for substance use reduction in young refugees with problematic use of alcohol and/or cannabis—Study protocol for a single-armed feasibility trial. *Frontiers in Public Health, 9.* https://doi.org/10.3389/fpubh.2021.557431

French, K., Golijani-Moghaddam, N., & Schröder, T. (2017). What is the evidence for the efficacy of self-help acceptance and commitment therapy? A systematic review and meta-analysis. *Journal of Contextual Behavioral Science, 6*(4), 360–374.

Giacco, D. (2020). Identifying the critical time points for mental health of asylum seekers and refugees in high-income countries. *Epidemiology and Psychiatric Sciences, 29*, e61

Grant, M. J., & Booth, A. (2009). A typology of reviews: An analysis of 14 review types and associated methodologies. *Health Information & Libraries Journal, 26*(2), 91–108.

Greene, M. C., Andersen, L. S., Leku, M. R., Au, T., Akellot, J., Upadhaya, N., Odokonyero, R., White, R., Ventevogel, P., Garcia-Moreno, C., & Tol, W. A. (2024a). Combining a guided self-help and brief alcohol intervention to improve mental health and reduce substance use among refugee men in Uganda: A cluster-randomized feasibility trial. *Global Mental Health, 11*, e106. https://doi.org/10.1017/gmh.2024.103

Greene, M. C., Busse, A., Ventevogel, P., Kane, J., & Ezard, N. (2024b). Moving from feasible to essential: Progress and future directions for promoting the implementation of substance use services for forcibly displaced populations in humanitarian settings. *Addiction, 119*(3), 408–410.

Greene, M. C., Haddad, S., Busse, A., Ezard, N., Ventevogel, P., Demis, L., Inoue, S., Gumm, J.-C., Campello, G., & Tol, W. A. (2021). Priorities for addressing substance use disorder in humanitarian settings. *Conflict and Health, 15*(1), 1–10.

Greene, M. C., Kane, J. C., Khoshnood, K., Ventevogel, P., & Tol, W. A. (2018). Challenges and opportunities for implementation of substance misuse interventions in conflict-affected populations. *Harm Reduction Journal, 15*(1), 1–10.

Greene, M. C., Ventevogel, P., & Kane, J. C. (2019). Substance use services for refugees. *Bulletin of the World Health Organization, 97*(4), 246.

Haar, K., El-Khani, A., Molgaard, V., Maalouf, W., & Nazir, A. (2020). Strong families: A new family skills training programme for challenged and humanitarian settings: A single-arm intervention tested in Afghanistan. *BMC Public Health, 20*, 1–16.

Harris, S., Dykxhoorn, J., Hollander, A. C., Dalman, C., & Kirkbride, J. B. (2019). Substance use disorders in refugee and migrant groups in Sweden: A nationwide cohort study of 1.2 million people. *PLoS medicine, 16*(11), e1002944.

Heim, E., Abi Ramia, J., Abi Hana, R., Burchert, S., Carswell, K., Cornelisz, I., Cuijpers, P., El Chammay, R., Noun, P., & van Klaveren, C. (2021). Step-by-step: Feasibility randomized controlled trial of a mobile-based intervention for depression among populations affected by adversity in Lebanon. *Internet Interventions, 24*, 100380.

Heinrichs, N., Kliem, S., & Hahlweg, K. (2014). Four-year follow-up of a randomized controlled trial of triple P group for parent and child outcomes. *Prevention Science, 15*(2), 233–245.

Hornfeck, F., Eglinsky, J., Garbade, M., Rosner, R., Kindler, H., Pfeiffer, E., & Sachser, C. (2023). Mental health problems in unaccompanied young refugees and the impact of post-flight factors on PTSS, depression and anxiety: A secondary analysis of the better care study. *Frontiers in Psychology, 14*, 1149634.

Horyniak, D., Melo, J. S., Farrell, R. M., Ojeda, V. D., & Strathdee, S. A. (2016). Epidemiology of substance use among forced migrants: A global systematic review. *PLoS One, 11*(7), e0159134.

Humeniuk, R., Henry-Edwards, S., Ali, R., Poznyak, V., Monteiro, M. G., & World Health Organization. (2010). The alcohol, smoking and substance involvement screening test (ASSIST): manual for use in primary care.

Husby, S. R., Carlsson, J., Mathilde Scotte Jensen, A., Glahder Lindberg, L., & Sonne, C. (2020). Prevention of trauma-related mental health problems among refugees: A mixed-methods evaluation of the MindSpring group programme in Denmark. *Journal of Community Psychology, 48*(3), 1028–1039.

Ingleby, D. (2019). Moving upstream: Changing policy scripts on migrant and ethnic minority health. *Health Policy, 123*(9), 809–817.

Kananian, S., Kip, A., Schumm, H., Giesebrecht, J., Nicolai, A., Schade-Brittinger, C., Reese, J.-P., Weise, C., Mewes, R., & Morina, N. (2022). Culturally adapted cognitive behavioural group therapy for mental disorders in refugees plus problem solving training (ReTreat): Study protocol for a multicentre randomised controlled trial. *BMJ Open, 12*(11), e061274.

Kane, J. C., & Greene, M. (2018). *Addressing alcohol and substance use disorders among refugees: A desk review of intervention approaches.* United Nations High Commissioner for Refugees.

Kane, J. C., Kamanga, M., Skavenski, S., Murray, L. K., Shawa, M., Bwalya, B., Metz, K., Paul, R., Mushabati, N., & Ventevogel, P. (2023). Testing a screening, brief intervention, and referral to treatment intervention approach for addressing unhealthy alcohol and other drug use in humanitarian settings: Protocol of the Ukuundapwa Chapamo randomised controlled trial. *Intervention Journal of Mental Health and Psychosocial Support in Conflict Affected Areas, 21*(1), 58–69.

Karyotaki, E., Sijbrandij, M., Purgato, M., Acarturk, C., Lakin, D., Bailey, D., Peckham, E., Uygun, E., Tedeschi, F., Wancata, J., Augustinavicius, J., Carswell, K., Valimaki, M., van Ommeren, M., Koesters, M., Popa, M., Leku, M. R., Anttila, M., & Churchill, R. (2023). Self-help plus for refugees and asylum seekers: An individual participant data meta-analysis. *BMJ Mental Health, 26*(1). https://doi.org/10.1136/bmjment-2023-300672

Kasten, S., van Osch, L., Candel, M., & de Vries, H. (2019). The influence of pre-motivational factors on behavior via motivational factors: A test of the I-change model. *BMC Psychology, 7*, 1–12.

Keynejad, R. C., Dua, T., Barbui, C., & Thornicroft, G. (2018). WHO Mental Health Gap Action Programme (mhGAP) intervention guide: A systematic review of evidence from low and middle-income countries. *Evidence Based Mental Health, 21*(1), 30–34.

Khan, R., Chatton, A., Nallet, A., Broers, B., Thorens, G., Achab-Arigo, S., Poznyak, V., Fleischmann, A., Khazaal, Y., & Zullino, D. (2011). Validation of the French version of the alcohol, smoking and substance involvement screening test (ASSIST). *European Addiction Research, 17*(4), 190–197.

Kip, A., Priebe, S., Holling, H., & Morina, N. (2020). Psychological interventions for posttraumatic stress disorder and depression in refugees: A meta-analysis of randomized controlled trials. *Clinical Psychology & Psychotherapy, 27*(4), 489–503.

Knefel, M., Kantor, V., Nicholson, A. A., Schiess-Jokanovic, J., Weindl, D., Schäfer, I., & Lueger-Schuster, B. (2020). A brief transdiagnostic psychological intervention for afghan asylum seekers and refugees in Austria: A randomized controlled trial. *Trials, 21*, 1–9.

Larsen, A., & Guler, J. (2024). Digital mental health approaches to improve Well-being of refugee families. *Psychiatric Services, 75*(2), 198–201. https://doi.org/10.1176/appi.ps.20230179

Lee, C.-T., Lin, C.-Y., Koós, M., Nagy, L., Kraus, S. W., Demetrovics, Z., Potenza, M. N., Ballester-Arnal, R., Batthyány, D., & Bergeron, S. (2023). The eleven-item alcohol, smoking and substance involvement screening test (ASSIST-11): Cross-cultural psychometric evaluation across 42 countries. *Journal of Psychiatric Research, 165*, 16–27.

Lemmens, P., Dupont, H., & Roosen, I. (2017). *Migrants, asylum seekers and refugees: An overview of the literature relating to drug use and access to services. Background paper commissioned by the EUDA for Health and Social Responses to Drug Problems: A European Guide.* EUDA. http://www.EUDA.europa.eu/system/files/attachments/6341/EuropeanResponsesGuide2017_BackgroundPaper-Migrants-Asylum-seekers-Refugees-Drug-use.pdf

Lorenz, M. H., Ensle, A., Taggert, J., Uricher, J., Heidenreich, T., & Laging, M. (2023). Professionals' perspectives on substance use among refugees in shared accommodations: A qualitative study. *Health & Social Work, 48*(3), 188–197. https://doi.org/10.1093/hsw/hlad017

Lorenz, M. H., Taggert, J., Laging, M., & Heidenreich, T. (2021). Prevention of hazardous substance use among refugees: A systematic review. *SUCHT, 67*(5), 255–271. https://doi.org/10.1024/0939-5911/a000732

Lorenz, M. H., Uricher, J., Michalak, J., Heidenreich, T., & Laging, A. M. (2024a). Hazardous substance use among refugees in shared accommodations: A mixed-methods study. *Zeitschrift für Klinische Psychologie und Psychotherapie, 53*(4), 187–204. https://doi.org/10.1026/1616-3443/a000778

Lorenz, M. H., Uricher, J., Pauzar, M. I., Michalak, J., Laging, M., & Heidenreich, T. (2024b). Evaluation of a multi-component prevention concept for hazardous substance use among refugees in shared accommodations: Study protocol for a cluster randomized controlled trial. *Trials, 25*(1), 770. https://doi.org/10.1186/s13063-024-08558-z

Lotzin, A., Lindert, J., Koch, T., Liedl, A., & Schäfer, I. (2021). STARC-SUD–adaptation of a transdiagnostic intervention for refugees with substance use disorders. *Clinical Psychology in Europe, 3*, e5329. https://doi.org/10.32872/cpe.532

Marth, S., Jakubauskiene, M., Schäfer, I., & Lindert, J. (2021). Substance use instruments for refugees: Systematic review. *European Journal of Public Health, 31*(Suppl_3), ckab164.055.

Menon, S., Katona, C., & Glover, N. (2024). The effectiveness and acceptability of culturally adapted cognitive behavioural therapy for traumatised refugees and asylum seekers: A systematic review. *Mental Health Science, 2*(4), e85.

Mrazek, P. J., & Haggerty, R. J. (1994). Treatment research and prevention research: A collaborative frontier. In *Reducing risks for mental disorders: Frontiers for preventive intervention research.* National Academies Press (US).

Murray, L. K., Kane, J. C., Glass, N., Skavenski van Wyk, S., Melendez, F., Paul, R., Kmett Danielson, C., Murray, S. M., Mayeya, J., & Simenda, F. (2020). Effectiveness of the common elements treatment approach (CETA) in reducing intimate partner violence and hazardous alcohol use in Zambia (VATU): A randomized controlled trial. *PLoS Medicine, 17*(4), e1003056.

Najdini, M., Mathieu, J., Shadili, G., Frigaux, A., Ménauges, M., Mouton, C., & Essadek, A. (2025). Substance use prevalence among immigrants by generational status in Europe: A systematic review and meta-analysis. *Alcohol: Clinical and Experimental Research, 49*(7), 1381–1391.

Nosè, M., Ballette, F., Bighelli, I., Turrini, G., Purgato, M., Tol, W., Priebe, S., & Barbui, C. (2017). Psychosocial interventions for post-traumatic stress disorder in refugees and asylum seekers resettled in high-income countries: Systematic review and meta-analysis. *PLoS One, 12*(2), e0171030.

Peltonen, K., Aalto, S., Vänskä, M., Lepistö, R., Punamäki, R.-L., Soye, E., Watters, C., de Wal Pastoor, L., Derluyn, I., & Kankaanpää, R. (2022). Effectiveness of promotive and preventive psychosocial interventions on improving the mental health of Finnish-born and immigrant adolescents. *International Journal of Environmental Research and Public Health, 19*(6), 3686.

Pluck, F., Ettema, R., & Vermetten, E. (2022). Threats and interventions on wellbeing in asylum seekers in The Netherlands: A scoping review. *Frontiers in Psychiatry, 13*, 829522. https://doi.org/10.3389/fpsyt.2022.829522

Priebe, S., Giacco, D., & El-Nagib, R. (2016). *Public health aspects of mental health among migrants and refugees: A review of the evidence on mental health care for refugees, asylum seekers, and irregular migrants in the WHO European region*. World Health Organization Regional Office Europe.

Prochaska, J. O., & Velicer, W. F. (1997). The transtheoretical model of health behavior change. *American Journal of Health Promotion, 12*(1), 38–48.

Purgato, M., Carswell, K., Acarturk, C., Au, T., Akbai, S., Anttila, M., Baumgartner, J., Bailey, D., Biondi, M., & Bird, M. (2019). Effectiveness and cost-effectiveness of self-help plus (SH+) for preventing mental disorders in refugees and asylum seekers in Europe and Turkey: Study protocols for two randomised controlled trials. *BMJ Open, 9*(5), e030259.

Purgato, M., Carswell, K., Tedeschi, F., Acarturk, C., Anttila, M., Au, T., Bajbouj, M., Baumgartner, J., Biondi, M., Churchill, R., Cuijpers, P., Koesters, M., Gastaldon, C., Ilkkursun, Z., Lantta, T., Nose, M., Ostuzzi, G., Papola, D., & Popa, M. (2021). Effectiveness of self-help plus in preventing mental disorders in refugees and asylum seekers in Western Europe: A multinational randomized controlled trial. *Psychotherapy and Psychosomatics, 90*(6), 403–414. https://doi.org/10.1159/000517504

Radu, I., Scheermesser, M., Spiess, M. R., Schulze, C., Händler-Schuster, D., & Pehlke-Milde, J. (2023). Digital health for migrants, ethnic and cultural minorities and the role of participatory development: A scoping review. *International Journal of Environmental Research and Public Health, 20*(20), 6962.

Reinhardt, I., Schmidt, L., Reske, D., Zielasek, J., Braun, G., Böttche, M., Boettcher, J., Burchert, S., Glaesmer, H., Knaevelsrud, C., Konnopka, A., Muntendorf, L., Nohr, L., Paskuy, S., Renneberg, B., Sierau, S., Stammel, N., Wagner, B., Wirz, T., & Gouzoulis-Mayfrank, E. (2023). Blended-ALMAMAR app for inpatient mental health care for refugees: Study protocol for a multicenter implementation study within the I-REACH consortium (internet-based REfugee mentAl healtH care). *BMC Health Services Research, 23*(1), 1409. https://doi.org/10.1186/s12913-023-10403-z

Röhr, S., Jung, F. U., Pabst, A., Grochtdreis, T., Dams, J., Nagl, M., Renner, A., Hoffmann, R., König, H.-H., & Kersting, A. (2021). A self-help app for Syrian refugees with posttraumatic stress (Sanadak): Randomized controlled trial. *JMIR mHealth and uHealth, 9*(1), e24807.

Rollnick, S., & Miller, W. R. (1995). What is motivational interviewing? *Behavioural and Cognitive Psychotherapy, 23*(4), 325–334.

Rosner, R., Sachser, C., Hornfeck, F., Kilian, R., Kindler, H., Muche, R., Müller, L. R. F., Thielemann, J., Waldmann, T., & Ziegenhain, U. (2020). Improving mental health care for unaccompanied young refugees through a stepped-care approach versus usual care+: Study protocol of a cluster ranomized controlled hybrid effectiveness implementation trial. *Trials, 21*(1), 1–13.

Schäfer, I., Heinz, A., Penka, S., Lindert, J., Klein, M., Albayrak, S., Lotzin, A., Hiller, P., Milin, S., & Raiser, P. (2023). Prevention and treatment of substance use disorders in refugees: The PREPARE network. *SUCHT, 69*(5), 235–242. https://doi.org/10.1024/0939-5911/a000832

Schäfer, I., Hiller, P., Milin, S., & Lotzin, A. (2022). A multicenter, randomized controlled trial to compare the effectiveness of STARC-SUD (skills training in affect regulation—A culture-sensitive approach) versus treatment as usual in trauma-exposed refugees with substance use problems. *Trials, 23*(1), 915. https://doi.org/10.1186/s13063-022-06761-4

Sever, C. A., Cuijpers, P., Dawson, K. S., Mittendorfer-Rutz, E., Akhtar, A., Bryant, R. A., & Sijbrandij, M. (2024). Addressing challenges faced by young refugees in The Netherlands: Adapting problem management plus (PM+) with an emotional processing module. *Cambridge Prisms: Global Mental Health, 11*, e80.

Sijbrandij, M., Acarturk, C., Bird, M., Bryant, R. A., Burchert, S., Carswell, K., de Jong, J., Dinesen, C., Dawson, K. S., & El Chammay, R. (2017). Strengthening mental health care systems for

Syrian refugees in Europe and the Middle East: Integrating scalable psychological interventions in eight countries. *European Journal of Psychotraumatology, 8*(sup2), 1388102.

Spaaij, J., Kiselev, N., Berger, C., Bryant, R. A., Cuijpers, P., De Graaff, A. M., Fuhr, D. C., Hemmo, M., McDaid, D., & Moergeli, H. (2022). Feasibility and acceptability of problem management plus (PM+) among Syrian refugees and asylum seekers in Switzerland: A mixed-method pilot randomized controlled trial. *European Journal of Psychotraumatology, 13*(1), 2002027.

Stöver, H., Grundmann, J., Mittel, K., Schneider, M., Zurhold, H., & Kuhn, S. (2018). *Behandlung geflüchteter Menschen mit Substanzgebrauchsstörungen–Erfahrungen und rechtliche Hintergründe der Finanzierung.* Institut für Suchtforschung Frankfurt am Main. https://www.researchgate.net/publication/332291091_Behandlung_gefluchteter_Menschen_mit_Substanzgebrauchsstorungen_-_Erfahrungen_und_rechtliche_Hintergrunde_der_Finanzierung

Stylianopoulos, P., Hertner, L., Heinz, A., Kluge, U., Schäfer, I., & Penka, S. (2024). Good practice in reaching and treating refugees in addiction care in Germany: A Delphi study. *BMC Public Health, 24*(1), 30. https://doi.org/10.1186/s12889-023-17446-1

Tucker, S., Baldonado, N., Ruina, O., Ratmann, O., Flaxman, S., Bryn, L., Lachman, J., Taradaika, E., Melendez-Torres, G. J., Vallance, I., Goldman, P., Cluver, L., & Hillis, S. (2024). Hope groups: A protocol for a cluster randomized controlled trial of psychosocial, mental health, and parenting support groups for Ukrainian caregivers during war and conflict. *Trials, 25*(1), 486. https://doi.org/10.1186/s13063-024-08233-3

Turrini, G., Purgato, M., Cadorin, C., Bartucz, M., Cristofalo, D., Gastaldon, C., Nosè, M., Ostuzzi, G., Papola, D., & Prina, E. (2025). Comparative efficacy and acceptability of psychosocial interventions for PTSD, depression, and anxiety in asylum seekers, refugees, and other migrant populations: A systematic review and network meta-analysis of randomised controlled studies. *The Lancet Regional Health–Europe, 48.*

Turrini, G., Purgato, M., Tedeschi, F., Acartürk, C., Anttila, M., Au, T., Carswell, K., Churchill, R., Cuijpers, P., & Friedrich, F. (2022). Long-term effectiveness of self-help plus in refugees and asylum seekers resettled in Western Europe: 12-month outcomes of a randomised controlled trial. *Epidemiology and Psychiatric Sciences, 31*, e39.

Uricher, J. (2025). Individual and contextual determinants of substance use among refugees in shared accommodations: A cross–sectional multilevel analysis. *European Addiction Research, 2025*(31), 384–395.

van der Boor, C. F., Taban, D., Tol, W. A., Akellot, J., Neuman, M., Weiss, H. A., Greco, G., Vassall, A., May, C., Nadkarni, A., Kinyanda, E., Roberts, B., & Fuhr, D. C. (2024). Effectiveness and cost-effectiveness of a transdiagnostic intervention for alcohol misuse and psychological distress in humanitarian settings: Study protocol for a randomised controlled trial in Uganda. *Trials, 25*(1), 148. https://doi.org/10.1186/s13063-024-07980-7

Weinreich, K. J., Frankova, I., Maksymets, N., Barbui, C., Klymchuk, V., Mooren, T., Olechno, E., Purgato, M., Sijbrandij, M., & Witteveen, A. B. (2025). Implementing scalable face-to-face and digital interventions among forcibly displaced persons from Ukraine in Europe: Protocol of the U-RISE project. *European Journal of Psychotraumatology, 16*(1), 2468117.

WHO. (2023). *WHO mhGAP guidelines update: Drug use disorder module—Evidence profile DRU1: Brief psychosocial interventions for people using cannabis or stimulants.* WHO. https://cdn.who.int/media/docs/default-source/mental-health/mhgap/drug-use-disorders/dru1_evidence_profilev3_0(17062024).pdf?sfvrsn=57fb114b_3

Widmann, M., Apondi, B., Musau, A., Warsame, A. H., Isse, M., Mutiso, V., Veltrup, C., Ndetei, D., & Odenwald, M. (2017). Comorbid psychopathology and everyday functioning in a brief intervention study to reduce khat use among Somalis living in Kenya: Description of baseline multimorbidity, its effects of intervention and its moderation effects on substance use. *Social Psychiatry and Psychiatric Epidemiology, 52*(11), 1425–1434. https://doi.org/10.1007/s00127-017-1368-y

Wiechers, M., Strupf, M., Bajbouj, M., Böge, K., Karnouk, C., Goerigk, S., Kamp-Becker, I., Banaschewski, T., Rapp, M., Hasan, A., Falkai, P., Jobst-Heel, A., Habel, U., Stamm, T., Heinz, A., Hoell, A., Burger, M., Bunse, T., & Hoehne, E. (2023). Empowerment group therapy for refugees with affective disorders: Results of a multicenter randomized controlled trial. *European Psychiatry, 66*(1), e64. https://doi.org/10.1192/j.eurpsy.2023.2431

Woodward, A., Burchert, S., Barry, A. S., Broerse, J. E., Sondorp, E., Bold, A., Ruberl, A., Hessling, J. M., Knaevelsrud, C., & Roberts, B. (2023). Scalability of digital psychological innovations for refugees: A comparative analysis in Egypt, Germany, and Sweden. *SSM-Mental Health, 4*, 100231.

Wright, J. H., Mishkind, M., Eells, T. D., & Chan, S. R. (2019). Computer-assisted cognitive-behavior therapy and mobile apps for depression and anxiety. *Current Psychiatry Reports, 21*, 1–9.

Zagha, K., Konietzny, K., Brettschneider, C., Chehadi, O., Chehadi-Köster, A., Chikhradze, N., Dababneh, N., Hegerath, F.-M., Heller, L., & Dehnen, A. (2024). Improve mental health (improve-MH) in refugee families using a culturally adapted, general practitioner-delivered psychotherapeutic intervention combined with triple P online parenting programme: Study protocol of a multicentre randomised controlled trial. *BMJ Open, 14*(9), e084080.

Chapter 12
Substance Use Among Refugees in Europe: Towards an Equity-Oriented Research and Policy Agenda

Charlotte De Kock

The World Health Organisation (WHO, 2021) defines health equity as the absence of unfair, avoidable or remediable differences in health among groups defined socially, economically, demographically or geographically. Health equity as a goal is a first step in the operationalisation of the European Union's (EU) objective to protect health across all EU policies (Art. 168 of Treaty on the Functioning of the EU). Based on the European Social Charter (ESC), the European Court of Human Rights ruled as early as 1998 that the failure to provide adequate reception conditions for an asylum seeker, including access to healthcare, amounted to inhuman and degrading treatment and is in violation of the ESC (Litins' ka, 2024).

The WHO's Health System Performance Framework (Papanicolas et al., 2022) identifies equity as one of the health system goals, alongside efficiency, people centredness, health improvement and financial protection. Access and quality are considered as the intermediate goals to achieve the former health system goals.

Whereas health system approaches to health equity vary—especially concerning what to consider as a function, intermediate or high-level goal—we choose to focus on equity as the main health system goal, which aligns with the WHO health system goal of Universal Health Coverage. This take is also in line with Savas and colleauges' (2024) call to prioritise accessibility, acceptability, quality and trust to achieve migrant-sensitive health care from a rights-based perspective.

Additionally, the WHO Health System approach allows us to identify governance, financing and resource generation as the underlying functions and prerequisites for the performance of service delivery. At the SUT level, this means that both the study and implementation of service provision for refugees should focus on equitable access and quality dimensions, while backed by coherent governance concerning financing and resource generation.

C. De Kock (✉)
Faculty of Law and Criminology, Institute for Social Drug Research, Ghent University, Ghent, Belgium
e-mail: Charlotte.DeKock@UGent.be

C. De Kock (ed.), *Substance Use Among Refugees in Europe*,
https://doi.org/10.1007/978-3-032-32399-6_12

Despite growing indications of disparities in mental health service provision for refugees and displaced populations (Daniel-Calveras et al., 2022; Satinsky et al., 2019), the specific domain of substance use-related phenomena and service delivery among these populations in Europe remains under-researched (Elkholy et al., 2023; EUDA & De Kock, 2022; Saleh et al., 2023; Solfrank et al., 2023).

This book argues that substance use should be understood ecosocially (Krieger, 2011/2024) as a product of the structural (macro), social (meso) and psychological (micro) pressures (De Kock, 2022b) experienced before, during and after displacement. By situating substance use within these intersecting contexts, the volume frames it as both a public health and social equity issue, calling for inclusive, evidence-informed interventions at macro (policy), meso (community) and micro (behavioural) levels in Europe.

12.1 Substance Use Prevalence, Risk Factors and Service Barriers

In line with the scarce literature on the prevalence of substance use among refugees in Europe (see, e.g. De Kock, 2022b), authors align with the consensus in the literature (Ezard et al., 2020) that substance use among refugees is caused by a complex interplay of pre-migration substance use or disposition for SU problems (Walg et al., 2024), the confrontation with new substance use patterns after migration and the culmination of individual and structural risk factors in combination with coping mechanisms.

Substance use can occur recreationally and without or limited harmful consequences for one's life domains. But whether substance use is self-defined as such non-problematic use, whether it is a coping strategy, or transitions into self-medication or into what the fifth diagnostic and statistical manual of mental disorders (DSM) has defined as a 'substance use disorder'—including physical dependence, risky use, social problems and impaired control—depends on multiple factors.

Several authors in this book document the complex interplay of substance use with individual mental health problems such as depressive symptoms (Petruželka et al., Chap. 2), suicidal thoughts (Uricher et al., Chap. 4), internalising behaviour among youth (Ivert and Magnusson, Chap. 8) and the combination with coping styles (Petruželka et al., Chap. 2), hinting at the importance of targeting the latter in interventions: How does one cope with adversity, in the absence of formal support?

Refugee youth, especially unaccompanied minors, have a high prevalence of PTSD, depression, anxiety and behavioural problems (Daniel-Calveras et al., 2022), mediated by degrees of social support. They are at higher risk of substance use-related problems because of these factors in combination with developmental dispositions and the absence of international protection if no formal request is made. Stallwitz et al. (2024) unpacks psychosocial functions of using and selling drugs among young Afghan men who came to Sweden as unaccompanied minors, attesting to 'not having a real life'. However, more prevalence research on substance use among (especially nomadic and unaccompanied) young refugees is necessary (Ivert & Magnusson, 2020; and in Chap. 8).

Structural factors, or upstream health risk factors such as the detrimental impact of a lengthy stay in a shared accommodation (Uricher et al., Chap. 4), instable housing (Pouille et al., Chap. 10) and economic instability (Petruželka et al., Chap. 2), were related in this book to changing substance use patterns. Additionally, although not discussed in this volume, the conditions in closed detention centres are harsh and can negatively impact refugee mental health (Van Hout et al., 2020).

These factors align with previous studies that demonstrate the impact of insecure housing (Horyniak et al., 2016) and economic status (Cook et al., 2021; Walg et al., 2024) on substance use in these populations. Previous studies also pointed out that unstable housing and low socio-economic status are significantly more prevalent among non-national clients in Belgian and German SUT (De Kock, 2022a, 2020b; López-Atanes et al., 2025) as compared to nationals, implying the importance of targeting these domains in recovery pathways.

Throughout the chapters, system hurdles were outlined as important intervention barriers to service provision and as risk factors for transitions in substance use. Most importantly, as pointed out by Setoodeh and colleagues (Chap. 3), the interpretation of the European right to urgent medical care in Denmark—as entrenched in the Reception Directive and the EU Charter of Fundamental Rights—varies and often excludes mental health service provision. This has been evidenced across Europe and goes directly against the WHO health system goal of reaching Universal Health Coverage.

Moreover, as outlined by Setoodeh, Uricher, Nikitin and colleagues (Chapters 3, 4 and 5), reception systems in Europe are often forced into crisis modes because of rapidly changing migration flows on the one hand, but importantly also because of changing political climates aimed at reducing reception capacity on the other. Indeed, resource limitations constrain quality service provision (Savas et al., 2024) both in reception and substance use treatment (SUT) contexts in Europe.

12.2 Prioritary Intervention Domains

In an ecosocial perspective, we distil three ways forward from the contributions in this volume. First, at the macro or policy level it is key to finance structural prevention by means of resilient reception systems with sufficient capacity, as well as to safeguard basic human needs and rights in the domains of housing and health by facilitating stable housing and increasing access to mental health services and SUT, in addition to accessible labour and education.

Second, at the meso level of the community it is vital to offer safe reception environments and capacitate professionals working in them, and to offer accessible, available and quality SUT. This requires equity-oriented governance, financing and resource generation.

Third, at the micro level, it is key to understand when and why substance use transitions occur and to intervene with appropriate, stepped evidence-based interventions accordingly, with a main focus on prevention and early intervention

12.2.1 Macro: Structural Prevention and Universal Health Coverage

First, European health policies must guarantee statutory recognition of healthcare entitlements—including essential services such as harm reduction, mental health and chronic care—for all migrants regardless of legal status. Legal and administrative safeguards should ensure what Setoodeh et al. in this volume (Chap. 3) termed 'firewalls' protecting migrants from immigration enforcement when accessing mental health care and during mental health interventions that take place in the reception setting.

The EU Temporary Protection Directive issued on 4 March 2022 capacitated member states to offer swift access to the health system for Ukrainian refugees, which illustrates that better and equitable access to health services for all refugees is possible in theory but strongly depends on political willingness. Although more SUT service level research is needed, scholars alert that mainly residential services remain largely inaccessible for refugee populations (De Kock, 2022a; Hertner et al., 2023; López-Atanes et al., 2025; Saleh et al., 2023).

Eliminating administrative, legal and financial barriers restricting access to prevention, treatment, harm reduction and social services is vital to uphold refugee health rights (Nikitin et al., Chapters 5 and 10). Accelerating asylum procedures and expediting access to (private) housing can further reduce stress and barriers to successful intervention in reception contexts (Uricher et al., Chap. 4).

Second, considering the key health principle that prevention is more cost-effective than disease reduction, and acknowledging that refugees face hardships before, during and after migration, it is primordial—as posited by the WHO (2023)—to fulfil basic needs related to food security, protection, accommodation and general subsistence (Setoodeh, Pouille et al., Chapters 3 and 10). Limiting detention, challenging harmful stereotyping of refugee populations and promoting social integration are essential strategies to reduce both health inequities and discrimination, which in itself poses a serious mental health risk.

Acknowledging the intrinsic link between these policy domains and the social determinants of mental health and upstream health factors (Ingleby, 2019) is a first step in structural prevention. Access to employment, daily structure and social integration further contribute positively to mental health and resilience among refugees, as exemplified by Pouille (Chap. 10) through the SEMID-EU project in this volume.

Recognising and addressing the social determinants of mental health thus stands as the most critical mental health intervention for refugees in Europe. Nationwide interventions like the Swedish PIA (Promoting Integration and Adjustment of Newly

Arrived Adolescents and their Families) model likely influence refugee mental health positively, though more rigorous studies are needed to evidence their impact. Migration governance thus influences health system equity for these populations. Moreover, structural prevention strategies addressing upstream factors—such as access to stable housing, healthcare, education and social integration opportunities—are essential complements to behavioural interventions aimed at reducing substance use vulnerability.

Third, facilitating system-level coordination across organisations is necessary to bridge service fragmentation and ensure continuity of care encompassing mental health, SUT and social support (de Jonge et al., Chap. 9). Moreover, accelerating asylum procedures and facilitating quicker transitions to private housing can materially reduce stress and prevent escalation of substance use risks arising from prolonged stays in collective reception conditions (Uricher et al., Chap. 4).

Lastly, to safeguard equitable SUT and interventions for refugee populations, it is key that European national health systems build robust monitoring systems—complying with necessary privacy measures to reduce the risk of data-related harm—to evaluate health and migration system capacity in achieving equity. Further development of the European Treatment Demand Indicator (TDI) by the European Drugs Agency could play an important role in this development by, for example, reintroducing a nationality-related indicator in its protocol (De Kock, 2021).

12.2.2 *Meso: Environmental Prevention, Prevention Infrastructure, Service Access and Quality*

Considering that substance use and related problems are influenced by both the length of stay in shared accommodations—as pointed out by Uricher and colleagues in Chap. 4—and the quality of accommodation (Horyniak et al., 2016), it is key to factor these conditions in environmental prevention strategies that transform reception environments into spaces that make healthy choices easier (Burkhart et al., 2022).

First, reception facilities should be safe environments to capacitate residents to foster the trust and resilience needed to build up their lives and as a prerequisite to successful mental health interventions.

Second, reception settings should equally be equipped with inclusive prevention infrastructures, meaning that they integrate capacity-building, for example by creating a drug policy and by offering professional training. This is a prerequisite for the implementation of context-sensitive, trauma-informed evidence-based approaches to prevention and early intervention. Existing professional trainings in Europe were identified by De Kock in Chap. 11. While the identified professional trainings are promising, future cross-country and sectoral collaboration is needed to scale these interventions up, strengthen their theoretical basis and evaluate them.

Third, reception facilities should be well embedded in the community and incorporated into mental health networks enabling them to tap into the expertise of services in the community as well as to intervene or refer in a timely and effective manner. This allows reception facilities to take a cross-sectoral approach and support refugees in their broader needs (education, housing, labour, health, etc.) that underlie the social determinants of (mental) health. This type of community engagement and partnerships are part of and partial to the prerequisites of striving for health equity (Prentice et al., 2024). Indeed, coordination across organisations in reception on the one hand, and treatment on the other, is needed to bridge service fragmentation and facilitate continuity of care in mental health, SUT and social support services (de Jonge et al., Chap. 9).

Fourth, as outlined in the macro interventions, SUT services should in turn be accessible, independent of nationality and refugee status. Moreover, whereas most research is focussed on inequity at the level of accessing mental health care services and SUT, more attention is needed from a health system perspective on the quality of care, retention in and outcomes of treatment, as these factors jointly compound equitable (mental) health care (Dauvrin et al., 2019; De Kock et al., 2020a, 2020b). Whereas access largely depends on formal requirements and procedures (macro), quality, retention and outcomes rather relate to organisational factors (meso) such as acceptability and trust.

Indeed, as alerted by the European Psychiatric Association (EPA) in its position paper on psychiatric care of refugees in Europe, refugees have an increased risk for treatment discontinuation and for incorrect diagnoses and treatments, leading to inequities.

Fifth, in the harm reduction domain, Nikitin and colleagues (Chap. 5) highlight the necessity of adapting opioid agonist therapy (OAT) and HIV-related services for (Ukrainian) refugee populations in Europe. Policy-level recommendations to permit task-shifting—such as allowing general practitioners to prescribe OAT, as is the case in Belgium, Pre-Exposure Prophylaxis (PrEP) and Antiretroviral Therapy (ART)—and enabling take-home OAT doses have proven effective in improving availability without exacerbating stigma (Nikitin, Chap. 5).

12.2.3 Micro: Behavioural Preventive Interventions and Early Intervention

Uricher and colleagues (Chap. 4) note that preventive interventions often do not align well with the 'energy sapping asylum process', higlighting that interventions can only be succesful if the underlying prerequisites are fulfilled. These prerequisitis include refugees' safety, living conditions, resource availability and temporal proximity to distressing events (Calam et al., 2022). These conditions influence intervention readiness and should subsequently feed into the logical models underlying the interventions.

Giacco and colleagues (2020) identify critical time points for refugee mental health—before, during and after travel, and importantly at initial settlement, during integration efforts and in the face of immigration status challenges. These critical time points—especially the latter, after migration—can guide the timing and tailoring of interventions.

These insights illustrate that interventions must not only be evidence-based but also developmentally appropriate, time specific and context-sensitive. Premature or ill-suited interventions, such as one-off 'just say no' poster campaigns, risk unintended negative consequences like sparking curiosity about substance use among youth. Evidence-based interventions must be built on theoretical insights in the mechanisms of change that underlie substance use transitions.

Throughout the chapters in this volume some preconditions for implementing interventions were outlined by the authors. Pouille and colleagues emphasise in Chap. 10 that non-judgmental, low-threshold, outreach-based models of care that integrate psychosocial support, harm reduction principles and culturally responsive practices to build trust and engagement are key. Interventions should of course also overcome language barriers (Nikitin, Chap. 5)—an important factor in SUT inequities in Europe (De Kock 2021). Health care-specific platforms such as S-MINDS, X-prompt, iTranslate and virtual tele-interpreters are promising as well as translated intervention materials such as ASSIST and mhGAP materials.

The insights on risk factors and barriers in this book, in combination with what we know from previous research (Greene et al.,2024a, 2024b), can only lead us to conclude that prevention and early intervention to prevent harmful transitions in substance use are key in the reception context. However, compared to universal prevention strategies, more attention is needed to the prerequisites of safety and stability, context and time specification, in addition to an evidence-based developmental focus.

In this line of research, US-based researchers Salas-Wright and Schwartz (2018) developed the cultural stress theoretical model which posits that cultural stress (discrimination, negative reception context, bicultural stress) influences both alcohol and other drug misuse and family functioning (parental involvement, communication, family coherence). It is an interesting hypothesis worth refining in future European research with an eye on creating and testing logical intervention models.

In Chap. 12 De Kock established, in line with the existent literature (Aleer et al., 2024; EUAA and EUDA 2023; Greene et al., 2018; Stylianopoulos et al., 2024), that the availability and implementation of evidence-based substance use prevention interventions in the reception setting is limited in Europe. Nevertheless, promising practices were identified in the domains of brief early intervention based on substance use assessment and in mental health interventions. In the absence of robust evidence on substance use prevention interventions, it is key to further develop, implement and test existing assessment and brief interventions.

In the past decade research on, and the implementation of, mental health interventions for refugees and displaced populations has grown substantially, infused by various (inter)national funding such as the EU's Horizon2020 as well as the United Nations Office on Drugs and Crime (UNODC), the UN Refugee Office (UNHCR), the WHO's Mental Health Gap Action Program (mhGAP) as well as the Interagency Standing Committee and the subgroup on substance use (cochaired by UNHCR, WHO and UNODC) and national bodies such as the German Federal Ministry of Education and Research and the Belgian Federal Agency for the Reception of Asylum Applicants (Fedasil).

Evidence-based interventions such as ASSIST, Self-Help Plus (SH+), Problem Management Plus (PM+), Step-by-Step (SbS) and Strong Families have been studied extensively (Acarturk et al., 2024, 2022; Barbui et al., 2023; Burchert et al., 2019; Carswell et al., 2018; de Graaff et al., 2022; de Graaff et al., 2024; El-Khani et al., 2023; El-Khani et al., 2021; Greene et al. 2024a, 2024b; Haar et al., 2020; Heim et al., 2021; Karyotaki et al., 2023; Lee et al., 2023; Mwangala et al., 2024; Purgato et al., 2019; Sever et al., 2024; Sijbrandij et al., 2017; Spaaij et al., 2022; Turrini et al., 2019; Turrini et al., 2022; van der Boor et al., 2024; Weinreich et al., 2025).

From reviewing this growing literature on mental health interventions for refugees in Europe, the following four conclusions emerge (also see Chap. 11).

12.2.3.1 The Need to Include Substance Use(rs) in Mental health Interventions

First, more often than not, substance users as a target population and substance use as a characteristic are excluded from intervention evaluations trials. Mental health and substance use are inextricably intertwined as substance use often serves as coping or self-medication for unmet mental health needs among refugees (Pouille, De Kock et al., Chapters 10 and 11)., although much remains unknown about the directionality of the relation (Harris et al., 2019).

Indeed, Okulicz-Kozaryn and Dzielska in Chap. 6 and De Kock in Chap. 11 alert that mental health interventions, where possible, should explicitly incorporate substance use components and outcomes to avoid exclusionary practices and advance the domain. Trauma-informed care and approaches that strengthen coping and resilience are essential components of behavioural interventions targeting substance use prevention in these populations (Okulicz-Kozaryn and Dzielska, Chap. 6).

Problem Management Plus for instance (de Graaff et al., 2024) shows positive outcomes in Europe, such as the reduction in psychological distress and anxiety at 1-year follow-up, rendering it an intervention for further evaluation and replication in European reception settings. Indeed, the WHO's scalable and evidence-based interventions for low-and middle-income settings gain relevance due to the increasing limitation of resources in European reception facilities (Spaaij et al., 2022).

Moreover, there is growing evidence for the implementation of stepped-care models to reduce mental health problems based on problem assessment and subsequent diversified interventions, as demonstrated in the literature (Böge et al., 2022; Zagha et al., 2024) and illustrated in Chap. 9 by de Jonge and colleagues. The CHANGE project in Uganda and Ukraine (Problem Management Plus with additional substance use modules) as well as ASSIST implementations in Zambia could be adapted, implemented and evaluated in European contexts.

Additionally, culturally adapted cognitive behavioural therapy (CA-CBT) and motivational strategies-inspired interventions show growing effectiveness as brief interventions adaptable to low-resource settings typical of refugee reception settings (WHO, 2023; de Jonge et al., Chap. 9).

12.2.3.2 Evidence-Based Prevention and Early intervention in Reception

As evidenced in humanitarian settings outside Europe (Ezard et al., 2020; Greene et al. 2024a, 2024b), evidence-based prevention and early intervention are equally key in the European reception settings and among displaced populations residing outside them. Interventions targeting families (such as UNODC's Strong Families), youth and multiple cultural groups, delivered with sensitivity to diverse backgrounds and past experiences, are necessary to maximise acceptability and effectiveness (Wanke et al., De Kock, Chapters 7 and 11). Additionally, interventions targeting displaced unaccompanied youth, particularly those outside formal schooling, are important to prevent risk behaviours and substance use initiation (Wanke, de Jonge et al., Chapters 7 and 9). Lastly, preventive interventions should be timed and tailored according to refugees' (migration) trajectories, critical mental health time points and psychological readiness (Giacco, 2020; Calam et al., 2022; Uricher et al., Chap. 4). Premature or simplistic interventions (such as one-shot information dissemination) should of course be avoided, while developmental appropriateness to prevent unintended harm, is key (Uricher et al., De Kock, Chapters 4 and 11; Calam et al., 2022).

Prevention is of course broader than delaying or postponing substance use. Including harm reduction approaches adapted to refugee-specific needs, with pragmatic policy support is equally important for OAT, PrEP and ART delivery (Nikitin et al., Chap. 5).

12.2.3.3 Training Reception and Treatment Staff

Third, the importance of training reception and treatment staff in trauma-informed, culturally and structurally competent behavioural preventive interventions is reiterated by multiple authors (de Jonge, Pouille, De Kock, Chapters 9, 10 and 11). As alerted in a recent EUDA/EUAA study (2023), European reception staff are in need of more training concerning substance use-related problems, including prevention and incident management. The intervention review in Chap. 11 demonstrates that such trainings do exist in Europe, but that conveners would benefit from upscaling with specific attention to skills training and case discussion in addition to knowledge-oriented trainings. The Finnish TAVATA project aimed at capacitating reception workers—discussed in Chap. 11—with the skills for motivational techniques is promising in that context (Peltonen et al., 2022).

12.2.3.4 Digital Advances as Bridges Towards Services

Fourth, digital interventions can complement live support but must not replace personal contact. Rigorous evaluation and careful integration of digital tools, including conversational agents and AI-supported approaches, are key for reaching mobile and hard-to-reach refugee populations (De Kock, Nikitin et al., Chapters 5 and 11). Indeed, as pointed out in Chap. 11, digital advances can help bridge towards, but not replace, services.

12.3 New Political Contexts and Underexplored Research Territories

Besides the need for aetiological, epidemiological and intervention research, we cannot but also call to look into political drivers that influence substance use and service delivery in both the countries of origin and reception. This entails collaborative research that bridges public health, political sciences, criminology and conflict studies to understand multi-factorial causal patterns linking war, trauma and substance use (Molina-Fernández et al., 2025).

In countries mainly perceived as reception countries, the growing 'securitisation' discourse of migration (Bureš & Stojanov, 2023) inevitably influences both the demand and supply side of substance use service provision. From the perspective of refugees or the 'demand side', it influences the fear of being stigmatised or outright excluded from reception, asylum and international protection among refugees (Douglass et al., 2023). On the 'supply side', it can influence professional's attitudes towards these populations. Indeed, conscious and unconscious 'hierarchising' of migrants (Koppel & Jakobson, 2023), or exclusionary deservingness categories (Borrelli, 2022), can seep into health service provision, resulting in inequitable quality of care (Savas et al., 2024).

In the countries of origin, political upheaval and war affect service provision and the availability and use of substances, which inevitably influence substance use phenomena observed in Europe. Nikitin in this volume (Chap. 5) and in previous work (Nikitin et al., 2023) confirmed reports (Bloswick et al., 2022; Dubov et al., 2024) that revealed the detrimental impact of the Russian invasion on OAT service delivery in Ukraine.

Moreover, migration can also be used to pressurise national health systems politically, as was the case when Belarusian authoritarian leader Alexander Lukashenko announced that he would 'flood the EU with migrants and drugs" (Broks et al., 2024, p. 205) via the Latvia–Belarus border, effectively leading to a sudden albeit limited increase in border crossings. Outside Europe, there are reports of migrants being forced into illegal activities in drug markets to get to their destination, as documented in Libya, for instance (Daniel et al., 2022). More research is needed to understand and act upon the relation between drug and human trafficking.

Moreover, specific substances that are mainly used medically in one country may be used in a different way in other contexts due to differing regulatory practices and drug policies, or lack of guidance. In this context Cleaver (2007), for instance, established that buprenorphine—used for OAT in European countries—became a substance of choice in Georgia due to smuggling routes from Europe in combination with the criminalisation and related stigma of overt heroin use in Georgia and the limited availability of methadone in certain regions. Rayes et al. (2022) in turn point to the rising use of Captagon among internally displaced populations in Syria, while SUT service capacity remains limited because of political instabilities.

Alemi et al. (2023) further alerted an exponential rise in opioid use among Afghan adults between 2005 and 2009, leading to adult opioid use prevalence rates that are more than twice the global average, while OAT—especially after the Taliban offensive in 2021—is rare and politically sensitive in Afghanistan. In Europe the use of pregabalin, a gabapentinoid-based medication—prescribed variably across member states—is on the rise among refugee and non-refugee populations alike and is raising concerns in concert with the use of benzodiazepines in opioid-based medication such as tramadol (Dufau, 2020; Fonseca et al., 2021; Servais et al., 2023; Transit, 2022).

Indeed, it is important to study how both the securitisation and the criminalisation of refugees as well as the situation in home countries and the availability of substances impact both substance use and service delivery, because these (political) mechanisms are parts of the puzzles that underlie substance use phenomena observed among refugees in Europe. It is key to do so from a perspective that does not harm the studied populations, but contrarily aims for reciprocal benefit (De Kock et al., 2025), without scapegoating already scapegoated populations (De Kock et al., 2017; Hunt & Kolind, 2017).

Moreover, the language we use as professionals and academics is key: observing 'unmet health needs', versus ascertaining the 'unavailability of services' and 'lack of response to basic health needs' (e.g., Petruželka, Setoodeh et al., Chapters 2 and 3) are distinct phrasing referring, respectively, to the demand versus supply side, or micro versus meso and macro barriers. As pointed out by Dumke and colleagues (2024) in their review on barriers to accessing mental health, studies tend to focus on migrant-specific characteristics that influence their involvement and quality of care (cultural understanding, fear of stigma, awareness, language and attitudes), while demand-side factors, or macro issues, remain under-researched. They point out that supply-side barriers are mostly related to the quality of care, while demand-side barriers are key determinants of access, which de facto precedes the adequacy of care in a health equity perspective (Dauvrin et al., 2019). Indeed, micro-or client-level factors are more often than not closely intertwined with organisational and policy factors at meso and macro levels (De Kock 2021). It is therefore imperative to distinguish between, and study the intersection of demand-and supply-side factors in assessing SUT equity.

Problem framing inevitably influences where to locate responses to overcome identified disparities and inequities (De Kock, 2020). That is why applying an ecosocial framework in understanding needs and responses, supply and demand, comes in: some responses are located mainly at the policy levels (macro), some rather at the community and reception facility level (meso) and some at the intervention (micro) level, targeting individual factors, but all are intertwined.

From a health equity and prevention infrastructure perspective it is key to invest in the supply side of access, in parallel but also prior to intervention quality and outcome investment. Subsequently, it is key to analytically study access as a goal that precedes quality to expand the current WHO Health System Assessment approach (Papanicolas et al., 2022).

12.4 Methodological Challenges and Ways Forward

Several methodological challenges and research caveats became apparent in this volume. Importantly, recruitment of participants for research among refugees is often hindered by issues such as low trust in health care professionals (de Jonge et al., Chap. 9), distrust towards state organisations (Setoodeh, Uricher et al., Chapters 3 and 4), but also because of the fear that partaking in research will influence the asylum procedure. Refugees, especially those who have not (yet) been granted international protection, are often considered 'hard-to-reach populations'. Moreover, retaining participants in evaluation trials can prove particularly challenging when people are transiting a country or when their circumstance change after having received a decision concerning their application for international protection.

In both quantitative and qualitative research it is quintessential to, in the research design phase, establish why and in which ways the study is a win-win from both a research and a participant perspective. Establishing reciprocal benefit in combination with creating genuine trust (e.g. by means of participatory observation, interview techniques and non-intrusive recruitment) and ensuring privacy safeguards precedes willingness to partake in research and a truly informed consent (De Kock et al., 2025). It is equally important to create watertight data environments with clear safeguards concerning the privacy of participants to avoid data-related harm.

Concerning quantitative research in this domain, different research needs arose in this volume. First, it is necessary to better understand and monitor the prevalence of substance use, problems and 'disorders' in representative samples comparing migration or displacement backgrounds and other factors such as socio-economic and housing factors and in cross-national designs. Data from cross-national comparisons are needed to analyse how migration-related lifestyle changes and host population lifestyles and circumstances (Agyemang & van den Born, 2019) influence substance use-related problems. Purposive sampling in these populations in the European national health surveys as well as targeted new surveys in representative samples could be a first step in reaching this goal.

Importantly, this research should allow for understanding the weight, function and direction of factors that mechanically underlie substance use transitions among varying displaced populations, implying that targeted surveys must not only focus on migration backgrounds and substance use but equally include potential moderators with special attention to housing and socio-economic status. Indeed, hypothesis-driven fundamental research is needed to understand how risk and protective as well as promotive factors at varying migration stages and among specific populations interact in substance use outcomes to inform intervention logical models.

This volume, in concert with recent literature, highlights that post-migration factors should be nuanced by distinguishing between reception conditions, integration and asylum decision-related factors in time and that special attention is needed for housing and socio-economic factors.

Second, in evaluation research, overrecruiting with an eye on adequately powered sample sizes is warranted as the research discussed in this volume demonstrates high drop-out rates. Additionally, as pointed out by Okulicz-Kozaryn and Dzielska and De Kock (Chapters 6 and 11), research instruments should be properly validated among these populations. Third, it is warranted that evidence-based mental health interventions include substance use-related mediators, moderators and outcomes and include refugees who use substances or with diagnosed substance use disorders in evaluation designs.

Lastly, while in this volume we deliberately used a broad interpretation of substance use and related problems, it will be key to distinguish between types of substances and their use in future research as well to monitor how specific (new) substances affect these populations with special attention to medication such as pregabalin and opioid-based medications as well as new psychoactive substances (NPS).

Moreover, female non-nationals have been documented to be gravely underrepresented in comparison to both their presence in the population and national treatment populations in Belgium and Germany (De Kock et al., 2020a, 2020b; López-Atanes et al., 2025), highlighting that gender-specific inquiries are urgently needed. Contrarily, experts in countries bordering Ukraine report that the majority of clients accessing drug services are women (EUDA, 2022), highlighting a changing treatment demand which requires further inquiry.

As this is an emerging research domain, qualitative research can additionally provide rich, in-depth insights on under-researched topics such as life trajectories and their relation to substance use transitions, as well as specific migration-related and other triggers at micro, meso and macro levels. Moreover, participatory approaches that ensure equity and reciprocal benefit may help overcome some of the barriers in this type of research (Uricher, De Kock et al., Chapters 4 and 11), but it requires time and resources as demonstrated in Uricher and colleagues' Chap. 4.

12.5 A Research and Policy Agenda for Substance Use Among Refugees in Europe

The contributions in this volume, together with recent literature on substance use among refugees in Europe, provide a basis for developing a first European research agenda (Table 12.1). The agenda is subdivided per topic, including social epidemiology, aetiology, intervention and implementation research, sociological and criminological perspectives, while taking into account methodological and ethical considerations presented (Table 12.1).

Table 12.1 An agenda for researching the migration substance use nexus in Europe

1. Social Epidemiology and Aetiologic research
1.1. Develop (cross-)national substance use prevalence studies including representative samples, distinguishing not only between migrants and non-migrants but allowing for differentiation by migration stage, legal status, gender and socio-economic indicators as well as per European policy contexts and in comparison to home country (drug and other) policy contexts 1.2. Develop (cross-)national studies among representative samples on substance use treatment service use that focus not only on access (presence in treatment) but also on retention and treatment outcomes and thus acceptability and quality (Savas et al., 2024) as components of equitable service provision 1.3. Integrate housing (Horyniak et al., 2016; Uricher et al., 2025), socio-economic status (Cook et al., 2021) and integration variables (Giacco, 2020) in addition to migration-related indicators as moderators in statistical models of prevalence and aetiological studies to understand transitions in substance use trajectories to feed into intervention and recovery recommendations 1.4. Conduct longitudinal cohort studies to identify causal mechanisms relating pre, during and post-migration stressors, coping, substance use onset and critical time points for transitions 1.5. Examine under-researched female and nomadic youth populations, including gender-based and life-course stressors to address service needs
2. Intervention and implementation research
2.1. Macro level: Structural Prevention and policy impact
2.1.1. Assess the impact of healthcare entitlement reforms (e.g. universal access models) on substance use treatment uptake among migrants 2.1.2. Evaluate the effects of reception and migration policy on resilience, housing and in relation to mental health and substance use (related problems or disorders) 2.1.3. Test structural prevention frameworks that integrate stable housing, labour access and education as health interventions 2.1.4. Implement system-level coordination trials connecting health, social and legal sectors from a prevention infrastructure perspective
2.2. Meso level: Environmental and Organisational responses
2.2.1. Test environmental prevention measures and interventions in reception contexts (e.g. reception centre drug policies, harm reduction readiness training) 2.2.2. Establish European multi-country implementation studies on professional training concerning substance use-related responses in reception settings 2.2.3. Evaluate community partnership models that embed refugee-led and local mental health actors in prevention systems 2.2.4. Monitor and map retention and quality-of-care outcomes to complement access equity indicators in substance use treatment research

(continued)

(continued)

2.3. Micro level: Behavioural preventive interventions
2.3.1. Develop developmentally timed early interventions informed by fundamental research including psychological readiness, migration phase and critical time points in displacement 2.3.2. Validate and scale stepped-care mental health models (e.g. CA-CBT and motivational strategies, problem management plus, strong families, ASSIST) integrating mental health and substance use outcomes 2.3.3. Co-design youth and family-based prevention programmes addressing coping, resilience and bicultural stress 2.3.4. Conduct comparative trials of digital and hybrid interventions, ensuring refugee-related adaptations (migration stage, age, etc.)
3. Sociological and criminological studies
3.1. Investigate political drivers of securitisation and their impact on both demand and supply of treatment in European host countries (e.g. 'undeserving migrant' rhetoric) 3.2. Explore the nexus between human trafficking / smuggling and drug economies along migration routes 3.3. Examine criminalisation effects on help-seeking behaviour and treatment provisions for undocumented migrants 3.4. Analyse professional attitudes and institutional discrimination patterns shaping differential access to, quality in and outcomes of substance use treatment services 3.5. Analyse the impact of war (economies) on substance use and their markets in home countries. 3.6. Analyse the impact of European drug policies and prescription policies on substance use trajectories in life-course perspectives
4. Methodological and ethical considerations
4.1. Invest in trust-building recruitment and retention strategies, including non-intrusive, participant-benefit-centred designs 4.2. Oversample in quantitative research and consider alternative experimental designs 4.3. Validate psychometric instruments for substance use and mental health assessment among multilingual refugee populations 4.4. Mainstream equity, reciprocity and privacy safeguards across research protocols to mitigate data-related harm 4.5. Adopt participatory research frameworks that operationalise equity and power-sharing in study design 4.6. Integrate both a do-no-harm and reciprocity perspective into the research design

The considerations in this volume and of recent literature equally allow us to identify eight policy recommendations presented in Table 12.2 (see e.g. Barbui et al., 2023; Daniel-Calveras et al., 2022; Dauvrin et al., 2012; Elkholy et al., 2023; EUAA and EUDA 2023; Hertner et al., 2023; Ingleby, 2019; Nikitin et al., 2023; Stylianopoulos et al., 2024; van Selm et al., 2024).

The eight policy recommendations align with and expand on recent guidance from the European Drugs Agency and the European Asylum Agency (EUAA & EUDA, 2023), the Pompidou Group, the Migration Policy Group, the SEMID-EU project (van Selm et al., 2024) and Caritas International. There is no distinction between European-level and member state recommendations for the sake of clarity and because these domains are inherently interconnected.

Table 12.2 Policy recommendation in the domain of substance use among refugees in Europe

1. Ensure equitable access to health services including mental health and substance use interventions (prevention, treatment, harm reduction), regardless of residence status or any other ground of discrimination, by removing legal limitations and simplifying administrative procedures
2. Ensure monitoring of population-level substance use and service use
2.1. Monitor SUT service use (access, quality, outcomes) by introducing nationality and migration indicators into monitoring tools (e.g. EUDA's TDI) to capture structural inequities more precisely, while safeguarding clients' privacy and -conform GDPR- explicitly including health equity monitoring as a data gathering goal in registration protocols. (De Kock, 2021) 2.2. Introduce targeted sampling to the European health surveys while safeguarding the inclusion of sufficient substance use-related questions (e.g. including medication such as pregabalin) and ensuring safety and trust throughout the survey process 2.3. Implement WHO's robust health system performance assessment in the SUT domain
3. Apply an inclusive *health in all* policy perspective by recognising the social determinants of health and upstream health factors, especially in integration and migration policy, as well as labour, housing and education policies, e.g. by establishing interministerial conferences
3.1. Safeguard the housing first principle for all refugees and applicants of international protection 3.2. Provide transitional low-threshold housing for young refugees who do not apply for international protection with the goal of meeting basic needs and allowing professionals to build trust with vulnerable youth
4. Prioritise durable structural and behavioural (mental health) prevention and early intervention in the reception setting
4.1. Apply an intervention pyramid (MHPSS) approach to substance use-related phenomena, implying that, e.g. basic services and security, community and family-strengthening mental health approaches should precede and influence implementing targeted substance use-related interventions 4.2. Apply a public health and intervention spectrum (from prevention to harm reduction) approach, implying that investments in structural and behavioural prevention are cost-effective measures 4.3. Implement behavioural interventions targeting critical mental health moments across the migration journey with special attention to early reception, the integration phase and the asylum decision phase 4.4. Foresee evidence-based training for reception workers, adapted to their own background 4.5. Integrate mental health and psychosocial support (MHPSS) into all humanitarian aid programmes to address trauma-driven substance use, prioritising evidence-based interventions, specifically ASSIST(-BI), problem management plus and other (CA-)CBT-related interventions, life skills training, strong families, early intervention, e.g. motivational interviewing and harm reduction strategies such as opioid agonist treatment 4.6. Mainstream training modules that exist across the member states in accordance with existing evidence-based professional training modules (e.g. mhGAP, EUAA training)
5. Sensitise generalist and specialist substance use treatment services concerning migration-related specificities by means of training structural competence and competences related to trauma and violence, loss and instability, transit, resettlement, acculturation, legal issues, trust and discrimination
6. Facilitate and fund language mediation and translation in service use

(continued)

(continued)

7. Facilitate durable cross-sectoral, cross-region and cross-national networks to share expertise, scale-up evidence-based interventions and monitor new substance use-related phenomena
7.1. Create a European network of reception Centre workers involved in substance use-related training to upscale and mainstream this type of training (adapted per staff category) and monitor new phenomena in this setting informed by expertise built up by EUDA, EUAA and the interagency standing committee (subgroup on substance use) cochaired by UNHCR, WHO and UNODC in concert with state of the art literature 7.2. Create a European network of substance use-related professionals who work with homeless migrants to monitor, share and disseminate expertise and respond to new phenomena and to inform the reception setting network 7.3. Promote collaboration between the reception setting and drug-related settings in the member states. 7.3.1. Include reception centres in existing mental health networks 7.3.2. Prioritise outreach work for homeless refugees as well as mobile teams that can reach remote reception settings and hard-to-reach refugees
8. Support the restoration and reinforcement of healthcare infrastructure in war-affected regions (e.g. Ukraine, Syria, Gaza) with a priority on mental health, SUT and continuity of care

These research and policy agendas represent only an initial effort to consolidate current knowledge in the field and will require further refinement to address the many challenges involved in both studying and governing this complex domain. The research agenda will be further developed within the European Migration and Substance Use research network (EUMISU), established in parallel with this publication.

12.6 Conclusion

As pointed out by Greene and colleagues (2021), epidemiological, intervention and implementation research as well as operational guidance are needed to improve access to SUT and substance use related interventions in humanitarian and reception settings.

For the European reception setting this implies a focus on inclusive mental health interventions that do not exclude substance use(rs), a priority focus on prevention and early intervention while digital advances cannot replace but can bridge towards services. Moreover, experimental evaluations are needed in Europe to scale interventions up while knowledge and skills transfer in and across the European reception settings can strengthen and capacitate reception workers.

Finally, the implementation and monitoring of inclusive prevention infrastructures and structural prevention (in concert with, behavioural interventions) are imperative to address upstream health risk factors.

In addition to Greene et al. (2021) outlined research needs, we add the need to also focus on politicological and criminological perspectives to understand how macro factors feed into the mechanisms that underlie substance use patterns and transitions as well as service delivery.

We additionally posit that it is high time to apply a health equity perspective to substance use-related service provision for refugees and displaced populations in Europe. This implies that in policy, research and practice the social determinants of substance use, access to services, quality and outcomes of services (Dauvrin et al., 2012) are considered. This equity lens requires the consideration of the prerequisites of equitable services provision such as community engagement and partnerships, institutional transformations, performance measures, a whole-society and health-in-all-policies perspective (Prentice et al., 2024) as well as inclusive evaluation trial designs.

The rationale of this volume also serves as its conclusion. As Claire Greene and colleagues argue, it is essential to move beyond questioning whether substance use services for displaced populations are feasible, and instead promote their adoption as essential components of humanitarian response (Greene et al. 2024a, 2024b, p. 408), from a rights-based, ecosocial and health equity perspective.

Competing Interests The authors declare that they have no competing interests. The author is funded by a postdoctoral fellowship from the Research Foundation—Flanders (FWO) [12AFB24N-7028].

References

Acarturk, C., Kurt, G., İlkkurşun, Z., de Graaff, A. M., Bryant, R., Cuijpers, P., Fuhr, D., McDaid, D., Park, A.-L., & Sijbrandij, M. (2024). Effectiveness of group problem management plus in distressed Syrian refugees in Türkiye: A randomized controlled trial. *Epidemiology and Psychiatric Sciences, 33*, e43.

Acarturk, C., Uygun, E., Ilkkursun, Z., Carswell, K., Tedeschi, F., Batu, M., Eskici, S., Kurt, G., Anttila, M., Au, T., Baumgartner, J., Churchill, R., Cuijpers, P., Becker, T., Koesters, M., Lantta, T., Nose, M., Ostuzzi, G., Popa, M., et al. (2022). Effectiveness of a WHO self-help psychological intervention for preventing mental disorders among Syrian refugees in Turkey: A randomized controlled trial. *World Psychiatry, 21*(1), 88–95. https://doi.org/10.1002/wps.20939

Agyemang, C., & van den Born, B.-J. (2019). Non-communicable diseases in migrants: An expert review. *Journal of Travel Medicine, 26*(2), tay107.

Aleer, E., Alam, K., & Rashid, A. (2024). A systematic literature review of substance-use prevention programs amongst refugee youth. *Community Mental Health Journal*, 1–20.

Alemi, Q., Panter-Brick, C., Oriya, S., Ahmady, M., Alimi, A. Q., Faiz, H., Hakim, N., Sami Hashemi, S. A., Manaly, M. A., Naseri, R., Parwiz, K., Sadat, S. J., Sharifi, M. Z., Shinwari, Z., Ahmadi, S. J., Amin, R., Azimi, S., Hewad, A., Musavi, Z., et al. (2023). Afghan mental health and psychosocial Well-being: Thematic review of four decades of research and interventions [review]. *BJPsych Open, 9*(4), e125. https://doi.org/10.1192/bjo.2023.50

Barbui, C., Tedeschi, F., Acarturk, C., Anttila, M., Au, T., Baumgartner, J., Carswell, K., Churchill, R., Cuijpers, P., Karyotaki, E., Klein, T., Koesters, M., Lantta, T., Nose, M., Ostuzzi, G., Pasquini, M., Prina, E., Sijbrandij, M., Tarsitani, L., et al. (2023). Risk factors for mental disorder development in asylum seekers and refugees resettled in Western Europe and Turkey: Participant-level analysis of two large prevention studies. *International Journal of Social Psychiatry, 69*(3), 664–674. https://doi.org/10.1177/00207640221132430

Batthyány, D., & Bergeron, S. (2023). The eleven-item Alcohol, Smoking and Substance Involvement Screening Test (ASSIST-11): Cross-cultural psychometric evaluation across 42 countries. *Journal of Psychiatric Research, 165*, 16–27

Bloswick, A., Mustra, D., Harasymiv, O., & Dubov, A. (2022). Facilitating Ukrainian refugees' continued participation in clinical trials [note]. *Hastings Center Report, 52*(3), 6–8. https://doi.org/10.1002/hast.1390

Böge, K., Karnouk, C., Hoell, A., Tschorn, M., Kamp-Becker, I., Padberg, F., Übleis, A., Hasan, A., Falkai, P., & Salize, H.-J. (2022). Effectiveness and cost-effectiveness for the treatment of depressive symptoms in refugees and asylum seekers: A multi-centred randomized controlled trial. *The Lancet Regional Health–Europe, 19.*

Borrelli, L. M. (2022). Should (S)he stay or should (S)he go?–street-level suspicion and the construction of the '(un)deserving migrant'. *Geopolitics, 27*(4), 1093–1116.

Broks, E., Buka, A., Buka, L., & Kučs, A. (2024). Limiting the right to access asylum: A case study of Latvia's response to the migration crisis on the Latvia-Belarus border. *Baltic Yearbook of International Law Online, 22*(1), 201–232.

Burchert, S., Alkneme, M. S., Bird, M., Carswell, K., Cuijpers, P., Hansen, P., Heim, E., Shehadeh, M. H., Sijbrandij, M., & van't Hof, E., & Knaevelsrud, C. (2019). User-centered app adaptation of a low-intensity e-mental health intervention for Syrian refugees. *Frontiers in Psychiatry, 9*. https://doi.org/10.3389/fpsyt.2018.00663

Bureš, O., & Stojanov, R. (2023). Securitization of immigration in The Czech Republic and its impact on the Czech migration policy: Experts' perceptions. *Problems of Post-Communism, 70*(6), 679–689.

Burkhart, G., Tomczyk, S., Koning, I., & Brotherhood, A. (2022). Environmental prevention: Why do we need it now and how to advance it? *Journal of Prevention, 43*(2), 149–156.

Calam, R., El-Khani, A., & Maalouf, W. (2022). Editorial perspective: How can we help the children of Ukraine and others affected by military conflict? *Child and Adolescent Mental Health, 27*(3), 294–296. https://doi.org/10.1111/camh.12581

Carswell, K., Harper-Shehadeh, M., Watts, S., et al. (2018). Step-by-step: A new WHO digital mental health intervention for depression. *Mhealth, 4*, 34.

Cleaver, H. (2007). Georgian drug misusers switch to Western heroin substitute. *BMJ. British Medical Journal, 334*(7598), 821.

Cook, W. K., Li, X., Sundquist, K., Kendler, K. S., Sundquist, J., & Karriker-Jaffe, K. J. (2021). Drinking cultures and socioeconomic risk factors for alcohol and drug use disorders among first- and second-generation immigrants: A longitudinal analysis of Swedish population data. *Drug and Alcohol Dependence, 226*, 108804.

Daniel, M. I., Oluwakemi, O., & Oluwasola, Y. V. (2022). Irregular migration, drug use and drug trafficking in sub-Saharan Africa; Libya and Nigeria. In I. Muenstermann (Ed.), *The changing tide of immigration and emigration during the last three centuries* (pp. 131–148). IntechOpen.

Daniel-Calveras, A., Baldaquí, N., & Baeza, I. (2022). Mental health of unaccompanied refugee minors in Europe: A systematic review. *Child Abuse & Neglect, 133*, 105865.

Dauvrin, M., Derluyn, I., Coune, I., Verrept, H., & Lorant, V. (2012). Towards fair health policies for migrants and ethnic minorities: The case-study of ETHEALTH in Belgium. *BMC Public Health, 12*(1), 726.

Dauvrin, M., Detollenaere, J., De Laet, C., Roberfroid, D., & Vinck, I. (2019). *Asylum seekers in Belgium: Options for a more equitable access to health care.* A stakeholder consultation, Belgian Health Care Knowledge Centre.

de Graaff, A. M., Cuijpers, P., Acarturk, C., Akhtar, A., Alkneme, M. S., Aoun, M., Awwad, M., Bawaneh, A. Y., Brown, F. L., Bryant, R., Burchert, S., Carswell, K., Drogendijk, A., Engels, M., & Fuhr, D. C. (2022). Scalable psychological interventions for Syrian refugees in Europe and the Middle East: STRENGTHS study protocol for a prospective individual participant data meta-analysis. *BMJ Open, 12*(4), e058101. https://doi.org/10.1136/bmjopen-2021-058101

de Graaff, A. M., Cuijpers, P., Elsawy, M., Hunaidy, S., Kieft, B., Gorgis, N., Twisk, J. W., Zakarian, Y., Bouman, T. K., & Lommen, M. J. (2024). The effectiveness of problem management plus at 1-year follow-up for Syrian refugees in a high-income setting. *Epidemiology and Psychiatric Sciences, 33*, e50.

De Kock, C. (2020). Cultural competence and derivatives in substance use treatment for migrants and ethnic minorities: What's the problem represented to be? *Social Theory & Health, 18*(4), 358–394.

De Kock, C. (2021). Migration and ethnicity related indicators in European drug treatment demand (TDI) registries. *Journal of Ethnicity in Substance Abuse, 20*(3), 444–470.

De Kock, C. (2022a). *Responding to drug-related problems among migrants, refugees and ethnic minorities in Europe.* European Union Drugs Agency. https://www.euda.europa.eu/drugs-library/responding-drug-related-problems-among-migrants-refugees-and-ethnic-minorities-europe_en

De Kock, C. (2022b). Equitable substance use treatment for migrants and ethnic minorities in Flanders, Belgium: Service coordinator and expert perspectives. *Substance Abuse: Research and Treatment, 16*, 11782218221097390.

De Kock, C., Blomme, E., & Antoine, J. (2020). Non-national clients in Belgian substance use treatment. *Drugs & Alcohol Today, 20*(2), 157–171.

De Kock, C., Decorte, T., Vanderplasschen, W., Derluyn, I., & Sacco, M. (2017). Studying ethnicity, problem substance use and treatment: From epidemiology to social change. *Drugs: Education, Prevention and Policy, 24*(3), 230–239.

De Kock, C., Toyinbo, L., Laudens, F., Alexandre, S., Hensgens, P., Marscia, C., Leclerq, S., Janssens, S., Jacobs, D., & Decorte, T. (2020). *Migrants et minorités ethniques: Receuil sur l'accesibilité et l'interculturalité des services pour usagers de drogues/Wegwijzer voor een toegankelijke en interculturele drughulpverlening.* Gompel & Svacina.

De Kock, C., Verhaeghe, F., Linthout, L., Orsini, G., Uzureau, O., Casteleyn, L., Pavic, G. L., Remue, L., Jacobs, M., Hest, E., & v. (2025). Ethics in qualitative migration and refugee studies in Europe: From "doing no harm" to reciprocity and equity. *International Journal of Qualitative Methods, 24*, 16094069251362965.

Douglass, C. H., Win, T. M., Goutzamanis, S., Lim, M. S., Block, K., Onsando, G., Hellard, M., Higgs, P., Livingstone, C., & Horyniak, D. (2023). Stigma associated with alcohol and other drug use among people from migrant and ethnic minority groups: Results from a systematic review of qualitative studies. *Journal of Immigrant and Minority Health, 25*(6), 1402–1425.

Dubov, A., Basenko, A., Dymaretskyi, O., & Shoptaw, S. (2024). Impact of the Russian invasion on opioid agonist therapy programs in Ukraine: A qualitative study. *Drug and Alcohol Dependence, 255*, 111069. https://doi.org/10.1016/j.drugalcdep.2023.111069

Dufau, M. (2020). *Le mésusage de la prégabaline chez les toxicomanes* (Publication Number 149) (Master's thesis). Université de Bordeaux, Bordeaux.

Dumke, L., Wilker, S., Hecker, T., & Neuner, F. (2024). Barriers to accessing mental health care for refugees and asylum seekers in high-income countries: A scoping review of reviews mapping demand and supply-side factors onto a conceptual framework. *Clinical Psychology Review, 113*, 102491.

El-Khani, A., Calam, R., & Maalouf, W. (2023). The role of faith in parenting: Considerations when implementing family skills interventions with families affected by armed conflict or displacement. *Frontiers in Psychiatry, 14*, 1118662. https://doi.org/10.3389/fpsyt.2023.1118662

El-Khani, A., Haar, K., Stojanovic, M., & Maalouf, W. (2021). Assessing the feasibility of providing a family skills intervention, "strong families", for refugee families residing in reception centers in Serbia. *International Journal of Environmental Research and Public Health, 18*(9), 4530.

Elkholy, H., Teck, T. W., Arunogiri, S., Asaad, M. R., Baessler, F., Bhad, R., Borghi, E. N., Busse, A., Ekhtiari, H., & Dave, S. (2023). Substance use disorders among forcibly displaced people: A narrative review. *Current Addiction Reports, 10*(2), 341–352.

EUAA & EUDA. (2023). *Professionals working in reception centres in Europe: An overview of drug-related challenges and support needs.* EUAA & EUDA. https://www.euda.europa.eu/publications/technical-reports/professionals-working-reception-centres-europe_en

EUDA. (2022). *Responsiveness and preparedness in addressing drug-related needs of displaced Ukrainians in EU countries bordering with Ukraine*. EU Publications Office.

EUDA & De Kock, C. (2022). *Responding to drug-related problems among migrants, refugees and ethnic minorities in Europe*. European Union Drugs Agency. https://www.euda.europa.eu/drugs-library/responding-drug-related-problems-among-migrants-refugees-and-ethnic-minorities-europe_en

Ezard, N., Manji, H., & Busse, A. (2020). Substance use disorders in conflict-displaced populations. In *Textbook of addiction treatment: International perspectives* (pp. 1463–1475). Springer.

Fonseca, F., Lenahan, W., Dart, R. C., Papaseit, E., Dargan, P. I., Wood, D. M., Guareschi, M., Maremmani, I., Auriacombe, M., & Farré, M. (2021). Non-medical use of prescription gabapentinoids (gabapentin and Pregabalin) in five European countries. *Frontiers in Psychiatry, 12*, 676224.

Giacco, D. (2020). Identifying the critical time points for mental health of asylum seekers and refugees in highincome countries. *Epidemiology and psychiatric sciences, 29*, e61.

Greene, M. C., Andersen, L. S., Leku, M. R., Au, T., Akellot, J., Upadhaya, N., Odokonyero, R., White, R., Ventevogel, P., Garcia-Moreno, C., & Tol, W. A. (2024). Combining a guided self-help and brief alcohol intervention to improve mental health and reduce substance use among refugee men in Uganda: A cluster-randomized feasibility trial. *Global Mental Health, 11*, e106. https://doi.org/10.1017/gmh.2024.103

Greene, M. C., Busse, A., Ventevogel, P., Kane, J., & Ezard, N. (2024). Moving from feasible to essential: Progress and future directions for promoting the implementation of substance use services for forcibly displaced populations in humanitarian settings. *Addiction, 119*(3), 408–410. https://doi.org/10.1111/add.15869

Greene, M. C., Haddad, S., Busse, A., Ezard, N., Ventevogel, P., Demis, L., Inoue, S., Gumm, J.-C., Campello, G., & Tol, W. A. (2021). Priorities for addressing substance use disorder in humanitarian settings. *Conflict and Health, 15*(1), 1–10.

Greene, M. C., Kane, J. C., Khoshnood, K., Ventevogel, P., & Tol, W. A. (2018). Challenges and opportunities for implementation of substance misuse interventions in conflict-affected populations. *Harm Reduction Journal, 15*(1), 1–10.

Harris, S., Dykxhoorn, J., Hollander, A. C., Dalman, C., & Kirkbride, J. B. (2019). Substance use disorders in refugee and migrant groups in Sweden: A nationwide cohort study of 1.2 million people. *PLoS medicine, 16*(11), e1002944

Haar, K., El-Khani, A., Molgaard, V., Maalouf, W., & Nazir, A. (2020). Strong families: A new family skills training programme for challenged and humanitarian settings: A single-arm intervention tested in Afghanistan. *BMC Public Health, 20*, 1–16.

Heim, E., Abi Ramia, J., Abi Hana, R., Burchert, S., Carswell, K., Cornelisz, I., Cuijpers, P., El Chammay, R., Noun, P., & van Klaveren, C. (2021). Step-by-step: Feasibility randomized controlled trial of a mobile-based intervention for depression among populations affected by adversity in Lebanon. *Internet Interventions, 24*, 100380.

Hertner, L., Stylianopoulos, P., Heinz, A., Kluge, U., Schäfer, I., & Penka, S. (2023). Substance (mis) use among refugees as a matter of social ecology: insights into a multi-site rapid assessment in Germany. *Conflict and health, 17*(1), 1

Horyniak, D., Melo, J. S., Farrell, R. M., Ojeda, V. D., & Strathdee, S. A. (2016). Epidemiology of substance use among forced migrants: A global sys-tematic review. *PloS One, 11*(7), e0159134.

Hunt, G., & Kolind, T. (2017). Researching ethnicity and substances: A contested arena. *Drugs: Education, Prevention and Policy, 24*(3), 227–229

Ivert, A. K., & Magnusson, M. M. (2020). Drug use and criminality among unaccompanied refugee minors: a review of the literature. *International Journal of Migration, Health and Social Care, 16*(1), 93–107.

Karyotaki, E., Miguel, C., Panagiotopoulou, O. M., Harrer, M., Seward, N., Sijbrandij, M., Araya, R., Patel, V., & Cuijpers, P. (2023). Digital interventions for common mental disorders in low-and middle-income countries: A systematic review and meta-analysis. *Cambridge Prisms: Global Mental Health, 10*, e68

Karyotaki, E., Sijbrandij, M., Purgato, M., Acarturk, C., Lakin, D., Bailey, D., Peckham, E., Uygun, E., Tedeschi, F., Wancata, J., Augustinavicius, J., Carswell, K., Valimaki, M., van Ommeren, M., Koesters, M., Popa, M., Leku, M. R., Anttila, M., Churchill, R., ... Barbui, C. (2023). Self-Help Plus for refugees and asylum seekers: An individual participant data me-ta-analysis. *BMJ Mental Health, 26*(1). https://doi.org/10.1136/bmjment-2023-300672

Koppel, K., & Jakobson, M. L. (2023). Who is the worst migrant? Migrant hierarchies in populist radical-right rhetoric in Estonia. In *Anxieties of Migration and Integration in Turbulent Times* (pp. 225–241). Cham: Springer International Publishing.

Krieger, N. (2011/2024). *Epidemiology and the people's health: theory and context.* Oxford University Press

Lee, C.-T., Lin, C.-Y., Koós, M., Nagy, L., Kraus, S. W., Demetrovics, Z., Potenza, M. N., Ballester-Arnal, R., Batthyány, D., & Bergeron, S. (2023). The eleven-item Alcohol, Smoking and Substance Involvement Screening Test (ASSIST-11): Cross-cultural psychometric evaluation across 42 countries. *Journal of Psychiatric Research, 165*, 16–27.

Litins' ka, Y. (2024). Healthcare services for asylum-seekers: Untangling the European Social Charter. *Medical law review, 32*(1), 1–19.

López-Atanes, M., Rosenkranz, M., Erkoreka, L., Recio-Barbero, M., Bari, M., Hiller, P., Penka, S., Lindert, J., Martens, M., & Schäfer, I. (2025). Special needs of refugees with substance use disorders from conflict-affected countries: a comparison with German-born individuals. *Social Psychiatry and Psychiatric Epidemiology, 60*(7), 1563–1572.

Molina-Fernández, A. J. M., Ayllón-Alonso, E., & Mena-García, B. (2025). *Wars, substances and addictions: Perspectives and solutions from public health to a global problem* [Preprint]. https://www.preprints.org/manuscript/xxxx.

Mwangala, P. N., Makandi, M., Kerubo, A., Nyongesa, M. K., & Abubakar, A. (2024). A scoping review of the literature on the application and usefulness of the Problem Management Plus (PM+) intervention around the world. *BJPsych Open, 10*(3), e91

Nikitin, B. M., Bromberg, D. J., Pykalo, I., Ivasiy, R., Islam, Z., & Altice, F. L. (2023). Early disruptions to syringe services programs during the Russian invasion of Ukraine. *Frontiers in Public Health, 11*, 1229057

Papanicolas, I., Rajan, D., Karanikolos, M., Soucat, A., & Marimont, J. F. (2022). *Health system performance assessment: A framework for policy analysis.* WHO.

Peltonen, K., Aalto, S., Vänskä, M., Lepistö, R., Punamäki, R.-L., Soye, E., Watters, C., de Wal Pastoor, L., Derluyn, I., & Kankaanpää, R. (2022). Effectiveness of promotive and preventive psychosocial interventions on improving the mental health of Finnish-born and immigrant adolescents. *International Journal of Environmental Research and Public Health, 19*(6), 3686.

Prentice, K. R., Beitelshees, M., Hill, A., & Jones, C. H. (2024). Defining health equity: A modern US perspective. *iScience, 27*(12).

Purgato, M., Carswell, K., Acarturk, C., Au, T., Akbai, S., Anttila, M., Baumgartner, J., Bailey, D., Biondi, M., & Bird, M. (2019). Effectiveness and cost-effectiveness of self-help plus (SH+) for preventing mental disorders in refugees and asylum seekers in Europe and Turkey: Study protocols for two randomised controlled trials. *BMJ Open, 9*(5), e030259.

Rayes, D., Almoshmosh, N., El-Khani, A., Alkhalil, M., Basha, S., Fouad, F., Hilal, M. A., & Abbara, A. (2022). *The epidemics of substance misuse and suicide in Syria: Casualties of protracted conflict and political instability.* Preprint. https://doi.org/10.21203/rs.3.rs-2070143/v1

Salas-Wright, C. P., Vaughn, M. G., Goings, T. C., Miller, D. P., & Schwartz, S. J. (2018). Immigrants and mental disorders in the United States: New evidence on the healthy migrant hypothesis. *Psychiatry research, 267*, 438–445

Saleh, E. A., Lazaridou, F. B., Klapprott, F., Wazaify, M., Heinz, A., & Kluge, U. (2023). A systematic review of qualitative research on substance use among refugees. *Addiction, 118*(2), 218–253.

Satinsky, E., Fuhr, D. C., Woodward, A., Sondorp, E., & Roberts, B. (2019). Mental health care utilisation and access among refugees and asylum seekers in Europe: A systematic review. *Health Policy, 123*(9), 851–863.

Savas, S. T., Knipper, M., Duclos, D., Sharma, E., Ugarte-Gurrutxaga, M. I., & Blanchet, K. (2024). Migrant-sensitive healthcare in Europe: Advancing health equity through accessibility, acceptability, quality, and trust. *The Lancet Regional Health–Europe, 41*.

Servais, L., Huberland, V., & Richelle, L. (2023). Misuse of Pregabalin: A qualitative study from a patient's perspective. *BMC Public Health, 23*(1), 1339.

Sever, C. A., Cuijpers, P., Dawson, K. S., Mittendorfer-Rutz, E., Akhtar, A., Bryant, R. A., & Sijbrandij, M. (2024). Addressing challenges faced by young refugees in The Netherlands: Adapting problem management plus (PM+) with an emotional processing module. *Cambridge Prisms: Global Mental Health, 11*, e80.

Sijbrandij, M., Acarturk, C., Bird, M., Bryant, R. A., Burchert, S., Carswell, K., de Jong, J., Dinesen, C., Dawson, K. S., El Chammay, R., van Ittersum, L., Jordans, M., Knaevelsrud, C., McDaid, D., Miller, K., Morina, N., Park, A. L., Roberts, B., & van Son, Y. (2017). Strengthening mental health care systems for Syrian refugees in Europe and the Middle East: Integrating scalable psychological interventions in eight countries. *European Journal of Psychotraumatology, 8*(2). https://doi.org/10.1080/20008198.2017.1388102

Solfrank, M., Nikendei, C., Zehetmair, C., Friederich, H.-C., & Nagy, E. (2023). The burden of substance use and (mental) distress among asylum seekers: A cross sectional study. *Frontiers in Psychiatry, 14*, 1258140.

Spaaij, J., Kiselev, N., Berger, C., Bryant, R. A., Cuijpers, P., De Graaff, A. M., Fuhr, D. C., Hemmo, M., McDaid, D., & Moergeli, H. (2022). Feasibility and acceptability of problem management plus (PM+) among Syrian refugees and asylum seekers in Switzerland: A mixed-method pilot randomized controlled trial. *European Journal of Psychotraumatology, 13*(1), 2002027.

Stallwitz, A., Nordgren, J., & Richert, T. (2024). 'Not having a real life': Psychosocial functions of using and selling drugs among young afghan men who came to Sweden as unaccompanied minors. *Journal of Ethnic and Migration Studies, 50*(14), 3570–3590. https://doi.org/10.1080/1369183X.2023.2290984

Stylianopoulos, P., Hertner, L., Heinz, A., Kluge, U., Schäfer, I., & Penka, S. (2024). Good practice in reaching and treating refugees in addiction care in Germany: A Delphi study. *BMC Public Health, 24*(1), 30. https://doi.org/10.1186/s12889-023-17446-

Transit. (2022). *Prégabaline—Etat des lieux en Région de Bruxelles-Capitale*. Transit. http://fr.transitasbl.be/documents-internes/

Turrini, G., Purgato, M., Acarturk, C., Anttila, M., Au, T., Ballette, F., Bird, M., Carswell, K., Churchill, R., & Cuijpers, P. (2019). Efficacy and acceptability of psychosocial interventions in asylum seekers and refugees: Systematic review and meta-analysis. *Epidemiology and Psychiatric Sciences, 28*(4), 376–388.

Turrini, G., Purgato, M., Tedeschi, F., Acarturk, C., Anttila, M., Au, T., Carswell, K., Churchill, R., Cuijpers, P., Friedrich, F., Gastaldon, C., Klein, T., Kosters, M., Lantta, T., Nose, M., Ostuzzi, G., Papola, D., Popa, M., Sijbrandij, M., et al. (2022). Long-term effectiveness of self-help plus in refugees and asylum seekers resettled in Western Europe: 12-month outcomes of a randomised controlled trial. *Epidemiology and Psychiatric Sciences, 31*, e39. https://doi.org/10.1017/S2045796022000269

Uricher, J. (2025). Individual and contextual determinants of substance use among refugees in shared accommodations: A cross-sectional multi-level analysis. *European Addiction Research, 2025*(31), 384–395

van der Boor, C. F., Taban, D., Tol, W. A., Akellot, J., Neuman, M., Weiss, H. A., Greco, G., Vassall, A., May, C., Nadkarni, A., Kinyanda, E., Roberts, B., & Fuhr, D. C. (2024). Effectiveness and cost-effectiveness of a transdiagnostic intervention for alcohol misuse and psychological distress in humanitarian settings: Study protocol for a randomised controlled trial in Uganda. *Trials, 25*(1), 148. https://doi.org/10.1186/s13063-024-07980-7

Van Hout, M.-C., Lungu-Byrne, C., & Germain, J. (2020). Migrant health situation when detained in European immigration detention centres: A synthesis of extant qualitative literature. *International Journal of Prisoner Health, 16*(3), 221–236.

van Selm, L., White, T. M., Picchio, C. A., Requena-Méndez, A., Busz, M., Perez Gayo, R., et al. (2024). A call to create integrated services to better address the needs of migrants who use drugs in Europe. *Harm Reduction Journal, 21*(1), 9.

Walg, M., Rosenbusch, S., Bender, S., & Hapfelmeier, G. (2024). Unhealthy substance use among unaccompanied refugees in Germany. *Drugs: Education, Prevention and Policy, 31*(5), 584–594. https://doi.org/10.1080/09687637.2023.2260548

Weinreich, K. J., Frankova, I., Maksymets, N., Barbui, C., Klymchuk, V., Mooren, T., Olechno, E., Purgato, M., Sijbrandij, M., & Witteveen, A. B. (2025). Implementing scalable face-to-face and digital interventions among forcibly displaced persons from Ukraine in Europe: Protocol of the U-RISE project. *European Journal of Psychotraumatology, 16*(1), 2468117.

World Health Organization. (2021). *Health equity*. https://www.who.int/health-topics/health-equity

WHO. (2023). *WHO mhGAP guidelines update: Drug use disorder module—Evidence profile DRU1: Brief psychosocial interventions for people using cannabis or stimulants*. WHO.

Zagha, K., Konietzny, K., Brettschneider, C., Chehadi, O., Chehadi-Köster, A., Chikhradze, N., Dababneh, N., Hegerath, F.-M., Heller, L., & Dehnen, A. (2024). Improve mental health (improve-MH) in refugee families using a culturally adapted, general practitioner-delivered psychotherapeutic intervention combined with triple P online parenting programme: Study protocol of a multicentre randomised controlled trial. *BMJ Open, 14*(9), e084080.

Index

C. De Kock (ed.), *Substance Use Among Refugees in Europe*,
https://doi.org/10.1007/978-3-032-32399-6

The manufacturer's authorised representative in the EU is Springer Nature Customer Service Centre GmbH, Europaplatz 3, 69115 Heidelberg, Germany. If you have any concerns regarding our products, please contact ProductSafety@springernature.com

Printed and bound by CPI Group (UK) Ltd, Croydon, CR0 4YY
09/10/2026
02231214-0003